Primate Models of Children's Health and Developmental Disabilities

To the monkeys who, in the service of science, helped to make the world a better place for children.

Primate Models of Children's Health and Developmental Disabilities

Thomas M. Burbacher
Gene P. Sackett
Kimberly S. Grant

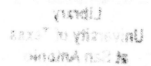

AMSTERDAM • BOSTON • HEIDELBERG • LONDON
NEW YORK • OXFORD • PARIS • SAN DIEGO
SAN FRANCISCO • SINGAPORE • SYDNEY • TOKYO
Academic Press is an imprint of Elsevier

Academic Press is an imprint of Elsevier
360 Park Avenue South, New York, NY 10010-1710
84 Theobald's Road, London WC1X 8RR, UK
30 Corporate Drive, Suite 400, Burlington, MA 01803, USA
525 B Street, Suite 1900, San Diego, CA 92101-4495, USA

First edition 2008

Library of Congress Catalog Number
2007932578

British Library Cataloguing in Publication Data
A catalogue record for this book is available from the British Library

ISBN: 978-0-123-73743-4

For information on all Academic Press publications
visit our web site at www.books.elsevier.com

Typeset by Charon Tec Ltd (A Macmillan Company), Chennai, India
www.charontec.com
Printed and bound in the United States of America

08 09 10 11   10 9 8 7 6 5 4 3 2 1

Working together to grow libraries in developing countries

www.elsevier.com | www.bookaid.org | www.sabre.org

ELSEVIER   BOOK AID International   Sabre Foundation

Contents

Preface

For more than half a century, the nonhuman primate model has been used in the service of the biological and behavioral sciences. The rich body of information that has been collected from decades of research has provided key insights on human health and development and transformed our most basic understanding of how we fit in the natural world. As greater emphasis is placed on the integration of scientific discoveries with clinical practices, it is important to remember the historical and sometimes revolutionary contributions made from primate studies.[1] These contributions have provided the impetus for key advances in contemporary pediatric medicine and the identification, prevention, and treatment of developmental disabilities.

In 2006, the Centers for Disease Control and Prevention published a report indicating that developmental disabilities affect 1 in 17 children aged 18 or under. These disabilities range from minor to severe and a broad range of educational and medical services are required to effectively treat these children. Although some families report that having a disabled child brought them closer together, other studies have found higher levels of stress, separation, and divorce in families with disabled children. The level of psychosocial stress that is placed on families with special-needs children can be weighty. As such, research on the prevention and potential causes of early childhood disabilities is urgently needed and macaque monkeys provide one important pathway to elucidation. Learning more about the causes of abnormal development in monkeys has and will continue to provide important insights into mechanisms underlying neurodevelopmental disabilities in human infants.

When considering the major scientific breakthroughs associated with monkeys, two historical cases jump to the forefront. In 1937, Landsteiner and Wiener's work with rhesus monkeys resulted in the discovery of the rhesus (Rh) blood group system. Incompatability of the maternal and fetal Rh factors is one important basis of erythroblastosis fetalis – hemolytic disease of the newborn – and was a serious problem in the past. Recognition of this blood antigen allowed, among many things, early identification of Rh incompatibility and the opportunity to prevent complications such as severe anemia, jaundice, brain damage, and heart failure in affected

---

[1]In an effort to be parsimonious, we exercise our literary license to use the term primates in a restricted sense. This book is based solely on work with monkeys and does not address the contributions of the great apes. In this book, we use the term primate to indicate both old and new world monkeys but not apes or humans. While this may offend the strict taxonomist, it is intended to make the information in this book accessible to readers with broadly varying backgrounds.

infants. The Rh test for immunocompatability is now one of the most widely conducted and important prenatal tests in the world.

From a psychological perspective, work by Harry Harlow with rhesus macaque monkeys revolutionized our understanding of love and nurturing, separation, and depression. Harlow's work with infant monkeys and maternal surrogates provided the foundation for sweeping changes in policies related to the handling of human neonates in hospital nurseries. Until the 1960s, neonatal handling procedures in hospital nurseries dictated the swift separation of the mother–infant pairs. Newborns were whisked away to nurseries where contact was discouraged and germ prevention was paramount. Research findings from the Harlow laboratory helped to persuade physicians that early contact comfort is vital to mother–infant bonding and long-term emotional health. Owing in large part to the visionary aspects of Harlow's laboratory work with monkeys, changes were made in birthing practices such that most mothers and babies, within the first few hours or even minutes after birth, were reunited, infants were allowed to sleep in their mother's room, and close physical contact between mother and infant was encouraged.

Pioneering laboratory and field work has provided the foundation for understanding the important role these intelligent animals play in understanding the causes and consequences of pediatric disease and disability. Much of what has been learned has come from studies of animals within the *Macaca* monkey genus. Macaques are Old World monkeys and share a common evolutionary history with apes and humans, including basic aspects of reproduction and development. Macaques split off from the chimpanzee–human lineage about 26 million years ago and share about 93% of their DNA with humans. Macaque species have lengthy pregnancies (5–6 months), allowing for protracted central nervous system development during gestation. At birth, monkeys and humans share certain limitations and abilities, particularly during the first months of life. Early neurobehavioral parallels (learning, memory, vision) and basic parameters of physiology, neurochemistry, and immunology have been well established in the developing macaque, offering the unique opportunity to study advanced biological and behavioral systems in a controlled, laboratory setting.

This book, a compilation of scholarly writings from global experts, seeks to bring the depth of the primate literature into focus and stresses the translational aspects of the research in relation to human infants and children. In this book, contributions from primate work on the origins of developmental psychopathology, visual disabilities and self-injurious behavior are presented to facilitate insight into the origins and treatments of these conditions in affected children. Developmental studies with monkeys addressing the consequences of pediatric AIDS, prenatal stress, maternal medications, drugs of abuse, and environmental chemicals are examined in detail, addressing some of the most pressing issues in contemporary pediatric research. This book also features the accomplishments of progressive research programs on (1) autoimmune diseases and (2) stem cell therapy for the effective treatment of genetically based developmental disabilities such as the fragile X syndrome. These programs have the capacity to make revolutionary contributions to our understanding of life, disease and disability.

To acknowledge our gratitude to others, we extend our thanks to the authors who contributed their time and talent to this book. Without their collective dedication this book would have simply remained a possibility, not a plausible reality. In recognition of his pioneering work with infant monkeys, we also salute the life's work of the late Mr Gerald Ruppenthal, who was the supervisor of our Infant Primate Research Laboratory at the University of Washington for over three decades. Gerry was truly a primate of excellent origins. We would also like to thank the staff of the Infant Primate Research Laboratory who have loved and cared for infant monkeys for over 35 years. We are grateful to the sustained support of the Center on Human Development and Disability (P30 HD02274) and the Washington National Primate Research Center (P51 RR00166) at the University of Washington as well as The National Institute of Environmental Health Sciences (R01 ES03745, R01 ES06673). Finally, we thank our families and friends for their endless encouragement of our research pursuits.

Thomas Burbacher, Gene Sackett, and Kimberly Grant
University of Washington
Seattle

Abbreviations

5-HIAA	5-hydroxyindoleacetic acid
6-OHDA	6-hydroxydopamine
ACTH	adrenocorticotropic hormone
ADEM	acute disseminated encephalomyelitis
ADHD	attention deficit hyperactivity disorder
AFP	alpha-fetoprotein
AIA	antigen-induced arthritis
AP	alkaline phosphatase
APCs	antigen-presenting cells
ART	antiretroviral treatment
ARTs	assisted reproductive technologies
ASD	autism spectrum disorder
CFA	complete Freund's adjuvant
CIA	collagen-induced arthritis
CMV	cytomegalovirus
CRH	corticotropin releasing hormone
CRP	C-reactive protein
CSF	cerebrospinal fluid
CTLs	cytotoxic T cells
DA	dopamine
DES	diethylstilbestrol
DHA	docosahexaenoic acid
DHEAS	dehydroepiandrosterone sulfate
DMTS	delayed matching-to-sample
DRI	differential reinforcement of incompatible behavior
DRL	differential reinforcement of low rate
DRO	differential reinforcement of other behavior
EAE	experimental autoimmune encephalomyelitis
FAL	$[^{18}F]$-fallypride
FI	fixed interval
FI/FR	fixed interval/fixed ratio
fMRI	functional magnetic resonance imaging
FMT	6-$[^{18}F]$-fluoro-m-tyrosine
gd	gestation day

GnRH	gonadotropin-releasing hormone
GR	glucocorticoid receptor
HAART	highly active antiretroviral therapy
HIV	human immunodeficiency virus
HLA	human leukocyte antigen
HPA	hypothalamic-pituitary-adrenal
HPG	hypothalamic-pituitary-gonadal
HPLC	high-performance liquid chromatography
HVA	homovanillic acid
ICSI	intracytoplasmic sperm injection
IOL	intraocular lenses
IRT	inter-response time or
IVF	*in vitro* fertilization
JRA	juvenile rheumatoid arthritis
LBW	low birth weight
LGN	lateral geniculate nucleus
LH	luteinizing hormone
LHPA	limbic-hypothalamic-pituitary-adrenal
LTP	long-term potentiation
MAO	monoamine oxidase
MBP	myelin basic protein
m-CPP	meta-chlorophenylpiperazine
MeHg	methylmercury
MeOH	methanol
MHC	major histocompatibility complex
MHPG	3-methoxy-4-hydroxyphenylglycol
MOG	myelin/oligodendrocyte glycoprotein
MPF	maternal–placental–fetal
MR	mineralocorticoid receptor
MRI	magnetic resonance imaging
MTCT	mother to child transmission
MTL	medial temporal lobe
MXC	methoxychlor
NBAS	Neonatal Behavioral Assessment Scale
NCR	noncontingent reinforcement
NIH	National Institutes of Health
NMDA	n-methyl-D-aspartate
NREM	nonrapid eye movement
NT	nuclear transfer
NTDs	neural tube defects
OSEM	Ordered Subset Estimation Method
OVA	ovalbumin
PBDEs	polybrominated diphenyl ethers

PCBs	polychlorinated biphenyls
PCP	phencyclidine
PCR	polymerase chain reaction
PET	positron emission tomography
PHT	phenytoin
PLP	proteolipid protein
PNNA	Primate Neonatal Neurobehavioral Assessment
RI	random interval
ROI	regions of interest
SCW	streptococcal cell walls
SHBG	sex hormone-binding globulin
SHIV	simian–human immunodeficiency viruses
SIB	self-injurious behavior
SIDS	sudden infant death syndrome
SIV	simian immunodeficiency virus
SLE	systemic lupus erythematosus
SSRI	selective serotonin reuptake inhibitor
TAC	time–activity
TcR	T cell receptor
THC	delta-9-tetrahydrocannabinol
TRD	temporal response differentiation
UADD	undifferentiated attention deficit disorder
UGTs	uridinyl-glucuronosyltransferases
UW	University of Washington
WCST	Wisconsin Card Sort Test
WGTA	Wisconsin General Test Apparatus
WISC	Wechsler Intelligence Scale for Children

CHAPTER 1

Developmental Disabilities and Primate Models Defined

Gene P. Sackett

The term "developmental disabilities" is used more as a political and economic category than a class of scientific studies. To be useful in research on animal models of human health and behavior this term needs to be defined operationally, as well as in its more governmental context. Furthermore, the phrase "animal models of human conditions" itself needs to be defined. To individuals opposed to animal research, the term is a call to battle. Scientifically, there are also a number of meanings that require definition. The purpose of this chapter is to set the stage for much of the remainder of the book by defining these terms in a way that is both scientific and compatible with translating primate research into application in the cure and prevention of human developmental disorders.

INTRODUCTION

Childhood diseases and developmental disabilities afflict millions of children worldwide. Many diseases, such as polio and malnutrition, are scientifically understood and completely preventable when given sufficient political and economic support. Other diseases, such as malaria and HIV/AIDS, are awaiting advances in immunology and vaccination science for eradication. On the other hand, the causes of many developmental physical and psychological conditions, such as learning disabilities, social behavior pathologies, and abnormal motor coordination, are often unknown. Prevention of these disabilities is difficult without knowing their causes. Cures often consist of preventing current symptoms, as opposed to reversing or blocking causal processes. For example, hyperactivity and attentional disorders in children are associated with many potential causes, but the primary cure often involves treating symptoms with drugs (see Anderson and Keating, 2006, for a review), symptoms often disappearing as the child matures.

The economic scope of disabilities in the United States is considerable. Braddock (2002) estimated that public support for all disabilities resulting from mental retardation, mental illness, and physical abnormalities in 2002 was 426 billion dollars. The Centers for Disease Control (CDC) 2007 cost estimates, in billions of dollars, were 51.2 for mental retardation, 11.5 for cerebral palsy, and 4.6 for sensory loss or impairment. This 67 billion dollar estimate did not include the considerable cost of education for individuals with these conditions. Developmental exposure to environmental contaminants has been associated with asthma, cancer, congenital malformations, and neurobehavioral disorders. In 2004, Washington State spent an estimated 1.6 billion dollars on services for children exposed to environmental chemicals (Davies, 2006) and Minnesota spent a similar 1.5 billion for children affected by pollution (Mincenter, 2006). The costs of child disabilities due to other causes such as genetic defects, accidents, abuse, and neglect are unknown. Besides money, of course, the emotional and social costs of child disease and disability to those affected and their families are incalculable.

Scientific understanding of the causes and cures of child disease and disabilities depends on research. Animal experimentation has generated much of our knowledge about normal life processes. Both preventive and curative medicine has also depended on animal research to identify causes leading to prevention and cure of human diseases. However, animal testing has been controversial in the United States and Europe for the past three decades. The pros and cons of this controversy are well illustrated by material on the World Wide Web (e.g. Wiki, 2007).

Although invertebrates such as fruit flies and various rodent species are used most often as animal models, the most controversial experimental species have been primates – monkeys and great apes – as well as dogs and cats. It is an irrefutable fact that basic mechanisms of anatomical structure, physiology, and bio-chemistry – from molecules to whole organ systems – exhibit continuity from single cell animals to humans. Less clear is exactly how this continuity relates to the development of behavioral characteristics of humans. How can an animal species model deviant human development and the complexity of language, social behavior, and societal structures of people? Advocates against animal research argue that important aspects of human development and behavior have unique properties that cannot be modeled by any animals. Animal models of human genetic abnormalities, organ transplantation and immunity, viral diseases, environmental pollutants, and drug effects, much of this work done using nonhuman primates, belies this argument.

Science progresses by observation, experimentation, and theory. An important aspect of this enterprise concerns definitions. Clear and objective definitions of concepts, variables, and methods are required for communicating scientific procedures and results. This book addresses the question above – how primate models are clarifying our understanding about ill-health and childhood disability. The purpose of this chapter is to define what is meant by the terms developmental disability and primate models.

DEVELOPMENTAL DISABILITY DEFINED?

The United States Developmental Disabilities Assistance and Bill of Rights Act of 2000, Public Law 106-402, states that developmental disability is a severe, chronic disability of an individual having five defining properties. The disability is (1) attributable to mental or physical impairment or a combination of mental and physical impairments; (2) manifested before the age of 22; (3) likely to continue indefinitely; (4) results in substantial functional limitations in three or more of the following areas of activity, self-care, receptive and expressive living, learning, mobility, self-direction, capacity for independent living, and economic self-sufficiency; and (5) reflects the need for special, interdisciplinary, or generic services, individualized support, or other forms of assistance that are of lifelong or extended duration and are individually planned and coordinated. When applied to children, developmental disability includes individuals from birth to age 9, who have a substantial developmental delay or specific congenital or acquired condition, and may be disabled without meeting three or more of the criteria above if, without services and supports, there is a high probability of meeting those criteria later in life.

Every state in the United States has a developmental disability definition similar to PL 106-402, although they may differ markedly in emphasis on specific areas of disability. For example, some definitions actually refer to mental retardation, characterized by subaverage intellectual functioning and concurrent limitations in communication, self-care, home-living, social skills, community use, self-direction, health and safety, functional academics, leisure, or work (American Association on Mental Retardation, 1992). Like PL 106-402, most definitions require some number of these concurrent limitations to be present in order to fit the definition. The width or narrowness of these definitions and the minimum number of limitation areas is very important, as they determine who is eligible for developmental disability services (Biersdorff, 1999). For example, a requirement of subaverage intelligence would eliminate many individuals with cerebral palsy or epilepsy from receiving aid. As seems apparent, these legal definitions serve political and economic ends as well as potential guides to scientific study by animal models.

Given such legal definitions, how are they operationalized in actual measurement? Intellectual functioning is assessed by standard IQ tests such as the Wechsler Intelligence Scale for Children, with substandard performance defined by some arbitrary cut-off score. This may cause problems, as updates and revisions to tests may change the score meanings and test difficulty. On the political–economic side, however, defining score cut-offs provides a convenient way for affecting budgets, especially on the reduction side.

The second dimension of measuring the presence and extent of disability concerns adaptive behavior skills and abilities. Biersdorff (1999) provides a useful summary of the adaptive behavior dimension, which is meant to assess what many call "practical" and "social" intelligence. Her list of these skill areas needed for coping with everyday life include the following: (1) Communication – understanding and expressing information through words, symbols or gestures; (2) Self-care – toileting, eating, dressing, and hygiene; (3) Home-living – household chores, budgeting, shopping, and home safety; (4) Social – managing social interactions and relationships; (5) Community use – getting around in the community and accessing public facilities and services; (6) Self-direction – making choices, self-advocacy, problem-solving, and accessing help when needed; (7) Health and safety – preventing, recognizing, and addressing health and safety issues through good habits; (8) Functional academics – reading, writing and handling math well enough to function in the community; (9) Leisure – being aware of and participating in leisure and recreational activities that reflect personal preferences; and (10) Work – specific job skills, good work habits and taking direction well. These adaptive skills are usually assessed by observation of behavior during daily activities or ratings by caregivers or teachers.

Many of the chapters in this book present a primate model addressing one or more of these cognitive or adaptive behavior areas. Aspects of most of these areas can be found in the behavior of wild living primates, while some are only studied in captive primates. Some of this work concerns normal developmental processes. As discussed below, normative information is often critical in order to determine how and when a developmental process has become deviant. Most primate development models use macaque monkeys, baboons, or apes as subjects. This is not a choice of convenience, as primate development research is expensive, time consuming, and requires special veterinary medicine and husbandry methods. These species are used because of similarities to humans. Their physiology, reproductive processes, cognitive and sensory abilities, social behavior, and in some instances specific gene alleles often make them the most appropriate animal models for studying a specific human process or ability.

PRIMATE MODELS DEFINED

In 1991, I published a paper with Patricia Gould concerning primate models of developmental psychopathology (Sackett and Gould, 1991). We presented a history of relevant models, discussed the characteristics of behavioral animal models, and described how a primate model can relate to a system for classifying human child behavior problems. My remarks here are a summary of this discussion, as I have not been able to improve on our thinking about this topic in the 16 years since this publication.

Stephens (1986), an important antivivesectionist opposed to animal research in general, and primate research in particular, stated his conclusion about primate behavioral models that can be paraphrased as follows. Such studies have almost no clinical application and little potential for future impact. They are simply trivial replications or attempts to identify in animals facts already known about humans. The fundamental criterion for an animal model is that the results must have direct and immediate application to a human health problem. Furthermore, a valid model must have the same causes, symptoms, biological mechanisms, and cures as the human disorder being studied. By Stephens' criteria there are probably few, if any, valid or useful primate or non-primate animal models of human behavior. But his criteria are unrealistic and unattainable for a variety of reasons.

For their development, human behavior systems involve interactions among biological, cognitive, social, emotional, communicative, and ecological processes occurring between generations and during the lifespan of individuals (Gottlieb and Halpern, 2002). These processes produce quantitative and qualitative changes as the individual matures. It is rarely possible to manipulate or control in humans more than a few of the potential causal factors operating longitudinally to affect these interactions. Most human longitudinal studies of behavior disability measure correlations among many variables, with any causal implications often unclear. In research relevant to developmental disabilities, such as birth defects due to drug use, there are often many uncontrolled confounding variables clouding interpretation. For example, human studies can rarely find subjects that only use the drug under study. The participants often smoke, drink alcohol, and/or take multiple drugs. Laboratory primate research can control some, or all, of an individual's total life history. It can produce knowledge about the actual processes by which genetic mechanisms, prenatal and perinatal factors, and postnatal conditions produce typical development, a range of normal individual differences, or deviant developmental paths. Such studies can serve as animal models of a human condition, but unlike Stephenson's criteria, the model may not apply to every aspect of the problem.

The purpose of a behavioral primate model is *to aid* in identifying causal processes affecting human behaviors, and *to assist* in specifying etiological factors, symptoms, therapies, and lifespan effects involved in abnormal behavior (Sackett, 1988). The need for an animal model implies ignorance about one or more aspects of a human problem. It does not imply Stephenson's unattainable demand that the human condition be exactly duplicated in the animal. A useful model might apply to only a single aspect of a disorder, etiology, symptoms, therapy, or outcomes, not necessarily to all aspects. In our 1991 paper, we suggested five steps for designing and applying a primate model. Some of these steps may have already been done, being available in a researcher's prior studies or in the scientific literature. Other steps may require new data and concepts, which for many developmental problems may need years of longitudinal study. I repeat these steps here. The chapters of this book each represent one or more of these steps in developing a primate model of human disability.

1. **Describe the human phenomenon**. This step is critical for modeling. It is necessary to have detailed knowledge about a target human condition in order to know what is to be modeled. In a sense, this step is actually generating a human model for a primate developmental phenomenon; a process that was recognized and described in some detail by Harlow and Mears (1979). It is also possible for primate research to identify phenomena not yet known to occur in humans, stimulating a search for that process in human research. This aspect of "modeling" will be discussed below.

2. **Identify an appropriate species**. The model should use a primate species that has one or more concordant characteristics of the target condition. This may involve genetic factors, prenatal or postnatal environmental variables, anatomical or physiological characteristics, specific behaviors, social relationships, reactivity to chemicals, or behavioral therapy procedures. After demonstrating concordance, some models, such as drug tests, may be ready for study. Other models may require more steps before modeling research commences.

3. **Identifying causal processes and mechanisms**. Studying processes rather than outcomes may require extended research before an actual model becomes feasible. This involves studies designed to test or generate concepts and theories; namely, the "basic research" that is rejected as a legitimate use of animals by many animal rights advocates. The purpose of such studies is to guide the course of human studies that can lead to future applications. A great deal of laboratory primate development research has been designed to study normal and abnormal developmental processes, not designed to be models of specific human conditions. Such basic information was essential to most of the models in this book.

4. **Assessing generality to humans**. Human clinical trials are required before a potential disease cure or preventative procedure is made available to the general population. Before clinical trials are done, preclinical human studies may need to be conducted guided by primate research findings. This assesses the generality of the model results. Because of individual differences in human risk factors and reactivity, these studies may also determine the range of potential application within a target human population. Given the current emphasis on multidisciplinary research and the funding emphasis at the National Institutes of Health (NIH) on "translational" research – application of results to clinical problems on a timely basis – this step in the modeling process may become more prevalent than in the past.

5. **Application to clinical problems**. The final step is actual application of the findings from an animal model. This application may be no more, nor no less, than the generation of valid principles about human conditions that lead to human research and clinical applications (step 3). It could also be an actual clinical practice based directly on the primate model. Either of these application directions will, of course, depend on communication between primate researchers, researchers studying basic processes of human development, and clinicians. A primary aim of this book is to make more of these dialogs happen.

NATURAL PRIMATE MODELS OF DEVELOPMENTAL DISABILITY

Although most of the primate models described in this book are experimental, fit at least steps 1 and 2 of our definitions, and purposely produce the disability situation, some models occur spontaneously in wild or captive populations. One of the most interesting examples concerns limb deformities in Japanese macaques (Nakamichi,

1986). Infants in a number of free-ranging groups in various parts of Japan were born with shortened or deformed limbs or digits. Although attempts to trace these abnormalities to herbicides and other poisons were made, no official etiology has been identified. However, study of mother–infant interaction and social behavior revealed that these infants received caregiving well beyond the normal age and, like normal infants, carried the social status of their mothers and her kin. They also managed to engage in aggressive and sexual behavior, often overcoming their postural and motor disabilities with highly creative methods. In addition to a potential model of human limb birth defects, these observations show that special care of the disabled is not a uniquely human activity and might make an interesting model for aspects of therapy for human limb and motor disability. Other disability models in free-ranging or wild primates await only detection by motivated researchers conducting studies in these environments.

In ending this chapter I would like to make a special plea to managers and directors of captive primate colonies, such as the National Primate Research Centers and the large commercial primate breeding colonies. These colonies house numerous cases of spontaneous disability, especially among newborns and young infants. Because these individuals require more caregiving than normal animals, they are usually euthanized, discarding their potential value as a human disorder model. I believe that their scientific value outweights economic liabilities. As examples of the value of spontaneous disability, I will cite some of our own work.

Each year from 1970 to 1996, 10–15% of the pigtailed monkey births at our Medical Lake colony occurred prematurely and/or resulted in low birth weight (LBW) babies. When left with their mother, up to 50% of these neonates died. Rather than lose them, we instituted a "save-a-baby" program in which LBW, premature, injured, or abandoned newborns were brought to our Infant Primate Laboratory. Almost all survived when reared under special protocols developed in collaboration with neonatologists from our medical school (Ruppenthal and Sackett, 2006). A number of studies compared development of these infants with normally developing animals. Among other effects, we found that LBW monkeys, whether premature or not, were developmentally delayed in sensorimotor development and self-feeding age (Kroeker *et al.*, 2007), social development throughout infancy (Worlein and Sackett, 1997), and acquisition of object permanence (Ha *et al.*, 1997). Tests of learning ability as juveniles revealed poor performance on difficult learning problems (Fredrickson *et al.*, 1987). Although persistent neurological effects in humans are often found among very low birth weight individuals, low birth weight itself is a risk factor for many developmental disabilities (Wolf *et al.*, 2002).

We followed up on our LBW primate model by studying parents from our breeding colony who had an excess of poor pregnancy outcomes – excessive fetal losses, neonatal deaths, and LBW babies – in their breeding histories. These were compared with breeders who rarely if ever had poor pregnancy outcomes or LBW offspring (Sackett, 1984). These groups were identified by studying our computer colony records, an important, but often overlooked, source of primate developmental disability models. We selectively bred over 300 pregnancies within and between the high-risk and low-risk groups. Beside females, the high-risk group consisted of males who produced excessive rates of poor pregnancy outcomes. When females bred to these males were mated to males with good pregnancy outcomes, their poor outcome rates were normal. Although common knowledge in human medicine and primate husbandry stated that male factors in pregnancy outcome were unimportant after conception, our results suggested that many poor pregnancy outcomes were due to male, not female, factors.

Our selective breeding results confirmed this suggestion (Sackett, 1990). High-risk males had a higher rate of LBW offspring, regardless of female risk, than low-risk males. Furthermore, high-risk males had over a 3.5 times higher probability of producing an aborted or stillborn offspring than low-risk males. And the high-risk male fetal loss probability was statistically higher than that of the high-risk female probability of 2.5. Thus, our breeding colony had not only spontaneously produced a potentially important model for understanding prenatal factors producing LBW infants, but also a more general model for studying fetal death as well.

This story ends with our attempts to identify specific factors producing risk for poor reproductive outcomes in both male and female breeders. Work on high-risk males failed to identify any sperm or chromosome-related causes. Unfortunately, these males aged and died before the dawn of DNA studies of reproductive outcome became available. Furthermore, our colony managers came to believe that male factors could actually be responsible for reproductive failure due to fetal loss. Rather than give new females to these males, as they had done in the past, they now removed males with poor reproductive histories from harem breeding. The result was that we could no longer find any male breeders with poor histories. Managers at other primate breeding colonies may not be so enlightened, so these colonies may still contain high-risk males to serve as models of male factors of poor reproductive outcomes.

Female studies fared better. Experiments were conducted combining our work on monkey reproductive outcome with teratogenic effects on rat embryos. When blood sera from our female pigtail monkeys were put into rat embryo cultures, abnormal growth was found in sera from high-risk but not low-risk individuals (Klein et al., 1982). Subsequent studies identified antibodies to laminin, a large protein important for cell adhesion, as the molecular cause of the high-risk monkey sera effect (Weeks et al., 1986). Unfortunately, funding could not be obtained to continue this primate model work. The NIH recommendation concluded that, although the proposed studies were excellent science, the work did not merit a primate model because there were no human reproductive abnormalities known to be caused by antibodies to laminin. This seemed to us as rather ironic, as one purpose of NIH support for primate colonies is to discover and utilize animal models of human health. Perhaps now that the NIH is emphasizing "translational studies," primate research can be more readily used to discover models of phenomena that may exist in humans but are as yet unknown.

THE FUTURE OF PRIMATE MODELS

A basic goal of primate models in developmental science is to maximize the physical and mental health of children in both current and future generations. Attaining this goal involves the study of environmental factors and genetic and non-genetic intergenerational effects on prenatal, perinatal, and postnatal development. Research in this endeavor spans all of the life sciences, many of the social sciences, and increasingly physics and chemistry. This multidisciplinary task is illustrated by the wide range of subject matter and scientists presented in the chapters of this book. These chapters also illustrate many of the variables that serve as sources of ill-health during development that can affect an individual's total lifespan. The book also shows how primate models are supplying critical information for preventing or curing effects of these variables.

Advances in genetics, pharmacology, immunology and endocrinology, reproductive biology, and neuroscience offer many potential new clinical applications. However, these advances also pose potential new developmental risks. Gene manipulation, stem cell transplantation, new assisted reproduction methods, and brain implants are just some examples of new technologies that have unknown potential for harm as well as good. Studies of rodents and other non-primate mammals offer important models indicating potential risks of these new applications. But, only primates are sufficiently similar to humans – biologically and developmentally and cognitively and in some species, even socially – to serve as preclinical models of potential harm to people. Given the many unknowns, both within and between generations, it seems clear that primate models will be required more than ever to maximize child health and well-being as scientific advances become translated into clinical and societal applications.

REFERENCES

American Association on Mental Retardation (1992). *Mental Retardation: Definition, Classification and Systems of Supports*. Washington, DC: American Association on Mental Retardation.

Anderson, V. R. and Keating, G. M. (2006). Methylphenidate controlled-delivery capsules (EquasymXL, Metadate CD): a review of its use in the treatment of children and adolescents with attention-deficit hyperactivity disorder. *Paediatr Drugs* 8, 319–333.

Biersdorff, K. K. (1999). Dueling definitions: Developmental disabilities, mental retardation and their measurement. *Rehabil Rev* 10, June.

Braddock, D. (2002). Public financial support for disability at the dawn of the 21st century. *Am J Ment Retard* 107, 478–489.

Centers for Disease Control (CDC) (2007). www.cdc.gov/ncbddd/ddsurv.htm.

Davies, K. (2006). Economic costs of childhood diseases and disabilities attributed to environmental contaminants in Washington State, USA. *Eco Health* 3, 86–94.

Fredrickson, W. T., Gould, P. L., Gunderson, V. M., and Grant–Webster, K. S. (1987). Complex learning by low-birth-weight and normal-birth-weight juvenile pigtailed macaques (*Macaca nemestrina*). *Dev Psychol* 23, 483–489.

Gottlieb, G. and Halpern, C. T. (2002). A relational view of causality in normal and abnormal development. *Dev Psychopathol* **14**, 421–435.

Ha, J. C., Kimpo C. L., and Sackett G. P. (1997). Multiple-spell discrete-time survival analysis of developmental data: object concept in pigtailed macaques. *Dev Psychol* **33**, 1054–1059.

Harlow, H. F. and Mears, C. (1979). *The Human Model: Primate Perspectives*. New York: John Wiley and Sons.

Klein, N. J., Plenefisch, J. D., Carey, S. W. *et al.* (1982). Serum from monkeys with histories of fetal wastage causes abnormalities in cultured rat embryos. *Science* **215**, 66–69.

Kroeker, R., Sackett, G., and Reynolds, J. (2007). Statistical methods for describing evelopmental milestones with censored data: effects of birth weight status and sex in neonatal pigtailed macaques. *Am J Primatol* (in press).

Mincenter (2006). Minnesota Center for Environmental Adequacy. www.mincenter.org, June.

Nakamichi, M. (1986). Behavior of infant Japanese monkeys (*Macaca fuscata*) with congenital limb malformations during their first three months. *Dev Psychobiol* **19**, 335–341.

Ruppenthal, G. C. and Sackett, G. P. (2006). Nursery care of at-risk nonhuman primates. In Sackett, G. P., Ruppenthal, G. C. and Elias, K. eds. *Nursery Rearing of Nonhuman Primates in the 21st Century*. New York: Kluwer Academic Publishers, pp. 371–390.

Sackett, G. P. (1984). A nonhuman primate model of risk for deviant development. *Am J Ment Defic* **88**, 469–476.

Sackett, G. P. (1988). Animal rights, human rights, scientific rights: Who's right? *Contemp Psychol* **33**, 23–25.

Sackett, G. P. (1990). Sires influence fetal death in pigtailed macaques (*Macaca nemestrina*). *Am J Primatol* **20**, 13–22.

Sackett, G. P. and Gould, P. (1991). What can primate models of human developmental psychology model? In Cichetti, D. and Toth, S. eds. *Rochester Symposium on Developmental Psychopathology*, Vol. 2: *Internalizing and Externalizing Expressions of Dysfunction*. Hillsdale, NJ: Erlbaum Associates, pp. 265–292.

Stephens, M. L. (1986). Maternal deprivation experiments in psychology: A critique of animal models. Jenkintown, PA: American Antivivisection Society.

Weeks, B., Klein, N., Kleinman, H., Fredrickson, W. T., and Sackett, G. P. (1986). Sera from monkeys immunized with laminin are teratogenic to cultured rat embryos. *Teratology* **33**, 62c.

Wiki (2007). Animal testing. http://en.wikipedia.org/wiki/animal_testing.

Wolf, M.-J., Koldewijn, K., Beelen, A., Smit, B., Hedlund, R., and de Groot, I. J. M. (2002). Neurobehavioral and developmental profile of very low birthweight preterm infants in early infancy. *Acta Paediatr* **91**, 930–938.

Worlein, J. M. and Sackett, G. P. (1997). Social development in nursery-reared pigtailed macaques (*Macaca nemestrina*). *Am J Primatol* **41**, 23–36.

CHAPTER 2

The Origin of Developmental Psychopathologies: Insights from Nonhuman Primate Studies

Anne-Pierre Goursaud and Jocelyne Bachevalier

Human psychopathologies with childhood onset, such as autism spectrum disorders and Williams syndrome, are frequently associated with profound socio-emotional deficits persisting into adulthood and can severely impair the life of affected individuals. Although there is increasing knowledge about the phenotypic characterization of such disorders, their biological origins are not well defined. Several brain regions, including the amygdala and orbital frontal cortex, have been identified as part of the primate social brain network underlying social cognition processes, but their respective roles in early-onset psychopathologies remain unclear. This chapter will show that neonatal lesions targeted to specific brain structures known to mediate social skills in primates can provide an excellent model to investigate the neural substrates of behavioral and cognitive deficits found in childhood psychopathologies. We begin with an overview of the contribution of the amygdala and orbital frontal cortex to social cognition. We then illustrate that social skills and their neural substrates develop in a similar sequence from infancy through adulthood in macaques and humans. Then, behavioral outcomes after early lesions of the macaque amygdala, adjacent mid-temporal areas, or orbital frontal cortex are reviewed. Next, data on social cognition deficits are summarized, as well as recent findings on dysfunction of the amygdala and orbital frontal cortex in the early-onset psychopathologies of autism spectrum disorders and Williams syndrome. The final section assesses the relevance of specific early lesions in monkeys for a better understanding of the neural substrates underlying human neurodevelopmental disorders.

INTRODUCTION

Early-onset psychopathologies, such as autism spectrum disorder (ASD), Williams syndrome, and schizophrenia, are severe disorders of human development often associated with profound social disabilities. Their biological origin is poorly understood for several reasons. First, these disorders show considerable variation between individuals in specific symptoms and in their development during childhood and early adolescence. Second, our knowledge of the mechanisms underlying the development of normal social cognition is incomplete, making it even more difficult to understand abnormal development of social cognitive processes. Third, many pre- and postnatal factors, such as genetic predispositions, hormonal influences, and early social experiences, might influence the development of the brain leading to abnormal functioning and early-onset psychopathologies. Finally, while there has been an unprecedented effort using an array of techniques for studying brain–behavior relationships to elucidate neural mechanisms underlying social cognition, much remains to be learned of the brain regions critically implicated in the emergence of basic social skills in childhood.

The difficulty mainly resides in the paucity of childhood cases with congenital or acquired damage to brain regions underlying social skills (Pelphrey *et al.*, 2004), and in the inability of using functional neuroimaging in early infancy when the basic social skills necessary for development of adaptive social relationships are laid out. Although case studies of developmental syndromes associated with social impairment provide critical information on specific neural substrates responsible for social impairment and brain systems contributing to social cognition in general, clearer knowledge will likely emerge from experimental studies. In this regard, nonhuman primates are excellent candidates because they display complex cognitive abilities and social skills, and many of these skills and brain structures develop in a sequence similar to that of humans. Thus, nonhuman primate mechanistic studies can show how dysfunction in a specific neural structure at a given developmental stage results in a characteristic behavioral phenotype.

In this chapter we first summarize recent progress in identifying brain systems underlying social cognition in primates. We focus on two key brain structures: the amygdala and orbital frontal cortex. We review what is known for monkeys about (1) the contribution of each structure to social cognition, (2) the maturation of these brain structures, and (3) the links of these structures to specific social and behavioral changes at critical periods from infancy through adolescence. Then, we review experimental investigations assessing effects of neonatal medial temporal lobe lesions, including the amygdala or orbital frontal cortex, on social cognition processes in rhesus macaques. Finally, we will examine the relevance of these nonhuman primate models for understanding the neural systems involved in developmental psychopathologies, with a specific focus on ASD and Williams syndrome.

SOCIAL COGNITION AND THE SOCIAL BRAIN

Social cognition refers to the capacity to guide and modulate behaviors in response to socially relevant stimuli from conspecifics (Brothers, 1990; Adolphs, 2001, 2003a,

2003b). It encompasses a set of abilities that includes the perception, identification, and interpretation of relevant social signals, as well as evaluation and modulation of one's own behavior in relation to that of others based on internal contingencies, emotion, and motivation. This perception–action cycle is a fundamental adaptive process. It begins early in life in humans and many animal species. It permits individuals to effectively achieve appropriate goals in an ever-changing social environment (Cicchetti and Tucker, 1994; Loveland, 2001). Recent progress towards understanding the neural structures or networks underlying social cognition has identified a set of interconnected brain regions that play a critical role (reviewed by Adolphs, 2001, 2003b; Bachevalier and Meunier, 2005). The amygdala, cortex within the superior temporal sulcus, fusiform gyrus, orbital frontal cortex, and anterior cingulate cortex have all been strongly implicated. For the purpose of this review, we focus on the primate amygdala and orbital frontal cortex because they are the only two structures for which we currently have information about postnatal maturation and about the behavioral and cognitive effects of their dysfunction early in development.

The primate amygdala (Figure 2.1b) consists of 13 interconnected nuclei that have extensive reciprocal connections with other subcortical and cortical structures (review by Amaral *et al.*, 1992; Aggleton and Saunders, 2000; Amaral, 2002). It receives highly processed sensory information from multimodal cortical areas, which can be reciprocally modulated through widespread feedback projections reaching as far as primary sensory cortical areas. It also modulates basic autonomic, hormonal, and motor functions, some linking perception to emotional response via connections to the hypothalamus, brainstem, and ventral striatum. It also links to higher cognitive processes involved in attention, memory, and executive functions through interactions with the hippocampus and prefrontal cortical areas.

Earlier behavioral studies in monkeys with large bilateral temporal lobe damage were the first to associate the amygdala with social cognition (Klüver and Bucy, 1938, 1939; Rosvold *et al.*, 1954). These operated monkeys displayed an array of symptoms including a tendency to explore and interact compulsively with every stimulus in the environment (often with the mouth), an inability to detect the meaning of objects by sight only (visual agnosia or psychic blindness), a transient loss of emotional reactions, occasional changes in alimentary habits involving eating meat or feces, excessive or aberrant sexuality, and disturbances of behavior such as unusual, repetitive motor behaviors. Refinement of the specific contribution of the amygdala to social cognition emerged from several lines of research, including selective lesions and electrophysiological studies in monkeys (reviewed by Bachevalier and Meunier, 2005), studies of human patients with circumscribed amygdala damage, and neuroimaging studies in normal humans (reviewed by Zald, 2003). These experiments showed that the amygdala is a critical structure for the perception and recognition of socially salient stimuli, such as faces (Leonard *et al.*, 1985; Fried *et al.*, 1997, 2002), facial and vocal expressions of emotion (Adolphs *et al.*, 1994, 1995; Breiter *et al.*, 1996; Morris *et al.*, 1996; Young *et al.*, 1996; Whalen *et al.*, 1998; Phillips *et al.*, 1998; Adolphs and Tranel, 2004), detection of gaze

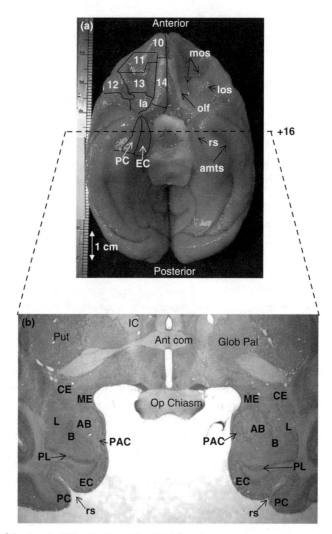

FIGURE 2.1   Anatomical localization of the orbital frontal cortex and amygdala in the rhesus macaque (*Macaca mulatta*) brain. Photograph of a ventral view of a macaque brain (a) identifying the borders (black lines) of the orbital frontal cortex cytoarchitectonic fields (e.g. Broadman areas 10, 11, 12, 13, and 14 from Carmichael and Price, 1994; Barbas, 1995; Öngür and Price, 2000; Petrides and Pandya, 2002) on the right hemisphere (left on the photograph). The borders of the entorhinal (EC) and perirhinal (PC) cortices in the temporal lobe are also shown on the right hemisphere. The sulci on the orbital and temporal surfaces of the brain are indicated by arrows on the left hemisphere (right on the photograph). (b) Photomicrograph of a Nissl-stained coronal section through the medial temporal lobe (at +16 mm from the interaural plane) of a macaque brain, showing the amygdala nuclei and the entorhinal and perirhinal cortices. Amts, anterior medial temporal sulcus; Ant com, anterior commissure; AB, accessory basal nucleus; B, basal nucleus; CE, central nucleus; Glob Pal, globus pallidus; Ia, Insular agranular cortex; IC, internal capsule; L, lateral nucleus; los, lateral orbital sulcus; ME, medial nucleus; mos, medial orbital sulcus; olf, olfactory sulcus; Op Chiasm, optic chiasm; PAC, periamygdaloid nucleus; PL, paralaminar nucleus; Put, putamen; rs, rhinal sulcus. (See Plate 1 for the color version of this figure.)

direction or body movements (Brothers, 1990; Brothers and Ring, 1993; Kawashima *et al.*, 1999) and identification of the salience of social signals (Adolphs, 2003c; Phillips *et al.*, 2003; Phelps and Ledoux, 2005).

The amygdala may also influence the type of visual information involving social versus non-social cues that our eyes spontaneously seek in the environment. Adolphs and colleagues (2005) observed that impairment in recognizing fear in facial expressions in a patient with early bilateral amygdala damage (S.M.) was associated with changes in spontaneous face scanning patterns. Thus, unlike normal subjects who spent more time scanning the eye region of the face, S.M. looked preferentially at other regions of the face such as nose and mouth. Interestingly, when explicitly instructed to focus on the eyes of a face stimulus, S.M. was able to identify facial expressions of fear. The amygdala is also involved in linking social information detected in faces, such as fear or trust, to internal representations involving the concept of fear or trust. This function involves higher cognitive processes, including social judgment (Adolphs *et al.*, 1994, 1998; Winston *et al.*, 2002; Stone *et al.*, 2003). Thus, when normal subjects looked at a video-clip displaying animated geometric shapes moving around a box, they immediately made social attributions and described the shapes as characters with emotions and intentions toward each others (Heider and Simmel, 1944). In contrast, patients with bilateral amygdala damage were unable to infer social intentions or emotional reactions to the animated shapes, describing them in geometrical terms (Heberlein and Adolphs, 2004; Shaw *et al.*, 2004).

Finally, the amygdala has been implicated in learning about the biological value of stimuli, such as associating stimuli to their reward value (reviewed by Baxter and Murray, 2002). Since social signals can be viewed as conditioned reinforcers or punishers (reviewed by Rolls, 1999, 2000, 2004; Schultz *et al.*, 2000a; Martin-Soelch *et al.*, 2001), the ability to regulate one's own behavior by suppressing responses that are no longer appropriate or by strengthening advantageous choices can be critical for social modulation and integration. In support for a role of the amygdala in such self-regulatory processes, human patients with amygdala damage, like amygdala-operated monkeys, display inappropriate and irrational social behavior and social disinhibition (see Emery *et al.*, 2001; Adolphs, 2003b; Bechara *et al.*, 2003; Machado and Bachevalier, 2006; Mason *et al.*, 2006).

The orbital frontal cortex (Figure 2.1a), located just above the orbit, is a mesio-cortical area that shares great similarities among primates, including analogous cytoarchitectonic fields, such as Broadmann's areas 11, 13, 12, and 14 (Carmichael and Price, 1994; Barbas, 1995; Öngür and Price, 2000; Petrides and Pandya, 2002). Like the amygdala, the orbital frontal cortex receives highly processed multisensory information, and has a vast field of reciprocal connections with many structures. These include the brainstem, hypothalamus, amygdala, hippocampus, cingulate gyrus, as well as other regions of the prefrontal cortex (reviewed by Cavada *et al.*, 2000; Rolls, 2004). The first indication of a role of this cortical area in social cognition was the description of a railroad worker who had had an accident in which an iron pole had passed through his orbit and cranium, predominantly damaging the ventral, medial, and orbital parts of the frontal lobes (Harlow, 1848, republished in Harlow, 1999; also Mesulam, 2002 for a more detailed description). Following his accident, this patient became socially irresponsible, irreverent, impulsive, and unstable, despite preserved general cognitive and motor abilities (Harlow, 1848).

More recent evidence in both human and nonhuman primates has identified specific roles of the orbital frontal cortex in social cognition (reviewed by Rolls, 2004; Bachevalier and Meunier 2005). Thus, neurophysiological, functional imaging, and lesion studies suggest that the orbital frontal cortex monitors and alters learned behavioral responses based on changes in stimulus contingencies (reward value) or current motivational states (Thorpe et al., 1983; Bechara et al., 1994, 1998; Rolls et al., 1996; O'Doherty et al., 2001; Rolls, 2000, 2004; Arana et al., 2003), even in the case of uncertain outcomes (Critchley et al., 2001).

The orbital frontal cortex also contributes to the anticipation of rewards (O'Doherty et al., 2002). For instance, orbital frontal neurons in monkeys respond differentially to sensory stimuli, such as odors, tastes, or faces (Thorpe et al., 1983; Ó Scalaidhe et al., 1997; Booth et al., 1998). These neurons modify their activity depending on actual or expected reward values (Thorpe et al., 1983; Rolls et al., 1996). Similarly, in humans, orbital frontal cortex activity is selectively increased when participants have to judge their level of emotion when watching emotional faces, but it is decreased when judging non-emotional features of the face such as a wide nose (Monk et al., 2003).

In an experimental model of social interaction, Kringelbach and Rolls (2003) demonstrated that normal people showed specific activation of the orbital frontal cortex during the reversal learning phase of a task requiring changes in behavioral responses based on facial expressions of emotion. This activation suggests a role of orbital frontal region in reappraisal of the affective or emotional value of stimuli. In addition, while sparing intellectual abilities, damage to the orbital frontal cortex in humans produces severe impairment in emotion and social behaviors, including euphoria, irresponsibility, impulsivity, and lack of affect, as well as difficulties in real-life decision-making (Damasio, 1994; Rolls et al., 1994; Kolb and Whishaw, 1996; Hornak et al., 1996, 2003; Rolls, 1999, 2004; Tranel, 2002; Berlin et al., 2004). These patients tend to make decisions based on short-term outcomes, disregarding long-term, but potentially more advantageous, choices (Eslinger and Damasio, 1985; Anderson et al., 1999; Bechara et al., 2000). Taken together, these data suggest that the orbital frontal cortex controls and adjusts behavioral responses by correcting choices when they become inappropriate. This probably occurs through its interactions with medial temporal lobe structures, thus contributing to higher cognitive processes involved in social and moral judgments and decoding or reasoning about mental (theory of mind) and emotional (empathy) states of others (Baron-Cohen et al., 1994; Stone et al., 1998; Baxter et al., 2000; Brunet et al., 2000; Farrow et al., 2001; Moll et al., 2002a, 2002b; Sabbagh, 2004).

In summary, the amygdala appears to critically code and process facial movements, eye-gaze directions, body postures, and gestures that are potent signals for the production and modulation of appropriate social and emotional responses towards other individuals (Adolphs, 1999, 2003c). The orbital frontal cortex makes use of this information by guiding goal-directed behaviors and adjusting behavior appropriately in accordance with changing conditions (Bechara *et al.*, 1999; Holland and Gallagher, 2004; Bachevalier and Loveland, 2006).

Given our current understanding of the amygdala and orbital frontal cortex functions, how could we best characterize their contribution to the development of social skills? We believe that the answer to this question is critical for a better understanding of the role of these brain regions in the symptoms associated with developmental psychopathologies. Unfortunately, our knowledge in this area is limited. Although we have a good understanding of the nature and time-course of the development of social skills in both human and nonhuman primates (reviewed by Machado and Bachevalier, 2003), the brain areas that support these skills in infancy and adolescence remain unknown. In addition, there exist only a handful of studies in monkeys that have systematically assessed the long-term behavioral outcomes of early dysfunction of neural structures mediating social cognition. The next three sections provide an updated account of what is known about these outcomes.

DEVELOPMENT OF SOCIAL SKILLS IN MACAQUES

Similarly to humans, macaque monkeys are highly social animals living in complex and dynamic social organizations that are maintained through a variety of social relationships between members of the group (Byrne and Whiten, 1988; de Waal, 1989; Cheney and Seyfarth, 1990). To maintain these multilevel relationships and group cohesion, monkeys must be able to recognize and remember each other as well as perceive and interpret the social cues and emotional behaviors displayed by other individuals. In addition, they must compare this information about others with what they know about themselves, such as their social rank (e.g. lower ranking infant versus dominant, alpha male) and their level of agonistic behavior. Monkeys must be able to respond appropriately to these social signals depending upon who they are interacting with and maintain a fitting course of social interaction when in pursuit of goals such as finding the appropriate mate, avoiding aggression, or maintaining their rank within the social hierarchy (see Ghazanfar and Santos, 2004, for a recent review).

In monkeys, these social skills develop progressively during infancy and follow a sequence similar to that found in humans, although the developmental process is faster in monkeys than in humans (Machado and Bachevalier, 2003, for review). Thus, during the first few postnatal weeks, infant monkeys have an exclusive relationship with their mother, characterized by face-to-face interactions, ventro-ventral contacts and grooming (Hinde and Spencer-Booth, 1967). During this early neonatal period, infant monkeys progressively learn to discriminate and recognize the social cues present in faces as well as to respond to them appropriately. In an earlier study, Mendelson and colleagues (1982) showed that during the first post-natal week, infant monkeys, although very interested by faces, looked indiscriminately at faces displaying different gaze directions. By the end of the second week of age, however, they displayed more gaze aversions toward faces staring at them than to faces looking away. Because staring faces and faces looking away convey different social signals (dominant and submissive signals, respectively), the abilities to discriminate gaze directions in the first weeks of life and to respond to it appropriately (averting gaze) suggest that by this age, monkeys are able to attribute social meaning to faces. Perception of gaze direction is a basic process necessary for the development of other critical social skills, such as gaze following and joint attention (Emery, 2000), that are known to be present in adult monkeys (Emery et al., 1997), although the exact timing of their emergence in infancy is still unknown. Concomitant with the emergence of gaze aversion, infant monkeys start to display species-typical facial expressions that appear to emerge at different ages (Mason, 1985). Thus, although infant monkeys first respond to faces (e.g. pictures or mirror-images of both humans and monkeys) with both gaze aversion and friendly/submissive facial expressions, such as lipsmacks (Mendelson, 1982), it is only by the third week of life that they also began to display the fear grimace (Kenney et al., 1979).

By the end of the first month and during the second month of life, infant monkeys become more independent of their mother and explore their social and non-social environment (Hinde et al., 1964; Hinde and Spencer-Booth, 1967). Thus, it is not surprising that by that age they are able to recognize their mother (Rosenblum and Paully, 1980) as well as to discriminate the calls of their mother from that of other familiar adult monkeys (Masataka, 1985).

Between 4 and 6 months of age, monkeys can adaptively modulate their defensive reactions to meet changing environmental demands (Kalin and Shelton, 1989; Kalin et al., 1991). It is also at this age that they respond with different emotions to specific facial expressions, and display fear of strangers (Suomi, 1984), suggesting that the innate wiring and/or learned skills needed to discriminate threatening cues are in place. Nonetheless, it is not until the second half of their first year, which corresponds to the period of weaning by the mother (Hinde et al., 1964; Hinde and Spencer-Booth, 1967) and of increasing interactions with peers, that infant monkeys display agonistic behaviors and begin to modulate their aggression in relation to specific situations (Suomi, 1984; Bernstein and Ehardt, 1985). This self-control of agonistic behavior, which is critical for their integration in the social hierarchy of the group, is not adult-like until one year of age (Hinde and Spencer-Booth, 1967). Thus, yearling infant monkeys have the ability to link their own actions to that of others and adapt their behavior, using self-regulation processes, in accordance with contingencies of the social environment.

Like humans, monkeys appear to progressively develop sophisticated cognitive abilities and social skills that will permit them to interpret and respond appropriately to social actions from their conspecifics (de Waal, 1989; Brothers, 1989, 1995; Cheney and Seyfarth, 1990). This progressive development of affective, affiliative,

and agonistic responses suggests that the maturation of the neural circuits supporting social skills progresses in stages, as different components of the circuit become
fully mature. As summarized below, the experimental data to support this proposal
are meager, but certainly offer a point of departure to initiate further investigations
of the development of the neural network supporting primate social cognition.

DEVELOPMENT OF THE SOCIAL BRAIN IN MACAQUES

As recently reviewed (Machado and Bachevalier, 2003), the amygdala is one of the
earliest developing structures in the primate telencephalon. Neurogenesis in the
rhesus macaque amygdala (Kordower *et al.*, 1992) occurs smoothly in all nuclei, at
approximately the same developmental time (i.e. between days 30 and 50 of the
165 days of gestation) and with a sequence and pattern similar to humans (Humphrey,
1968). This maturation progresses until weeks 13–16 of gestation for developing
neurons in the lateral nucleus (Nikolić and Kostović, 1986). Connectivity, from
and toward the amygdala, is present at birth and almost adult-like at two weeks
(Amaral and Bennett, 2000), although some amygdala afferents are still in their
immature form, such as the projections from posterior visual temporal areas
(Webster *et al.*, 1991).

The development of neuronal myelination in the amygdala is largely unknown,
but seems to begin around the end of the first postnatal month and continues during the first 3 years of life (Gibson, 1991). A similar postnatal progression in the
maturation of the amygdala was also found in a recent *in vivo* neuroimaging study
indicating that, in both male and female monkeys, amygdala volumes increased
from 1 to 115 weeks (i.e. 2 years) of age, although males maintained a larger amygdala size relative to brain volume throughout this developmental period compared
with females (Payne *et al.*, 2006). Finally, the few studies that have investigated the
neurochemical development of the amygdala in monkeys have shown that whereas
the distribution of some components, such as opioid receptors, seems to be adult-
like at birth (Bachevalier *et al.*, 1986), some other components, such as the sero-
toninergic fibers, continue to expand and differentiate during the first few postnatal
months (Bauman and Amaral, 2005). Thus, although the morphological development of the primate amygdala appears to be complete relatively early after birth, its
connectional and neurochemical development continues progressively within the
first two years of life.

Much less is known on the maturation of the orbital frontal cortex in monkeys
(for a complete review, see Machado and Bachevalier, 2003). Although there are no
specific reports on its embryologic development, the establishment of its connections
seems to continue during the postnatal period. Thus, cortico-cortical fibers between
the left and the right orbital frontal cortex are well organized by the end of the gestation (Goldman and Nauta, 1977) and its connectivity with the temporal cortical

areas appears complete shortly after birth (Webster *et al.*, 1994). By contrast, the reciprocal connections between the orbital frontal cortex and several visual temporal cortical areas reach the adult-like pattern only during the third postnatal month (Rodman and Consuelos, 1994). Myelination within the orbital frontal cortex is slow and apparently continues during the first four postnatal months (Gibson, 1991). Neurochemical organization of the orbital frontal cortex is also not completely achieved at birth, but continues to develop during the six first postnatal months (Hayashi and Oshima, 1986). Thus, although the dopaminergic system attains adult-like distribution very rapidly, during the first few days after birth, some reorganization in its pattern of innervations continues during the second postnatal month (Berger *et al.*, 1990). In contrast, the cholecystokininergic neurons within the orbital frontal cortex begin to regress in the first postnatal month to reach the neuronal number seen in the adult around the fifth month after birth (Oeth and Lewis, 1993). Gender differences in the functional development of the orbital frontal cortex, with the males showing earlier maturation than the females, also exist (see for review Overman, 2004). Thus, as for the amygdala, the primate orbital frontal cortex continues to develop postnatally and is not fully functional before 1–2 years of age.

In sum, with the early morphological development of the amygdala in the first postnatal month, infant monkeys should be able to discriminate affective cues from faces of their mother and other conspecifics, and possibly recognize intonations of vocal communications as well. However, with the refinement of the cortico-amygdala projections during the first three months of life, infants may gain increasingly detailed information about the perceptual characteristics of social signals. This refinement could well be at the origin of the emergence of the ability to adapt and modulate defensive responses towards threatening stimuli. The emergence of fear and defensive responses around the third postnatal month corresponds to the age at which rhesus mothers generally allow their infants to venture off with their peers. This affective development indicates that, by this age, infant monkeys respond with different emotional displays to specific facial expressions from other conspecifics, suggesting that the innate wiring and learned skills needed to discriminate threatening cues are in place. It also suggests that some important changes in the neural organization of the network assuring defensive responses have occurred. It is likely that these changes encompass a refinement of connectivity not only within the amygdala but also between the amygdala and other areas of the brain.

Given the participation of the orbital frontal cortex in the interpretation of sensory stimuli and in the suppression of maladaptive responses in favor of appropriate ones, one would assume that important changes could occur between amygdala-orbital frontal cortex interactions around this postnatal age. Very little is known in this respect, except that it is around this age that the ability to perform object reversal tasks emerges in monkeys (Goldman, 1971). Since this learning skill is known to depend on the integrity of the orbital frontal cortex in adult monkeys, the maturation of the orbital frontal cortex and of its connections with the amygdala around 3–4 months would permit the animal to modulate their affective responses according to constant changes in social cues provided by others and to contend successfully with danger.

Finally, increasingly complex social skills such as accurately identifying emotional and intention states and selecting the most appropriate behavioral responses emerge at an age (approximately 1 year) when the orbital frontal cortex, namely its most posterior portion, attains adult level of myelination (Gibson, 1991) and shows changes in its neurochemistry (Oeth and Lewis, 1993).

BEHAVIORAL OUTCOMES FOLLOWING SELECTIVE NEONATAL LESIONS

Kling and colleagues (Kling and Green, 1967; Kling, 1972) followed the development of four monkeys that had received an amygdalectomy during infancy. When returned to their mothers, these operated infant monkeys displayed normal nipple orientation, sucking, and grasping, with a somatic and affective development in the normal range. In addition, following repeated presentations of inedible objects, these operated animals did not display the typical compulsive oral behavior seen in amygdalectomized adult monkeys (Bachevalier and Meunier, 2005). This apparent normal behavioral repertoire after neonatal amygdalectomy is consistent with a number of studies showing that the behavioral effects of brain damage are minimized when the injury occurs early in life and can be accounted for by incomplete maturation of the brain at the time of the insult (Goldman, 1971). Nevertheless, the normal behavioral responses after early amygdala lesions could have resulted from the lack of specific quantification of behavioral responses and from the few aspects of amygdala functions investigated in these studies.

More systematic and detailed investigation of the effects of neonatal amygdala lesions in rhesus monkeys clearly show that bilateral amygdalectomy does not leave the subject unharmed, even when the surgery is performed during infancy (Thompson et al., 1969, Thompson and Towfighi, 1976, Thompson et al., 1977, Thompson, 1981). Aspiration lesions of the amygdala at 2–3 months of age, including all amygdaloid nuclei, the entorhinal and perirhinal cortices (see Figure 2.1a) and all fibers coursing within and around the amygdala, yielded significant behavioral and emotional changes. These changes varied according to whether the environment was social or non-social and/or familiar or unfamiliar and the age at which behavioral testing was performed. Peer-reared operated monkeys were tested at 3–5 months while interacting with familiar age-matched normal monkeys. They showed enhanced fear reactions, such as grimaces, withdrawals, rigid postures, screams and rocking movements during social interactions, but less fear than the normal controls toward novel objects when tested alone (Thompson et al., 1969). As adolescents at 3.5 years or adults at 6.5 years, the operated monkeys still displayed increased fear responses towards familiar conspecifics (Thompson and Towfighi, 1976; Thompson et al., 1977). In addition, as adults they showed less fearful behaviors than normal controls when paired with unfamiliar aggressive normal monkeys. They also displayed inappropriate behaviors, such as staring at the unfamiliar monkey, immediately after an attack from the later (Thompson et al., 1977). These results suggest that it is not the emergence of fear responses that is altered by neonatal amygdala lesions, but rather the appropriate modulation of fear responses according to the social or nonsocial environmental context. Thus, neonatal amygdala lesions may have hampered the ability to evaluate the significance of social cues expressed by conspecifics (Adolphs, 2001).

The operated monkeys also had a tendency to change behaviors more frequently than controls and this phenomenon was most evident when the animals were placed in a novel environment prior to 13 months of age, as well as in social situations later on (Thompson, 1969; Thompson et al., 1977). Thus, neonatal amygdala damage resulted in behavioral changes that intensified over time and appeared to be similar to those found in adult monkeys that had acquired the same lesions in adulthood (Thompson et al., 1977). Thus, beginning early in infancy, the primate amygdala appears to play a critical role in the modulation of emotional responses and in the regulation of social behavior.

Another series of developmental studies in monkeys replicated and extended Thompson's findings (Bachevalier 1991, 1994; Bachevalier et al., 1999a, 2001). Peer-reared infant monkeys received neonatal bilateral aspiration lesions that were more extensive than those used in Thompson's studies. They included not only the amygdala and rhinal cortex but also the hippocampus and parahippocampal cortex. This was intended to reproduce the brain damage inflicted in the well-known amnesic case of H.M. (Scoville and Milner, 1957). The major goal was to investigate whether neonatal medial temporal lobe (MTL) lesions would, like H.M., result in an amnesic syndrome or whether memory functions would be spared and mediated by other neural systems due to plasticity of the brain at the time of the lesions.

Neonatal MTL lesions yielded a profound anterograde and global amnesia, but they were also associated with socio-emotional changes (Bachevalier and Malkova, 2000). When tested at two months of age during social interactions with a same-age familiar peer in a familiar environment, the operated infants initiated less social approach than controls, but did accept approaches. They were also more passive and more irritable than the controls. At six months of age, the amount of social interaction by operated animals dramatically decreased, presumably because of their increased withdrawal from social interactions coupled with an increase in aggressive approaches on the part of the control subjects. Operated infants also showed unexpressive faces and had little eye contact, and during social exchanges exhibited more repetitive motor behaviors and self-directed activities than controls (Bachevalier et al., 2001). As adults, the MTL-operated animals had a negligible amount of social interaction. All of the social and emotional disturbances observed at younger ages were still present (Malkova et al., 1997), and even more severe than those observed after MTL lesions acquired in adulthood (Malkova et al., 1997).

Further investigations suggested that most of these emotional and social abnormalities could have resulted, as in the case of Thompson's studies (Thompson, 1969,

1981; Thompson et al., 1969, 1977; Thompson and Towfighi, 1976), from damage to the amygdala and not from additional damage to the hippocampus (Bachevalier, 1994). Thus, neonatal bilateral aspiration lesions restricted to the amygdala, sparing the hippocampus and parahippocampal cortex, yielded social and emotional disturbances similar to those of the more widespread neonatal MTL lesions. Although the nature of emotional and social changes resulting from neonatal MTL and amygdala lesions was similar, their magnitude was less after the neonatal amygdala lesions than the larger neonatal MTL lesions (Bachevalier, 1994; Meunier et al., 1999). Like MTL-operated infants during social interactions with their normal age-matched peers at two months of age, amygdala-operated infants displayed more inactivity than controls. But unlike the MTL infants, the amygdala-operated monkeys showed no impairments in initiation of social contacts. However, by six months of age, both MTL-operated and amygdala-operated infants displayed less initiation of social contact and more social withdrawal than controls, as well as an increased amount of stereotyped behaviors. The amygdala-operated animals also displayed an inability to modulate fear vocalizations when briefly separated from their familiar conspecifics (Newman and Bachevalier, 1997). Nonetheless, no neonatal amygdala-operated monkey showed the severe memory deficits found after neonatal MTL lesions (Bachevalier et al., 1999a).

When compared with the MTL and amygdala lesions, neonatal lesions of the hippocampus, which spared the amygdala, had little effect on socio-emotional behavior at two and six months. However, hippocampal lesions did yield decreased social interaction and increased locomotor stereotypy at a later age (Beauregard et al., 1995). In addition, unlike neonatal amygdala lesions, those involving the hippocampus did result in significant memory deficits (Beauregard et al., 1995; Bachevalier et al., 1999a, 1999b). Taken together, these earlier studies indicated that neonatal damage to the amygdala results in socio-emotional changes that seem to intensify with age. With more extended damage to adjacent brain structures, such as the medial temporal cortical areas and the hippocampus, these socio-emotional behavioral changes became more severe and memory loss was profound.

Two issues from these studies remain unresolved. First, it was found in adult monkeys that the magnitude of emotional changes after amygdala aspiration or electrolytic lesions including fibers of passage and adjacent entorhinal and perirhinal cortical areas is greater than after neurotoxic lesions which spared these cortical structures (Meunier et al., 1999, also see Figure 2.2). In addition, selective damage to the rhinal cortical areas alone resulted in emotional changes of opposite direction from amygdala damage. These changes included heightened defensiveness and attenuated submission and approach responses (Meunier and Bachevalier, 2002; Meunier et al., 2006). Like lesions acquired in adulthood, these findings suggest that the socio-emotional effects found after neonatal amygdala aspiration lesions in the earlier studies could be ascribed to combined damage to the amygdala and rhinal cortex. Second, recent evidence indicates that nursery peer-rearing in monkeys results in deviant emotional reactivity and physiology compared with mother-rearing

(a) Normal amygdala

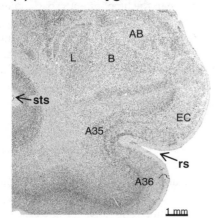

(c) Electrolytic lesion

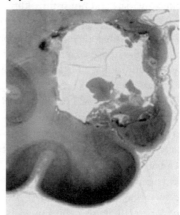

(b) Normal amygdala

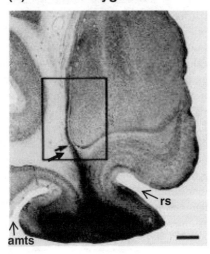

(d) Ibotenic acid lesion

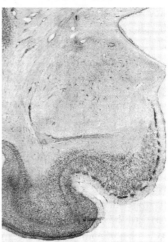

FIGURE 2.2   Photomicrographs of Nissl-stained sections through the amygdala (at +16 mm from the interaural plane) in macaque brains. (a) Amygdaloid nuclei and entorhinal and perirhinal cortices in a normal macaque brain. (b) Injection site of tritiated amino acid (blackened area) centered in the perirhinal cortex on the lateral bank of the rhinal sulcus and efferent fiber bundle traveling just lateral to the lateral nucleus of the amygdala (black arrow). (c,d) Extent of damage produced by electrolytic and neurotoxic lesions of the amygdala, respectively. Note that most of the fibers from the medial temporal cortex traveling through the amygdala and along its lateral border are damaged by electrolytic, but not neurotoxic, lesions. AB, accessory basal nucleus of the amygdala; A35 and A36, areas 35 and 36 of the perirhinal cortex; amts, anterior medial temporal sulcus; B, basal nucleus of the amygdala; EC, enthorhinal cortex; L, lateral nucleus of the amygdala; rs, rhinal sulcus; sts, superior temporal sulcus. Photomicrograph in (b) is from Murray (1991).

(Mason, 2000; Sanchez et al., 2001; Capitanio et al., 2005). Thus, it is possible that the peer-rearing conditions used in the earlier lesion studies could have contributed to the observed behavioral effects. However, in studies using peer-rearing techniques, the behavioral abnormalities that were observed in neonatally amygdala or MTL-operated monkeys were absent in normal controls infants and those with neonatal lesions of visual temporal cortex (Malkova et al., 1997; Bachevalier et al., 2001).

The issues of lesion extent and rearing conditions have been addressed in a series of developmental lesion studies in monkeys. Amaral and colleagues re-evaluated the long-term effects of selective neonatal amygdala and hippocampal lesions, using neuroimaging techniques to produce selective neurotoxic lesions (Prather et al., 2001; Bauman et al., 2004a, 2004b, 2006). These procedures spared adjacent cortical areas and fibers of passage. They also used a more natural rearing condition involving mother-rearing in small social groups.

Two-week-old monkeys received neurotoxic lesions of the amygdala, hippocampus or sham-operations, and were returned to their mother for rearing in individual cages (Prather et al., 2001) or small social groups (Bauman et al., 2004a, 2004b). Amygdala-operated infants displayed increased physical contact with their mother during the first six postnatal months. They did not differ from age-matched hippocampus-operated or sham-operated infants in their maternal interactions and showed recognition and attachment to their mother at six months (Bauman et al., 2004a). However, compared with age-matched controls and hippocampus-operated monkeys, they displayed increased affiliative/submissive responses during peer social interactions after weaning at 9–12 months (Bauman et al., 2004b) and lower social dominance as adolescents at 18 months (Bauman et al., 2006). In addition, amygdala-operated infants displayed more fear grimaces, screams and withdrawals during familiar and unfamiliar peer social interactions than sham-operated controls and hippocampus-operated monkeys, but the groups did not differ when interacting with novel objects (Prather et al., 2001; Bauman et al., 2004b). These data suggest that neonatal amygdala lesions do not alter the development of a normal social repertoire and typical emergence of species-specific fear responses, but do alter modulation of fear responses depending on whether the context is a social or non-social situation. In addition, both neonatal hippocampal and amygdala lesions resulted in an increase in stereotypes (Babineau et al., 2005).

Although these data are in agreement with the earlier observations described above, it is unknown whether the behavioral changes produced by these selective lesions will intensify with further maturation. In addition, the cognitive processes responsible for these behavioral changes have not been carefully investigated. For example, the lack of modulation of fear responses after neonatal amygdala lesions could result from an inability to evaluate the significance of social signals, such as facial expressions, eye gaze direction, or body postures, an ability necessary for selecting appropriate responses in complex social situations. Also, the behavioral deficits after neonatal amygdala lesions found in the studies by Amaral suggest that effects may not be directly linked to amygdala damage. These may be indirect effects of other neural structures, such as the orbital frontal cortex, a structure with strong connections to the amygdala (Barbas, 2000; Cavada et al., 2000; Amaral, 2002) and more protracted anatomical and functional development (Goldman-Rakic et al., 1983). Thus, neonatal damage to the amygdala could indirectly hamper the normal maturation and functioning of the orbital frontal cortex.

An indirect atrophic effect on distant neural structures has been demonstrated for neonatal MTL lesions. Monkeys with these early lesions displayed a striatal-prefrontal dopamine dysregulation (Saunders et al., 1998) and an arrest in maturation of the dorsolateral prefrontal cortex (Bertolino et al., 1997; Chlan-Fourney et al., 2000, 2003). Interestingly, neonatal lesions of the amygdala and hippocampus, separately or in combination, yielded an increase in stereotypies presumably associated with the dysregulation of the striatal-prefrontal dopamine system.

Despite its involvement in social cognition, few studies have assessed the role of the orbital frontal cortex in the development of primate social skills. Bowden and colleagues (1971) did observe the behavior of mother- or peer-reared 10-month-old monkeys who received lesions of the orbital frontal cortex or dorsolateral prefrontal cortex at two months of age. When observed in a familiar social group, orbital-operated monkeys were less active, spent more time huddling alone and initiated fewer behaviors than normal controls. They also touched peers less frequently, but were more often in ventral contact with peers. When alone in a novel environment, infants with orbital frontal cortex lesions were more active than controls, but displayed less environmental exploration. This study supports a role of the orbital frontal cortex in initiation of social behavior, as well as self-regulation of behavioral responses.

These behavioral effects in monkeys are consistent with the impairments in social behavior that have been reported for patients with acquired prefrontal damage in infancy (Anderson et al., 1999; Eslinger et al., 2004). Thus, both the amygdala and orbital frontal cortex apparently play a role in the development of affect at a critical period of primary socialization. In humans, a similar period begins at the end of the second year of life (Tucker et al., 1986; Schore, 1994, 1996; Thatcher, 1994).

IMPLICATION FOR DEVELOPMENTAL DISABILITIES IN HUMANS

This summary of primate developmental studies raises the question of how the pattern of behavioral and cognitive deficits produced by selective neonatal lesions of the amygdala or orbital frontal cortex relate to behavioral and cognitive deficits found in human developmental psychopathologies. Can the data obtained in these animal studies shed light on childhood developmental psychopathology? In this section we discuss the relevance of these findings for two disorders of human development known to severely affect social cognition processes, namely, autism spectrum disorders and Williams syndrome.

Autism spectrum disorder

Autism spectrum disorder (ASD) was first described by Kanner in 1943. By current criteria, ASD is a developmental disorder with a prevalence rate ranging from 2.5 to 30.8 in 10 000 children worldwide, with four times more males than females being affected (see Fombonne, 1999, 2003 for reviews). ASD is characterized by impairment in reciprocal social interactions and relationships, verbal and non-verbal communication, unusual and repetitive behaviors, and restrictive and obsessive interests (see Grossman *et al.*, 1997; Baron-Cohen *et al.*, 2000; Frith and Hill, 2003; Volkmar and Pauls, 2003; Sigman *et al.*, 2004; Baron-Cohen and Belmonte, 2005; Volkmar *et al.*, 2005; Loveland, 2005; Bachevalier and Loveland, 2006; DiCicco-Bloom *et al.*, 2006, for reviews). Although some individuals with autism have high intellectual abilities, most have some degree of mental retardation.

The core deficit is believed to be abnormal socio-emotional development. Young children with autism may develop an attachment to their mother early in life (Ainsworth *et al.*, 1978; Dissanayake and Crossley, 1997; Dissanayake and Sigman 2001; Rutgers *et al.*, 2004; Sigman *et al.*, 2004). This is thought to be critical for development of social competence (see Goursaud and Bachevalier, 2006, for review). However, ASD children have difficulties in establishing and maintaining relationships and reciprocal social interactions later in life.

Many studies have shown that social and emotional deficits in autism can be traced to basic cognitive skills that normally emerge in the first and second years of life (Klin, 1991; Klin *et al.*, 1992, 1999; Adrien *et al.*, 1993; Osterling and Dawson, 1994; Werner *et al.*, 2000). People with autism may not spontaneously seek social information (e.g. Dawson *et al.*, 1998; Klin, 2000). They also show severe impairment in social processing skills, such as face recognition, identification of facial expressions and gestures, or discrimination and memorization of faces (Grelotti *et al.*, 2002; Pelphrey *et al.*, 2002). When they do respond to faces or scenes of social situations, they display atypical patterns of visual scanning (Klin *et al.*, 2002a, 2002b). This might explain their impairments in gaze monitoring, eye contact, gaze following, eye-gaze alternation, and joint attention (Mundy *et al.*, 1986; Adrien *et al.*, 1993; Osterling and Dawson, 1994; Baron-Cohen *et al.*, 1997; Stone, 1997; Leekam *et al.*, 1998, 2000; Baird *et al.*, 2000; Howard *et al.*; 2000; Mundy and Neal, 2001; Charman, 2003; Leekam and Ramsden, 2006), as well as their difficulties in social monitoring (Klin *et al.*, 2002a, 2002b), imitation processes (Smith and Bryson, 1994; Williams *et al.*, 2001, 2004, 2006; McIntosh *et al.*, 2006), and understanding other people's mental and emotional states from their facial expressions (Baron-Cohen, 1995, 2003; Baron-Cohen *et al.*, 1999; Brent *et al.*, 2004) or voices (Klin, 1991; Loveland *et al.*, 1995; Rutherford *et al.*, 2002). Finally, individuals with autism show a higher incidence of anxiety or unusual fears, mania, and depression than matched individuals without autism (Kim *et al.*, 2000; Bradley *et al.*, 2004).

Although the neural origin of ASD is unknown, several anatomical and functional abnormalities have been located within brain systems critical for social skills.

These include not only the amygdala and orbital frontal cortex but also the superior temporal sulcus, cingulate cortex, and fusiform gyrus (reviewed by Pelphrey *et al.*, 2004; Baron-Cohen and Belmonte, 2005; Bachevalier and Loveland, 2006). Morphometric studies have shown abnormal amygdala volume, some studies finding enlargement (Howard *et al.*, 2000; Sparks *et al.*, 2002; Brambilla *et al.*, 2003) and others reduction (Abell *et al.*, 1999; Aylward *et al.*, 1999; Courchesne *et al.*, 2001; Schumann *et al.*, 2004). Another study suggests that the right, but not the left, amygdala is enlarged in autism and that the enlargement is proportional to and predictive of social and communication impairments in early childhood (Munson *et al.*, 2006).

Histopathological studies have demonstrated decreased numbers of neurons, reduced dendritic arborization and increased cell packing density within the amygdala and anterior cingulate cortex (Bauman and Kemper, 1985, 1993). Functional neuroimaging studies consistently report changes in activation in neural structures mediating social skills (Baron-Cohen *et al.*, 2000; Schultz *et al.*, 2003; Bachevalier and Loveland, 2003, 2006; Pelphrey *et al.*, 2004; Schultz, 2005, for reviews). Thus, during face processing, individuals with autism exhibited hypoactivation of the amygdala and fusiform gyrus (e.g. Critchley *et al.*, 2000; Schultz *et al.*, 2000b; Pierce *et al.*, 2001; Hubl *et al.*, 2003; Wang *et al.*, 2004), which was proportionally related to their decreased fixation toward the eye region (e.g. Dalton *et al.*, 2005). They also displayed dysfunction within the frontal lobe, including the orbital frontal cortex (Kawasaki *et al.*, 1997; Harrison *et al.*, 1998; Minshew *et al.*, 1999; Schultz *et al.*, 2000b; Carper and Courchesne, 2000). During processing of voices, but not non-social sounds, there was failure to activate the superior temporal sulcus region in people with autism (Gervais *et al.*, 2004). When making inferences on mental states of others using information conveyed by their eyes, people with autism displayed no amygdala activation and less frontal activity than normal subjects (Baron-Cohen *et al.*, 1997, 1999). During imitation of facial emotional expressions, children with autism compared with typically developing children had lower amygdala and frontal activity. But autistic children had increased activation in neural structures not activated in controls (Dapretto *et al.*, 2006). The latter observation suggests that compensatory brain systems and/or functional reorganization occur in the autistic brain.

Williams syndrome

Williams syndrome is a rare disorder of genetic origin involving 1 in 30 000 births. It is caused by a microdeletion of one copy of a small set of genes, including the gene for elastine and LIM1 kinase, on chromosome 7 (7q11.23) (Ewart *et al.*, 1993). The syndrome is characterized by cognitive and behavioral abnormalities that include mild to moderate mental retardation, delayed language and motor development, and exceedingly poor visuo-spatial skills (Bellugi and St George, 2001; Bhattacharjee, 2005; Meyer-Lindenberg *et al.*, 2006). Other cognitive abilities are relatively spared or even heightened, including expressive language abilities, face and sound perception, recognition and memory (Bellugi *et al.*, 2001).

The most striking characteristic of individuals with Williams syndrome is hypersociality. In contrast to ASD, individuals with this syndrome tend to be overly friendly and engage easily in social interactions, even with strangers. Infants with Williams syndrome show more positive than negative emotional verbal and facial expressions, and an extremely high level of eye contact behavior (Bellugi *et al.*, 2001; Jones *et al.*, 2001; Mervis *et al.*, 2003). Individuals with Williams syndrome gave more positive ratings when judging approachability in faces of unfamiliar people than normal subjects. This suggests an abnormally high motivation to interact with others compared with patients with acquired amygdala damage and people with ASD (Adolphs *et al.*, 1998; Pelphrey *et al.*, 2004). They appear to rely on superficial signals from face stimuli that are typically viewed positively, such as smiling faces, but overlook subtle social cues, such as furrowed eyebrows. Adolescent and adult patients with Williams syndrome process faces differently than other people, and their pattern of facial processing deficits is opposite to that of patients with autism (Rose *et al.*, 2006).

During separation from parents, children with Williams syndrome displayed less frequent negative expressions, lower intensity of vocal and facial distress and negativity, and fewer frustration behaviors, even if they were aware of being alone. When reunited, they resumed play quickly and searched for comfort less frequently than normally developing children (Jones *et al.*, 2001). Thus, it appears that either the quality of the relationship with the caregiver is less intense and/or social isolation is not perceived as traumatic or dangerous in children with Williams syndrome than in typically developing children. Thus, Mervis and colleagues (2003) showed that children with Williams syndrome spent more time looking at familiar and unfamiliar adults during social interactions than typically developing children or children with other genetic syndromes. Also, the duration of their gazes, especially when looking at strangers, was unusually long compared with that of normally developing infants.

Despite their strong attraction for social interaction and fascination with faces, patients with Williams syndrome are impaired in the same aspects of theory of mind tasks as individuals with autism (Sullivan and Tager-Flusberg, 1999; Tager-Flusberg and Sullivan, 2000). Although they show no social fear and no frustration behaviors when unable to perform cognitive tasks (Jones *et al.*, 2001), patients with Williams syndrome display higher non-social anxiety and are more often diagnosed with generalized anxiety disorder than normally developing children (Dykens, 2003).

A few studies investigated neural correlates underlying Williams syndrome social cognition strengths and deficits (reviewed by Meyer-Lindenberg *et al.*, 2006). Both anatomical and functional studies indicate that frontal, cerebellar, and superior temporal structures involved in social behavior are relatively preserved (Reiss *et al.*, 2001). This may contribute to the relative strength of language processing and face and sound perception in Williams syndrome (e.g. Bellugi *et al.*, 2001).

However, other areas, including the amygdala and orbital frontal cortex, are abnormal. Disproportionate increases in volume and gray matter density are observed in
the amygdala, and also in the medial prefrontal, anterior cingulate, insular cortices, and
superior temporal gyrus in Williams syndrome (Meyer-Lindenberg et al., 2004).
Similarly, structural abnormalities, such as increase (Reiss et al., 2004) or decrease
(Meyer-Lindenberg et al., 2004) in gray matter volume in the orbital frontal cortex, have been reported in patients with Williams syndrome with both normal IQ
and mental retardation. In addition, patients with Williams syndrome show a disproportionate reduction in cerebral white matter compared with normal subjects,
suggesting abnormalities in connectivity between neural structures.

Although individuals with Williams syndrome have a relative preserved ability
to process faces, anomalous patterns of brain activation were found in the fusiform
gyrus and frontal and temporal cortex, all areas involved in face processing (Mobbs
et al., 2004). Meyer-Lindenberg et al. (2005) used functional magnetic resonance
imaging (fMRI) to compare brain activation and functional connectivity between
normal-intelligence adult patients with Williams syndrome and normal subjects
during matching tasks requiring processing of angry/fearful faces and threatening/
fearful scenes. Although task performance was similar, significant group differences
were observed in activation of the amygdala and orbital frontal cortex and in their
reciprocal connectivity. The amygdala and orbital frontal cortex were more activated during the faces than scenes conditions in normal controls, whereas patients
with Williams syndrome exhibited the opposite pattern. Furthermore, there was
no functional connectivity between the amygdala and orbital frontal cortex in
patients with Williams syndrome, indicating the existence of abnormal regulatory
interactions between these two structures. These amygdala and orbital frontal
cortex abnormalities may contribute to the hypersociality and social disinhibition
of patients with Williams syndrome, as well as their elevated anxiety to non-social
stimuli.

In summary, ASD and Williams syndrome are developmental disorders characterized by social and emotional behavioral abnormalities starting early in infancy.
Neural abnormalities affecting structures of the social brain (e.g. amygdala and
orbital frontal cortex), are correlated with these behavioral characteristics and suggest that the underlying brain dysfunction in these disorders might be related to
dysfunction of these structures (Machado and Bachevalier, 2003; Bachevalier and
Loveland, 2006). However, these developmental disorders lead to opposite social
phenotypes. Whereas individuals with autism are not interested in social interactions, individuals with Williams syndrome proactively seek social interactions and
even interact happily with strangers.

The reasons for these differences in clinical outcome are unknown and speculative at this point. One possibility is that the two syndromes could show similar dysfunction of amygdala and orbital frontal cortex structures, but differences in
dysfunction of other neural systems, such as temporal cortical areas, hippocampus,
superior temporal sulcus, or cingulate cortex. This type of pattern has been shown

in adult monkeys with medial temporal lobe damage. In adults, lesions of the amygdala reduced fear and increased submission, whereas lesions of the rhinal cortex result in an opposite pattern of heightened defensiveness, attenuated affiliation and compulsive behaviors. Surprisingly, combined lesions of the two structures enhanced the emotional effects found after selective amygdala lesions (Meunier *et al.*, 1999, 2006; Meunier and Bachevalier, 2002).

Similarly, our earlier developmental studies demonstrated that large neonatal lesions of the medial temporal lobe resulted in social and emotional effects and memory deficits much greater than those seen after neonatal amygdala damage alone (Bachevalier, 1994). Interestingly, memory deficits resembling those found in temporal lobe amnesia are also reported in individuals with ASD (Ben Shalom, 2003; Salmond *et al.*, 2005) but not in those with Williams syndrome (Vicari *et al.*, 1996; Vicari, 2001; Majerus *et al.*, 2003; Devenny *et al.*, 2004; Brock *et al.*, 2006). Thus, different degrees of dysfunction within a network including temporal lobe structures and their interactions with the orbital frontal cortex could explain both the heterogeneity of symptoms in ASD and the divergent social phenotypes of development psychopathologies such as ASD and Williams syndrome.

CONCLUDING REMARKS AND FUTURE STUDIES

The previous speculative discussion underscores the need for further developmental studies in nonhuman primates. These studies could aim to (1) obtain information regarding the contribution of particular neural structures to development of normal social cognition abilities, (2) better characterize the behavioral abnormalities produced by specific lesions and follow their development over time, and (3) explore the impact that dysfunctional structures may have on the development of other brain systems. Nonhuman primate models might also provide information on how factors such as social experience or hormonal influences concomitant with early life lesions influence the heterogeneous and divergent phenotypes found in developmental psychopathologies.

However, there are several limitations with primate developmental models. First, human developmental psychopathologies have not been associated with specific brain lesions, although there are reports of medial temporal lobe damage in children that result in autistic-like behaviors (Chutorian and Antunes, 1981; DeLong *et al.*, 1981; Tonsgard *et al.*, 1987; Rossitch and Oakes, 1989; Lanska and Lanska, 1994). On the other hand, nonhuman primate neurodevelopmental studies that approximate the psychopathology observed in ASD and Williams syndrome could provide neural models for the study of these disorders.

Second, in addition to the neural origin of developmental psychopathologic disorders, other pre- and postnatal factors, such as maternal hormones, early social environment, and genetic predisposition, probably influence how a disordered brain develops during infancy and childhood. Some of these other factors can be assessed

using nonhuman primate models by comparing peer- versus mother-reared operated animals, as was done in the studies described above. However, factors such as
genetic influences on individual predispositions will require models in which
genetic modification can be produced. Preliminary rodent experiments will be
needed before such studies are feasible with primates. For instance, Ruiz-Opazo
and Tonkiss (2006) recently localized chromosomal regions in rats linked to social
recognition memory. These regions occur on two or more loci of the same chro-
mosomes that have been linked to ASD in humans (Chudley, 2004). Thus, manipulation of these genes in rodents could provide the information needed to perform
genetic developmental studies in monkeys.

Finally, although monkeys are the closest existing animals in which empirical
and invasive studies can ethically be performed, they still differ significantly from
humans. Developmental nonhuman primate models may only reproduce some of the
social and emotional symptoms found in human developmental psychopathologies.
Nevertheless, given the many similarities in perception and behavior across primate
species, research in monkeys and humans can proceed in parallel, each informing
and complementing the other with theoretical and empirical contributions. Such a
multidisciplinary approach offers a foundation for determining the specific neuropathological bases of many human developmental psychopathologies and, ultimately, for developing therapies to alleviate these disorders.

Acknowledgements

We are grateful to Dr G.P. Sackett for helpful comments on the manuscript. Prepara-
tion of this chapter was supported in part by grants from the National Institute of
Mental Health, MH58846; National Institute of Child and Human Development,
HD35471, The Robert W. Woodruff Health Sciences Center Fund, Inc., Emory
University, and The National Alliance for Autism Research Mentor-Based
Postdoctoral Fellowship to JB; the National Institute of Mental Health MH076031
and Center for Behavioral Neuroscience (CBN) Postdoctoral Fellowship to APG;
and the Yerkes Base Grant NIH RR00165 and the CBN grant NSF IBN-9876754.

REFERENCES

Abell, F., Krams, M., Ashburner, J. *et al.* (1999). The neuroanatomy of autism: a voxel-based whole
    brain analysis of structural scans. *NeuroReport* **10**, 1647–1651.
Adolphs, R. (1999). Social cognition and the human brain. *Trends Cogn Sci* **3**, 469–479.
Adolphs, R. (2001). The neurobiology of social cognition. *Curr Opin Neurobiol* **11**, 231–239.
Adolphs, R. (2003a). Investigating the cognitive neuroscience of social behavior. *Neuropsychologia* **41**,
    119–126.
Adolphs, R. (2003b). Cognitive neuroscience of human social behaviour. *Nat Rev Neurosci* **4**, 165–178.
Adolphs, R. (2003c). Is the human amygdala specialized for processing social information? *Ann NY
    Acad Sci* **985**, 326–340.

Adolphs, R. and Tranel, D. (2004). Impaired judgments of sadness but not happiness following bilateral amygdala damage. *J Cogn Neurosci* **16**, 453–462.

Adolphs, R., Tranel, D., Damasio, H., and Damasio, A. (1994). Impaired recognition of emotion in facial expressions following bilateral damage to the human amygdala. *Nature* **372**, 669–672.

Adolphs, R., Tranel, D., Damasio, H., and Damasio, A. R. (1995). Fear and the human amygdala. *J Neurosci* **15**, 5879–5891.

Adolphs, R., Tranel, D., and Damasio, A. R. (1998). The human amygdala in social judgement. *Nature* **393**, 470–474.

Adolphs, R., Gosselin, F., Buchanan, T. W., Tranel, D., Schyns, P., and Damasio, A. R. (2005). A mechanism for impaired fear recognition after amygdala damage. *Nature* **433**, 68–72.

Adrien, J. L., Lenoir, P., Martineau, J. *et al.* (1993). Blind ratings of early symptoms of autism based upon family home movies. *J Am Acad Child Adolesc Psychiatry* **32**, 617–626.

Aggleton, J. P. and Saunders, R. C. (2000). The amygdala – What's happened in the last decade? In Aggleton, J.P. ed. *The Amygdala: A Functional Analysis*. New York: Oxford University Press, pp. 1–30.

Ainsworth, M., Blehar, M., Waters, E., and Wall, S. (1978). *Patterns of Attachment*. Hillsdale, NJ: Erlbaum Associates.

Amaral, D. G. (2002). The primate amygdala and the neurobiology of social behavior: implications for understanding social anxiety. *Biol Psychiatry* **51**, 11–17.

Amaral, D. G. and Bennett, J. (2000). Development of amygdalo-cortical connections in the macaque monkey. Program No. 644.10. *Abstract Viewer/Itinerary Planner*. Washington, DC: Society for Neuroscience, 2000. Online.

Amaral, D. G., Price, J. L., Pitkanen, A., and Carmichael, S. T. (1992). Anatomical organization of the primate amygdaloid complex. In Aggleton, J. P. ed. *The Amygdala: Neurobiological Aspects of Emotion, Memory, and Mental Dysfunction*. New York: Wiley-Liss, Inc., pp. 1–66.

Anderson, S. W., Bechara, A., Damasio, H., Tranel, D., and Damasio A. R. (1999). Impairment of social and moral behavior related to early damage in human prefrontal cortex. *Nat Neurosci* **2**, 1032–1037.

Arana, F. S., Parkinson, J. A., Hinton, E., Holland, A. J., Owen, A. M., and Roberts, A. C. (2003). Dissociable contributions of the human amygdala and orbitofrontal cortex to incentive motivation and goal selection. *J Neurosci* **23**, 9632–9638.

Aylward, E. H., Minshew, N. J., Goldstein, G. *et al.* (1999). MRI volumes of amygdala and hippocampus in non-mentally retarded autistic adolescents and adults. *Neurology* **53**, 2145–2150.

Babineau, B. A., Bauman, M. D., Toscana, J. E., Mason, W. A., and Amaral, D. G. (2005). Juvenile macaque monkeys with neonatal lesions of the amygdala and hippocampus display higher frequencies of stereotypies than control subjects. Program No. 323.13. *Abstract Viewer/Itinerary Planner*. Washington, DC: Society for Neuroscience, 2005. Online from http://www.sfn.org/index.cfm?pagename=abstracts_ampublications&section=publications

Bachevalier, J. (1991). An animal model for childhood autism: memory loss and socioemotional disturbances following neonatal damage to the limbic system in monkeys. In Tamminga, C.A. and Schulz, S.C. eds. *Advances in Neuropsychiatry and Psychopharmacology*: Vol. 1: *Schizophrenia Research*. New York: Raven Press, pp. 129–140.

Bachevalier, J. (1994). Medial temporal lobe structures and autism: a review of clinical and experimental findings. *Neuropsychologia* **32**, 627–648.

Bachevalier, J. and Loveland, K. A. (2003). Early orbitofrontal-limbic dysfunction and autism. In Cicchetti, D. and Walker, E. F. eds. *Neurodevelopmental Mechanisms in the Genesis and Epigenesis of Psychopathology: Future Research Directions*. New York: Cambridge University Press, pp. 215–236.

Bachevalier, J. and Loveland, K. A. (2006). The orbitofrontal-amygdala circuit and self-regulation of social-emotional behavior in autism. *Neurosci Biobehav Rev* **30**, 97–117.

Bachevalier, J. and Malkova, M. (2000). Behavioral indices of early medial temporal lobe dysfunction in nonhuman primates. In Levin, H.S. and Grafman, J. eds. *Neuroplasticity and Reorganization of Function after Brain Injury*. Oxford: Oxford University Press, pp. 27–48.

Bachevalier, J. and Meunier, M. (2005). Neurobiology of socio-emotional cognition in primates. In: Eaton, A. and Emery, N.J. eds. *Cognitive Neuroscience of Social Behaviour.* London: Psychology Press, pp. 19–58.

Bachevalier, J., Ungerleider, L. G., O'Neill, J. B., and Friedman, D. P. (1986). Regional distribution of [^{3}H]naloxone binding in the brain of a newborn rhesus monkey. *Brain Res* **390**, 302–308.

Bachevalier, J., Beauregard, M., and Alvarado, M. (1999a). Long-term effect of neonatal damage to the hippocampal formation and amygdaloid cortex on object discrimination learning and object recognition memory in monkeys. *Behav Neurosci* **113**, 1127–1151.

Bachevalier, J., Alvarado, M. C., and Malkova, L. (1999b). Memory and socioemotionel behavior in monkeys after hippocampal damage incurred in infancy or in adulthood. *Biol Psychiatry* **46**, 329–339.

Bachevalier, J., Malkova, L., and Mishkin, M. (2001). Effects of selective neonatal temporal lobe lesions on sociemotional behavior in infant rhesus monkeys. *Behav Neurosci* **115**, 545–560.

Baird, G., Charman, T., Baron-Cohen, S., Cox, A., Swettenham, J., Wheelwright, S., and Drew, A. (2000). A screening instrument for autism at 18 months of age: a 6-year follow-up study. *J Am Acad Child Adolesc Psychiatry* **39**, 694–702.

Barbas, H. (1995). Pattern in the cortical distribution of prefrontally directed neurons with divergent axons in the rhesus monkey. *Cereb Cortex* **5**, 158–165.

Barbas, H. (2000). Connections underlying the synthesis of cognition, memory, and emotion in primate prefrontal cortices. *Brain Res Bull* **52**, 319–330.

Baron-Cohen, S. (1995). *Mindblindness: An Essay on Autism and Theory of Mind.* Cambridge, MA: MIT Press.

Baron-Cohen, S. (2003). Theory of mind and autism: a fifteen year review. In Baron-Cohen, S., Tager-Flusberg, H., and Cohen, D.J. eds. *Understanding Other Minds: Perspectives From Developmental Cognitive Neuroscience.* Oxford, UK: Oxford University Press, pp. 3–20.

Baron-Cohen, S. and Belmonte, M. K. (2005). Autism: a window onto the development of the social and the analytic brain. *Annu Rev Neurosci* **28**, 109–126.

Baron-Cohen, S., Ring, H., Moriarty, J., Schmitz, B., Costa, D., and Ell, P. (1994). Recognition of mental state terms. Clinical findings in children with autism and a functional neuroimaging study of normal adults. *Br J Psychiatry* **165**, 640–649.

Baron-Cohen, S., Jolliffe, T., Mortimore, C., and Robertson, M. (1997). Another advanced test of theory of mind: evidence from very high functioning adults with autism or asperger syndrome. *J Child Psychol Psychiatry* **38**, 813–822.

Baron-Cohen, S., Ring, H. A., Wheelwright, S. *et al.* (1999). Social intelligence in the normal and autistic brain: an fMRI study. *Eur J Neurosci* **11**, 1891–1898.

Baron-Cohen, S., Ring, H. A., Bullmore, E. T., Wheelwright, S., Ashwin, C., and Williams, S. C. R. (2000). The amygdala theory of autism. *Neurosci Biobehav Rev* **24**, 355–364.

Bauman, M. D. and Amaral, D. G. (2005). The distribution of serotonergic fibers in the macaque monkey amygdala: An immunohistochemical study using antisera to 5-hydroxytryptamine. *Neuroscience* **136**, 193–203.

Bauman, M. D., Lavenex, P., Mason, W. A., Capitanio, J. P., and Amaral, D. G. (2004a). The development of mother-infant interactions after neonatal amygdala lesions in rhesus monkeys. *J Neurosci* **24**, 711–721.

Bauman, M. D., Lavenex, P., Mason, W. A., Capitanio, J. P., and Amaral, D. G. (2004b). The development of social behavior following neonatal amygdala lesions in rhesus monkeys. *J Cogn Neurosci* **16**, 1388–1411.

Bauman, M. D., Toscano, J. E., Mason, W. A., Lavenex, P., and Amaral, D. G. (2006). The expression of social dominance following neonatal lesions of the amygdala or hippocampus in rhesus monkeys. *Behav Neurosci* **120**, 749–760.

Bauman, M. L. and Kemper, T. L. (1985). Histoanatomic observations of the brain in early infantile autism. *Neurology* **35**, 866–874.

Bauman, M. L. and Kemper, T. L. (1993). Cytoarchitectonic changes in the brain of people with autism. In Bauman, M.L. and Kemper, T.L. eds. *The Neurobiology of Autism*. Baltimore, MD: John Hopkins, pp. 119–145.

Baxter, M. G. and Murray, E. A. (2002). The amygdala and reward. *Nat Rev Neurosci* **3**, 563–573.

Baxter, M. G., Parker, A., Lindner, C. C. C., Izquierdo, A. D., and Murray E. A. (2000). Control of response selection by reinforcer value requires interaction of amygdala and orbital prefrontal cortex. *J Neurosci* **20**, 4311–4319.

Beauregard, M., Malkova, L., and Bachevalier, J. (1995). Stereotypies and loss of social affiliation after early hippocampectomy in primates. *NeuroReport* **6**, 2521–2526.

Bechara, A., Damasio, A. R., Damasio, H., and Anderson, S. W. (1994). Insensitivity to future consequences following damage to human prefrontal cortex. *Cognition* **50**, 7–15.

Bechara, A., Damasio, H., Tranel, D., and Anderson, S. W. (1998). Dissociation of working memory from decision making within the human prefrontal cortex. *J Neurosci* **18**, 428–437.

Bechara, A., Damasio, H., Damasio, A. R., and Lee, G. P. (1999). Different contributions of the human amygdala and ventromedial prefrontal cortex to decision-making. *J Neurosci* **19**, 5473–5481.

Bechara, A., Tranel, D., and Damasio, H. (2000). Characterization of the decision-making deficit of patients with ventromedial prefrontal cortex lesions. *Brain* **123** (Pt 11), 2189–2202.

Bechara, A., Damasio, H., and Damasio, A. R. (2003). Role of the amygdala in decision-making. *Ann NY Acad Sci* **985**, 356–369.

Bellugi, U. and St George, M. (2001). *Journey from Cognition to Brain to Gene: Perspectives from Williams Syndrome*. Cambridge, MA: The MIT Press.

Bellugi, U., Lichtenberger, L., Jones, W., Lai, Z., and St.George, M. (2001). The neurocognitive profile of Williams syndrome: a complex pattern of strengths and weaknesses. In Bellugi, U. and St George, M. eds. *Journey from Cognition to Brain to Gene: Perspectives from Williams Syndrome*. Cambridge, MA: The MIT Press, pp. 1–41.

Ben Shalom, D. (2003). Memory in autism: review and synthesis. *Cortex* 39, 1129–1138.

Berger, B., Febvret, A., Greengard, P., and Goldman-Rakic, P. S. (1990). DARPP-32, a phosphoprotein enriched in dopaminoceptive neurons bearing dopamine D1 receptors: distribution in the cerebral cortex of the newborn and adult rhesus monkey. *J Comp Neurol* **299**, 327–348.

Berlin, H. A., Rolls, E. T., and Kischka, U. (2004). Impulsivity, time perception, emotion and reinforcement sensitivity in patients with orbitofrontal cortex lesions. *Brain* **127**, 1108–1126.

Bernstein, I. S. and Ehardt, I. S. (1985). Age-sex differences in the expression of agonistic behavior in rhesus monkey (*Macaca mulatta*) groups. *J Comp Psychol* **99**, 115–132.

Bertolino, A., Saunders, R. C., Mattay, V. S., Bachevalier, J., Frank, J. A., and Weinberger, D. R. (1997). Altered development of prefrontal neurons in rhesus monkeys with neonatal mesial temporo-limbic lesions: a proton magnetic resonance spectroscopic imaging study. *Cereb Cortex* **7**, 740–748.

Bhattacharjee, Y. (2005). Friendly faces and unusual minds. *Science* **310**, 802–804.

Booth, M. C. A., Rolls, E. T. Critchley, H. D., Browning, A. S., and Hernadi, I. (1998). Face selective neurons in the primate orbital frontal cortex. *Soc Neurosci Abstr* **24**, 898.

Bowden, D. M., Goldman, P. S., Rosvold, H. E., and Greenstreet, R. L. (1971). Free behavior of rhesus monkeys following lesions of the dorsolateral and orbital prefrontal cortex in infancy. *Exp Brain Res* **12**, 265–274.

Bradley, E. A., Summers, J. A., Wood, H. L., and Bryson, S. E. (2004). Comparing rates of psychiatric and behavior disorders in adolescents and young adults with severe intellectual disability with and without autism. *J Autism Dev Dis* **34**, 151–161.

Brambilla, P., Hardan, A., di Nemi, S. U., Perez, J., Soares, J. C., and Barale, F. (2003). Brain anatomy and development in autism: review of structural MRI studies. *Brain Res Bull* **61**, 557–569.

Breiter, H. C., Etcoff, N. L., Whalen, P. J. *et al.* (1996). Response and habituation of the human amygdala during visual processing of facial expressions. *Neuron* **17**, 875–887.

Brent, E., Rios, P., Happe, F., and Charman, T. (2004). Performance of children with autism spectrum disorder on advanced theory of mind tasks. *Autism* **8**, 283–299.

Brock, J., Brown, G. D. and Boucher. J. (2006). Free recall in Williams syndrome: is there a dissociation between short- and long-term memory? *Cortex* 42, 366–375.

Brothers, L. (1989). A biological perspective on empathy. *Am J Psychiatry* **146**, 10–19.

Brothers, L. A. (1990). The social brain: A project for integrating primate behaviour and neurophysiology in a new domain. *Conc Neurosci* **1**, 27–51.

Brothers, L. (1995). Neurophysiology of the perception of intention by primates. In Gazzaniga, M.S. ed. *The Cognitive Neurosciences.* Cambridge, MA: The MIT Press, pp. 1107–1117.

Brothers, L. and Ring, B. (1993). Mesial temporal neurons in the macaque monkey with responses selective for aspects of social stimuli. *Behav Brain Res* **57**, 53–61.

Brunet, E., Sarfati, Y., Hardy-Bayle, M. C., and Decety, J. (2000). A PET investigation of the attribution of intentions with a nonverbal task. *NeuroImage* **11**, 157–166.

Byrne, R. and Whiten, A. (1988). *Machavellian Intelligence: Social Expertise and the Evolution of Intellect in Monkeys, Apes and Humans.* Oxford: Clarendon Press.

Capitanio, J. P., Mendoza, S. P., Mason, W.A., and Maninger, N. (2005). Rearing environment and hypothalamic-pituitary-adrenal regulation in young rhesus monkeys (*Macaca mulatta*). *Dev Psychobiol* **46**, 318–330.

Carmichael, S. T. and Price, J. L. (1994). Limbic connections of the orbital and medial prefrontal cortex in macaque monkeys. *J Comp Neurol* **363**, 615–641.

Carper, R. A. and Courchesne, E. (2000). Inverse correlation between frontal lobe and cerebellum sizes in children with autism. *Brain* **123**, 836–844.

Cavada, C., Compañy, T., Tejedor, J., Cruz-Rizzolo, R. J., and Reinoso-Suárez, F. (2000). The anatomical connections of the macaque monkey orbitofrontal cortex. A review. *Cereb Cortex* **10**, 220–242.

Charman, T. (2003). Why is joint attention a pivotal skill in autism? *Philos Trans R Soc Lond B Biol Sci* **358**, 315–324.

Cheney, D. L. and Seyfarth, R. M. (1990). *How Monkeys See the World.* Chicago: University of Chicago Press.

Chlan-Fourney, J., Webster, M. J., Felleman, D. J., Bachevalier, J. (2000). Neonatal medial temporal lobe lesions alter the distribution of tyrosine hydroxylase immunoreactive varicosities in the macaque prefrontal cortex. Program No. 228.18. *Abstract Viewer/Itinerary Planner.* Washington, DC: Society for Neuroscience. Online from http://www.sfn.org/index.cfm?pagename=abstracts_ampublications&section=publications

Chlan-Fourney, J., Webster, M. J., Jung, J., Bachevalier, J. (2003). Neonatal medial temporal lobe lesions decrease GABAergic interneuron densities in macaque prefrontal cortex: Implications for schizophrenia and autism. Program No. 315.9. *Abstract Viewer/Itinerary Planner.* Washington, DC: Society for Neuroscience. Online from http://www.sfn.org/index.cfm?pagename=abstracts_ampublications&section=publications

Chudley, A. E. (2004). Genetic landmarks through philately – autism spectrum disorders: a genetic update. *Clin Genet* **65**(5), 352–357.

Chutorian A. M. and Antunes., J. L. (1981). Kluver-Bucy syndrome and herpes encephalitis: case report. *Neurosurgery* **8**, 388–390.

Cicchetti, D. and Tucker, D. (1994). Development and self-regulatory structures of the mind. *Dev Psychopathol* **6**, 533.

Courchesne, E., Karns, C. M., Davis, H. R. *et al.* (2001). Unusual brain growth patterns in early life in patients with autistic disorder: an MRI study. *Neurology* **57**, 245–254.

Critchley, H. D., Simmons, A., Daly, E. M. *et al.* (2000). Prefrontal and medial temporal correlates of repetitive violence to self and others. *Biol Psychiatry* **47**, 928–934.

Critchley, H. D., Mathias, C. J., and Dolan, R. J. (2001). Neural activity in the human brain relating to uncertainty and arousal during anticipation. *Neuron* **29**, 537–545.

Dalton, K. M., Nacewicz, B. M., Johnstone, T. *et al.* (2005). Gaze fixation and the neural circuitry of face processing in autism. *Nat Neurosci* **8**, 519–526.

Damasio, A. R. (1994). The somatic-marker hypothesis. In Damasio, A. R., ed. *Descartes' Error-Emotion, Reason and the Human Brain*. New York: Avon Book Inc., pp. 165–201.

Dapretto, M., Davies, M. S., Pfeifer, J. H. *et al.* (2006). Understanding emotions in others: mirror neuron dysfunction in children with autism spectrum disorders. *Nat Neurosci* **9**, 28–30.

Dawson, G., Meltzoff, A. N., Osterling, J., Rinaldi, J., and Brown, E. (1998). Children with autism fail to orient to naturally occurring social stimuli. *J Autism Dev Disord* **28**, 479–485.

de Waal, F. B. M. (1989). *Peacemaking Among Primates*. Cambridge, MA: Harward University Press.

DeLong, G. R., Bean, S. C., and Brown III, F. R. (1981). Acquired reversible autistic syndrome in acute encephalopathic illness in children. *Arch Neurol* **38**, 191–194.

Devenny, D. A., Krinsky-McHale, S. J., Kittler, P. M., Flory, M., Jenkins, E., and Brown W. T. (2004). Age-associated memory changes in adults with williams syndrome. *Dev Neuropsychol* **26**, 691–706.

DiCicco-Bloom, E., Lord C., Zwaigenbaum, L. *et al.* (2006). The developmental neurobiology of autism spectrum disorder. *J Neurosci* 26, 6897–6906.

Dissanayake, C. and Crossley, S. A. (1997). Autistic children's responses to separation and reunion with their mothers. *J Autism Dev Disord* **27**, 295–312.

Dissanayake, C. and Sigman, M. (2001). Attachment and emotional responsiveness in children with autism. *Int Rev Res Ment Retard* **23**, 239–266.

Dykens. E. M. (2003). Anxiety, fears, and phobias in persons with Williams syndrome. *Dev Neuropsychol* **23**(1–2), 291–316.

Emery, N. J. (2000). The eyes have it: the neuroethology, function and evolution of social gaze. *Neurosci Biobehav Rev* **24**, 581–604.

Emery, N. J., Lorincz, E. N., Perrett, D. I., Oram, M. W., and Baker, C. I. (1997). Gaze following and joint attention in rhesus monkeys (*Macaca mulatta*). *J Comp Psychol* **111**, 286–293.

Emery, N. J., Capitanio, J. P., Mason, W. A., Machado, C. P., Mendoza, S. P., and Amaral, D. G. (2001). The effects of bilateral lesions of the amygdala on dyadic social interactions in rhesus monkeys (*Macaca mulatta*). *Behav Neurosci* **115**, 515–544.

Eslinger, P. J. and Damasio, A. R. (1985). Severe disturbance of higher cognition after bilateral frontal lobe ablation: patient EVR. *Neurology* **35**, 1731–1741.

Eslinger, P. J., Flaherty-Craig, C. V., and Benton, A. L. (2004). Developmental outcomes after early prefrontal cortex damage. *Brain Cogn* **55**, 84–103.

Ewart, A. K., Morris, C. A., Atkinson, D. *et al.* (1993). Hemizygosity at the elastin locus in a developmental disorder, Williams syndrome. *Nat Genet* **5**, 11–16.

Farrow, T. F., Zheng, Y., Wilkinson, I. D. *et al.* (2001). Investigating the functional anatomy of empathy and forgiveness. *NeuroReport* **12**, 2433–2438.

Fombonne, E. (1999). The epidemiology of autism: a review. *Psychol Med* **29**, 769–786.

Fombonne, E. (2003). Epidemiological surveys of autism and other pervasive developmental disorders: an update. *J Autism Dev Disord* **33**, 365–382.

Fried, I., Mac Donald, K. A., and Wilson, C. L. (1997). Single neuron activity in human hippocampus and amygdala during recognition of faces and objects. *Neuron* **18**, 753–765.

Fried, I., Cameron, K. A., Yashar, S., Fong, R., and Morrow, J. W. (2002). Inhibitory and excitatory responses of single neurons in the human medial temporal lobe during recognition of faces and objects. *Cereb Cortex* **12**, 575–584.

Frith, U. and Hill, E. L. (2003). Autism: mind and brain. *Philos Trans Lond R Soc Biol Sci* **358**, 277–280.

Gervais, H., Belin, P., Boddaert, N. *et al.* (2004). Abnormal cortical voice processing in autism. *Nat Neurosci* **7**, 801–802.

Ghazanfar, A. A. and Santos, L. R. (2004). Primate brains in the wild: the sensory bases for social interactions. *Nat Rev Neurosci* **5**, 603–616.

Gibson, K. R. (1991). Myelination and behavioral development: A comparative perspective on questions of neoteny, altriciality and intelligence. In Gibson, K. R. and Peterson, A. C. eds. *Brain Maturation and Cognitive Development: Comparative and Cross-cultural Perspectives*. New York: Aldine De Gruyter, pp. 29–63.

Goldman, P. S. (1971). Functional development of the prefrontal cortex in early life and the problem of neuronal plasticity. *Exp Neurol* **32**, 366–387.

Goldman, P. S. and Nauta, W. J. (1977). Columnar distribution of cortico-cortical fibers in the frontal association, limbic, and motor cortex of the developing rhesus monkey. *Brain Res* **122**, 393–413.

Goldman-Rakic, P. S., Isseroff, A., Schwartz, M. L., and Bugbee, N. M. (1983). The neurobiology of cognitive development. In Mussen, P. ed. *Handbook of Child Psychology and Biology: Infancy and Development*. New York: John Wiley and Sons, pp. 281–344.

Goursaud, A. P. and Bachevalier, J. (2006). Social attachment in juvenile monkeys with neonatal lesion of the hippocampus, amygdala and orbital frontal cortex. *Behav Brain Res* **176**, 75–93.

Grelotti, D. J., Gauthier, I., and Schultz, R. T. (2002). Social interest and the development of cortical face specialization: what autism teaches us about face processing. *Dev Psychobiol* **40**, 213–225.

Grossman, J. B., Carter, A., and Volkmar, F. R. (1997). Social behavior in autism. *Ann NY Acad Sci* **807**, 440–454.

Harlow, J. M. (1848). Passage of an iron rod through the head. *Boston Med Surg J* **39**, 389–393.

Harlow, J. M. (1999). Passage of an iron rod through the head. 1848. *J Neuropsychiatry Clin Neurosci* **11**, 281–283.

Harrison, D. W., Demaree, H. A., Shenal, B. V., and Everhart, D. E. (1998). QEEG assisted neuropsychological evaluation of autism. *Int J Neurosci* **93**, 133–140.

Hayashi, M. and Oshima, K. (1986). Neuropeptides in cerebral cortex of macaque monkey (*Macaca fuscata fuscata*): regional distribution and ontogeny. *Brain Res* **364**, 360–368.

Heberlein, A. S. and Adolphs, R. (2004). Impaired spontaneous anthropomorphizing despite intact perception and social knowledge. *Proc Natl Acad Sci USA* **101**, 7487–7491.

Heider, F. and Simmel, M. (1944). An experimentasl study of apparent behavior. *Am J Psychol* **57**, 243–259.

Hinde, R. A. and Spencer-Booth, Y. (1967). The behaviour of socially living rhesus monkeys in their first two and a half years. *Anim Behav* **15**, 169–196.

Hinde, R. A., Rowell, T. E., and Spencer-Booth, Y. (1964). Behaviour of socially living rhesus monkeys in their first six months. *Proc Zoo Soc Lond* **143**, 609–649.

Holland, P. C. and Gallagher, M. (2004). Amygdala-frontal interactions and reward expectancy. *Curr Opin Neurobiol* **14**, 148–155.

Hornak, J., Rolls, E. T., and Wade, D. (1996). Face and voice expression identification in patients with emotional and behavioural changes following ventral frontal lobe damage. *Neuropsychologia* **34**, 247–261.

Hornak, J., Bramham, J., Rolls, E. T. *et al.* (2003). Changes in emotion after circumscribed surgical lesions of the orbitofrontal and cingulate cortices. *Brain* **126**, 1691–1712.

Howard, M. A., Cowell, P. E., Boucher, J. *et al.* (2000). Convergent neuroanatomical and behavioural evidence of an amygdala hypothesis of autism. *NeuroReport* **11**, 2931–2935.

Hubl, D., Bolte, S., Feineis-Matthews, S. *et al.* (2003). Functional imbalance of visual pathways indicates alternative face processing strategies in autism. *Neurology* **61**, 1232–1237.

Humphrey, T. (1968). The development of the human amygdala during early embryonic life. *J Comp Neurol* **132**, 135–165.

Jones, W., Bellugi, U., Lai, Z. *et al.* (2001). Hypersociability: the social and affective phenotype of Williams Syndrome. In Bellugi, U. and St.George, M. eds. *Journey from Cognition to Brain to Gene: Perspectives from Williams Syndrome*. Cambridge, MA: The MIT Press, pp. 43–71.

Kalin, N. H. and Shelton, S. E. (1989). Defensive behaviors in infant rhesus monkeys: environmental cues and neurochemical regulation. *Science* **243**, 1718–1721.

Kalin, N. H., Shelton, S. E., and Takahashi, L. K. (1991). Defensive behaviors in infant rhesus monkeys: ontogeny and context-dependent selective expression. *Child Dev* **62**, 1175–1183.

Kawasaki, Y., Yokota, K., Shinomiya, M., Shimizu, Y., and Niwa, S. (1997). Brief report: electroencephalographic paroxysmal activities in the frontal area emerged in middle childhood and during adolescence in a follow-up study of autism. *J Autism Dev Disord* **27**, 605–620.

Kawashima, R., Sugiura, M., Kato, T. *et al.* (1999). The human amygdala plays an important role in gaze monitoring. A PET study. *Brain* **122**, 779–783.

Kenney, M. D., Mason, W. A., and Hill, S. D. (1979). Effects of age, objects, and visual experience on affective responses of monkeys to strangers. *Dev Psychol* **15**, 176–184.

Kim, J. A., Szatmari, P., Bryson, S. E., Streiner, D. L., and Wilson, F. J. (2000). The prevalence of anxiety and mood problems among children with autism and asperger syndrome. *Autism* **4**, 117–132.

Klin, A. (1991). Young autistic children's listening preferences in regard to speech: a possible characterization of the symptom of social withdrawal. *J Autism Dev Disord* **21**, 29–42.

Klin, A. (2000). Attributing social meaning to ambiguous visual stimuli in higher-functioning autism and Asperger syndrome: The Social Attribution Task. *J Child Psychol Psychiat* **41**, 831–846.

Klin, A., Volkmar, F. R., and Sparrow, S. S. (1992). Autistic social dysfunction: some limitations of the theory of mind hypothesis. *J Child Psychol Psychiat* **33**, 861–876.

Klin, A., Sparrow, S. S., de Bildt, A., Cicchetti, D. V., Cohen, D. J., and Volkmar, F. R. (1999). A normed study of face recognition in autism and related disorders. *J Autism Dev Disord* **29**, 499–508.

Klin, A., Jones, W., Schultz, R., Volkmar, F., and Cohen, D. (2002a). Visual fixation patterns during viewing of naturalistic social situations as predictors of social competence in individuals with autism. *Arch Gen Psychiat* **59**, 809–816.

Klin, A., Jones, W., Schultz, R., Volkmar, F., and Cohen, D. (2002b). Defining and quantifying the social phenotype in autism. *Am J Psychiat* **159**, 895–908.

Kling, A. S. (1972). Effects of amygdalectomy on social-affective behavior in nonhuman primates. In Eleftheniou, B. E. ed. *The Neurobiology of the Amygdala*. New York: Plenum Press, pp. 511–536.

Kling, A. and Green, P. C. (1967). Effects of neonatal amygdalectomy in the maternally reared and maternally deprived monkey. *Nature* **213**, 742–743.

Klüver, H. and Bucy, P. C. (1938). An analysis of certain effects of bilateral temporal lobectomy in the rhesus monkey, with special reference to "psychic blindness". *J Psychol* **5**, 33–54.

Klüver, H. and Bucy, P. C. (1939). Preliminary analysis of functions of the temporal lobes in monkeys. *Arch Neurol Psychiat* **42**, 979–1000.

Kolb, B. and Whishaw, I. Q. (1996). *Fundamental of Human Neuropsychology*. New York: Freeman Press.

Kordower, J. H., Piecinski, P., and Rakic, P. (1992). Neurogenesis of the amygdaloid nuclear complex in the rhesus monkey. *Dev Brain Res* **68**, 9–15.

Kringelbach, M. L. and Rolls, E. T. (2003). Neural correlates of rapid reversal learning in a simple model of human social interaction. *NeuroImage* **20**, 1371–1383.

Lanska, D. J. and Lanska, M. J. (1994). Klüver-Bucy syndrome in juvenile neuronal ceroid lipofuscinosis. *J Child Neurol* **9**, 67–69.

Leekam, S. R. and Ramsden, C. A. (2006). Dyadic orienting and joint attention in preschool children with autism. *J Autism Dev Disord* **36**, 185–197.

Leekam, S. R., Hunnisett, E., and Moore, C. (1998). Targets and cues: gaze-following in children with autism. *J Child Psychol Psychiat* **39**, 951–962.

Leekam, S. R., Lopez, B., and Moore, C. (2000). Attention and joint attention in preschool children with autism. *Dev Psychol* **36**, 261–273.

Leonard, C. M., Rolls, E. T., Wilson, F. A., and Baylis, G. C. (1985). Neurons in the amygdala of the monkey with responses selective for faces. *Behav Brain Res* **15**, 159–176.

Loveland, K. (2001). Toward an ecological theory of autism. In Burack, J. A., Charman, T., Yirmiya, N. and Zelazo, P. R. eds. *The Development of Autism: Perspectives from Theory and Research*. Hillsdale, NJ: Erlbaum Press, pp. 17–37.

Loveland, K. A. (2005). Social-emotional impairment and self-regulation in Autism spectrum-disorders, In Nadel, J. and Muir, D. eds. *Typical and Impaired Emotional Development*. Oxford: Oxford University Press, pp. 365–382.

Loveland, K. A., Tunali-Kotoski, B., Chen, R., Brelsford, K. A., Ortegon, J., and Pearson, D. A. (1995). Intermodal perception of affect in persons with autism or Down syndrome. *Dev Psychopathol* **7**, 409–418.

Machado, C. J. and Bachevalier, J. (2003). Nonhuman primate models of childhood psychopathology: the promise and limitations. *J Child Psychol Psychiat* **44**, 64–87.

Machado, C. J. and Bachevalier, J. (2006). The impact of selective amygdala, orbital frontal cortex, or hippocampal formation lesions on established social relationships in rhesus monkeys (*Macaca mulatta*). *Behav Neurosci* **120**, 761–86.

Majerus, S., Barisnikov, K., Vuillemin, I., Poncelet, M., and van der. Linden M. (2003) An investigation of verbal short-term memory and phonological processing in four children with Williams syndrome. *Neurocase* **9**, 390–401.

Malkova, L., Mishkin, M., Suomi, S. J., and Bachevalier, J. (1997). Socioemotional behavior in adult rhesus monkeys after early versus late lesions of the medial temporal lobe. *Ann NY Acad Sci* **807**, 538–540.

Martin-Soelch, C., Leenders, K.L., Chevalley, A.-F. *et al.* (2001). Reward mechanisms in the brain and their role in dependence: evidence from neurophysiological and neuroimaging studies. *Brain Res Rev* **36**, 139–149.

Masataka, N. (1985). Development of vocal recognition of mothers in infant Japanese macaques. *Dev Psychobiol* **18**, 107–114.

Mason, W. A. (1985). Experiential influences on the development of expressive behaviors in rhesus monkeys. In Zivin, G. ed. *The Development of Expressive Behavior: Biology-Environment Interactions.* New York: Academic Press, pp. 117–152.

Mason, W. A. (2000). Early development influences of experience on behaviour, temperament and stress, In Moberg, G. P. and Mench, J. A. eds. *The Biology of Animal Stress. Basic Principles and Implications for Animal Welfare.* New York: CABI, pp. 269–290.

Mason, W. A., Capitanio, J. P., Machado, C. J., Mendoza, S. P., and Amaral, D. G. (2006). Amygdalectomy and responsiveness to novelty in rhesus monkeys (*Macaca mulatta*): generality and individual consistency of effects. *Emotion* **6**, 73–81.

McIntosh, D. N., Reichmann-Decker, A., Winkielman, P., and Wilbarger, J. L. (2006). When the social mirror breaks: deficits in automatic, but not voluntary, mimicry of emotional facial expressions in autism. *Dev Sci* **9**, 295–302.

Mendelson, M. J. (1982). Visual and social responses in infant rhesus monkeys. *Am J Primatol* **3**, 333–340.

Mendelson, M. J., Haith, M. M., and Goldman-Rakic, P. S. (1982). Face scanning and responsiveness to social cues in infant rhesus monkeys. *Dev Psychol* **18**, 658–662.

Mervis, C. B. Morris, C. A. Klein-Tasman, B. P. *et al.* (2003). Attentional characteristics of infants and toddlers with Williams syndrome during triadic interactions. *Dev Neuropsychol* **23**, 243–268.

Mesulam, M. M. (2002). The human frontal lobes: transcending the default mode through contingent encoding. In Stuss, D. T. and Knight, R. T. eds. *Principles of Frontal Lobe Function.* New York: Oxford University Press, pp. 8–50.

Meunier, M. and Bachevalier, J. (2002). Comparison of emotional responses in monkeys with rhinal cortex or amygdala lesions. *Emotion* **2**, 147–161.

Meunier, M., Bachevalier, J., Murray, E. A., Malkova, L., and Mishkin, M. (1999). Effects of aspiration versus neurotoxic lesions of the amygdala on emotional responses in monkeys. *Eur J Neurosci* **11**, 4403–4418.

Meunier, M., Cirilli, L., and Bachevalier, J. (2006). Responses to affective stimuli in monkeys with entorhinal or perirhinal cortex lesions. *J Neurosci* **26**, 7718–7722.

Meyer-Lindenberg, A., Kohn, P., Mervis, C. B. *et al.* (2004). Neural basis of genetically determined visuospatial construction deficit in Williams syndrome. *Neuron* **43**, 623–631.

Meyer-Lindenberg, A., Hariri, A. R., Munoz, K. E. *et al.* (2005). Neural correlates of genetically abnormal social cognition in Williams syndrome. *Nat Neurosci* **8**, 991–993.

Meyer-Lindenberg, A., Mervis, C. B., and Faith Berman, K. (2006). Neural mechanisms in Williams syndrome: a unique window to genetic influences on cognition and behaviour. *Nat Rev Neurosci* **7**, 380–393.

Minshew, N. J., Luna, B., and Sweeney, J. A. (1999). Oculomotor evidence for neocortical systems but not cerebellar dysfunction in autism. *Neurology* **52**, 917–922.

Mobbs, D., Garrett, A. S., Menon, V., Rose, F. E., Bellugi, U., and Reiss, A. L. (2004). Anomalous brain activation during face and gaze processing in Williams syndrome. *Neurology* **62**, 2070–2076.

Moll, J., Oliveira-Souza, R., Bramati, I. E., and Grafman, J. (2002a). Functional networks in emotional moral and nonmoral social judgments. *NeuroImage* **16**, 696–703.

Moll, J., Oliveira-Souza, R., Eslinger, P. J. *et al.* (2002b). The neural correlates of moral sensitivity: a functional magnetic resonance imaging investigation of basic and moral emotions. *J Neurosci* **22**, 2730–2736.

Monk, C. S., McClure, E. B., Nelson, E. E. *et al.* (2003). Adolescent immaturity in attention-related brain engagement to emotional facial expressions. *NeuroImage* **20**, 420–428.

Morris, J. S., Frith, C. D., Perrett, D. I. *et al.* (1996). A differential neural response in the human amygdala to fearful and happy facial expressions. *Nature* **383**, 812–815.

Mundy, P. and Neal, A. R. (2001). Neural plasticity, joint attention, and a transactional social-orienting model of autism. In Gliden, L. M. ed. *International Review of Research in Mental Retardation*, Vol 23. New York: Academic Press, pp. 139–168.

Mundy, P., Sigman, M., Ungerer, J., and Sherman, T. (1986). Defining the social deficits of autism: the contribution of non-verbal communication measures. *J Child Psychol Psychiat* **27**, 657–669.

Munson, J., Dawson, G., Abbott, R. *et al.* (2006). Amygdalar volume and behavioral development in autism. *Arch Gen Psychiat* **63**, 686–693.

Murray, E. A. (1991). Medial temporal lobe structures contributing to recognition memory: The amygdaloid complex versus the rhinal cortex. In Aggleton, J. P. ed. *The Amygdala: Neurobiological Aspects of Emotion, Memory and Mental Dysfunction*. New York: Wiley-Liss Inc., pp. 453–470.

Newman, J. D. and Bachevalier, J. (1997). Neonatal ablations of the amygdala and inferior temporal cortex alter the vocal response to social separation in rhesus macaques. *Brain Res* **758**, 180–186.

Nikolić, I. and Kostović, I. (1986). Development of the lateral amygdaloid nucleus in the human fetus: Transient presence of discrete cytoarchitectonic units. *Anat Embryol* **174**, 355–360.

Ó Scalaidhe, S. P., Wilson, F. A., and Goldman-Rakic, P. S. (1997). Areal segregation of face-processing neurons in prefrontal cortex. *Science* **278**, 1135–1138.

O'Doherty, J., Kringelbach, M. L., Rolls, E. T., Hornak, J., and Andrews, C. (2001). Abstract reward and punishment. *Nat Neurosci* **4**, 95–102.

O'Doherty, J. P., Deichmann, R., Critchley, H. D., and Dolan, R. J. (2002). Neural responses during anticipation of a primary taste reward. *Neuron* **33**, 815–826.

Oeth, K. M. and Lewis, D. A. (1993). Postnatal development of the cholecystokinin innervation of monkey prefrontal cortex. *J Comp Neurol* **336**, 400–418.

Öngür, D. and Price, J. L. (2000). The organization of networks within the orbital and medial prefrontal cortex of rats, monkeys and humans. *Cereb Cortex* **10**, 206–219.

Osterling, J. and Dawson, G. (1994). Early recognition of children with autism: a study of first birthday home videotapes. *J Autism Dev Disord* **24**, 247–257.

Overman, W. H. (2004). Sex differences in early childhood, adolescence, and adulthood on cognitive tasks that rely on orbital prefrontal cortex. *Brain Cogn* **55**, 134–147.

Payne, C. D., Machado, C. J., Jackson, E. F., and Bachevalier, J. (2006). The maturation of the nonhuman amygdala: a magnetic resonance imaging study. Program No. 718.9. *Abstract Viewer/Itinerary Planner*. Washington, DC: Society for Neuroscience. Online.

Pelphrey, K. A., Sasson, N. J., Reznick, J. S., Paul, G., Goldman, B. D., and Piven, J. (2002). Visual scanning of faces in autism. *J Autism Dev Disord* **32**, 249–261.

Pelphrey, K., Adolphs, R., and Morris, J. P. (2004). Neuroanatomical substrates of social cognition dysfunction in autism. *Ment Retard Dev Disabil Res Rev* **10**, 259–271.

Petrides, M. and Pandya, D. N. (2002). Comparative cytoarchitectonic analysis of the human and the macaque ventrolateral prefrontal cortex and corticocortical connection patterns in the monkey. *Eur J Neurosci* **16**, 291–310.

Phelps, E. A. and LeDoux, J. E. (2005). Contributions of the amygdala to emotion processing: from animal models to human behavior. *Neuron* **48**, 175–187.

Phillips, M. L., Young, A. W., Scott, S. K. *et al.* (1998). Neural responses to facial and vocal expressions of fear and disgust. *Proc Biol Sci* **265**, 1809–1817.

Phillips, M. L., Drevets, W. C., Rauch, S. L., and Lane, R. (2003). Neurobiology of emotion perception I: the neural basis of normal emotion perception. *Biol Psychiat* **54**, 504–514.

Pierce, K., Muller, R. A., Ambrose, J., Allen, G., and Courchesne, E. (2001). Face processing occurs outside the fusiform 'face area' in autism: evidence from functional MRI. *Brain* **124**, 2059–2073.

Prather, M. D., Lavenex, P., Mauldin-Jourdain, M. L. *et al.* (2001). Increased social fear and decreased fear of objects in monkeys with neonatal amygdala lesions. *Neuroscience* **106**, 653–658.

Reiss, A. L., Eliez, S., Schmitt, J. E., Straus, E., Lai, Z., Jones, W., and Bellugi, U. (2001). Neuroanatomy of Williams syndrome: a high-resolution MRI study. In Bellugi, U. and St. George, M. eds. *Journey from Cognition to Brain to Gene: Perspectives from Williams Syndrome.* Cambridge, MA: The MIT Press, pp. 105–122.

Reiss, A. L., Eckert, M. A., Rose, F. E. *et al.* (2004). An experiment of nature: brain anatomy parallels cognition and behavior in Williams syndrome. *J Neurosci* **24**, 5009–5015.

Rodman, H. R. and Consuelos, M. J. (1994). Cortical projections to anterior inferior temporal cortex in infant macaque monkeys. *Vis Neurosci* **11**, 119–133.

Rolls, E. T. (1999). *The Brain and Emotion.* Oxford: Oxford University Press.

Rolls, E. T. (2000). The orbitofrontal cortex and reward. *Cereb Cortex* **10**, 284–294.

Rolls, E. T. (2004). The functions of the orbitofrontal cortex. *Brain Cogn* **55**, 11–29.

Rolls, E. T., Hornak, J., Wade, D., and McGrath, J. (1994). Emotion-related learning in patients with social and emotional changes associated with frontal lobe damage. *J Neurol Neurosurg Psychiat* **57**, 1518–1524.

Rolls, E. T., Critchley, H. D., Mason, R., and Wakeman, E. A. (1996). Orbitofrontal cortex neurons: role in olfactory and visual association learning. *J Neurophysiol* **75**, 1970–1981.

Rose, F. E., Lincoln, A. J., Lai, Z., Ene, M., Searcy, Y. M., and Bellugi, U. (2006). Orientation and affective expression effects on face recognition in Williams syndrome and autism. *J Autism Dev Disord* **4**, 1–10.

Rosenblum, L. A. and Paully, P. W. (1980). The social milieu of the developing monkey: studies of the development of social perception. *Reprod Nutr Dev* **20**, 827–841.

Rossitch, E. Jr. and Oakes, W. J. (1989). Klüver-Bucy syndrome in a child with bilateral arachnoid cysts: report of a case. *Neurosurgery* **24**, 110–112.

Rosvold, H. E., Mirsky, A. F., and Pribam, K. H. (1954). Influence of amygdalectomy on social behavior in monkeys. *J Comp Physiol Psychol* **47**, 173–178.

Ruiz-Opazo, N. and Tonkiss, J. (2006). Genome-wide scan for quantitative trait loci influencing spatial navigation and social recognition memory in Dahl rats. *Physiol Genomics* **26**, 145–151.

Rutgers, A. H., Bakermans-Kranenburg, M. J., van IJzendoorn, M. H., and Berckelaer-Onnes, I. A. (2004). Autism and attachment: a meta-analytic review. *J Child Psychol Psychiat* **45**, 1123–1134.

Rutherford, M. D., Baron-Cohen, S., and Wheelwright, S. (2002). Reading the mind in the voice: a study with normal adults and adults with Asperger syndrome and high functioning autism. *J Autism Dev Disord* **32**, 189–194.

Sabbagh, M. A. (2004). Understanding orbitofrontal contributions to theory-of-mind reasoning: Implications for autism. *Brain Cogn* **55**, 209–219.

Salmond, C. H., Ashburner, J., Connelly, A., Friston, K. J., Gadian, D. G., and Vargha-Khadem, F. (2005). The role of the medial temporal lobe in autistic spectrum disorders. *Eur J Neurosci* **22**, 764–772.

Sanchez, M. M., Ladd, C. O., and Plotsky, P. M. (2001). Early adverse experience as a developmental risk factor for later psychopathology: evidence from rodent and primate models. *Dev Psychopathol* **13**, 419–449.

Saunders, R. C., Kolachana, B. S., Bachevalier, J., and Weinberger, D. R. (1998). Neonatal lesions of the medial temporal lobe disrupt prefrontal cortical regulation of striatal dopamine. *Nature* **393**, 169–171.

Schore, A. N. (1994). *Affect Regulation and the Origin of the Self: the Neurobiology of Emotional Development.* Hillsdale, NJ: Lawrence Erlbaum.

Schore, A. N. (1996). The experience-dependent maturation of a regulatory system in the orbital prefrontal cortex and the origin of developmental psychopathology. *Dev Psychopathol* **8**, 59.

Schultz, R. T. (2005). Developmental deficits in social perception in autism: the role of the amygdala and fusiform face area. *Int J Dev Neurosci* **23**, 125–141.

Schultz, W., Tremblay, L., and Hollerman, J. R. (2000a). Reward processing in primate orbitofrontal cortex and basal ganglia. *Cereb Cortex* **10**, 272–283.

Schultz, R. T., Gauthier, I., Klin, A. *et al.* (2000b). Abnormal ventral temporal cortical activity during face discrimination among individuals with autism and Asperger syndrome. *Arch Gen Psychiat* **57**, 331–340.

Schultz, R. T., Grelotti, D. J., Klin, A. *et al.* (2003). The role of the fusiform face area in social cognition: implications for the pathobiology of autism. *Philos Trans R Soc Lond B Biol Sci* **358**, 415–427.

Schumann, C. M., Hamstra, J., Goodlin-Jones, B. L. *et al.* (2004). The amygdala is enlarged in children but not adolescents with autism; the hippocampus is enlarged at all ages. *J Neurosci* **24**, 6392–6401.

Scoville, W.B. and Milner, B. (1957). Loss of recent memory after bilateral hippocampal lesions. *J Neurol Neurosurg Psychiat* **20**, 11–21.

Shaw, P., Lawrence, E. J., Radbourne, C., Bramham, J., Polkey, C. E., and David, A. S. (2004). The impact of early and late damage to the human amygdala on 'theory of mind' reasoning. *Brain* **127**, 1535–1548.

Sigman, M., Dijamco, A., Gratier, M., and Rozga, A. (2004). Early detection of core deficits in autism. *Ment Retard Dev Disabil Res Rev* **10**, 221–233.

Smith, I. M. and Bryson, S. E. (1994). Imitation and action in autism: a critical review. *Psychol Bull* **116**, 259–273.

Sparks, B. F., Friedman, S. D., Shaw, D. W. *et al.* (2002). Brain structural abnormalities in young children with autism spectrum disorder. *Neurology* **59**, 184–192.

Stone, W. L. (1997). Autism in infancy and early childhood. In Cohen, D. and Vokmar, F. R. eds. *Handbook of Autism and Pervasive Developmental Disorders*, 2nd edn. New York: Wiley and Sons Inc.

Stone, V. E., Baron-Cohen, S., and Knight. R. T. (1998). Frontal lobe contributions to theory of mind. *J Cogn Neurosci* **10**, 640–656.

Stone, V. E., Baron-Cohen, S., Calder, A. J., Keane, J., and Young, A. W. (2003). Acquired theory of mind impairments in individuals with bilateral amygdala lesions. *Neuropsychologia* **41**, 209–220.

Sullivan, K. and Tager-Flusberg, H. (1999). Second-order belief attribution in Williams syndrome: intact or impaired? *Am J Ment Retard* **104**, 523–532.

Suomi, S. J. (1984). The development of affect in rhesus monkeys. In Fox, N. A. and Davidson, R. J. eds. *The Psychobiology of Affective Development*. Hillsdale, NJ: Lawrence Erlbaum Associates, Inc, pp. 119–159.

Tager-Flusberg, H. and Sullivan, K. A. (2000). Componential view of theory of mind: evidence from Williams syndrome. *Cognition* **76**, 59–90.

Thatcher, R. W. (1994). Psychopathology of early frontal lobe damage: Dependence on cycles of development. *Dev Psychopathol* **6**, 565–596.

Thompson, C. I. (1969). Time in test cage and behavior after amygdalectomy in infant rhesus monkeys. *Physiol Behav* **4**, 249–254.

Thompson, C. I. (1981). Long-term behavioral development of rhesus monkeys after amygdalectomy in infancy. In Ben-Ari, Y., ed. *Conference Proceeding of Biomedical Press*. North-Holland: Elsevier, pp. 259–270.

Thompson, C. I. and Towfighi, J. T. (1976). Social behavior of juvenile rhesus monkeys after amygdalectomy in infancy. *Physiol Behav* **17**, 831–836.

Thompson, C. I., Schwartzbaum, J. S., and Harlow, H. F. (1969). Development of social fear after amygdalectomy in infant rhesus monkeys. *Physiol Behav* **4**, 249–254.

Thompson, C. I., Bergland, R. M., and Towfighi, J. T. (1977). Social and nonsocial behaviors of adult rhesus monkeys after amygdalectomy in infancy or adulthood. *J Comp Physiol Psychol* **91**, 533–548.

Thorpe, S. J., Rolls, E. T., and Maddison, S. (1983). The orbitofrontal cortex: neuronal activity in the behaving monkey. *Exp Brain Res* **49**, 93–115.

Tonsgard, J. H., Harwicke, N., and Levine S. C. (1987). Kluver-Bucy syndrome in children. *Pediatr Neurol* **3**, 162–165.

Tranel, D. (2002). Emotion, decision making, and the ventromedial prefrontal cortex. In Stuss, D. T. and Knight, R. T. eds. *Principles of Frontal Lobe Function*. Oxford: Oxford University Press, pp. 338–353.

Tucker, G. J., Price, T. R., Johnson, V. B., and McAllister, T. (1986). Phenomenology of temporal lobe dysfunction: a link to atypical psychosis – a series of cases. *J Nerv Ment Dis* **174**, 348–356.

Vicari. S. (2001). Implicit versus explicit memory function in children with Down and Williams syndrome. *Downs Syndr Res Pract* **7**, 35–40.

Vicari, S. Brizzolara, D. Carlesimo, G. A. Pezzini, G., and Volterra V. (1996). Memory abilities in children with Williams syndrome. *Cortex* **32**, 503–514.

Volkmar, F. R. and Pauls, D. (2003). Autism. *The Lancet* **362**, 1133–1141.

Volkmar, F., Chawarska, K., and Klin, A. (2005). Autism in infancy and early childhood. *Annu Rev Psychol* **56**, 315–336.

Wang, A. T., Dapretto, M., Hariri, A. R., Sigman, M., and Bookheimer, S. Y. (2004). Neural correlates of facial affect processing in children and adolescents with autism spectrum disorder. *J Am Acad Child Adolesc Psychiat* **43**, 481–490.

Webster, M. J., Ungerleider, L. G., and Bachevalier, J. (1991). Connections of inferior temporal areas TE and TEO with medial temporal-lobe structures in infant and adult monkeys. *J Neurosci* **11**, 1095–1116.

Webster, M. J., Bachevalier, J., and Ungerleider, L. G. (1994). Connections of inferior temporal areas TEO and TE with parietal and frontal cortex in macaque monkeys. *Cereb Cortex* **4**, 470–483.

Werner, E., Dawson, G., Osterling, J., and Dinno, N. (2000). Recognition of autism spectrum disorder before one year of age: a retrospective study based on home videotapes. *J Autism Dev Disord* **30**, 157–162.

Whalen, P. J., Rauch, S. L., Etcoff, N. L., McLnerney, S. C., Lee, M. B., and Jenike, M. A. (1998). Masked Presentations of emotional facial expressions modulate amygdala activity without explicit knowledge. *J Neurosci* **18**, 411–418.

Williams, J. H., Whiten, A., Suddendorf, T., and Perrett, D. I. (2001). Imitation, mirror neurons and autism. *Neurosci Biobehav Rev* **25**, 287–295.

Williams, J. H., Whiten, A., and Singh, T. (2004). A systematic review of action imitation in autistic spectrum disorder. *J Autism Dev Disord* **34**, 285–299.

Williams, J. H. G., Waiter, G. D., Gilchrist, A., Perrett, D. I., Murray, A. D., and Whiten, A. (2006). Neural mechanisms of imitation and 'mirror neuron' functioning in autistic spectrum disorder. *Neuropsychologia* **44**, 610–621.

Winston, J. S. Strange, B. A. O'Doherty, J., and Dolan, R. J. (2002). Automatic and intentional brain responses during evaluation of trustworthiness of faces. *Nat Neurosci* **5**, 277–283.

Young, A. W., Hellawell, D. J., VanDeWal, C., and Johnson, M. (1996). Facial expression processing after amygdalotomy. *Neuropsychologia* **34**, 31–39.

Zald, D. H. (2003). The human amygdala and the emotional evaluation of sensory stimuli. *Brain Res Rev* **41**, 88–123.

CHAPTER 3

Macaque Models of Visual Development and Disability

Lynne Kiorpes

Beginning in the 1960s with the work of David Hubel and Torsten Wiesel, Jennifer Lund, Anita Hendrickson, and others, great strides were made in our understanding of visual system organization (see Friedlander and Tootle, 1990). The earliest studies employed the cat as the primary animal model. These studies were followed by physiological and anatomical investigation into the visual system of the macaque monkey. Those ground-breaking studies showed that visual system organization in nonhuman primates, the Old World macaque monkeys in particular, closely mirrors that of humans (see Kaas, 2004; Van Essen, 2004). Since that time the macaque monkey has become the animal model of choice for human vision. Hundreds of studies have used the macaque as a model system for understanding visual system function in normal adults and for studying the origins of dysfunction. To learn how developmental visual disabilities arise, it is important to first understand how the visual system normally develops and to establish that the model system that is best for adults is also appropriate for infants.

NORMAL DEVELOPMENT OF VISION IN MACAQUE MONKEYS

In 1975 Davida Teller, Ronald Boothe, and their colleagues began to document the remarkable similarity between human and macaque monkey infants in the development of vision (see Boothe et al., 1985). They studied visual acuity in both species using the forced-choice preferential looking technique developed by Teller (Teller et al., 1974). They concluded that vision in monkeys develops with the same progression as humans, although the process proceeds four times faster in macaques (Teller and Boothe, 1979). Hence, visual development as measured behaviorally is comparable in monkey and human infants if age is expressed in weeks for monkeys

Primate Models of Children's Health and Developmental Disabilities

and in months for humans. This relationship is shown in Figure 3.1 (also see Teller, 1997). Figure 3.1 (upper data set, open symbols) plots development of grating acuity (similar to acuity as measured with a Snellen eye chart) as a function of age in weeks for monkeys (circles) and as a function of age in months for humans (open triangles). Clearly, the data can be described by the same developmental profile; the weeks-to-months translation is often called the four-to-one rule (see Boothe *et al.*, 1985).

While this four-to-one relationship is a useful metric, it is important to realize it cannot be assumed to necessarily hold for *all* visual processes. Subsequent studies have examined a variety of other measures of spatial vision to see if the rule holds. Two measures that reflect sensitivity to spatial position are Vernier acuity and stereoacuity. These acuities are based on fine spatial positional judgments, the former for co-planar judgments and the latter for localization in depth. Kiorpes (1992a) showed that Vernier acuity is less mature than grating acuity near birth in

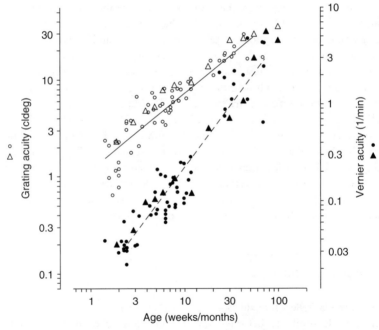

FIGURE 3.1   The development of visual acuity in macaque monkeys and humans. Two measures of visual acuity are plotted together as a function of age, in weeks for monkey data and in months for human data. Grating acuity is referenced to the left ordinate (open symbols) and Vernier acuity is referenced to the right ordinate (filled symbols). The two ordinates are normalized to adult levels of performance for monkeys, and so reflect the relative maturation of Vernier and grating acuity. Monkey data (circles) are from Kiorpes (1992a) with additional unpublished data from the author; human data are from Zanker *et al.* (1992). The lines are regression fits to the monkey data.

macaques, but develops more quickly so that the two functions approach adult levels at similar ages. However, recent studies of Vernier acuity development in children have shown a longer, later developmental profile for Vernier acuity compared with grating acuity (Zanker *et al.*, 1992; Carkeet *et al.*, 1997; Skoczenski and Norcia, 1999, 2002).

The relative development of grating and Vernier acuity is shown in Figure 3.1. The filled symbols represent Vernier acuity data for the same groups of infants from which the grating acuity data were obtained. The scales are normalized to align at adult levels on the log–log plot. Thus the profiles represent the relative maturation of the two visual functions. Once again the developmental profiles match well between the two species, suggesting that the four-to-one rule holds for Vernier acuity as well as grating acuity. Also, although human studies generally conclude that Vernier acuity develops over a longer time-course, the four data sets plotted in Figure 3.1 appear to converge at similar ages. In line with the four-to-one rule, stereoacuity tested using identical techniques across species shows an abrupt onset at 3–4 weeks in macaques (O'Dell and Boothe, 1997) and 3–4 months in humans (Birch *et al.*, 1982). Interestingly, development thereafter appears to proceed at a similar *absolute* rate. This suggests slower relative development of stereoacuity in monkeys than in humans (O'Dell and Boothe, 1997). In neither species is it clear when adult levels of stereoacuity are reached, so the relative rates of development remain to be completely quantified.

The most common and complete descriptor of spatial vision is the contrast sensitivity function. This function describes the sensitivity of the visual system across all spatial scales within the visible range from coarse to fine, describing the ability to detect luminance variations at various spatial scales. Contrast sensitivity functions for monkeys and humans at various ages are shown in Figure 3.2. With age the function shifts from low to high spatial frequency and low to high levels of sensitivity in both species. Adult levels of sensitivity are reached between 40 and 60 weeks in monkeys (Boothe *et al.*, 1988; Kiorpes, 1996) and between 48 and 72 months in humans (Ellemberg *et al.*, 1999). On balance, then, the four-to-one rule seems to be a good metric of relative rates of spatial visual development in macaques and humans.

These studies of basic visual development provide reasonable support for the weeks-equals-months relationship for spatial vision, although complete data sets are sometimes unavailable. Most typical day-to-day visual functioning relies less on fine acuity or threshold level vision, and more on global integration of visual information over space and time. Therefore, it is worth examining whether this rule is also obeyed for so-called higher level visual performance. Examples of higher level vision are figure–ground segmentation and motion and form integration. The most commonly studied global ability is motion perception, which requires integration of information over space and time.

There have been many studies of sensitivity to visual motion in human infants, but few that reveal a complete developmental time-course (Braddick *et al.*, 2003).

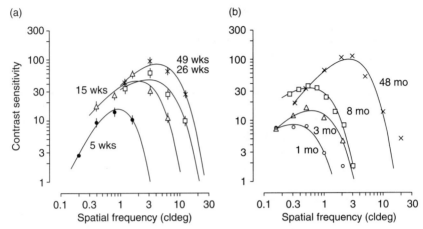

FIGURE 3.2   Development of contrast sensitivity in macaque monkeys and humans.
(a) Contrast sensitivity as a function of spatial frequency is plotted for individual monkeys tested at the
ages noted in the figure. Data are from Boothe *et al.* (1988). (b) Average contrast sensitivity is plotted
for groups of infants tested at the spatial frequencies and ages noted in the figure. Data are from Banks
and Salapatek (1978) (1 and 3 months); Peterzell *et al.* (1995) (8 months); Ellemberg *et al.* (1999) (48
months). The smooth curves fit to the data are described in Williams *et al.* (1981) or Kozma and
Kiorpes (2003).

Gunn *et al.* (2002) showed a slow maturation of sensitivity for motion integration
that reached asymptote around age 10–11 years. A related measure, global form
integration ability, had an earlier asymptote at age 6–7 years. Interestingly, Kiorpes
and Movshon (2004b) found a similarly long developmental time-course for
motion integration in macaque infants. They found that motion sensitivity reached
adult levels between 2 and 3 years, which would translate to a maturation rate of
9–13 years in humans by the four-to-one rule. This rate is consistent with the findings of Gunn *et al.* (2002). In macaque monkeys, Kiorpes and Bassin (2003) found
earlier asymptotic performance in the range of 1.5–2 years on a form integration
task using figure–ground segmentation. These results suggest a slightly earlier maturation of form than motion integration in macaques as well as humans. Thus, the
overall pattern of development of integrative visual function, which presumably
underlies the ability to extract figures from a visual scene and discriminate common
motion among elements in a scene, is similar in macaques and humans and seems
to also follow a four-to-one age translation.

VISUAL DISABILITY IN CHILDHOOD

The most common cause of vision loss in children is amblyopia. Amblyopia, literally
"blunt sight," is classically defined as a loss of visual acuity in one eye with no obvious

accompanying pathology (von Noorden, 1980). In other words, the child has poor visual performance but there is no obvious impediment to clear vision. On inspection the eye looks normal. However, it is important to realize that vision is accomplished not by the eye alone, but by the visual brain. The eye gathers light from the environment, processes that light energy, and transmits the information to the brain. The estimated incidence of amblyopia ranges from 1% to 6% across many studies, but it is most often in the range of 3–4% in western populations (von Noorden, 1980; Chua and Mitchell, 2004; see also, Simons, 2005).

Amblyopia is typically associated with three primary conditions: congenital cataract, dense opacity in one or both eyes; anisometropia, unequal refractive error in the two eyes; and strabismus, misalignment of the two eyes. These conditions are associated with amblyopia when they occur in infancy and early childhood. It is important to note that these conditions do not result in loss of visual function when they occur in adults. Thus, amblyopia is a disorder of visual development and there is some period of susceptibility, a "critical period," for its development. Although amblyopia was initially considered to affect only visual acuity and binocular function, it is now clear that many other visual abilities are compromised.

A good deal of attention has been paid to the effect of childhood vision loss on the academic and psychosocial development of children (Packwood et al., 1999; Holmes and Clarke, 2006; Koklanis et al., 2006; Williams and Harrad, 2006). Specific effects on reading and math performance have been reported, as well as a general sense that amblyopia interferes with work, school, and sports performance. The poor stereopsis that is associated with amblyopia also affects a child's ability to participate in sports and compromises some motor skills. Although survey results are somewhat inconsistent, amblyopia appears to have a secondary effect on self-esteem. Most recent studies have shown that amblyopia *treatment* is responsible for the greatest negative psychological effects on the child (Choong et al., 2004; Koklanis et al., 2006; Williams and Harrad, 2006), whereas the amblyopia itself has greater long-term consequences for performance. As discussed below, the most common treatment involves eye patching, which itself affects the child's psycho-social well-being. In studying effects on adults, Chua and Mitchell (2004) found that people with amblyopia were less likely to hold university degrees. However, they found no significant effect of amblyopia on occupational choice, although certain occupations such as flying commercial aircraft are closed to those with vision disorders.

One often overlooked consequence of life-long amblyopia is an increased risk of losing sight in the fellow eye. Recent studies have highlighted the increased risk of vision loss in the fellow eye in the amblyopic population (Rahi et al., 2002; Chua and Mitchell, 2004). Taken together, these concerns increase the importance of early childhood vision screening and serious efforts to treat the condition prior to school-age (Williams and Harrad, 2006).

In summary, the normal development of visual function proceeds in a systematic way in both human and nonhuman primates. Three decades of comparative research shows that the macaque monkey provides an excellent model system for studying the normal development of visual function and mechanisms that underlie visual immaturity in infants (see Kiorpes and Movshon, 2004a). The development of visual function is compromised by abnormal ocular and ocular motor conditions that exist during infancy and early childhood. These conditions result in amblyopia, which is a significant source of concern for pediatric ophthalmologists and compromises many aspects of a child's life in addition to their vision. Research with animal models presents a significant advantage for understanding the processes that underlie the development of amblyopia. In particular, the causal relationship between visual impediment and amblyopia can be studied prospectively, the natural progress of amblyopia development can be studied without the complication of treatment history, age of onset of visual impediment can be completely specified, and studies can be undertaken to directly assess the underlying neural substrate.

With this background I next review the visual disabilities that have been investigated using the nonhuman primate as a model system. In each disability I highlight the clinical relevance of the work. I also emphasize results that provide insight into the underlying mechanisms, as they are the aspect of our work with animal models that provide unique and otherwise unattainable knowledge. The review is not intended to be exhaustive. Instead, the goal is to illustrate the important contributions that nonhuman primate research has made to our understanding of, and treatment strategies for, developmental sensory disability.

EFFECTS OF VISUAL EXPERIENCE ON VISUAL DEVELOPMENT

A defining moment for understanding the role played by visual experience in visual development came with the early studies of Wiesel and Hubel in kittens (Wiesel and Hubel, 1963, 1965; Hubel and Wiesel, 1965). They found that closing one eye to impose form deprivation, or misaligning one eye to create a strabismus, significantly altered the physiological and anatomical organization of the primary visual cortex (V1, the first cortical area in the visual system hierarchy). They noted anecdotally that after eye closure the kittens appeared blind when using the formerly closed eye following a period – sometimes quite short – of monocular deprivation. Subsequent studies in macaque monkeys showed similar alteration of the structure of V1 (e.g. Hubel and Wiesel, 1977; Wiesel, 1982). Behavioral monkey studies confirmed a devastating loss of visual function (von Noorden et al., 1970; Harwerth et al., 1983).

The normal visual cortex has a balanced representation of the two eyes, known as eye dominance, with regular modulation of binocular and monocular zones. This organization is present at birth in infant monkeys. With normal visual experience it is then refined to some degree over the first few postnatal weeks (Horton and Hocking, 1996). This organization is disrupted following deprivation. The deprived eye zones are minimized and binocularity is severely compromised (see LeVay *et al.*, 1980; Horton and Hocking, 1997). On the basis of these studies, the authors proposed that impediments to normal visual experience during early post-natal development caused a reduction in the influence of the deprived eye in V1, which in turn led to poor visual function in the adult (see Movshon and van Sluyters, 1981; Movshon and Kiorpes, 1990 for reviews). These findings formed the foundation for a body of work using the macaque monkey as a model system for understanding childhood developmental visual disorders.

Models of amblyopia

Beginning in the 1970s, behavioral studies of macaque monkeys raised under visual conditions that mimic human developmental visual disorders were conducted to determine how well the monkey model reflected the visual losses found in human amblyopia and to explore the underlying neural mechanisms. As mentioned above, three primary conditions are associated with poor visual development in children. In congenital *cataract*, ocular opacities result in form deprivation amblyopia. In *anisometropia*, blur in one eye results in anisometropic amblyopia. In *strabismus*, ocular motor misalignment of the two eyes results in strabismic amblyopia. These conditions are associated with permanent visual loss only when they occur in infancy and early childhood.

Initially, it was not known whether there was a causal relationship between the physical disorders and the behavioral loss of vision. It was only known that there was a correlation. The nature of the association between early visual abnormality and amblyopia was unclear because only about 40–60% of those with strabismus or anisometropia develop amblyopia. The relationship is much stronger for depriva-tion amblyopia. Furthermore, the condition that the child presents with at the time of diagnosis may not be the same as the original precipitating disorder. For exam-ple, anisometropia can cause strabismus. The strabismus is obvious to the parent, but the anisometropia is often not noticed until vision screening at school age.

Animal studies showed direct causality between visual impediment and the devel-opment of amblyopia and provided definitive information on the nature of the criti-cal period for vision. They also provided insight into the neural basis of amblyopia and had a direct impact on the way in which amblyopia is treated in children.

Monocular deprivation

The earliest behavioral visual deprivation studies were conducted by von Noorden and colleagues in 1970 (von Noorden *et al.*, 1970; von Noorden, 1973). They showed that early visual deprivation by lid suture, a monkey model for congenital cataract, resulted in a loss of visual acuity in the deprived eye. They closed one eye of young monkeys for various durations and tested acuity using a clinical Landolt-C test, comparable to letter chart acuity. Amblyopia occurred in all animals deprived prior to the age of nine weeks, even when the period of deprivation was as short as one or two weeks. The data suggested that the critical period for amblyopia development was the first three postnatal months, as only animals deprived before 12 weeks failed to achieve normal visual acuity when tested as adults. It is important to note that in these studies and most others of this kind, the vision was not assessed immediately following the end of the deprivation period. Instead, vision was assessed 1–2 years after the period of deprivation, so it was unclear whether the outcome was purely the result of the early deprivation or reflected much later recovery of function.

Later, more extensive behavioral studies showed that the effect of visual deprivation from lid suture was in fact quite dramatic and largely refractory to recovery following eye opening (Harwerth et al., 1983, 1989). Animals reared with only a few weeks of deprivation, followed by years of normal binocular vision, often developed only limited visual function. Figure 3.3a shows contrast sensitivity data from an animal that was monocularly deprived from the age of 4 months until approximately 18 months (Harwerth et al., 1990). The sensitivity of the deprived eye following early deprivation is substantially poorer than would be expected from even a very young normal infant. This is seen by comparing the deprived eye function to the functions in Figure 3.2. It shows that visual experience is required for normal development of visual function and it is essential to maintain even the rudimentary vision of newly born infants.

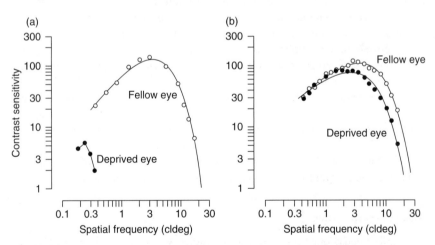

FIGURE 3.3   The effect of monocular deprivation on contrast sensitivity in monkeys. Contrast sensitivity is plotted as a function of spatial frequency for each eye of a monkey monocularly deprived for 18 months from the age of 4 months (a) or 12 months (b). Filled symbols represent data from the deprived eye. Data are from Harwerth et al. (1990), figures 5 and 6. The smooth curves fit to the data are described in Williams et al. (1981) or Kozma and Kiorpes (2003).

Figure 3.3b shows comparable data for an animal that was monocularly deprived for a similarly long period of time, but beginning at the later age of 12 months. Note that sensitivity at middle and high spatial frequencies is depressed for the deprived eye, but only moderately so compared to the fellow non-deprived eye. Thus, the visual system of the monkey is vulnerable to deprivation well beyond the first three months after birth, the period originally proposed by von Noorden. Furthermore, there is a gradation in susceptibility with age. This work had a direct impact on management of infants born with congenital cataracts. It led to a dramatic reduction in the age at surgery to remove the cataract and stimulated prospective studies on the effect of age at surgery on visual outcome in humans (Birch and Stager, 1996).

The lid suture model was instrumental in establishing the nature of the critical period for the development of amblyopia. The initial work of von Noorden and colleagues identified the early postnatal weeks as a period of extreme vulnerability to abnormal visual experience. This period of susceptibility declines gradually over the succeeding year. Harwerth *et al.* (1986, 1989, 1990) systematically charted the period of vulnerablility to deprivation of spatial, temporal, and chromatic visual functions over the first two postnatal years in monkeys. They clearly showed that different visual functions have different critical periods. Similarly, different levels in the visual pathway have different critical periods. Subcortical structures show less vulnerability than cortical levels (Levitt *et al.*, 2001) and cortical layer IV shows a shorter period of susceptibility to deprivation than other layers (LeVay *et al.*, 1980; Horton and Hocking, 1997).

These and similar studies of monkeys and humans, as well as kittens, revealed that the concept of a critical period needs to be refined. This is because there are different sensitive periods for normal development, for the disruptive effects of deprivation, and for recovery from deprivation (Daw, 1998; Mitchell and MacKinnon, 2002; Lewis and Maurer, 2005). As argued by Daw (1998), there are different, but not mutually exclusive, critical periods for the disruptive effects of abnormal visual experience on development and for the efficacy of treatment. In neither case is the critical period completely coincident with the period of normal visual development. This principle is illustrated clearly in a publication showing different but overlapping sensitive periods for the susceptibility of stereopsis to abnormal binocular visual experience in humans (Fawcett *et al.*, 2005). Thus, these distinctions hold true for humans as well as for animal models and for binocular as well as spatial vision.

The lid suture model has been very important for our understanding of constraints on visual development and the nature of critical periods in vision. Neurophysiological and anatomical investigation of the visual pathways and properties of single neurons following lid suture have shown shrinkage of cells associated with the deprived eye at the level of the lateral geniculate nucleus (LGN) and a nearly complete loss of influence by the deprived eye in primary visual cortex. The degree of the abnormality reflects the amount and timing of the deprivation (e.g. von Noorden and Crawford, 1978; LeVay *et al.*, 1980; Horton and Hocking, 1997). However, because the deep amblyopia that results from lid suture occurs relatively infrequently in human clinical practice, and because the representation of the deprived eye in cortex following lid suture is minimal at best, the lid suture model is not the best one for understanding the development of and neural basis for amblyopia. More clinically relevant models for amblyopia are those that are associated with moderate visual loss and permit maintained representation of the deprived eye in the primary visual pathways.

Anisometropia and strabismus

Models of amblyopia that create or simulate strabismus or anisometropia are preferred over lid suture because they are associated with more moderate visual loss. Early studies of vision following surgically induced strabismus in young monkeys established a clear, causal relationship between strabismus onset and the development of amblyopia in the otherwise normal visual system (von Noorden and Dowling, 1970; Kiorpes and Boothe, 1980; Harwerth *et al.*, 1983; Kiorpes *et al.*, 1987, 1989). These studies showed that strabismus created surgically, or anisometropia produced by unilateral blur, reliably resulted in amblyopia when imposed during the height of the critical period. Longitudinal studies, easily conducted in monkeys but difficult to conduct in humans, showed that amblyopia develops over time as a gradual set-back or slowing of the developmental program. This is followed later by a resumption of development. Figure 3.4 illustrates one pattern, showing acuity development in each eye of one strabismic monkey. Interestingly, prospective and retrospective studies using these animal models have

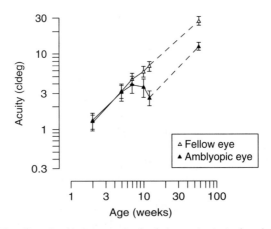

FIGURE 3.4   The effect of strabismus on acuity development. Acuity is plotted as a function of age for each eye of a monkey made strabismic by surgery at 3 weeks of age. Filled symbols represent data from the strabismic eye. Data are from Kiorpes *et al.* (1989), figure 2b.

shown not only that strabismus and anisometropia cause amblyopia, but also that amblyopia can cause strabismus and anisometropia (Quick *et al.*, 1989; Kiorpes and Wallman, 1995; Smith, Hung and Harwerth, 1999). It is important to note that, similar to humans, macaque monkeys naturally develop strabismus, anisometropia, and cataracts, allowing study of the natural history of these disorders (see Kiorpes, 1989, 2002; Horton *et al.*, 1997).

In addition to the acuity loss in amblyopia, sensitivity to contrast across spatial scales from coarse to fine is compromised. The fine spatial scales representing sensitivity to fine detail are affected most deeply (Kiorpes, 1996). Contrast sensitivity functions for each eye of two amblyopic monkeys, one strabismic and one anisometropic, are shown in Figure 3.5. Note the relatively greater loss of sensitivity at the high spatial frequency ranges near the acuity limit, represented by the extrapolation of the curves to the abscissa. The range of visual deficits following experimental strabismus is similar to that found in the human population and experimentally produced amblyopia occurs with similar frequency to natural amblyopia. Thus, somewhat surprisingly, only about 60% of those with experimental strabismus actually develop amblyopia (Kiorpes *et al.*, 1989; Kiorpes, 2002). Experimentally produced anisometropia created by rearing with defocus of one eye either by spectacle lenses, contact lenses, or dilation of the pupil, also results in clinically relevant depths of amblyopia (Boothe *et al.*, 1982; Smith *et al.*, 1985; Kiorpes *et al.*, 1987; Kiorpes *et al.*, 1993; Smith *et al.* 1999). Taken together, this work

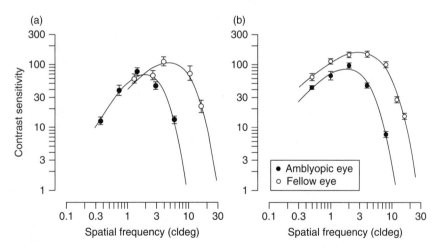

FIGURE 3.5   The effect of strabismus and anisometropia on contrast sensitivity in monkeys. Contrast sensitivity is plotted as a function of spatial frequency for each eye of a monkey (a) made strabismic at 3 weeks of age or (b) made anisometropic at 3 weeks of age. Filled symbols represent data from the deprived eye. Data in (a) are from Kiper and Kiorpes (1994), figure 1d; data in (b) are from Kozma and Kiorpes (2003), figure 5c. The smooth curves fit to the data are described in Kozma and Kiorpes (2003).

established experimental amblyopia in macaque monkeys as an excellent model for human amblyopia, and identified many of the constraints on its development.

Neural mechanisms in amblyopia

To identify the neural basis for amblyopia, Movshon *et al.* (1987) and Kiorpes *et al.* (1998) evaluated the response properties of neurons in the primary visual cortex of monkeys with behaviorally documented amblyopia. Both studies revealed losses of neuronal "acuity" in cells responding to stimulation of the amblyopic eye, results which were reminiscent of those seen behaviorally. No loss was found at earlier levels of the visual pathway (Movshon *et al.*, 1987), even following severe form deprivation (Blakemore and Vital-Durand, 1986; Levitt *et al.*, 2001). These studies established for the first time that, in addition to disruption of the binocular organ-ization of the visual cortex, there were effects of abnormal visual experience on the spatial response properties of neurons.

Acuity loss at the neuronal level was reflected in the tuning properties of the cells in V1 that are driven by the amblyopic eye. These cells responded to lower ranges of spatial frequency compared with cells driven by the fellow eye. There were varying degrees of loss in contrast sensitivity of individual neurons driven by the amblyopic eye in addition to the reduction in acuity, but these were not consistent across animals and studies. Other properties of these cells, such as their selectivity for orientation and direction of motion, were uniformly normal. A direct comparison between the degree of behaviorally measured amblyopia and the extent of the neural deficit showed a strong correlation, supporting the conclusion that the neural deficits were actually related to the behavioral losses (Kiorpes *et al.*, 1998; Kiorpes and Movshon, 2004a). However, the cortical losses tended to be smaller than the behavioral ones and did not explain the contrast sensitivity deficit. Thus, the properties of ambly-opic neurons at this early cortical stage cannot completely account for even the basic loss in spatial vision. These studies established that the primary visual cortex is the first site in the visual pathway that reflects developmental disruption related to amblyopia and that abnormalities early in the visual system may be amplified in downstream visual areas.

While the effect of abnormal visual experience on the spatial properties of V1 neu-rons is more modest than might be expected, amblyopic V1 does reflect dramatic abnormalities of binocularity similar to those found following lid suture (e.g. Movshon *et al.*, 1987; Crawford *et al.*, 1996a; Kiorpes *et al.*, 1998). Anisometropic rearing results in a shift of ocular dominance away from the defocused eye, but strabismic rearing generally results in relatively balanced ocular dominance as measured physiologically. In all cases, regardless of the type of model used, there is a reduction in the number of binocularly driven neurons (see Kiorpes and Movshon, 2004a). Amblyopic neurons appeared to be monocular with the standard procedure of testing each eye independ-ently. However, Smith *et al.* (1997) showed that residual binocular interaction could be demonstrated in a large proportion of amblyopic neurons when the cells were tested dichoptically by stimulating both eyes at the same time.

These interactions were more often than not suppressive rather than excitatory, particularly following strabismic rearing. Suppressive interactions developed quickly following the onset of abnormal binocular visual experience. They are present following as little as 3 days of binocular decorrelation (Zhang *et al.*, 2005) and correlate well with deficits of binocular vision assessed behaviorally (Smith *et al.*, 1997; Wensveen *et al.*, 2001, 2003; Zhang *et al.*, 2003). These findings serve as a caution to clinicians that infants with strabismus should be treated as early as possible in order to preserve normal binocular function.

To summarize, neurophysiological investigation into the neural correlates of amblyopia show that V1 is the first site along the visual pathway reflecting behaviorally documented abnormalities of vision. In the case of binocular function, the neural abnormalities at the level of V1 closely correlate with those measured behaviorally. However, in the case of spatial vision, the neural deficits are qualitatively similar but not quantitatively sufficient to account for the vision losses. The inevitable conclusion is that the neural basis for the spatial visual deficits that characterize amblyopia lies further along the visual pathway in higher order processing areas. If that is the case, there should be a range of perceptual deficits in amblyopes that reflect processing disruption at higher levels of the visual pathways.

Perceptual disorder in amblyopia

Behavioral studies of amblyopia in nonhuman primates and psychophysical studies of adult human amblyopes have shown that amblyopia affects far more than acuity and contrast sensitivity (see Kiorpes, 2006; Levi, 2006). There is a disruption of the position sense, as exemplified by measurements of Vernier acuity (Kiorpes, 1992b). There is also a loss of binocular vision, in particular stereopsis, in amblyopic monkeys (Crawford *et al.*, 1996b; Wensveen *et al.*, 2003). Moreover, there is disruption of higher level perception in amblyopes that cannot be understood only on the basis of the acuity loss. An example of such a function is figure–ground segregation as measured by contour integration (see Kozma and Kiorpes, 2003). Contour integration is the ability to extract a coherent structured form from a field of background noise elements. It is disrupted in strabismic and anisometropic amblyopia in both monkeys and humans. Whether this task relies on areas beyond V1, or on V1 itself, is a matter of controversy, but performance is clearly not predictable from knowledge of the depth of the acuity loss.

Another example of higher level processing is motion perception. This requires integration of motion signals over time and space and is thought to depend on a visual area downstream from V1 known as MT, the middle temporal area (Newsome and Pare, 1988; Britten *et al.*, 1992). Kiorpes *et al.* (2006) studied motion sensitivity of amblyopic monkeys and found substantial losses when viewing with the amblyopic eye. The deficits were apparent in both the spatial and temporal domains. The spatial losses could be ascribed to the reduced range of spatial frequency sensitivity of the amblyopic eye, but the temporal losses could not be related to any known V1 abnormality. This finding strongly supports the idea that additional amblyopic processing deficits arise in downstream visual areas.

A now common finding in studies of higher order perception in amblyopia is that the perceptual losses identified for the amblyopic eye extend to the fellow "normal" eye (e.g. Giaschi et al., 1992; Kozma and Kiorpes, 2003). Performance using the fellow eye is poorer than for normal controls, but not as poor as the amblyopic eye. In the past, it was typically assumed that the fellow eye was unaffected in amblyopia. The combination of the findings of subnormal performance with the fellow eye in monkey models and abnormal performance with the fellow eye in human studies stimulated caution in the clinical community. Simons (2005) makes this point and urges reference to the fellow eye not as "normal" or "sound" but as the "better" eye.

To summarize, investigations into the ability of amblyopes to perform higher order perceptual tasks have found substantial deficits that cannot be predicted from contrast sensitivity and acuity deficits and often extend to the fellow eye. This behavioral profile is consistent with the neurophysiological findings discussed above, suggesting that the development of visual cortical areas well beyond V1 is disrupted by abnormal postnatal visual experience. To date, no studies of neuronal sensitivity in extrastriate areas have been conducted in amblyopic macaque monkeys, although one study has noted abnormal binocular organization in an extrastriate area following early monocular defocus (Movshon et al., 1987). Nevertheless, the nonhuman primate work is consistent with recent psychophysical studies of human amblyopes showing high order perceptual losses that are not explained by losses in contrast sensitivity (Simmers et al., 2003; Simmers et al., 2005; Levi, 2006). Also, functional imaging studies show abnormal activity in brain areas beyond V1 in amblyopes (Anderson and Swettenham, 2006).

Treatment of amblyopia

Patching has been the treatment of choice for amblyopia in children for more than a century (see von Noorden, 1980; Simons, 2005). Patching therapy involves occlusion of the fellow eye with an eye patch, forcing use of the amblyopic eye. One important corollary of the lid suture studies discussed above is that deprivation amblyopia can result from this common treatment. In the animal model, recovery from early deprivation was typically effected by "treatment" likened to patching, a procedure called reverse occlusion. This involves closure of the previously non-deprived eye with concurrent opening of the initially deprived eye. Monkey studies showed that the visual "recovery" of the initially deprived eye occurred at the expense of the fellow eye (Harwerth et al., 1989).

Examples of the consequences of reverse suture on contrast sensitivity are shown in Figure 3.6. Harwerth *et al.* (1989) closed one eye of monkey subjects at about 1 month of age, then performed the reverse occlusion at various time points thereafter. The data in Figure 3.6a are from a monkey "treated" after 60 days of monocular deprivation. The filled symbols represent data from the *initially* deprived eye. Clearly there has been a complete reversal of the deprivation effect, with the initially deprived eye showing almost normal contrast sensitivity and the initially open, fellow eye, showing deep amblyopia. The data in Figure 3.6b reflect "treatment" at a later age after 90 days of deprivation. In this case, contrast sensitivity is similar in the two eyes, but not normal for either eye. The treatment has resulted in a bilateral loss of visual function.

These data are reminiscent of findings from a longitudinal study in kittens as a model of patching therapy (Mitchell, 1991; Mitchell and MacKinnon, 2002). The study revealed a gradual trade-off of acuity between the initially amblyopic eye and the initially "normal" eye resulting from reverse occlusion. Similarly, studies of recovery of vision following removal of the lens of the eye in monkeys were conducted to explore treatment options for children with congenital cataract. This work documents a dramatic trade-off of acuity in nonhuman primates when the fellow eye is continuously occluded (see Boothe, 1996). Neurophysiological

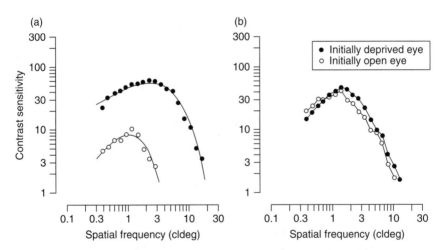

FIGURE 3.6   The effect of "treatment" of amblyopia on contrast sensitivity in monkeys. Contrast sensitivity is plotted as a function of spatial frequency for each eye of two monkeys monocularly deprived at the age of 4 weeks. (a) The initially deprived eye was opened after 60 days of deprivation and the initially open eye was closed for 120 days. (b) The initially deprived eye was opened after 90 days of deprivation and the initially open eye was closed for 120 days. Thereafter, both monkeys received normal binocular visual experience until tested at approximately one year of age. Filled symbols represent data from the initially deprived eye. Data are from Harwerth *et al.* (1989), figure 1c and d. The smooth curves fit to the data are described in Williams *et al.* (1981); the data in panel b could not be fit by our function.

recordings from monkey visual cortex neurons following reverse occlusion treatment confirm that the initially open eye, once continuously patched, loses dominance to the initially deprived eye (Blakemore et al., 1978; Wiesel, 1982; Crawford et al., 1989). Depending on the age of the reverse occlusion, the result is a greater or lesser takeover of cortical territory by the initially deprived eye. These animal studies clearly showed that covering the fellow eye can itself cause amblyopia to develop and often the long-term outcome is poor vision in both eyes.

The primary backup treatment for amblyopia is a procedure called penalization. Penalization involves instillation of a drop of atropine into the fellow eye daily. This dilates the pupil and paralyzes accommodation, thereby inducing blur. Penalization of the preferred fellow eye is intended to shift the child's fixation preference to the amblyopic eye. Unfortunately, this procedure also has been shown to induce amblyopia in young nonhuman primates (Boothe et al., 1982; Harwerth et al., 1983; Kiorpes et al., 1987). The resulting amblyopia is similar in character to anisometropic amblyopia following rearing with blur from defocusing lenses. The effect of penalization during development on cortical neurons is to reduce the acuity and contrast sensitivity of neurons driven by the treated eye (Movshon et al., 1987). Studies such as these alerted the clinical community to the negative effects of patching and penalization, generating a quest for better therapeutic options.

Amblyopia secondary to occlusion and penalization therapy continues to be a concern for treatment (Simons, 2005; Levi, 2006). Recent retrospective studies in treated and untreated amblyopic humans show that contrast sensitivity of the fellow eye is often compromised, but it is difficult to know for sure whether or not this is the result of patching (e.g. Lew et al., 2005; Chatzistefanou et al., 2005). One recent study in monkeys has shown a clear advantage of part-time occlusion strategies for prevention of occlusion amblyopia (Wensveen et al., 2006). It has recently become possible to conduct controlled randomized clinical studies of treatment effectiveness. Several large-scale prospective clinical studies have been implemented to assess the efficacy of alternative strategies such as part-time patching and penalization in amblyopic children (see Holmes and Clarke, 2006; PEDIG, 2005, 2006).

Another concern with typical treatment strategies is that they prolong the period of abnormal binocular visual experience. As described above, amblyopia not only affects spatial vision but also binocular vision. A lack of correlation between the information from the two eyes creates a rapid loss of binocular function at the level of the visual cortex. Patching and penalization further disrupt binocular vision, thereby preventing any opportunity for rescue of binocular vision. Treated human amblyopes often lack binocular function and the poor binocularity may in fact be primary in determining the nature of amblyopic adult spatial vision (McKee et al., 2003). Motivated by the findings in animals, prospective studies in human infants show that early surgery for strabismus and cataracts improve the chances of recovery of binocular function (Birch and Stager, 2006). Minimizing the amount of occlusion therapy further improves binocular outcome (Jeffrey et al., 2001). In addition to revealing the detrimental effects of common therapeutic strategies on the vision of the fellow eye and binocular function, one clear impact of animal work on clinical practice is demonstrating the importance of continued examination of visual acuity during and after treatment for amblyopia.

Treatment of congenital cataract

Cataracts are opacities of the lens that prevent form vision. Either bilateral or unilateral congenital cataracts have a devastating effect on development of vision (see Birch and Stager, 1996; Maurer et al., 1999; Sjöström et al., 1996). The parallels between visual outcomes in monkeys deprived of vision during infancy by lid suture and children deprived in infancy by cataract was obvious by the late 1970s. Since then it has been clearly demonstrated that amblyopia develops as a result of even more moderate levels of form deprivation than lid suture. Smith et al. (2000) raised monkeys with varying degrees of image degradation. They found that the resultant depth of amblyopia was directly related to the degree of image degradation. Work with animal models combined with accumulating evidence from human studies has revealed a strong correlation between duration and degree of form deprivation and depth of vision loss (see Mitchell and MacKinnon, 2002; Lewis and Maurer, 2005). It has now become standard practice to remove cataracts as early as possible in infancy to minimize the period and degree of early visual deprivation.

The primary difficulty with the management of cataracts in infancy is that removal of the cataract requires removal of the lens of the eye. This results in a condition called aphakia, in which the eye has no power to focus. Removal of the cataract thus results in continuing form deprivation after surgery. Prior to about 1980 spectacle lenses were typically prescribed to correct the defocus. There were two problems with this approach. First, it was difficult to keep glasses on young children. Second, the correction required high magnification to compensate for the missing lens. High magnification correction was sometimes difficult to achieve and created aniseikonia, unequal image size in the two eyes. The visual outcome for the aphakic eye was generally poor.

The introduction of contact lenses for use with infants presented a significant advantage over spectacle lenses, but a high degree of compliance and monitoring was required for successful therapy. Contact lenses also require relatively high magnification for proper correction, although less so than with glasses. However, the problem of aniseikonia remained and often the result was still a suboptimal visual outcome (Birch et al., 1986; Lambert et al., 1994). Contrast sensitivity data from each eye of a child with deprivation amblyopia are shown in Figure 3.7. This child had a unilateral congenital cataract that was removed at four months and wore contact lens correction essentially continuously thereafter. In spite of a substantial amount of patching therapy she had significant amblyopia when tested at age 6 years.

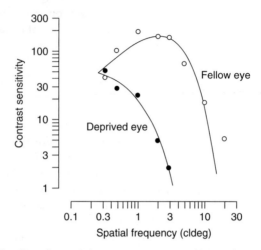

FIGURE 3.7   The effect of congenital cataract on contrast sensitivity in humans. Contrast sensitivity is plotted as a function of spatial frequency for each eye of a child who had a congenital cataract. The cataract was removed at about 4 months of age. Thereafter, the child's vision was corrected by contact lenses and patching therapy; testing took place when the child was about 6 years old. The data are from Tytla *et al.* (1988), figure 1, static gratings. The smooth curves fit to the data are described in Williams *et al.* (1981).

The problems associated with glasses and contact lenses are alleviated by use of intraocular lenses (IOL) following removal of the natural lens. An extensive series of studies by Lambert and colleagues in macaque monkeys was instrumental in evaluating the effect of aphakia on visual development and efficacy of various regimes of treatment following removal of the natural lens. They modeled treatment regimes involving lens removal followed by implantation of either monofocal or multifocal intraocular lenses, with or without subsequent full or part-time patching (Lambert *et al.*, 1994; Boothe, 1996; Boothe *et al.*, 1996, 2000). Grating acuity was longitudinally measured in each eye and assessed by Landolt-C acuity and contrast sensitivity after 1 year of age. The best visual outcomes were produced by a combination of IOL implantation of either kind and subsequent use of contact lenses for optical correction. Part-time patching further improved visual outcomes, but patching of less than 70% of the day produced subnormal grating acuity in the treated eye. Interestingly, although grating acuity reached normal adult levels under optimal treatment conditions, contrast sensitivity and Landolt-C acuity were never normal.

These studies demonstrated the advantage of IOL for good visual outcome, alone or in combination with extended wear contact lenses, over lens removal without subsequent IOL implantation. The results led directly to altered clinical practice. Subsequent clinical studies confirmed the benefit of this regime for visual outcome in human infants (Lambert *et al.*, 2001), although good compliance with contact lens wear can produce equivalently good outcomes (Birch *et al.*, 2005b).

To summarize, congenital cataracts present a significant challenge to the developing visual system. They leave devastating visual losses if left untreated, often resulting
in life-long deprivation amblyopia even if treated aggressively. Monkey studies have
been used to establish optimal treatment ages and strategies and have changed clinical
practice accordingly.

NUTRITION AND VISUAL DEVELOPMENT

Although it has long been known that diet and nutrition affect growth and development, it took primate research results to make specific recommendations on
amino acid and fatty acid content in infant formula. Taurine is an important amino
acid normally present at high levels in the retina, brain, and other tissues throughout the body. Some early soy-based infant formulas lacked taurine. A series of studies by Neuringer and colleagues evaluated the effect of feeding taurine-free soy
formula on visual development in macaque infants (Neuringer and Sturman, 1987;
Neuringer et al., 1987; Imaki et al., 1987). They found reduced visual acuity in
infants fed the taurine-poor diet. Infants fed a diet lacking taurine also had degeneration of cone photoreceptors in the retina and disorganization of the normally
regular photoreceptor matrix. These studies provided evidence that dietary taurine
is essential for normal visual system development. Soy-based infant formulas are
now enhanced to include several amino acids including taurine.

There is accumulating evidence that some lipids are important for normal
development of vision and the brain. Neuringer et al. (1986) studied the effect of
dietary $\omega 3$ fatty acid concentration on the developing retina and brain of macaque
monkeys. Pregnant monkeys were fed either control or $\omega 3$ fatty acid-deficient
diets. Following parturition, the presence or absence of $\omega 3$ fatty acids in the diet
was maintained in a manner consistent with the prenatal exposure. Biochemical
changes were found in the level of long-chain fatty acids in the brain and retina of
those fed deficient diets. Moreover, the infants deprived of $\omega 3$ fatty acids showed
poorer visual acuity and abnormal photoreceptor function evidenced by longer
times to recover from a bright flash of light. Infant formulas were in general lacking in $\omega 3$ fatty acids until the early 1990s, when manufacturers began to add specific ones to their formulas. Subsequent prospective studies of full-term human
infants showed the importance of docosahexaenoic acid (DHA), among others, for
supporting normal visual and cognitive function (see Neuringer, 2000; Auestad et al.,
2003; Birch et al., 2005a).

CONCLUSIONS

The Old World macaque monkey has been shown to provide an excellent model for
normal visual development in humans and for understanding clinically important

developmental disorders of vision. Animal studies in general have contributed greatly to our understanding of the vulnerability of the visual system to early abnormal visual experience.

While it has been known for over a century that conditions like strabismus are associated with poor vision in adults, no data existed to demonstrate a direct causal relationship prior to a longitudinal study in infant monkeys by Kiorpes and Boothe (1980). The work of Wiesel and Hubel identified, for the first time, anatomical and neurophysiological correlates of abnormal visual experience on the visual system. This work inspired many subsequent studies that revealed the existence and nature of critical periods in vision. In particular, studies of monocular deprivation during development illustrated the extreme devastation to visual system structure and function created by form deprivation. The work in aggregate identified the nature of the critical period for normal visual development, showing varying degrees of vulnerability over different age ranges and showing different periods of susceptibility for recovery after deprivation. Retrospective analyses of this literature led to a revision of the concept of the critical period, suggesting that there are three conceptually separate, but overlapping sensitive periods; namely for normal development, for disruption of function, and for recovery of function. The results of studies with the lid suture model led directly to a shift in clinical practice in two ways. First, they led to treatment of children with vision disorders, in particular those with cataracts, at the youngest possible ages. Second, they led to a major re-evaluation of classical treatment strategies such as full-time patching of the fellow eye. Current recommendations are to use part-time patching, if possible in combination with focused activity to improve the vision in the amblyopic eye.

Other macaque models of amblyopia, such as experimental strabismus and anisometropia, characterized the nature of amblyopia in relation to the losses in acuity and contrast sensitivity. This work revealed the extent of loss in spatial, temporal, and binocular vision and showed additional significant loss in perceptual vision. Macaque models have also been used to evaluate treatment strategies for recovery of function. The basic neural mechanisms underlying amblyopia have been identified in macaque monkeys. The unexpected finding was that in addition to correlates of amblyopia at the level of the primary visual cortex, there must be additional sites of dysfunction further along the visual pathways. This is surprising because since the early studies of Wiesel and Hubel it has been assumed that V1 is the primary site of developmental plasticity in the visual system. Future work must address the possibility of additional, perhaps escalating, deficiency at higher levels of the system. This idea has important implications for treatment. Given the clear impact of amblyopia on higher order perceptual visual functions, and finding that these problems remain even when acuity measures reflect successful treatment,we should be developing clinical tests for perceptual dysfunction and extending treatment over a longer time period than might be dictated by acuity measures alone (Simons, 2005).

One subtle but none-the-less important result of studies of visual development in cat and monkey models of amblyopia was to show the necessity of following visual function in children undergoing treatment. Longitudinal studies in animals showed the progression of visual acuity development in the presence of amblyogenic factors and revealed the gradual trade-off of good visual function between the two eyes during occlusion therapy. The use of quick visual assessment tools, such as the Teller Acuity Cards (Teller *et al.*, 1986), in the practitioner's office is becoming commonplace, thus improving the ability of clinicians to track visual acuity during treatment without a major investment of time and effort. Finally, this body of work in aggregate has led to increased attention to the importance of early childhood vision screening programs to identify and treat visual disorders with optimal success (Hartmann, 2000; Williams and Harrad, 2006).

The primary challenge remaining for future studies of visual dysfunction in macaque monkeys is to identify the nature of neural plasticity in areas of the visual system beyond V1. The critical periods for these downstream areas are likely to be longer than for V1. This may provide a better opportunity for the successful treatment of amblyopia.

REFERENCES

Anderson, S. J. and Swettenham, J. B. (2006). Neuroimaging in human amblyopia. *Strabismus* **14**, 21–35.

Auestad, N., Scott, D. T., Janowsky, J. S. *et al.* (2003). Visual, cognitive, and language assessments at 39 months: a follow-up study of children fed formulas containing long-chain polyunsaturated fatty acids to 1 year of age. *Pediatrics* **112**, e177–183.

Banks, M. S. and Salapatek, P. (1978). Acuity and contrast sensitivity in 1-, 2-, and 3-month-old human infants. *Invest Ophthalmol Vis Sci* **17**, 361–365.

Birch, E. E. and Stager, D. R. (1996). The critical period for surgical treatment of dense congenital unilateral cataract. *Invest Ophthalmol Vis Sci* **37**, 1532–1538.

Birch, E. E. and Stager, D. R., Sr. (2006). Long-term motor and sensory outcomes after early surgery for infantile esotropia. *J Aapos* **10**, 409–413.

Birch, E. E., Gwiazda, J., and Held, R. (1982). Stereoacuity development for crossed and uncrossed disparities in human infants. *Vision Res* **22**, 507–513.

Birch, E. E., Stager, D. R., and Wright, W. W. (1986). Grating acuity development after early surgery for congenital unilateral cataract. *Arch Ophthalmol* **104**, 1783–1787.

Birch, E. E., Castaneda, Y. S., Wheaton, D. H., Birch, D. G., Uauy, R. D., and Hoffman, D. R. (2005a). Visual maturation of term infants fed long-chain polyunsaturated fatty acid-supplemented or control formula for 12 mo. *Am J Clin Nutr* **81**, 871–879.

Birch, E. E., Cheng, C., Stager, D. R., Jr., and Felius, J. (2005b). Visual acuity development after the implantation of unilateral intraocular lenses in infants and young children. *J Aapos* **9**, 527–532.

Blakemore, C. and Vital-Durand, F. (1986). Effects of visual deprivation on the development of the monkey's lateral geniculate nucleus. *J Physiol* **380**, 493–511.

Blakemore, C., Garey, L. J., and Vital-Durand, F. (1978). Reversal of physiological effects of monocular deprivation in monkeys [proceedings]. *J Physiol* **276**, 47P–49P.

Boothe, R. G. (1996). Visual development following treatment of a unilateral infantile cataract. In Vital-Durand, F., Atkinson, J. and Braddick, O. J., eds. *Infant Vision*. Oxford: Oxford University Press, pp. 401–412.

Boothe, R. G., Kiorpes, L., and Hendrickson, A. (1982). Anisometropic amblyopia in *Macaca nemestrina* monkeys produced by atropinization of one eye during development. *Invest Ophthalmol Vis Sci* **22**, 228–233.

Boothe, R. G., Dobson, V., and Teller, D. Y. (1985). Postnatal development of vision in human and nonhuman primates. *Annu Rev Neurosci* **8**, 495–545.

Boothe, R. G., Kiorpes, L., Williams, R. A., and Teller, D. Y. (1988). Operant measurements of contrast sensitivity in infant macaque monkeys during normal development. *Vision Res* **28**, 387–396.

Boothe, R. G., Louden, T. M., and Lambert, S. R. (1996). Acuity and contrast sensitivity in monkeys after neonatal intraocular lens implantation with and without part-time occlusion of the fellow eye. *Invest Ophthalmol Vis Sci* **37**, 1520–1531.

Boothe, R. G., Louden, T., Aiyer, A., Izquierdo, A., Drews, C., and Lambert, S. R. (2000). Visual outcome after contact lens and intraocular lens correction of neonatal monocular aphakia in monkeys. *Invest Ophthalmol Vis Sci* **41**, 110–119.

Braddick, O., Atkinson, J., and Wattam-Bell, J. (2003). Normal and anomalous development of visual motion processing: motion coherence and 'dorsal-stream vulnerability'. *Neuropsychologia* **41**, 1769–1784.

Britten, K. H., Shadlen, M. N., Newsome, W. T., and Movshon, J. A. (1992). The analysis of visual motion: a comparison of neuronal and psychophysical performance. *J Neurosci* **12**, 4745–4765.

Carkeet, A., Levi, D. M., and Manny, R. E. (1997). Development of Vernier acuity in childhood. *Optom Vis Sci* **74**, 741–750.

Chatzistefanou, K. I., Theodossiadis, G. P., Damanakis, A. G., Ladas, I. D., Moschos, M. N., and Chimonidou, E. (2005). Contrast sensitivity in amblyopia: the fellow eye of untreated and successfully treated amblyopes. *J Aapos* **9**, 468–474.

Choong, Y. F., Lukman, H., Martin, S., and Laws, D. E. (2004). Childhood amblyopia treatment: psychosocial implications for patients and primary carers. *Eye* **18**, 369–375.

Chua, B. and Mitchell, P. (2004). Consequences of amblyopia on education, occupation, and long term vision loss. *Br J Ophthalmol* **88**, 1119–1121.

Crawford, M. L., de Faber, J. T., Harwerth, R. S., Smith, E. L., III, and von Noorden, G. K. (1989). The effects of reverse monocular deprivation in monkeys. II. Electrophysiological and anatomical studies. *Exp Brain Res* **74**, 338–347.

Crawford, M. L., Harwerth, R. S., Chino, Y. M., and Smith, E. L., III (1996a). Binocularity in prism-reared monkeys. *Eye* **10**(Pt 2), 161–166.

Crawford, M. L., Harwerth, R. S., Smith, E. L., and von Noorden, G. K. (1996b). Loss of stereopsis in monkeys following prismatic binocular dissociation during infancy. *Behav Brain Res* **79**, 207–218.

Daw, N. W. (1998). Critical periods and amblyopia. *Arch Ophthalmol* **116**, 502–505.

Ellemberg, D., Lewis, T. L., Liu, C. H., and Maurer, D. (1999). Development of spatial and temporal vision during childhood. *Vision Res* **39**, 2325–2333.

Fawcett, S. L., Wang, Y. Z., and Birch, E. E. (2005). The critical period for susceptibility of human stereopsis. *Invest Ophthalmol Vis Sci* **46**, 521–525.

Friedlander, M. J. and Tootle, J.S. (1990). Postnatal anatomical and physiological development of the visual system. In Coleman, J. R., ed. *Development of Sensory Systems in Mammals.* New York: John Wiley & Sons, pp. 61–124.

Giaschi, D. E., Regan, D., Kraft, S. P., and Hong, X. H. (1992). Defective processing of motion-defined form in the fellow eye of patients with unilateral amblyopia. *Invest Ophthalmol Vis Sci* **33**, 2483–2489.

Gunn, A., Cory, E., Atkinson, J., Braddick, O., Wattam-Bell, J., Guzzetta, A., and Cioni, G. (2002). Dorsal and ventral stream sensitivity in normal development and hemiplegia. *Neuroreport* **13**, 843–847.

Hartmann, E. (2000). Preschool vision screening: Summary of a task force report. *Pediatrics* **106**, 1105–1112.

Harwerth, R. S., Smith, E.L., III, Boltz, R.L., Crawford, M.L., and von Noorden, G.K. (1983). Behavioral studies on the effect of abnormal early visual experience in monkeys: spatial modulation sensitivity. *Vision Res* **23**, 1501–1510.

Harwerth, R. S., Smith, E. L., III, Duncan, G. C., Crawford, M. L., and von Noorden, G. K. (1986). Multiple sensitive periods in the development of the primate visual system. *Science* **232**, 235–238.

Harwerth, R. S., Smith, E. L., III, Crawford, M. L., and von Noorden, G. K. (1989). The effects of reverse monocular deprivation in monkeys. I. Psychophysical experiments. *Exp Brain Res* **74**, 327–347.

Harwerth, R. S., Smith, E. L., III, Crawford, M. L., and von Noorden, G. K. (1990). Behavioral studies of the sensitive periods of development of visual functions in monkeys. *Behav Brain Res* **41**, 179–198.

Holmes, J. M. and Clarke, M. P. (2006). Amblyopia. *Lancet* **367**, 1343–1351.

Horton, J. C. and Hocking, D. R. (1996). An adult-like pattern of ocular dominance columns in striate cortex of newborn monkeys prior to visual experience. *J Neurosci* **16**, 1791–1807.

Horton, J. C. and Hocking, D. R. (1997). Timing of the critical period for plasticity of ocular dominance columns in macaque striate cortex. *J Neurosci* **17**, 3684–3709.

Horton, J. C., Hocking, D. R., and Kiorpes, L. (1997). Pattern of ocular dominance columns and cytochrome oxidase activity in a macaque monkey with naturally occurring anisometropic amblyopia. *Vis Neurosci* **14**, 681–689.

Hubel, D. H. and Wiesel, T. N. (1965). Binocular interaction in striate cortex of kittens reared with artificial squint. *J Neurophysiol* **28**, 1041–1059.

Hubel, D. H. and Wiesel, T. N. (1977). Ferrier lecture. Functional architecture of macaque monkey visual cortex. *Proc R Soc Lond B Biol Sci* **198**, 1–59.

Imaki, H., Moretz, R., Wisniewski, H., Neuringer, M., and Sturman, J. (1987). Retinal degeneration in 3-month-old rhesus monkey infants fed a taurine-free human infant formula. *J Neurosci Res* **18**, 602–614.

Jeffrey, B. G., Birch, E. E., Stager, D. R., Jr., Stager, D. R., Sr., and Weakley, D. R., Jr. (2001). Early binocular visual experience may improve binocular sensory outcomes in children after surgery for congenital unilateral cataract. *J Aapos* **5**, 209–216.

Kaas, J. H. (2004). The Evolution of the Visual System in Primates. In Chalupa, L. and Werner, J., eds. *The Visual Neurosciences*, Vol. 2. Cambridge, MA: The MIT Press, pp. 1563–1572.

Kiorpes, L. (1989). The development of spatial resolution and contrast sensitivity in naturally strabismic monkeys. *Clin Vision Sci* **4**, 279–293.

Kiorpes, L. (1992a). Development of vernier acuity and grating acuity in normally reared monkeys. *Vis Neurosci* **9**, 243–251.

Kiorpes, L. (1992b). Effect of strabismus on the development of vernier acuity and grating acuity in monkeys. *Vis Neurosci* **9**, 253–259.

Kiorpes, L. (1996). Development of contrast sensitivity in normal and amblyopic monkeys. In Vital-Durand, F., Atkinson, J. and Braddick, O.J., eds. *Infant Vision*. Oxford: Oxford University Press, pp. 3–15.

Kiorpes, L. (2002). Sensory processing: animal models of amblyopia. In Moseley, M. and Fielder, A., eds. *Amblyopia: A Multidisciplinary Approach*. Oxford: Butterworth-Heinemann, pp. 1–18.

Kiorpes, L. (2006). Visual processing in amblyopia: animal studies. *Strabismus* **14**, 3–10.

Kiorpes, L. and Bassin, S. A. (2003). Development of contour integration in macaque monkeys. *Vis Neurosci* **20**, 567–575.

Kiorpes, L. and Boothe, R. G. (1980). The time course for the development of strabismic amblyopia in infant monkeys (*Macaca nemestrina*). *Invest Ophthalmol Vis Sci* **19**, 841–845.

Kiorpes, L. and Movshon, J.A. (2004a). Neural limitations on visual development in primates. In Chalupa, L. and Werner, J., eds. *The Visual Neurosciences*, Vol. 1. Cambridge: The MIT Press, pp. 159–173.

Kiorpes, L. and Movshon, J. A. (2004b). Development of sensitivity to visual motion in macaque monkeys. *Vis Neurosci* **21**, 851–859.

Kiorpes, L. and Wallman, J. (1995). Does experimentally-induced amblyopia cause hyperopia in monkeys? *Vision Res* **35**, 1289–1297.

Kiorpes, L., Boothe, R. G., Hendrickson, A. E., Movshon, J. A., Eggers, H. M., and Gizzi, M. S. (1987). Effects of early unilateral blur on the macaque's visual system. I. Behavioral observations. *J Neurosci* **7**, 1318–1326.

Kiorpes, L., Carlson, M., and Alfi, D. (1989). Development of visual acuity in experimentally strabismic monkeys. *Clin Vision Sci* **4**, 95–106.

Kiorpes, L., Kiper, D. C., and Movshon, J. A. (1993). Contrast sensitivity and vernier acuity in amblyopic monkeys. *Vision Res* **33**, 2301–2311.

Kiorpes, L., Kiper, D. C., O'Keefe, L. P., Cavanaugh, J. R., and Movshon, J. A. (1998). Neuronal correlates of amblyopia in the visual cortex of macaque monkeys with experimental strabismus and anisometropia. *J Neurosci* **18**, 6411–6424.

Kiorpes, L., Tang, C., and Movshon, J. A. (2006). Sensitivity to visual motion in amblyopic macaque monkeys. *Vis Neurosci* **23**, 247–256.

Kiper, D. C. and Kiorpes, L. (1994). Suprathreshold contrast sensitivity in experimentally strabismic monkeys. *Vision Res* **34**, 1575–1583.

Koklanis, K., Abel, L. A., and Aroni, R. (2006). Psychosocial impact of amblyopia and its treatment: a multidisciplinary study. *Clin Exp Ophthalmol* **34**, 743–750.

Kozma, P. and Kiorpes, L. (2003). Contour integration in amblyopic monkeys. *Vis Neurosci* **20**, 577–588.

Lambert, S. R., Fernandes, A., Drews-Botsch, C., and Boothe, R. G. (1994). Multifocal versus monofocal correction of neonatal monocular aphakia. *J Pediatr Ophthalmol Strabismus* **31**, 195–201.

Lambert, S. R., Lynn, M., Drews-Botsch, C. *et al.* (2001). A comparison of grating visual acuity, strabismus, and reoperation outcomes among children with aphakia and pseudophakia after unilateral cataract surgery during the first six months of life. *J Aapos* **5**, 70–75.

LeVay, S., Wiesel, T. N., and Hubel, D. H. (1980). The development of ocular dominance columns in normal and visually deprived monkeys. *J Comp Neurol* **191**, 1–51.

Levi, D. M. (2006). Visual processing in amblyopia: human studies. *Strabismus* **14**, 11–19.

Levitt, J. B., Schumer, R. A., Sherman, S. M., Spear, P. D., and Movshon, J. A. (2001). Visual response properties of neurons in the LGN of normally reared and visually deprived macaque monkeys. *J Neurophysiol* **85**, 2111–2129.

Lew, H., Han, S. H., Lee, J. B., and Lee, E. S. (2005). Contrast sensitivity function of sound eye after occlusion therapy in the amblyopic children. *Yonsei Med J* **46**, 368–371.

Lewis, T. L. and Maurer, D. (2005). Multiple sensitive periods in human visual development: evidence from visually deprived children. *Dev Psychobiol* **46**, 163–183.

Maurer, D., Lewis, T. L., Brent, H. P., and Levin, A. V. (1999). Rapid improvement in the acuity of infants after visual input. *Science* **286**, 108–110.

McKee, S. P., Levi, D. M., and Movshon, J. A. (2003). The pattern of visual deficits in amblyopia. *J Vis* **3**, 380–405.

Mitchell, D. E. (1991). The long-term effectiveness of different regimens of occlusion on recovery from early monocular deprivation in kittens. *Philos Trans R Soc Lond B Biol Sci* **333**, 51–79.

Mitchell, D. E. and MacKinnon, S. (2002). The present and potential impact of research on animal models for clinical treatment of stimulus deprivation amblyopia. *Clin Exp Optom* **85**, 5–18.

Movshon, J. A. and Kiorpes, L. (1990). The role of experience in visual development. In Coleman, J. R., ed. *Development of Sensory Systems in Mammals.* New York: John Wiley & Sons, pp. 155–202.

Movshon, J. A. and Van Sluyters, R. C. (1981). Visual neural development. *Annu Rev Psychol* **32**, 477–522.

Movshon, J. A., Eggers, H. M., Gizzi, M. S., Hendrickson, A. E., Kiorpes, L., and Boothe, R. G. (1987). Effects of early unilateral blur on the macaque's visual system. III. Physiological observations. *J Neurosci* **7**, 1340–1351.

Neuringer, M. (2000). Infant vision and retinal function in studies of dietary long-chain polyunsaturated fatty acids: methods, results, and implications. *Am J Clin Nutr* **71**, 256S–267S.

Neuringer, M. and Sturman, J. (1987). Visual acuity loss in rhesus monkey infants fed a taurine-free human infant formula. *J Neurosci Res* **18**, 597–601.

Neuringer, M., Connor, W. E., Lin, D. S., Barstad, L., and Luck, S. (1986). Biochemical and functional effects of prenatal and postnatal omega 3 fatty acid deficiency on retina and brain in rhesus monkeys. *Proc Natl Acad Sci USA* **83**, 4021–4025.

Neuringer, M., Imaki, H., Sturman, J. A., Moretz, R., and Wisniewski, H. M. (1987). Abnormal visual acuity and retinal morphology in rhesus monkeys fed a taurine-free diet during the first three postnatal months. *Adv Exp Med Biol* **217**, 125–134.

Newsome, W. T. and Pare, E. B. (1988). A selective impairment of motion perception following lesions of the middle temporal visual area (MT). *J Neurosci* **8**, 2201–2211.

O'Dell, C. and Boothe, R. G. (1997). The development of stereoacuity in infant rhesus monkeys. *Vision Res* **37**, 2675–2684.

Packwood, E. A., Cruz, O. A., Rychwalski, P. J., and Keech, R. V. (1999). The psychosocial effects of amblyopia study. *J Aapos* **3**, 15–17.

PEDIG. (2005). Two-year follow-up of a 6-month randomized trial of atropine vs patching for treatment of moderate amblyopia in children. *Arch Ophthalmol* **123**, 149–157.

PEDIG. (2006). A randomized trial to evaluate 2 hours of daily patching for strabismic and anisometropic amblyopia in children. *Ophthalmology* **113**, 904–912.

Peterzell, D. H., Werner, J. S., and Kaplan, P. S. (1995). Individual differences in contrast sensitivity functions: longitudinal study of 4-, 6- and 8-month-old human infants. *Vision Res* **35**, 961–979.

Quick, M. W., Tigges, M., Gammon, J. A., and Boothe, R. G. (1989). Early abnormal visual experience induces strabismus in infant monkeys. *Invest Ophthalmol Vis Sci* **30**, 1012–1017.

Rahi, J. S., Logan, S., Borja, M. C., Timms, C., Russell-Eggitt, I., and Taylor, D. (2002). Prediction of improved vision in the amblyopic eye after visual loss in the non-amblyopic eye. *Lancet* **360**, 621–622.

Simmers, A. J., Ledgeway, T., Hess, R. F., and McGraw, P. V. (2003). Deficits to global motion processing in human amblyopia. *Vision Res* **43**, 729–738.

Simmers, A. J., Ledgeway, T., and Hess, R. F. (2005). The influences of visibility and anomalous integration processes on the perception of global spatial form versus motion in human amblyopia. *Vision Res* **45**, 449–460.

Simons, K. (2005). Amblyopia characterization, treatment, and prophylaxis. *Surv Ophthalmol* **50**, 123–166.

Sjöström, A., Abrahamsson, M., Byhr, E., and Sjostrand, J. (1996). Visual development in children with congenital cataract. In Vital-Durand, F., Atkinson, J. and Braddick, O.J., eds. *Infant Vision*. Oxford: Oxford University Press, pp. 413–421.

Skoczenski, A. M. and Norcia, A. M. (1999). Development of VEP Vernier acuity and grating acuity in human infants. *Invest Ophthalmol Vis Sci* **40**, 2411–2417.

Skoczenski, A. M. and Norcia, A. M. (2002). Late maturation of visual hyperacuity. *Psychol Sci* **13**, 537–541.

Smith, E. L., III, Harwerth, R. S., and Crawford, M. L. (1985). Spatial contrast sensitivity deficits in monkeys produced by optically induced anisometropia. *Invest Ophthalmol Vis Sci* **26**, 330–342.

Smith, E. L., III, Chino, Y. M., Ni, J., Cheng, H., Crawford, M. L., and Harwerth, R. S. (1997). Residual binocular interactions in the striate cortex of monkeys reared with abnormal binocular vision. *J Neurophysiol* **78**, 1353–1362.

Smith, E. L., III, Hung, L. F., and Harwerth, R. S. (1999). Developmental visual system anomalies and the limits of emmetropization. *Ophthalmic Physiol Opt* **19**, 90–102.

Smith, E. L., III, Hung, L. F., and Harwerth, R. S. (2000). The degree of image degradation and the depth of amblyopia. *Invest Ophthalmol Vis Sci* **41**, 3775–3781.

Teller, D. Y. (1997). First glances: the vision of infants. the Friedenwald lecture. *Invest Ophthalmol Vis Sci* **38**, 2183–2203.

Teller, D. Y. and Boothe, R. (1979). Development of vision in infant primates. *Trans Ophthalmol Soc UK* **99**, 333–337.

Teller, D. Y., Morse, R., Borton, R., and Regal, D. (1974). Visual acuity for vertical and diagonal gratings in human infants. *Vision Res* **14**, 1433–1439.

Teller, D. Y., McDonald, M. A., Preston, K., Sebris, S. L., and Dobson, V. (1986). Assessment of visual acuity in infants and children: the acuity card procedure. *Dev Med Child Neurol* **28**, 779–789.

Tytla, M. E., Maurer, D., Lewis, T. L., and Brent, H. P. (1988). Contrast sensitivity in children treated for congenital cataract. *Clin Vision Sci* **4**, 251–264.

Van Essen, D. (2004). Organization of visual areas in macaque and human cerebral cortex. In Chalupa, L. and Werner, J., eds. *The Visual Neurosciences*, Vol. 1. Cambridge, MA: The MIT Press, pp. 507–521.

von Noorden, G. K. (1973). Experimental amblyopia in monkeys. Further behavioral observations and clinical correlations. *Invest Ophthalmol* **12**, 721–726.

Von Noorden, G. K. (1980). *Binocular Vision and Ocular Motility*. St. Louis: C.V. Mosby Co.

von Noorden, G. K. and Crawford, M. L. (1978). Morphological and physiological changes in the monkey visual system after short-term lid suture. *Invest Ophthalmol Vis Sci* **17**, 762–768.

Von Noorden, G. K. and Dowling, J. E. (1970). Experimental amblyopia in monkeys. II. Behavioral studies in strabismic amblyopia. *Arch Ophthalmol* **84**, 215–220.

Von Noorden, G. K., Dowling, J. E., and Ferguson, D. C. (1970). Experimental amblyopia in monkeys. I. Behavioral studies of stimulus deprivation amblyopia. *Arch Ophthalmol* **84**, 206–214.

Wensveen, J. M., Harwerth, R. S., and Smith, E. L., III (2001). Clinical suppression in monkeys reared with abnormal binocular visual experience. *Vision Res* **41**, 1593–1608.

Wensveen, J. M., Harwerth, R. S., and Smith, E. L., III (2003). Binocular deficits associated with early alternating monocular defocus. I. Behavioral observations. *J Neurophysiol* **90**, 3001–3011.

Wensveen, J. M., Harwerth, R. S., Hung, L. F., Ramamirtham, R., Kee, C. S., and Smith, E. L., III (2006). Brief daily periods of unrestricted vision can prevent form-deprivation amblyopia. *Invest Ophthalmol Vis Sci* **47**, 2468–2477.

Wiesel, T. N. (1982). The postnatal development of the visual cortex and the influence of environment. *Biosci Rep* **2**, 351–377.

Wiesel, T. N. and Hubel, D. H. (1963). Single-cell responses in striate cortex of kittens deprived of vision in one eye. *J Neurophysiol* **26**, 1003–1017.

Wiesel, T. N. and Hubel, D. H. (1965). Comparison of the effects of unilateral and bilateral eye closure on cortical unit responses in kittens. *J Neurophysiol* **28**, 1029–1040.

Williams, C. and Harrad, R. (2006). Amblyopia: Contemporary clinical issues. *Strabismus* **14**, 43–50.

Williams, R. A., Boothe, R. G., Kiorpes, L., and Teller, D. Y. (1981). Oblique effects in normally reared monkeys (*Macaca nemestrina*): meridional variations in contrast sensitivity measured with operant techniques. *Vision Res* **21**, 1253–1266.

Zanker, J., Mohn, G., Weber, U., Zeitler-Driess, K., and Fahle, M. (1992). The development of vernier acuity in human infants. *Vision Res* **32**, 1557–1564.

Zhang, B., Matsuura, K., Mori, T., Wensveen, J. M., Harwerth, R. S., Smith, E. L., III, and Chino, Y. (2003). Binocular deficits associated with early alternating monocular defocus. II. Neurophysiological observations. *J Neurophysiol* **90**, 3012–3023.

Zhang, B., Bi, H., Sakai, E., Maruko, I., Zheng, J., Smith, E. L., III, and Chino, Y. M. (2005). Rapid plasticity of binocular connections in developing monkey visual cortex (V1). *Proc Natl Acad Sci USA* **102**, 9026–9031.

CHAPTER 4

Spontaneous and Experimentally Induced Autoimmune Diseases in Nonhuman Primates

Michel Vierboom and Bert A. 't Hart

The advent of biotechnology has provided new tools for the identification of new therapeutic targets and the creation of safer and more specifically acting therapeutic agents. Especially for the immune-mediated inflammatory disorders, including autoimmune disease, biotechnology-based therapies hold great promise for more specific treatments. Autoimmune disorders affect 15–25 million people in the United States and strike both children and adults. Although they are less common in children than in adults, the clinical course is often more severe. The most prevalent autoimmune diseases in American children are juvenile idiopathic arthritis, type 1 diabetes, glomerulonephritis, and chronic active hepatitis. Research on autoimmune diseases has been limited because many new treatments showing promising effects in rodent models appear to be only marginally effective in clinical trials. A progressively decreasing percentage of new drug applications survive the clinical trials. This raises the question of whether the currently used rodent disease models may be poor predictors for clinical success of new therapies. This may be due to the wide evolutionary gap between rodents and humans. Given their phylogenetic proximity to humans, nonhuman primate models of autoimmune diseases are being developed to help bridge this gap. Primate models of two human autoimmune diseases, multiple sclerosis and arthritis, are being developed in the Netherlands. Experimental results have provided fundamental insights into the etiology and treatment of both diseases.

INTRODUCTION

Autoimmune diseases represent a group of immune-mediated inflammatory disorders that are driven by an unwanted hyperactivity of the immune system. The prevalence

Primate Models of Children's Health and Developmental Disabilities

of the different types of autoimmune disease differs (Table 4.1), but collectively they affect between 15 and 25 million individuals in the USA (Zerhouni, 2005). This is in the same range as cancer or heart disease. Women are more frequently affected by autoimmune disease than men (Cooper and Stroehla, 2003). Although the prevalence of autoimmune disease increases with older age these are not age-bound diseases. Juvenile forms of common autoimmune disease in adults, such as rheumatoid arthritis and multiple sclerosis, do exist, but may be distinct clinical entities. In general, the prevalence of autoimmune disease in juveniles is lower than in adults, but the diseases are often more severe. Although autoimmune disease can thus be considered as a serious health problem, scientists still know very little about the origin and pathogenic mechanisms underlying these diseases. Effective therapies are lacking.

Autoimmune diseases are often characterized by chronic inflammation which can either be systemic (i.e. affecting the whole body) or confined to one of a few organs. The chronic inflammation can lead to a spectrum of mild to severe clinical conditions depending on the organ/system targeted by the autoimmune response. The chronic nature of autoimmune disease and the often invalidating consequences result not only in personal tragedy but also high medical and socioeconomic costs. The last three decades of research have provided a wealth of information and new concepts on the pathogenic mechanisms operating in these diseases, as well as the identification of new targets for treatment. The advent of biotechnology has fueled the search for more specific drugs to overcome the considerable side-effects of currently available non-specifically acting anti-inflammatory and immunosuppressive drugs (Denton et al., 1999; Fishman and Rubin, 1998; Penn, 2000). Especially for immune-mediated inflammatory disorders, biotechnology-based therapies hold great promise for more specific treatments.

Substantial investments in scientific research has certainly led to a better understanding of pathogenic principles involved in immune-mediated inflammatory disorders. Moreover, impressive biotechnological developments have provided new tools for the identification of new therapeutic targets and the creation of safer and more specifically acting therapeutic agents. It is a great concern, however, that many new treatments showing promising effects in rodent models appear only marginally effective in clinical trials, or even show detrimental effects. A progressively decreasing percentage of new drug applications (NDA) survive clinical trials (Contag, 2002; Roses et al., 2005). This raises the question of whether the currently used rodent disease models may be poor predictors for clinical success of new therapies. As explained elsewhere, this may be due to the wide evolutionary gap between rodents and humans. Nonhuman primates, because of their phylogenetic proximity to humans, may help to bridge this gap ('t Hart et al., 2004a).

The burden of autoimmune diseases

The number of autoimmune diseases in the human population varies depending on the criteria used to identify them. In a recent report by the US National

TABLE 4.1   The most prevalent of autoimmune diseases in the United States

Disease	Prevalence (%)	Female/male ratio	Total number	Age of onset	Features
Autoimmune diseases (overall)	3.13	3.75	8.511.844		Fatigue, weight loss, tachycardia
Graves' disease	1.12	7.2	3.048.636	Usually middle age, but also in children and adolescents.	
Rheumatoid arthritis	0.86	2.96	1.736.099	Usually between 25 and 50 years	Painful swelling of joints, functional loss
Juvenile idiopathic arthritis	0.01–0.02[b]	F > M		<5 years (early onset)	
Oligoarthritis		M > F		>9 years (late onset)	
Polyarticular		Varies		1–3 years and 8–10 years (40%)	
Systemic		Varies		Between 5 and 10 years (10%)	
Vitiligo	0.4	1.1	1.059.560	Usually between 10 and 30 years	Skin depigmentation, socio-psychological burden
Pernicious anemia	0.15	2.0	399.455	>60 years	Fatigue and low muscle strength
Multiple sclerosis Childhood-onset MS	0.14	1.79	388.571	Between 20 and 40 years <16 years	Incontinence, cognitive dysfunction, ataxia, optic problems, muscle weakness
Type 1 diabetes	0.192	0.91	146.892	Between 0 and 15 years	Excessive thirst and urination, acidosis, wasting, optic and vascular problems
Glomerulonephritis[a]	0.04	0.46	105.902	Childhood onset is common	Fever, weakness, abdominal aches, joint ache
Systemic lupus erythematosus	0.024	7.4	63.052	<16 years (20%); Between 16 and 55 years (65%); >55 years (15%)	Fever, skin lesions, joint pain and anemia

(Continued)

TABLE 4.1 (*Continued*)

Disease	Prevalence (%)	Female/male ratio	Total number	Age of onset	Features
Sjögren's syndrome	0.014	15	38.108	Usually in the 4th to 5th decade.	Dry mouth and dry eyes
Addison's disease	0.005	12.3	13.335	At any age	Anemia, weakness, low blood pressure. Bronze-like pigmentation
Myasthenia gravis	0.005	2.66	13.589	2nd and 3rd decades (female predominance); 6th–8th decade (male predominance)	Muscular weakness
Polymyositis/dermatomyositis	0.005	2.0	13.462	Juvenile (5–10 years); Adult (peak incidence in the 5th decade)	Rash and muscle weakness
Primary biliary cirrhosis	0.0035	7.85	9232	Usually between 30 and 65 years	Fatigue, an itchy skin, jaundice
Scleroderma	0.004	11.8	8922	Between 30 and 50 years	Skin thickening and scarring
Uveitis	0.0017	1	4637	<16 years (±6% of total) side-effect of JCA/JRA	Inflammation of the eye
Chronic active hepatitis	0.0004	7.5	1.156	Type I mean ±10 years (<20 years; 40%); type II mean ±6.5 years (<20 years; 80%)	Malaise, anorexia, fever and fatigue

[a] Only primary glomerulonephritis.
[b] Based on prospective studies in well-defined Caucasian population.
JIA, juvenile idiopathic arthritis; JRA, juvenile rheumatoid arthritis.
Derived from Jacobsen (1997).

Institutes of Health (NIH) over 80 clinically distinct autoimmune diseases were listed (Zerhouni, 2005). In the current review we have limited ourselves to disorders that comply with criteria described by Rose and Bona (1993); namely, a disease is defined as an autoimmune disease only when direct or indirect proof of autoimmune pathogenesis is available. Direct proof implies that disease can be induced by transfer of autoantibodies or autoreactive T cells, the two major mediators of autoimmunity, in animal models or into *in vitro* systems. Indirect evidence may come from the induction of characteristic autoimmune disease features after immunization with implicated autoantigens or that autoantibodies or autoreactive T cells can be isolated from major target tissues implicated in the disease. From the 24 reviewed autoimmune diseases selected on those criteria, we have chosen those disorders for which epidemiological data were available for further discussion (Jacobson *et al.*, 1997; Table 4.1).

Overall it can be concluded that epidemiological data for most autoimmune diseases is scanty. For the few diseases where such data are present, they date back more than a decade, resulting in gross underestimation of the impact of autoimmune disease during development and on aging societies. Rheumatoid arthritis, including the developmental disorder juvenile idiopathic arthritis and multiple sclerosis are among the best-monitored diseases worldwide (Jacobson *et al.*, 1997). Juvenile idiopathic arthritis is a heterogeneous disease, which, for some forms, uniquely develops during childhood.

IMMUNE MECHANISMS IN IMMUNE-MEDIATED INFLAMMATORY DISORDERS

The human body has several layers of defense against invading pathogens. The first line of defense is formed by the skin as well as the epithelial and mucous surfaces of the lungs, gastrointestinal tract and gonads. When this first line of defense is breached, the body is armed with the immune system to deal with unwanted invaders or internal subversive elements. The immune system comprises the innate system and the adaptive system.

The innate immune system reaches full maturity about six months after birth. It is composed of effector cells and molecules that together neutralize, opsonize and phagocytose pathogens, without memory induction. Typical components of the innate immune system are neutrophils, monocytes, macrophages, natural killer (NK) cells, complement factors and acute phase proteins. Although the innate immune system acts in a relatively non-specific manner, it can distinguish between classes of pathogens (parasites, fungi, viruses, bacteria) but not between individual species or strains. Furthermore, each subsequent attack from a recurrent pathogenic infection is met with an immune reaction of equal strength.

The adaptive immune response, which generates a rapid and effective immune reaction against a recurrent infection, reaches maturity at a later stage than the innate system, at around the age of 12–15 years. The key players of the adaptive immune system are B and T lymphocytes. The adaptive immune system responds in a highly specific manner against antigenic components of pathogens, which are processed and presented by professional antigen-presenting cells (APCs). B cells produce antibodies mediating the humoral response. Antibodies bind to invading pathogens or extra-cellular structures of affected cells, marking them for disposal by components of the innate system (i.e. phagocytes). T lymphocytes recognize fragments of proteins (peptides) presented by the major histocompatibility complex (MHC) with their T cell receptor (TcR). CD8$^+$ cytotoxic T cells usually recognize peptides from endogenously expressed proteins in the context of MHC class I molecules and can attack virus-infected cells. Foreign cells, such as in a transplanted organ, are also attacked by CD8$^+$ T cells. Peptides derived from the extracellular environment are usually presented by MHC class II molecules and recognized by CD4$^+$ helper T cells, a cell type that supports various adaptive immune reactions (reviewed in Parkin and Cohen, 2001).

All immune cells originate from the bone marrow. During ontogeny the adaptive immune system is instructed not to respond to components of the own body (self- or autoantigens), a phenomenon called immune tolerance. The thymus, in which a large fraction (>90%) of the newly arising lymphocytes are deleted, has an important, albeit not exclusive, function in the induction of central immune tolerance by the physical elimination of autoreactive T cells and the induction of suppressor T cells. A fully developed thymus can already be found in the fetus after the third month of pregnancy, but is only fully populated with T cells after six months. Self-reactive T lymphocytes that have escaped deletion in the thymus because these self-antigens are expressed later in life or are sequestered in immune-privileged organs (eye, brain), are rendered unresponsiveness in the periphery (peripheral tolerance) by a complex of regulatory mechanisms including deletion, anergy, and the induction of regulatory cells.

Natural killer cells and natural killer T cells, which operate at the interphase of the innate and adaptive immune system, will not be discussed in this review, as little is known about their role in nonhuman primates autoimmune diseases.

From autoimmunity to autoimmune disease

Autoimmune diseases can be grouped on the basis of the location at which the autoimmune reaction takes place (i.e. organ-specific) (King and Sarvetnick, 1997) versus systemic (Davidson and Diamond, 2001). Diabetes is a typical organ-specific autoimmune disease as only pancreatic islets are affected, whereas systemic lupus erythematosus (SLE) is a prototypical systemic autoimmune disease, affecting multiple organs such as skin, kidneys, guts, and joints.

A sharp separation often does not exist, however. For example, rheumatoid arthritis and juvenile idiopathic arthritis are destructive inflammatory joint diseases, but patients often show extra-articular disease symptoms. Autoimmune disease can also be classified on the basis of the nature of the pathogenic process: antibody versus

T cell-mediated autoimmunity (Davidson and Diamond, 2001). A typical humoral autoimmune disease is myasthenia gravis, a neurological disease caused by auto-antibodies against acetylcholine receptors (De Baets and Stassen, 2002). Type I diabetes, one of the most common chronic childhood illnesses, and ankylosing spondilitis are examples of predominantly T cell-mediated autoimmune diseases. Often, however, humoral as well as cellular autoimmune reactions contribute to the disease, such as in rheumatoid arthritis and multiple sclerosis.

Autoreactive T and B cells are part of the normal immune repertoire. Weakening or failure of the central and peripheral tolerance mechanisms that keep these autoreactive cells in check can cause the induction of cellular and humoral autoimmune reactions, which under appropriate conditions can become clinically manifest as an autoimmune disorder. Animal models have been indispensable for the unraveling of the pathogenic mechanisms in autoimmune diseases.

Autoimmunity is thought to arise from a complex interplay of genetic and environmental factors. Moreover, aging (Nandy, 1981), pregnancy (Kaaja and Greer, 2005) and lifestyle factors are conditioning factors for the activation of autoimmune reactions and the expression of autoimmune diseases. Genetic linkage studies have demonstrated that some genetic defects can predispose to different autoimmune diseases, which is suggestive for common pathogenic pathways. As a working concept for the modeling of autoimmune disease we favor the "primary lesion hypothesis" by Wilkin (1989, 1990), which states that autoimmunity can be regarded as a dysregulated form of a physiological immune reaction to the sustained release of excess antigen from a diseased tissue (the primary lesion). Genes that predispose to an autoimmune disease may cause a hyperresponsiveness to certain self-peptides and/or may cause a weakening of immune regulatory mechanisms that normally counterbalance an ongoing response ('t Hart and van Kooyk, 2004). This response-to-damage hypothesis is compatible with the observation in several genome-wide screenings that the MHC emerges as a prominent source of genes predisposing to autoimmune disease.

Epidemiological studies point to environmental pathogens as a trigger of certain autoimmune diseases, whereas other factors, such as sun exposure, diet, and stress may affect the disease course. One of the mechanisms connecting pathogens with the induction of autoimmunity is molecular mimicry (Whitton and Fujinami, 1999; Fujinami et al., 2006). This phenomenon implies that certain viruses or bacteria can directly activate naturally occurring autoreactive T and B cells via the expression of immunologically similar antigenic structures (so-called mimicry motifs). The selection of antigenic peptides presented by APCs to T and B cells is made by MHC molecules. This may explain the strong influence of this polymorphic gene family on autoimmune disease. Probably the most impressive example is that transgenic rats expressing HLA-B27 develop ankylosing spondylitis after experimental infection with yersinia (Yu and Kuipers, 2003). Alternatively, infectious microorganisms may cause damage to body tissues and release of self-antigens. These may be recognized as foreign because they normally remain sequestered (cryptic) or because they have been modified by the pathological condition (altered self).

The activation of autoreactive T and B cells in peripheral lymphoid organs does not automatically lead to a clinically manifest autoimmune disorder, as pathogenic cofactors need to be involved. Binding of complement factors to a tissue-binding autoantibody may be needed to induce disease symptoms, such as in myasthenia gravis, Guillain–Barré syndrome or autoimmune thyroiditis. Clinical expression of T cell-dependent organ-specific autoimmune diseases, such as multiple sclerosis or autoimmune diabetes, requires the peripheral activation of autoreactive T cells and also activation of the APC within the target organ (Darabi *et al.*, 2004).

Although the vast majority of research is done in wild-type or genetically engineered mice, nonhuman primates are essential models for the translation of rodent research to the patient. Because of the genetic, physiological, immunological, and microbiological proximity to humans, nonhuman primates such as rhesus monkeys provide excellent models to study the impact of these factors on autoimmunity and disease (Roth *et al.*, 2004).

In the following section we will first discuss whether spontaneous autoimmunity and autoimmune disease occurs in nonhuman primates. Subsequently we will discuss experimentally induced models of autoimmune diseases in nonhuman primates, which are used as laboratory models of human autoimmune diseases. We have limited ourselves to the modeling of two prevalent diseases, namely multiple sclerosis and rheumatoid arthritis, including the developmental disorder juvenile idiopathic arthritis.

SPONTANEOUS AUTOIMMUNITY AND AUTOIMMUNE DISORDERS IN NONHUMAN PRIMATES

We have searched for articles on the prevalence of autoimmune diseases in nonhuman primates in the PubMed database using as search terms "nonhuman primates" combined with the most prevalent human autoimmune diseases (see Table 4.1). Our search yielded ±20 articles and these all referred to the modeling of autoimmune diseases and not to the natural occurrence of these diseases in nonhuman primates. Although this search was in no way exhaustive, it illustrates that the spontaneous occurrence of autoimmune diseases in nonhuman primates has been poorly investigated. In the following we have listed a number of clinical conditions observed in captive nonhuman primates colonies, which may have an autoimmune component.

Wasting disease in common marmosets (Brack and Rothe, 1981)

The common marmoset (*Callithrix jacchus*) is a laboratory nonhuman primate species that has its natural habitat in the Amazon region in South America. It is prone to a naturally occurring inflammatory condition (Ludlage and Mansfield, 2003). Marmoset wasting syndrome (MWS) is a systemic disorder that affects animals at any age and is characterized by inflammatory lesions in the skin, gastrointestinal tract, and kidneys. Although the cause is not known, low housing temperature, stress and protein-poor diet have been implicated as possible triggering factors. That MWS is similar to toxic wasting syndrome in rodents exposed to heavy metals (Fournie *et al.*, 2001) and to graft-versus-host disease, a serious complication in recipients of a bone marrow transplant, indicates that anti-self-immune responses may occur in MWS.

Idiopathic colitis in cotton-top tamarins (Mansfield *et al.*, 2001)

The cotton-top tamarin (*Saguinus oedipus*) is an endangered species from South America (Colombia and Panama) that does not adapt easily to captive conditions. Because of this it is a less favored laboratory primate. In captive conditions, a high proportion of cotton-top tamarins develop inflammatory bowel disease (IBD) resembling Crohn's disease and ulcerative colitis in the human population. As in MWS, the cause of this IBD is not known and has no age or gender bias, although the syndrome is more prevalent in colonies housed at temperatures below 23°C and receiving protein-poor diet. In the absence of an alternative explanation a possible autoimmune etiology of both MWS and IBD should not be overlooked.

Chronic polyarthritis in rhesus monkeys

There is little literature on the natural occurrence of autoimmune arthritis in monkeys. Anecdotal cases of several forms of arthritis have been described for rhesus monkeys (*Macaca mulatta*) and gorillas (Rothschild and Woods, 1989; Rothschild and Woods, 1991; Rothschild, 1994). Interestingly, arthritis has been observed more frequently in colonies housed outdoors than indoors.

Simian immunodeficiency virus in rhesus monkeys and sooty mangabeys

Lentivirus infection leads to a general dysfunction of the immune system in humans (human immunodeficiency virus, HIV) and in rhesus monkeys (simian immunodeficiency virus, SIV) (Ansari, 2004). The immune dysregulation leads to the production of autoantibodies and autoimmune responses contributing to the pathogenesis of acquired immune deficiency syndrome (AIDS) (Zandman-Goddard and Shoenfeld, 2002; Bourinbaiar and Abulafia-Lapid, 2005; Ansari, 2004). The mechanisms responsible for the dysfunction of the immune system are difficult to study in humans. Sooty mangabeys are naturally infected with SIV but do not develop the same AIDS-related phenomena observed in SIV-infected rhesus monkeys and HIV-infected humans (McClure et al., 1989; Ansari et al., 2003). This provides us with a unique opportunity to separate the pathogenic mechanism involving autoimmune phenomena and other pathogenic mechanisms caused by the infection. The observation that autoimmunity might contribute significantly to the pathogenesis of AIDS should make us reconsider the development of the current vaccines enhancing responses against HIV, while strategies aimed at inducing tolerance against autoantigens might provide new treatment options for AIDS patients (Zandman-Goddard and Shoenfeld, 2002).

Autoimmunity in chronic allograft rejection in rhesus monkeys (Jonker et al., 2005; Rose, 1998)

Chronic rejection of transplanted organs is believed to result mainly from alloimmune responses directed against the graft (Colvin, 2003). However, despite improved immunosuppression targeting those alloimmune responses, long-term graft survival has not improved. It is now believed that chronic allograft survival is limited by the induction of autoimmune reactions against the graft (Jonker et al., 2005). This is certainly true for lung transplants, where long-term graft survival is limited by the development of bronchiolitis obliterans (Sumpter and Wilkes, 2004).

Virus-induced diabetes mellitus (Yoon et al., 1987; Jun and Yoon, 2003)

With a concordance rate of only 40% in monozygotic twins (Barnett et al., 1981) non-genetic factors play a prominent role in the expression of type 1 diabetes, which results from the immune-mediated destruction of pancreatic beta islet cells. More than 10 different viruses have been implicated in the pathogenesis of the disease in both humans and various animal models (Jun and Yoon, 2003). Viruses could contribute to the pathology by inducing β-cell-specific autoimmunity or cytolytic infection of β cells and the subsequent development of autoimmunity. Most data supporting a role for viruses in the development of the disease come from rodent models. Nonhuman primate models to evaluate the role of viruses in type 1 diabetes should be developed to fill the gap between rodents and humans.

Lyme disease in Old World monkeys

Lyme borreliosis is caused by infection with the tick-borne spirochete *Borrelia burgdorfi*, resulting in a chronic variable inflammation. The spirochete invades the nervous system soon after the initial infection, giving rise to neurological symptoms, such as headache, fatigue, leg numbness or tingling, and chronic cognitive impairment when the infection persists. People with Lyme disease express autoantibodies directed against structures expressed in neural tissues such as axons, myelin, myelin basic protein, and neurons (Sigal and Tatum, 1988; Aberer *et al.*, 1989; Sigal, 1993; Pachner *et al.*, 2001). Infected patients can experience relapses of infection through antigenic variation. All these features of the disease show similarity with patients affected by multiple sclerosis. The anatomical similarities between the brains of humans and those of Old World monkeys are remarkable, making rhesus monkeys an ideal model to study immune responses in relation to the specific neurological deficits common in both Lyme disease and multiple sclerosis (Pachner *et al.*, 2001; Bolz and Weis, 2004).

EXPERIMENTALLY INDUCED AUTOIMMUNE DISORDERS IN NONHUMAN PRIMATES

Impressive developments in the field of biotechnology have fueled the search for animal models in which the safety and efficacy of new reagents can be tested before clinical trials are initiated. As biotechnology products are often highly species specific, reagents developed for use in humans cannot be tested in normal rodent strains, but should be evaluated in transgenic mice or nonhuman primates.

Ethical implications

The use of nonhuman primates for biomedical research is limited by legal constraints. The law on animal experimentation in the Netherlands prescribes the qualification of the experimenters and the conditions under which experiments in nonhuman primates can be considered and performed. In general terms, nonhuman primates can only be used for *in vivo* experimentation if there are no valid alternative methods to obtain crucial information on new therapies or mechanisms of disease. Alternatives that can be considered are *in vitro* experiments or experiments in rodent models of disease or in the patients themselves. Furthermore, lower ranking primate species that are evolutionary more distant are to be preferred over more closely related "higher" primate species to obtain pivotal information.

The evolutionary proximity of nonhuman primates to humans becomes more relevant in the development of treatments that use human-specific biological products (Jonker, 1990; Bach *et al.*, 1993; Kennedy *et al.*, 1997; Wierda *et al.*, 2001). It is of critical importance for preclinical safety testing that the selected animal model is sensitive to the pharmacological action of the tested drug and that the tissue distribution and pharmacological properties of the molecules targeted by the treatment are comparable to those observed in patients. The phylogenetic proximity between humans and nonhuman primates translates into a high degree of immunological similarity. This is also important for the analysis of the underlying pathophysiological processes in autoimmune diseases. It is remarkable that in transplantation research nonhuman primates are considered an essential preclinical model in the development of new therapies, whereas the selection of therapies for chronic immune-mediated diseases relies mainly on inbred rodent models (Sachs, 2003).

Experimental autoimmune encephalomyelitis in nonhuman primates as a preclinical model of multiple sclerosis

Hominoid primates (chimpanzee, gorilla, orangutan) are the closest living relatives of humans in nature. The common ancestor of chimpanzee and human dates back about 5 million years and the genomic overlap may be more than 98%. However, hominoid primates are highly endangered species and maintenance under captive conditions is difficult and very expensive. Hence, these valuable species have been used in biomedical research only for very specific purposes, such as safety tests of new therapeutic antibodies and to test vaccines against serious infectious diseases such as AIDS and hepatitis (Muchmore, 2001). Noteworthy though is the observation that chimpanzees injected with multiple sclerosis patient brain cells develop acute encephalomyelitis, possibly due to cytomegalovirus (CMV) in the inoculum (Wroblewska et al., 1979). This is an interesting observation in view of the possible involvement of CMV in the acute experimental autoimmune encephalomyelitis (EAE) model in rhesus monkeys (see below).

Macaque models of experimental autoimmune encephalomyelitis

The preferred nonhuman primates species in biomedical research are the rhesus and cynomolgus macaques (Macaca mulatta and Macaca fascicularis). Both species have often been used for the safety and efficacy assessment of new therapies. Despite the >35 million years separation from humans, macaques are characterized by strong anatomical, genetic, immunological, virological, and physiological similarity with humans (Bontrop, 2001; Roth et al., 2004; Herodin et al., 2005; 't Hart et al., 2005e).

Spontaneous occurrence of multiple sclerosis-like disease in hominoid primates has rarely been reported. We are aware of only one report on the occurrence of multiple sclerosis-like neurological signs in the macaque colony at the Oregon Primate Center, which are infected by a g-herpesvirus. As the lymphocryptovirus is related to Epstein–Bar virus (EBV) this interesting observation may shed light on the association of EBV with multiple sclerosis. This observation has only been reported as a conference abstract, which makes it difficult to test the validity of the observation.

The first successful attempt to induce multiple sclerosis-like disease in macaques was reported by Rivers in the 1930s (Rivers et al., 1933). Soon after this first observation, however, it was recognized that the EAE model is more like the acute clinical course and the serious inflammatory lesion pathology of acute disseminated encephalomyelitis (ADEM) than multiple sclerosis (Rivers and Schwenkter, 1935; Ravkina et al., 1979). It has taken over half a century for a more multiple sclerosis-like nonhuman primates EAE model to be developed using the common marmoset (*Callithrix jacchus*) (Massacesi et al., 1995). This model appears to resemble multiple sclerosis in many respects, including the clinical course and pathological presentation (see below).

Rhesus monkeys immunized with central nervous system (CNS) myelin or myelin antigens, such as myelin basic protein (MBP) or myelin/oligodendrocyte glycoprotein (MOG), develop a neurological disease associated with lesions, serving as foci of serious inflammation and destruction of myelin as well as axons within the CNS white matter (reviewed in Rose et al., 1994; Brok et al., 2001a; 't Hart et al., 2005b). Although neutrophilic granulocytes and macrophages are the most prevalent cell types in the lesions, lesion formation is probably primarily initiated by the CNS infiltration of myelin-specific $CD4^+$ precursor T cells. This is concluded from the suppressive effect of depleting anti-CD4 antibody (Van Lambalgen and Jonker, 1987). As could be expected on the basis of its outbred nature, rhesus monkeys show a variable T cell response to several MBP epitopes such as MBP 29–84 (Slierendregt et al., 1995), MBP 61–82 and MBP 80–105 (Meinl et al., 1997) and MBP 170–186 (Price et al., 1988). The EAE course in rhesus monkeys is determined by genetic factors encoded within the MHC class II region; monkeys positive for the *Mamu-DPB1*01* allele were found to be more susceptible to EAE induced with purified bovine MBP in complete Freund's adjuvant (CFA) (Slierendregt et al., 1995). However, no effect of this allele was found on EAE induced with a recombinant version of another myelin protein, namely human MOG (amino acids 1–125; rhMOG) in CFA (Kerlero de Rosbo et al., 2000).

The presence of potentially pathogenic MBP-reactive $CD4^+$ T cells in the normal rhesus monkey repertoire has been documented (Meinl et al., 1997). Although not formally proven, we assume that, similar to the situation in many rodent EAE models, the CNS-infiltrating T cells that cause lesions and neurological deficits are of the helper 1 phenotype, which means that they secrete proinflammatory cytokines such as IFNγ, IL-2 and TNFα. This assumption is supported by the observation that intra-CSF injection of rhesus monkeys with a herpes simplex virus-based vector engineered with the human IL-4 gene suppressed the development of EAE (Poliani et al., 2001).

Potentially pathogenic T and B cells present in the natural repertoire can be activated by inoculation with emulsified oil, together with a strong stimulant of the innate immune system. This forms the basis of autoimmune disease models. It is unknown, however, which factor triggers these cells in patients. We have analysed this in the rhesus monkey EAE model for autoreactive T cells specific for one of the immunodominant T cell epitopes of MOG, namely MOG_{34-56}. That the peptide by itself induces EAE underlines the pathogenic relevance. Alignment of the amino acid sequence of MOG_{34-56} with sequences of viral antigens published in the BLAST database revealed significant sequence similarity with the major capsid protein of human cytomegalovirus (CMVmcp) (Brok et al., 2006). We have demonstrated in the same publication that MOG_{34-56}-reactive $CD4^+$ T cells could be activated in vivo in rhesus monkeys by immunization with a 22-mer synthetic peptide based on the human CMVmcp. It is therefore tempting to speculate that recrudescence of a latent CMV infection may boost CNS inflammation via the activation of MOG_{34-56} reactive T cells.

It is still an unresolved question why rhesus monkeys develop such an aggressive form of EAE after inoculation of human CNS myelin or myelin protein, while with the same immunizing agents multiple sclerosis-like disease is induced in marmosets (Brok et al., 2001a; 't Hart et al., 2005a, 2004b). A detailed lesion analysis of pathogenic mechanisms revealed some interesting differences between both models. The destructive lesions in the rhesus monkey model are densely populated by neutrophils containing proinflammatory bacterial antigen (L. Visser, submitted for publication) and express less complement regulatory protein CD55/DAF on the neurons (van Beek et al., 2005). Moreover, rhesus monkey monocytes were found to produce more aggressive types of reactive oxygen species than those of marmosets (our own unpublished observation). It remains to be established whether this is also the case with CNS microglia cells, which share many similarities with blood-borne macrophages (Town et al., 2005).

The common marmoset model of experimental autoimmune encephalomyelitis

The common marmoset is a small-sized neotropical primate (300–400 g at adult age) that has its natural habitat in the Amazon forest. Although less known as laboratory animals than rhesus and java macaques, the common marmoset has been used for the modeling of a variety of disorders (Mansfield, 2003). A highly useful characteristic of this species for immune-mediated inflammatory disorders research is that marmosets are born as non-identical twins which have shared the placental bloodstream. Hence they have a chimeric immune system that contains bone marrow-derived elements originating from both siblings. This implies that immune cells can be exchanged between twins without the risk of allorejection (Haig, 1999). Just as in rhesus monkeys, T cells specific for CNS myelin antigens could be detected in the normal immune repertoire (Massacesi et al., 1995; Villoslada et al., 2001).

EAE could be induced in 100% of human myelin-immunized monkeys ($n > 50$) that we have analyzed thus far, although the disease course and severity of neurological deficit differed substantially between individual monkeys from this outbred species ('t Hart et al., 2000). The remarkably high susceptibility of the marmoset to EAE maps to the MHC class II region (see below). The clinical course, characterized by alternating episodes of neurological dysfunction and disease remission as well as the neuropathological presentation, shows strong similarity with multiple sclerosis ('t Hart et al., 2000, 2004b; Genain and Hauser, 2001). The severity of EAE is normally assessed using the disease scores in Table 4.2.

TABLE 4.2   Integrated clinical and discomfort scoring table for the primate EAE models

Discomfort score	Clinical signs	Monitoring	Maximal duration[a]
0	Asymptomatic No general discomfort signs	Daily	End of experiment
0.5	Reduced alertness, loss of appetite, altered walking pattern without ataxia	Daily	20 weeks
1	Lethargy and/or weight loss less than 15% from start weight	Daily	10 weeks
2	Ataxia (= reduced capacity to keep balance); visual disturbance, including optic neuritis	Daily	6 weeks
2.5	Incomplete paralysis: para- or monoparesis and/or sensory loss and/or brainstem syndrome	Daily	4 weeks
3.0	Complete paralysis hind part of the body one- (hemiplegia) or two-sided (paraplegia)	Daily	1 weeks
4	Complete paralysis all four limbs quadriplegia	Daily	<18 hours
5	Lack of reaction to external stimuli; incapacity to eat or drink without help, self mutilation, blindness more than 2 days, untreatable pain	Daily	<1 hour

[a] The discomfort time duration is used in a cumulative fashion.

The myelin-induced EAE model is typically characterized by the apparently random distribution through the white matter of brain and spinal cord of focal areas of primary demyelination, with a variable degree of inflammation, remyelination, gliosis, and axonal pathology ('t Hart *et al.*, 1998b). Using the staging criteria that have been defined for multiple sclerosis lesions (Brück *et al.*, 1995), we observed that all lesion stages present in multiple sclerosis patients (i.e. early active, late active, and chronically inactive) can also be found in the myelin-induced EAE model in marmosets ('t Hart *et al.*, 1998b).

Genetics and immunopathogenesis

The MHC class II genomic region of the common marmoset (indicated with *Caja*) is remarkably compressed (Antunes *et al.*, 1998). Thus far *Caja-DP* genes have not been found, while the *Caja-DQA* and *-DQB loci* seem to show very little allelic variation. The *Caja-DR* region contains three loci, one of which (*Caja-DRB*W12*) is monomorphic and two (*Caja-DRB1*03* and *Caja-DRB*W16*) are polymorphic. While RNA transcripts of all *Caja-DRB*W12* and *Caja-DRB*W16* alleles have been found, we initially observed that *Caja-DRB1*03* transcripts were absent, meaning that this locus contains pseudogenes. Interestingly, in some monkeys we have observed expression of exon 2 from *Caja-DRB1*03* as a recombination with exons 1 and 3 from *Caja-DRB*W16* (Doxiadis *et al.*, 2006).

As a first step towards the identification of myelin components critical to EAE induction we immunized marmoset twins with myelin isolated from C57/Bl6 mice: one sibling with myelin from wild-type mice and the other with myelin from the MOG-deficient mice generated by Pham-Dinh and co-workers (Delarasse *et al.*, 2003). The EAE course and lesion pathology in monkeys immunized with the wild-type mouse myelin strongly resembled the model induced with human myelin. The absence of MOG in the inoculum, however, led to a reduction of the brain lesion load as well as the EAE incidence from 5 out of 5 to only 1 out of 5 (S. Amor, manuscript in preparation). This experiment indicates that although MOG is a quantitatively minor CNS glycoprotein (Johns and Bernard, 1999), it may have a much more important pathogenic function in EAE than major myelin proteins such as MBP or proteolipid protein (PLP). To date, several EAE models have been established in the common marmoset.

MBP-induced experimental autoimmune encephalomyelitis

While immunization with MBP induces severe EAE in rhesus monkeys, MBP appears only weakly encephalitogenic in marmosets (Brok *et al.*, 2000). However, when administered with strong adjuvant stimulation, relapsing–remitting EAE can be induced (Massacesi *et al.*, 1995).

MOG-induced experimental autoimmune encephalomyelitis

We have investigated the pathogenic role of MOG in great detail. To this end, marmosets were immunized with recombinant human MOG_{1-125} (rhMOG) in commercial CFA. In the vast majority of immunized monkeys we observed that after an asymptomatic episode of variable length irreversible neurological deficit developed ('t Hart *et al.*, 2004b). Cases with a relapsing–remitting disease course were only rarely observed. A possible explanation for the discrepancy with the myelin-induced EAE model may be that the lesions in the rhMOG-induced EAE model seem to remain fixed in an early active state, although small numbers of late active and chronically inactive lesions were found to accumulate with time ('t Hart *et al.*, 2004c).

To investigate the immunological basis of the 100% EAE incidence in rhMOG-immunized monkeys we have determined the fine-specificity of T cell lines from the inguinal and axillary lymph nodes. For this analysis we used a panel of 22-mer synthetic peptides overlapping by 10 that covers the extracellular domain of human MOG (1–125). We observed a proliferative response against MOG_{24-36} in all monkeys and identified the monomorphic *Caja-DRB*W1201* allele as the domi-nant restriction element (Brok *et al.*, 2000). As anticipated, immunization/booster of four unrelated monkeys with the MOG_{14-36} peptide was found to induce clinical EAE and perivascular cuffs of inflammatory cells within the CNS white matter. Furthermore, adoptive transfer of a T cell clone specific for peptide 21–40 from rat MOG into an MHC-compatible naïve recipient was found to induce mild EAE and similar inflammatory cuffs (Villoslada *et al.*, 2001). These combined data war-rant the conclusion that the 100% EAE incidence may be caused by the *Caja-DRB*W1201*-restricted activation of T cells specific for MOG_{24-36}. Consequently, this MHC class II allele is likely the major risk factor to autoimmune encephalomyelitis in this species.

A second peptide of interest is MOG_{34-56}, as it appears to contain dominant T cell epitope(s) for autoreactive T cells and autoantibodies in multiple sclerosis patients and rhMOG-immunized marmosets (manuscript in preparation) and rhesus mon-keys (Kerlero de Rosbo *et al.*, 2000). The peptide was found to induce clinical EAE in 8 out of 8 tested marmosets following a relapsing–remitting course in some monkeys and a progressive course in others. At the time this chapter was written, the MHC restriction elements regulating the T cell response against this peptide had not yet been determined.

Magnetic resonance imaging and biomarkers

In comparison with rats and mice, the marmoset brain contains a higher propor-tion of compact myelin which is an obvious advantage for modeling the white mat-ter pathology of multiple sclerosis ('t Hart *et al.*, 2005a). We have used essentially the same magnetic resonance imaging (MRI) techniques as used in multiple scle-rosis patients for the visualization and characterization of brain white matter lesions in intact animals. With the 4.7 tesla spectrometer used for our analysis, lesions in the white matter as well as the leukocortex can be well visualized. However, it is rather difficult to distinguish lesions in subpial areas of the cerebral cortex from the surrounding CSF.

The standard imaging technique for lesion detection in the marmoset EAE model is T2W MRI, visualizing the size and spatial distribution of lesions. Blood–brain barrier leakage can be visualized by the signal change in T1W MRI where intravenous gadopentetate-dimeglumine (Gd-DTPA) extravasates. To be able to test the effect of therapies on existing lesions we have also implemented a set of (semi-)quantitative images that are created by plotting the T1 and T2 relax-ation times or the magnetization transfer ratios (MTR). A more detailed discussion of these techniques can be found in 't Hart *et al.* (2005f).

A key question in MRI analysis is the relation with pathomorphological aspects of the examined regions of interest (ROI). It was found that of the MRI parame-ters used in our studies, MTR most strongly correlates with lesion stages defined on the basis of expressed macrophage activity markers (Blezer *et al.*, 2007).

Pathology

The myelin- and rhMOG-induced models differ in their pathological presentation. The myelin-induced EAE model presents at MRI as large hyperintense areas around the ventral horns of the lateral ventricles and many (up to 900) isolated small hyperintense foci scattered through the white matter. Often large confluent hyperintense regions are observed. The histological examination of the MRI-detectable changes in the EAE-affected marmoset brain showed that these represent sharply edged foci of primary demyelination with a variable degree of inflammation, axonal pathology, remyelination, and gliosis ('t Hart et al., 1998b). Different stages of lesion development, including early active, late active, and chronic inactive, can be present in the same hemisphere. The early and late active lesions are areas of high humoral and cellular immune activity, where the dynamic interaction of infiltrated T cells with resident and infiltrated APCs induces pro- and anti-inflammatory cytokine production within lesions and by surrounding astrocytes (Laman et al., 1998). Moreover, antibody deposition on myelin sheaths and neurons together with complement components and complement regulatory proteins is clearly detected ('t Hart et al., 1998b; Raine et al., 1999; van Beek et al., 2005). A very important observation is that a significant proportion of the antibodies within areas of myelin disintegration and demyelination are directed against MOG peptides 1–20, 21–40, and 61–80 (Genain et al., 1999). Antibodies against these and overlapping peptides can be found in the serum of MOG-immunized monkeys (Genain et al., 1995; our own unpublished observations).

The rhMOG-induced experimental autoimmune encephalomyelitis model

This model has been investigated in much greater detail. Marmosets immunized with rhMOG develop many fewer brain lesions (1–20) than in the myelin-induced EAE model. In a large group of more than 50 rhMOG-immunized monkeys with serious clinical EAE at least four different patterns could be detected ('t Hart et al., 2005e) (Figure 4.1). The MRI pattern in (a) is by far the most frequently observed in this model, showing a large hyperintense area with Gd-DTPA enhancement that persists for several weeks. Histologically, the depicted lesion presents with intense inflammation and demyelination, which explains the strong hyperintense signal on the T2-RT image and the strong hypointense signal on the MTR image. The hypointense area within the lesion of the T2 image appears due to gliosis.

Pattern (b) is rarely found, showing large symmetrical hyperintense areas on the T2W and T2-RT images and more diffuse Gd-DTPA leakage than the lesion in (a). Also the MTR reduction is less than in pattern (a). These lesions may be areas with strong inflammatory activity.

Pattern (c) has only been found once, showing diffuse hyperintense areas on the T2W and T2-RT images that affect a large proportion of the white matter. In this pattern focal changes in the MTR and Gd-DTPA-enhanced T1W images are absent.

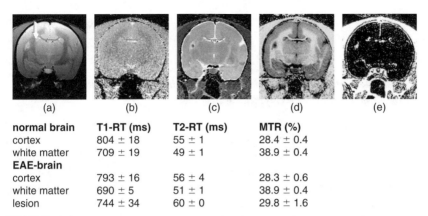

(a)	(b)	(c)	(d)	(e)

normal brain	T1-RT (ms)	T2-RT (ms)	MTR (%)
cortex	804 ± 18	55 ± 1	28.4 ± 0.4
white matter	709 ± 19	49 ± 1	38.9 ± 0.4
EAE-brain			
cortex	793 ± 16	56 ± 4	28.3 ± 0.6
white matter	690 ± 5	51 ± 1	38.9 ± 0.4
lesion	744 ± 34	60 ± 0	29.8 ± 1.6

FIGURE 4.1 Magnetic resonance images of a lesion in the experimental autoimmune encephalomyelitis (EAE)-affected marmoset brain. High-contrast T2-weighted images (a) are made to visualize a lesion (arrow) in the white matter. On T1-weighted images (e) leakage of intravenously injected contrast substance (Gd-DTPA) into the lesion can be observed, pointing at blood–brain barrier leakage. T1 (b) and T2 (c) relaxation time and magnetization ratio transfer images (d) are made to quantitate pathological changes. The tabular data give the quantification of T1 and T2 signal intensities (as relaxation times (RT) in milliseconds) and the actual magnetization transfer ratios (MTS) of cortex, (normal appearing) white matter, and lesions. Note the marked differences in the MRI values between lesions and white matter.

Around the ventral horn of the left lateral ventricle a region of several square millimeters is found that presents as a strong hyperintense region on the T2-RT images and hypointense on the MTR images. This pattern may represent the ubiquitous disintegration of the compact myelin structure, being an early pathological change in demyelination (Ohler, 2004) associated with anti-MOG antibody deposition (Genain et al., 1999).

In pattern (d), which is more commonly observed than patterns (b) and (c), but much less than pattern (a), multifocal small regions are found, which are hyperintense on T2W images and hypointense on MTR images. No marked changes were observed on the T2-RT and Gd-DTPA-enhanced T1W images, indicating that inflammatory activity in these lesions may be low.

Gray matter lesions

Most of our research thus far has been focused on the formation of white matter lesions, which can easily be visualized with standard MRI techniques. However, two independent publications reported the occurrence of dramatic demyelination in the gray matter of rhMOG-immunized monkeys (Pomeroy et al., 2005; Storch, personal communication). Based on the histological presentation, in particular the lower inflammatory cell content, both reports conclude that T cells may play a less prominent role in the formation of lesions in the gray matter than of those in the white matter. These findings complement observations in multiple sclerosis (Peterson *et al.*, 2001).

Experimental autoimmune encephalomyelitis in the common marmoset: a preclinical model for the development of new therapies

We have designed a new two-step strategy in the marmoset EAE model that may help to bridge the discrepancy between preclinical and clinical studies ('t Hart *et al.*, 2005f). The aim of step 1 is to confirm that the beneficial effect of a new therapy observed in rodents can be reproduced in a more complex animal model. This is an important step as rodent EAE models are more sensitive to suppression or deviation of immunopathogenic processes than the same models in nonhuman primates ('t Hart *et al.*, 2004a). Therapies that have successfully passed the step 1 test will be transferred to step 2, with the aim to test whether they are effective in ongoing disease using brain MRI as a primary, and progression of neurological deficit as a secondary, outcome parameter. In brief, MRI scans are made at two-week intervals recording the whole set of MRI parameters discussed in the previous paragraph. White matter high contrast T2W-images are used to determine the size and spatial distribution of pathological abnormalities in the brain. As soon as one or more focal hyperintense areas are detected, administration of the therapeutic or placebo preparation (often an equal volume of the solvent) is started. Then the MRI parameters of normal-appearing white matter and all focal hyperintense areas are separately recorded (see Figure 4.1). We have tested this novel preclinical approach using two monoclonal antibodies directed against co-stimulatory molecules of human APCs, one against the surface expressed CD40 (Boon *et al.*, 2001; 't Hart *et al.*, 2005c) and the other against the secreted p40 subunit of IL-12 and IL-23 (Brok *et al.*, 2002; 't Hart *et al.*, 2005d).

As discussed elsewhere, we believe that this new approach will help to bridge the gap between EAE models in rodents and the patient and the preclinical selection of the most promising therapeutics from the development pipeline ('t Hart *et al.*, 2004a; 't Hart *et al.*, 2005f).

Juvenile arthropathies

The syndrome juvenile idiopathic arthritis (JIA), formerly known as juvenile rheumatoid arthritis (JRA), comprises a heterogeneous group of arthropathies of children (Andersson Gare, 1999; Quarta *et al.*, 2005). Compared with rheumatoid arthritis in adults, the prevalence of JIA is relatively low, namely less than 1 per 10 000. Nevertheless, it is the most common form of juvenile arthritis and is among the most common forms of childhood disabilities in the United States (Lawrence *et al.*, 1998). JIA is usually monophasic and children can completely recover. However, in a substantial number of patients disease activity persists through adolescence and may ultimately develop into rheumatoid arthritis. Such patients may develop severe physical disability such as skeletal growth retardation, osteopenia, and increased risks of fractures. Furthermore, they can suffer the severe side-effects of the disease, such as uveitis.

Based on the number of involved joints and localization of the disease three major JIA forms are discerned. In oligoarticular JIA, formerly known as pauciarticular JIA, 1–4 joints are affected, while polyarticular JIA affects 5 or more joints. The third group, systemic JIA, is characterized by spiking fever and a salmon-pink rash and shows distinct extra-articular symptoms, as the name implies affecting other bodily systems next to the joints. Although JIA can occur in boys or girls of any age, girls are more frequently affected than boys. As discussed above for multiple sclerosis, valid models of juvenile and adult arthritis in nonhuman primates can help to better understand underlying pathogenic mechanisms as well as to develop more effective therapies.

ARTHRITIS MODELS IN NONHUMAN PRIMATES

The rhesus monkey model of collagen-induced arthritis (CIA) was originally developed as a preclinical model of rheumatoid arthritis in adults. However, the model shows distinct similarities with juvenile forms of arthritic disease, such as the heterogenic clinical presentation (Vierboom et al., 2005a), the monophasic course ('t Hart et al., 1998a; Bakker et al., 1991b), the prominent production of IL-6, a proinflammatory cytokine that is pivotal in the perpetuation of JIA (Rooney et al., 1995; Ou et al., 2002) and the pathogenic role of autoimmunity against type II collagen (Myers et al., 2001).

Nonhuman primates spontaneously develop several of the arthritic diseases that affect the human population ('t Hart et al., 2003, 2005e). However, we have only rarely observed spontaneous manifestations of arthritis in the large outbred population of rhesus monkeys (>1000 individuals) kept at the Biomedical Primate Research Centre in Rijswijk (The Netherlands). The low incidence and unpredictable nature of spontaneous arthritis prompted us to develop an experimental model that can be induced at will and that is suitable for testing new therapies for safety and efficacy.

We have initially tried to reproduce well-established arthritis models in rats and mice to test whether these were experimentally feasible and would be compatible with ethical and practical standards. However, the commonly used rat models, such as those induced with streptococcal cell walls (SCW) or mycobacteria, could not be reproduced in rhesus monkeys (Bakker et al., 1990).

A frequently used model of joint inflammation in rodents is antigen-induced arthritis (AIA) (van den Berg, 1991). In preliminary experiments intra-articular injection of methylated ovalbumin (OVA) into OVA-sensitized rhesus monkeys was found to induce macroscopic arthritis in monkeys that displayed both serum antibodies as well as a positive delayed-type hypersensitivity response against OVA (own unpublished observation). The AIA model may provide a useful model with less discomfort to the animals than systemic polyarthritis for the assessment of immunogenic properties of new products developed for the repair of the joint under local inflammatory conditions or of therapeutics that are administered locally to suppress inflammation.

While inbred rodent strains are genetically uniform and essentially represent a single individual in an outbred population, an outbred colony of rhesus macaques more closely resembles the heterogeneous human population. Predictably, we observed a similarly variable clinical presentation of CIA, as has been observed in human rheumatoid arthritis, in a random sample ($N > 50$) from the large rhesus monkey colony at our institute (more than 1200 animals). On the basis of these data we chose to develop the CIA model further in rhesus monkeys as a preclinical model of human rheumatoid arthritis.

The rhesus monkey model of collagen-induced arthritis

Collagen-induced arthritis (CIA) is routinely induced in rhesus monkeys by immunization with bovine type II collagen (b-CII) dissolved in CFA. One milliliter of this emulsion is injected into the dorsal skin distributed over 10 spots to reduce the formation of ulcerative skin lesions, which are rather serious in this species.

Clinical course

A randomly selected cohort of monkeys from our outbreed colony ($N > 1000$) were immunized with b-CII. Three disease patterns could be distinguished (Bakker et al., 1991b). In about 50% of the animals we were unable to induce any clinical signs. Immunologically these monkeys are characterized by a low ratio of anti-CII IgM versus IgG antibodies and absence of anti-CII T cell reactivity. In about 10% of the monkeys we observed a rapid onset of severe polyarthritis. These monkeys were characterized by a high ratio of anti-CII IgM versus IgG antibodies in their serum; these had to be sacrificed for ethical reasons before T cell reactivity could develop. In the remaining 40% of the monkeys a rather severe polyarthritis develops, which remits spontaneously. In these monkeys moderate levels of IgM and IgG antibodies as well as T cell proliferation against CII are detectable. Interestingly, in monkeys in which persistent T cell reactivity was measured, exacerbation of arthritis could be induced by a booster immunization with CII in IFA (Bakker et al., 1991a). In further experiments we could confirm that the ability to induce CIA correlated well with the monkey's capacity to produce IgM antibodies against CII ('t Hart et al., 1993).

Genetic influence on the development of collagen–induced arthritis in rhesus monkeys

The time of onset and severity of clinical signs varies, most likely reflecting the genetic heterogeneity in the colony. Whereas rheumatoid arthritis susceptibility, more precisely the disease severity, in the human population maps to the MHC class II alleles HLA-DR1/-DR4, thus far no apparent association with the MHC class II region has been observed in rhesus monkeys. This was rather unexpected because "shared epitopes" (QKRAA and QRRAA) that are associated with a high risk of rheumatoid arthritis in the human population are present at the correct location in several *Mamu-DRB1* alleles (see the IPD-MHC sequence database, EMBL-EBI 2007). In contrast, a strong influence of the MHC class I region on the susceptibility to CIA was found, mapping to the *Mamu-A26* serotype in Indian-origin rhesus monkey (Bakker *et al.*, 1992). *Mamu-A26* has recently been renamed *Mamu-B26* because molecular analysis revealed that the *Mamu-A26* typing sera recognize B-locus products (Otting *et al.*, 2005). While young *Mamu-B26*-positive Indian-origin animals from our colony appeared completely resistant to the disease even after several booster immunizations, mild arthritic signs could be induced in *Mamu-B26*-positive monkeys that were over 20 years old (Bakker *et al.*, 1992). Furthermore, the resistance is specific for the immunizing antigen since *Mamu-B26*-positive and *-B26*-negative monkeys are equally susceptible to EAE induced with human MBP (Table 4.3).

By selection of *B26*-negative rhesus monkeys, a reproducible CIA model of high incidence (>95%) could be established in monkeys of Indian origin. Notably, *Mamu-B26*-associated CIA resistance was not observed in rhesus monkeys of Chinese or Burmese origin (unpublished observations). As we do not understand the cellular basis for the *Mamu-B26*-associated CIA resistance, it is unclear whether resistance is defined by a particular combination of MHC class I molecules or by a closely linked gene. A female gender bias as observed in humans for the risk of developing rheumatoid arthritis was not found in the rhesus monkey CIA model, although a female prevalence has been found in the closely related cynomolgus macaque (Terato *et al.*, 1989).

An important genetic polymorphism has been established in human rheumatoid arthritis that confers the strongest genetic association with rheumatoid arthritis outside the human leukocyte antigen (HLA) region. A single-nucleotide polymorphism in

TABLE 4.3   Genetic susceptibility to collagen-induced arthritis (CIA) in rhesus monkeys

	CIA^{+ve}	CIA^{-ve}
Mamu B26 $^{+ve}$	2	3
Mamu B26 $^{-ve}$	25	9

the gene product protein tyrosine phosphatase non-receptor 22 encoded by *PTPN22* is strongly associated with human rheumatoid arthritis. *PTPN22* plays an important role in the negative regulation of T cells (Begovich *et al.*, 2004; Gregersen, 2005; Gregersen and Batliwalla, 2005). We are currently investigating whether a similar polymorphism is associated with the heterogeneous CIA expression in rhesus monkeys.

Biomarkers for inflammation and joint destruction

Several surrogate markers for CIA have been developed that reflect the different pathological aspects of the model; inflammation, bone degradation, and clinical signs of arthritis. These markers also aid in the efficacy assessment of a new treatment. Consistent improvement of a biomarker in the experimental group versus a control group, without a direct clinical effect, can reveal a therapeutic effect. The relation between various biomarkers, the clinical manifestation of arthritis in the model and the response to treatment is illustrated by data collected over the last decade.

Serum C-reactive protein as a biomarker of collagen-induced arthritis severity

The serum level of C-reactive protein (CRP), an acute phase protein produced in the liver under conditions of systemic inflammation, is increased in patients with clinically active rheumatoid arthritis (Wollheim, 2000). A low, albeit significant, increase of serum CRP concentration can be observed years before the onset of rheumatoid arthritis symptoms (Nielen *et al.*, 2004). CRP is a very useful marker of inflammation and a potential biomarker for the anti-inflammatory effect of a new therapy, as the serum half-life remains unchanged under conditions of health and disease. Moreover, the serum CRP concentration directly reflects the intensity of the joint inflammation. A small increase of serum CRP in the first week after CIA induction without overt clinical signs is followed by a second increase in CIA-sensitive animals which is more pronounced and precedes the onset of clinical arthritis.

Changes in serum CRP levels are not observed in CIA-resistant monkeys ('t Hart *et al.*, 1998a), illustrating that the CRP increment is due to the systemic arthritis and not caused by the inflammatory skin reaction to the inoculation of b-CII/CFA emulsion. In the CIA model CRP is elevated before macroscopic clinical signs are observed and can be used as an early marker for disease onset. Three types of CIA responders can be distinguished in *Mamu-B26*-negative monkeys on the basis of the serum CRP pattern. Early responders show a CRP increase above an arbitrary threshold of 50 mg/L before postsensitization day (psd) 14. Moderate responders show an increase in CRP above 50 mg/L between psd 14 and 21. Late responders show a CRP increase of more than 50 mg/L after psd 21. The highest peak CRP levels were observed in early responders (Figure 4.2a); the lowest in the late responders (Figure 4.2c).

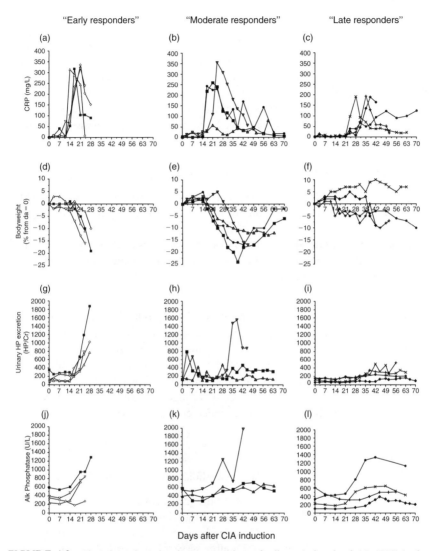

Days after CIA induction

FIGURE 4.2   Clinical, serological and urinary markers of collagen-induced arthritis (CIA) in the rhesus monkey. Early responders to challenge (a) demonstrate a sharp and larger increase in C-reactive protein (CRP) than observed for moderate (b) and late responders (c). This corresponds with an early weight loss in the early responders (d) compared with late responders (f), which demonstrate only minor weight loss after day 28. More acute and severe responders to induction (g) also show increased urinary excretion rates of hydroxylysylpyridinoline (HP) during the active phase of the disease compared to moderate and late responders (h and i). Alkaline phosphatase (AP) is mainly produced by liver and osteoblasts. With a normal liver function changes in AP can be indicative for bone remodeling processes as a result from bone degradation (j, k, l).

Bodyweight as a general disease marker

Early CIA responders display a rapid weight loss between days 14 and 28 (Figure 4.2d). In early experiments, monkeys were not sacrificed at the height of the disease. After a disease episode of variable length with substantial bodyweight loss in these experiments, CIA-affected monkeys displayed a bodyweight increase that coincided with remission of clinical arthritis (Figure 4.2e) such as pain or apathy. Hence, bodyweight is a useful objective biomarker of the general disease status.

Hematological and serological markers of disease

Once a week a complete hematological and serological analysis is performed, which provides additional information on disease status and general physical condition.

Neutrophils, platelets and hematocrit   Episodes of clinically active arthritis are marked by increased blood levels of platelets and neutrophils and decreased hematocrit values (data not shown).

Albumin and alkaline phosphatase   The production of serum protein albumin is affected by the induction of acute phase proteins such as CRP. Predictably, serum levels of albumin were found to be decreased during active joint inflammation. Alkaline phosphatase (AP) is a useful marker for the evaluation of bone metabolism. It is mainly produced in the liver and by osteoblasts in the skeleton. When liver enzymes are unaltered, changes in AP can be indicative of increased bone metabolism as a consequence of ongoing destructive joint erosion (Figure 4.2j–l).

Urinary excretion rates of collagen crosslinks as a biomarker of joint erosion

Joint tissues contain variable quantities of the major collagen crosslinks hydroxylysylpyridinoline (HP) and lysylpyridinoline (LP), which are degradation products of collagen contained in cartilage and bone and excreted into the urine. Urinary excretion rates of these metabolites can therefore serve as a biomarker of joint destruction. About 95% of the crosslinks in the rhesus monkey joint cartilage consist of HP (HP/LP ratio = 55), while the HP/LP ratio of bone is 3.8 ('t Hart et al., 1998a). As the excretion rate of the crosslink product varies during the day, urine samples for analysis were collected overnight and stored frozen at $-20°C$. Unhydrolysed urine samples are used for the measurement of collagen crosslinks using reversed-phase high-performance liquid chromatography (HPLC) (Black et al., 1988). Increased excretion rates of HP and LP, expressed relative to creatinine, were observed during the active phase of CIA. In particular the excretion rates of HP were associated with CIA severity (Figure 4.2g–i).

A mean fivefold increase relative to baseline values was observed in early responders (Vierboom *et al.*, 2005a). The LP excretion rate follows the same course but
increases only twofold, suggesting a prominence of cartilage degradation (Vierboom
et al., 2005a). The HP excretion rate correlates with the number of affected joints
(n.o.a.j.) per animal in each group. Early responders display a higher n.o.a.j. (>20)
relative to the moderate responders (±15), which was higher than the late responders who had a mean n.o.a.j. of 10 (Vierboom *et al.*, 2005a).

Histology of collagen–induced arthritis–affected joints

For routine histology the patellae of both knee joints and the proximal (PIP) and
distal interphalangeal (DIP) joints of the third digit of hand and foot are normally
processed and analyzed. Figure 4.3 shows the outward manifestation of joint
swelling in relation to the destruction of cartilage and subchondral bone observed
in the affected finger joint. We use the pathology grading system published by
Pettit *et al.* (2001) for histological quantitation of arthritis severity. This system
quantifies the degree of inflammation, bone destruction, and cartilage degradation
on an arbitrary scale from 0 to 5.

The arthritic joints of CIA-affected rhesus monkeys display essentially the same
histopathological hallmarks as rheumatoid arthritis joints. Hyperplasia of the synovium and pannus formation were already observed in the early phase of active
CIA. This preceded the dramatic destruction of cartilage and bone in advanced CIA.

Ethical management

The ethical management of the rhesus monkey CIA model relies on a semi-
quantitative clinical scoring system that represents the overall disease status of the

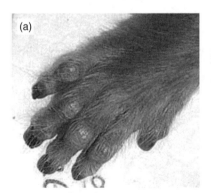
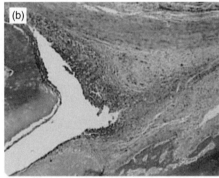

FIGURE 4.3   Clinical manifestation and histopathology of arthritic joints. (a) Outward clinical signs
of collagen-induced arthritis can be severe. (b) Histology of an affected proximal interphalangeal joint
shows a hyperplastic synovium resulting in pannus formation producing factors as cytokines and matrix
metalloproteinases (MMPs) mediating the destruction of the cartilage. (See Plate 2 for the color version
of this figure.)

TABLE 4.4   Clinical and ethical management scheme for collagen-induced arthritis (CIA) in rhesus monkeys

Disease score	Characteristics	Monitoring	Maximal duration[a]
0	No disease symptoms	daily	End of experiment
0.5	Fever (>0.5°C)	2× per week	12 weeks
1	Apathy; less mobility; loss of appetite	daily	10 weeks
2	Weight-loss; warm extremities[b]	2× per week	6 weeks
	Treatable pain without STS	Daily	
3	Redness of joints (with STS)[b]	2× per week	4 weeks
	Normal flexibility of extremities		
4	Severe STS of joints (+ redness) with joint stiffness[b]	2× per week	2 weeks
5	Untreatable pain; immobility of joints; weight loss > 25%	Daily 2× per week	18 hours

STS, soft tissue swelling.
[a] The discomfort time duration is used in a cumulative fashion.
[b] This can only be assessed in the sedated monkey, which cannot be done more than twice a week for ethical reasons.

animals (Table 4.4). Clinical signs that are monitored on a daily basis are bodyweight, body temperature, and the amount of pain relief used. Macroscopic signs of inflammation, the number of joints showing soft-tissue swelling, warmth, and redness, are recorded twice weekly. Medication to minimize the discomfort during the experiment is given at the indication of the institute's veterinarians. Pain relief medication consisted of buprenorfine (Temgesic, an opiate). Furthermore, ulcerative skin lesions developing at the immunization sites are sprayed daily with disinfecting wound spray to prevent further contamination.

Prophylactic treatment with a promising compound can result in a marked reduction of the clinical score, signifying improved clinical well-being. This was recently described for a small molecular weight CCR5 antagonist (Vierboom et al., 2005b).

All of these markers can be used to evaluate different aspects of the disease, allowing us to differentiate between disease-modifying drugs affecting bone degradation or therapies affecting inflammation.

Collagen-induced arthritis in the rhesus monkey: a preclinical model for the development of new therapies

The variety of intervention studies performed in the past decade have provided insight into the pathogenic mechanisms operating in the rhesus monkey CIA model. As proposed for rheumatoid arthritis by Choy and Panayi (2001), three phases are distinguished in the ethiopathogenesis of arthritis in the CIA model. In the presymptomatic phase the joint looks healthy. The "early phase" of rheumatoid arthritis is marked by synovitis, leading to the recruitment of leukocytes from the circulation and the development of a hyperplastic synovium resulting in over-growth and subsequent degradation of the cartilage (pannus formation). Many new treatments aim to control the disease in this early phase. In the late phase of rheumatoid arthritis, the joint cartilage and bone are usually so seriously damaged that repair of the damage is required for the restoration of function.

Synovitis

As in rheumatoid arthritis, a hyperplastic synovium staining positively for $CD3^+$- and $CD68^+$-infiltrated cells can be found in joints lacking macroscopic signs of arthritis (Kraan et al., 1998). Inflammation can be abolished by the removal of the hyperplastic synovium, for example by intra-articular injection of a thymidine kinase-expressing adenovirus followed by gancyclovir infusion (Goossens et al., 1999). This finding indicates that similar to rheumatoid arthritis, CIA starts with synovitis.

Leukocyte infiltration

Histological analysis of arthritic joints has revealed the presence of several leukocyte subsets such as T cells, B cells, macrophages, and neutrophils. Lymphocyte migra-tion to the site of inflammation is directed by chemokines. Effector T helper 1 (Th1) cells expressing chemokine receptors CCR5 and CXCR3 have been found to be enriched in synovial joints of rheumatoid arthritis patients. Ligands for both chemokine receptors are elevated in inflamed synovial tissue and synovial fluid (Wedderburn et al., 2000; Patel et al., 2001; Shadidi et al., 2003). A small molecu-lar CCR5 antagonist that prevents the binding of its ligand and hence the migra-tion of these destructive T cells was tested in the CIA model of rhesus monkeys. Prophylactic treatment with this compound resulted in a diminished disease sever-ity compared with non-treated controls (Vierboom et al., 2005b) and normaliza-tion of several disease markers.

T cells

The role of T cells in the onset of CIA in rhesus monkeys was demonstrated in two separate studies. Early treatment with cyclosporine A, a strong inhibitor of T cell immunity, prevented the development of CIA (Bakker et al., 1993). However, treat-ment of animals during clinically active CIA had no effect on the disease. In a separate study we showed a beneficial effect of daclizumab, a humanized antibody directed against the Tac antigen present on the IL-2 receptor alpha chain (Brok et al., 2001b). Both studies underline that T cells present in the early inflammatory synovium play an important role in the onset of arthritis. However, the poor proliferative response of rhesus monkey blood mononuclear cells to CII has hampered the generation of stable cell lines. Hence, the precise specificity analysis and MHC restriction of cellular autoimmune mechanisms has not been systematically evaluated.

Autoantibodies

A newly emerging target of therapy is the B cell. One example uses rituximab, a depleting antibody directed against CD20. Initially used for the treatment of B cell lymphomas, it was also effective in the treatment of rheumatoid arthritis (Edwards et al., 2004). That collagen-specific antibodies, in particular those of the IgM isotype, have a pivotal role in the rhesus monkey model of CIA appears from two findings: the absence of anti-CII IgM production in CIA-resistant monkeys (Bakker et al., 1992) and the protection against CIA of monkeys in which the capacity to produce anti-CII antibodies had been impaired by presensitization with heat-denatured b-CII ('t Hart et al., 1993).

Interferon beta (IFNβ)

The current state of the art biological treatment in rheumatoid arthritis uses inhibitors of proinflammatory cytokines such as TNFα and IL-1. We have not directly tested antagonists of these cytokines in the model, as treatments that have already been approved for usage in patients are not usually tested in nonhuman primates. However, we did test mammalian cell-derived interferon beta (IFNβ). IFNβ inhibits the production or the effects of proinflammatory cytokines such as IL-12. It also inhibits the secretion of TNFα and exerts a variety of immunomodulatory effects which underlie the therapeutic benefit in multiple sclerosis.

We have tested recombinant human IFNβ (REBIF, Ares-Serono) as a treatment for CIA in four rhesus monkeys. At the tested dose, 10^7 units per day administered via subcutaneous injection during one week, the cytokine showed a clear beneficial effect on clinically manifest arthritis in two monkeys and abolished arthritis in one monkey (Tak et al., 1999). A clinical trial in rheumatoid arthritis patients of fibroblast-derived IFNβ (Frone, Ares-Serono) combined with methotrexate failed to reproduce the promising effects of IFNβ observed in the monkeys (van Holten et al., 2005), but negative interactions between the medications cannot be excluded.

In the later stages of the disease the cartilage is severely damaged, requiring repair of the damage for restoration of function. We have little information about this stage of the disease because the monkeys are usually killed earlier for ethical reasons.

Future perspectives

CIA in rhesus monkeys is a very useful preclinical model of human arthritis, but is suboptimal in a number of respects. (1) The arthritis can be very severe. As an alternative the AIA-model can be used, which is less burdening for the animal and still provides important *in vivo* efficacy data. (2) The large size of the monkeys is advantageous with regard to the amount of blood that can be collected and the use of invasive techniques (arthroscopy). However, large amounts of test compound are required to observe a clinical effect. (3) Due to their aggressive nature rhesus monkeys usually have to be sedated for each handling, limiting the frequency of experimental interventions. (4) The model is acute and monophasic, although in some cases exacerbation could be induced by booster immunization (Bakker *et al.*, 1991b). (5) Due to the high susceptibility to mycobacterial components of adjuvant, rhesus monkeys develop severe ulcerating skin lesions where the CII/CFA inoculum is injected.

To overcome several of these issues we have started to develop a CIA model in a New World nonhuman primates species, the common marmoset. Whether we can successfully translate the CIA model into the common marmoset as a better model for rheumatoid arthritis in humans will become clear in the coming years.

To conclude, there is an increasing awareness that the occurrence of autoimmune diseases in children is a complex issue. Some autoimmune diseases, such as diabetes start at a young age and develop into adulthood. Other autoimmune diseases, such as juvenile multiple sclerosis and juvenile arthritis, may be distinct clinical entities, which may or may not develop into the adult form. This implies that juvenile forms of autoimmune disease may require different treatments than adult autoimmune disease. The elucidation of basic disease mechanisms from the multiple sclerosis and arthritis models described above may provide important insights into the spectrum of autoimmune diseases that affect children and young adults.

REFERENCES

Aberer, E., Brunner, C., Suchanek, G. *et al.* (1989). Molecular mimicry and Lyme borreliosis: a shared antigenic determinant between *Borrelia burgdorferi* and human tissue. *Ann Neurol* **26**, 732–737.

Andersson Gare, B. (1999). Juvenile arthritis – who gets it, where and when? A review of current data on incidence and prevalence. *Clin Exp Rheumatol* **17**, 367–374.

Ansari, A. A. (2004). Autoimmunity, anergy, lentiviral immunity and disease. *Autoimmun Rev* **3**, 530–540.

Ansari, A. A., Onlamoon, N., Bostik, P., Mayne, A. E., Gargano, L., and Pattanapanyasat, K. (2003). Lessons learnt from studies of the immune characterization of naturally SIV infected sooty mangabeys. *Front Biosci* **8**, s1030–1050.

Antunes, S. G., de Groot, N. G., Brok, H. *et al.* (1998). The common marmoset: a new world primate species with limited MHC class II variability. *Proc Natl Acad Sci USA* **95**, 11745–11750.

Bach, J. F., Fracchia, G. N., and Chatenoud, L. (1993). Safety and efficacy of therapeutic monoclonal antibodies in clinical therapy. *Immunol Today* **14**, 421–425.

Bakker, N. P., van Erck, M. G., Zurcher, C. *et al.* (1990). Experimental immune mediated arthritis in rhesus monkeys. A model for human rheumatoid arthritis? *Rheumatol Int* **10**, 21–29.

Bakker, N. P., van Erck, M. G., 't Hart, L. A., and Jonker, M. (1991a). Acquired resistance to type II collagen-induced arthritis in rhesus monkeys is reflected by a T cell low-responsiveness to the antigen. *Clin Exp Immunol* **86**, 219–223.

Bakker, N. P., van Erck, M. G., Botman, C. A., Jonker, M., and 't Hart, B. A. (1991b). Collagen-induced arthritis in an outbred group of rhesus monkeys comprising responder and nonresponder animals. Relationship between the course of arthritis and collagen-specific immunity. *Arthritis Rheum* **34**, 616–624.

Bakker, N. P., van Erck, M. G., Otting, N. *et al.* (1992). Resistance to collagen-induced arthritis in a nonhuman primate species maps to the major histocompatibility complex class I region. *J Exp Med* **175**, 933–937.

Bakker, N. P., Van Besouw, N., Groenestein, R., Jonker, M., and 't Hart, L. A. (1993). The anti-arthritic and immunosuppressive effects of cyclosporin A on collagen-induced arthritis in the rhesus monkey. *Clin Exp Immunol* **93**, 318–322.

Barnett, A. H., Eff, C., Leslie, R. D., and Pyke, D. A. (1981). Diabetes in identical twins. A study of 200 pairs. *Diabetologia* **20**, 87–93.

Begovich, A. B., Carlton, V. E., Honigberg, L. A. *et al.* (2004). A missense single-nucleotide polymorphism in a gene encoding a protein tyrosine phosphatase (PTPN22) is associated with rheumatoid arthritis. *Am J Hum Genet* **75**, 330–337.

Black, D., Duncan, A., and Robins, S. P. (1988). Quantitative analysis of the pyridinium crosslinks of collagen in urine using ion-paired reversed-phase high-performance liquid chromatography. *Anal Biochem* **169**, 197–203.

Blezer, E. L. A., Nicolay, K., Bauer, J., Brok, H. P. M., and 't Hart, B. A. (2007). Quantitative MRI-pathology correlations of brain white matter lesions developing in a non-human primate model of multiple sclerosis. *NMR Biomed* **20**, 90–103.

Bolz, D. D., and Weis, J. J. (2004). Molecular mimicry to *Borrelia burgdorferi*: pathway to autoimmunity? *Autoimmunity* **37**, 387–392.

Bontrop, R. E. (2001). Nonhuman primates: essential partners in biomedical research. *Immunol Rev* **183**, 5–9.

Boon, L., Brok, H. P., Bauer, J. *et al.* (2001). Prevention of experimental autoimmune encephalomyelitis in the common marmoset (*Callithrix jacchus*) using a chimeric antagonist monoclonal antibody against human CD40 is associated with altered B cell responses. *J Immunol* **167**, 2942–2949.

Bourinbaiar, A. S. and Abulafia-Lapid, R. (2005). Autoimmunity, alloimmunization and immunotherapy of AIDS. *Autoimmun Rev* **4**, 403–409.

Brack, M. and Rothe, H. (1981). Chronic tubulointerstitial nephritis and wasting disease in marmosets (*Callithrix jacchus*). *Vet Pathol* **18**, 45–54.

Brok, H. P., Uccelli, A., Kerlero De Rosbo, N. *et al.* (2000). Myelin/oligodendrocyte glycoprotein-induced autoimmune encephalomyelitis in common marmosets: the encephalitogenic T cell epitope pMOG24–36 is presented by a monomorphic MHC class II molecule. *J Immunol* **165**, 1093–1101.

Brok, H. P., Bauer, J., Jonker, M. *et al.* (2001a). Nonhuman primate models of multiple sclerosis. *Immunol Rev* **183**, 173–185.

Brok, H. P., Tekoppele, J. M., Hakimi, J. *et al.* (2001b). Prophylactic and therapeutic effects of a humanized monoclonal antibody against the IL-2 receptor (DACLIZUMAB) on collagen-induced arthritis (CIA) in rhesus monkeys. *Clin Exp Immunol* **124**, 134–141.

Brok, H. P., Van Meurs, M., Blezer, E. *et al.* (2002). Prevention of experimental autoimmune encephalomyelitis in common marmosets using an anti-IL-12p40 monoclonal antibody. *J Immunol* **169**, 6554–6563.

Brok, H. P. M., Boven, L. A., van Meurs, M. *et al.* (2006). Mobilisation of CNS-specific autoreactive T-cells in primates by a CMV-derived peptide *submitted*.

Brück, W., Porada, P., Poser, S. *et al.* (1995). Monocyte/macrophage differentiation in early multiple sclerosis lesions. *Ann Neurol* **38**, 788–796.

Choy, E. H. and Panayi, G. S. (2001). Cytokine pathways and joint inflammation in rheumatoid arthritis. *N Engl J Med* **344**, 907–916.

Colvin, R. B. (2003). Chronic allograft nephropathy. *N Engl J Med* **349**, 2288–2290.

Contag, P. R. (2002). Whole-animal cellular and molecular imaging to accelerate drug development. *Drug Discov Today* **7**, 555–562.

Cooper, G. S. and Stroehla, B. C. (2003). The epidemiology of autoimmune diseases. *Autoimmun Rev* **2**, 119–125.

Darabi, K., Karulin, A. Y., Boehm, B. O. *et al.* (2004). The third signal in T cell-mediated autoimmune disease? *J Immunol* **173**, 92–99.

Davidson, A. and Diamond, B. (2001). Autoimmune diseases. *N Engl J Med* **345**, 340–350.

De Baets, M. and Stassen, M. H. (2002). The role of antibodies in myasthenia gravis. *J Neurol Sci* **202**, 5–11.

Delarasse, C., Daubas, P., Mars, L. T. *et al.* (2003). Myelin/oligodendrocyte glycoprotein-deficient (MOG-deficient) mice reveal lack of immune tolerance to MOG in wild-type mice. *J Clin Invest* **112**, 544–553.

Denton, M. D., Magee, C. C., and Sayegh, M. H. (1999). Immunosuppressive strategies in transplantation. *Lancet* **353**, 1083–1091.

Doxiadis, G. M., van der Wiel, M., Brok, H. P. M. *et al.* (2006). Reactivation of a conserved HLA-DR3-like pseudogene segment in a New World primate species by exon shuffling. *Proc Natl Acad Sci USA* **103**, 5864–5868.

Edwards, J. C., Szczepanski, L., Szechinski, J. *et al.* (2004). Efficacy of B-cell-targeted therapy with rituximab in patients with rheumatoid arthritis. *N Engl J Med* **350**, 2572–2581.

EMBL-EBI. Immuno Polymorphism Database, IPD-MHC. Non-Human Primate (NHP) Sequence Alignments (http://www.ebi.ac.uk/ipd/mhc/nhp/align.html). Accessed May 2007.

Fishman, J. A. and Rubin, R. H. (1998). Infection in organ-transplant recipients. *N Engl J Med* **338**, 1741–1751.

Fournie, G. J., Mas, M., Cautain, B. *et al.* (2001). Induction of autoimmunity through bystander effects. Lessons from immunological disorders induced by heavy metals. *J Autoimmun* **16**, 319–326.

Fujinami, R. S., von Herrath, M. G., Christen, U., and Whitton, J. L. (2006). Molecular mimicry, bystander activation, or viral persistence: infections and autoimmune disease. *Clin Microbiol Rev* **19**, 80–94.

Genain, C. P. and Hauser, S. L. (2001). Experimental allergic encephalomyelitis in the New World monkey *Callithrix jacchus*. *Immunol Rev* **183**, 159–172.

Genain, C. P., Nguyen, M. H., Letvin, N. L. *et al.* (1995). Antibody facilitation of multiple sclerosis-like lesions in a nonhuman primate. *J Clin Invest* **96**, 2966–2974.

Genain, C. P., Cannella, B., Hauser, S. L., and Raine, C. S. (1999). Identification of autoantibodies associated with myelin damage in multiple sclerosis. *Nat Med* **5**, 170–175.

Goossens, P. H., Schouten, G. J., 't Hart, B. A. *et al.* (1999). Feasibility of adenovirus-mediated nonsurgical synovectomy in collagen-induced arthritis-affected rhesus monkeys. *Hum Gene Ther* **10**, 1139–1149.

Gregersen, P. K. (2005). Pathways to gene identification in rheumatoid arthritis: PTPN22 and beyond. *Immunol Rev* **204**, 74–86.

Gregersen, P. K., and Batliwalla, F. (2005). PTPN22 and rheumatoid arthritis: gratifying replication. *Arthritis Rheum* **52**, 1952–1955.

Haig, D. (1999). What is a marmoset? *Am J Primatol* **49**, 285–296.

Herodin, F., Thullier, P., Garin, D., and Drouet, M. (2005). Nonhuman primates are relevant models for research in hematology, immunology and virology. *Eur Cytokine Netw* **16**, 104–116.

Jacobson, D. L., Gange, S. J., Rose, N. R., and Graham, N. M. (1997). Epidemiology and estimated population burden of selected autoimmune diseases in the United States. *Clin Immunol Immunopathol* **84**, 223–243.

Johns, T. G., and Bernard, C. C. (1999). The structure and function of myelin oligodendrocyte glycoprotein. *J Neurochem* **72**, 1–9.

Jonker, M. (1990). The importance of non-human primates for preclinical testing of immunosuppressive monoclonal antibodies. *Semin Immunol* **2**, 427–436.

Jonker, M., Danskine, A., Haanstra, K. *et al.* (2005). The autoimmune response to vimentin after renal transplantation in nonhuman primates is immunosuppression dependent. **80**, 385–393.

Jun, H. S. and Yoon, J. W. (2003). A new look at viruses in type 1 diabetes. *Diabetes Metab Res Rev* **19**, 8–31.

Kaaja, R. J. and Greer, I. A. (2005). Manifestations of chronic disease during pregnancy. *JAMA* **294**, 2751–2757.

Kennedy, R. C., Shearer, M. H., and Hildebrand, W. (1997). Nonhuman primate models to evaluate vaccine safety and immunogenicity. *Vaccine* **15**, 903–908.

Kerlero de Rosbo, N., Brok, H. P. *et al.* (2000). Rhesus monkeys are highly susceptible to experimental autoimmune encephalomyelitis induced by myelin oligodendrocyte glycoprotein: characterisation of immunodominant T- and B-cell epitopes. *J Neuroimmunol* **110**, 83–96.

King, C. and Sarvetnick, N. (1997). Organ-specific autoimmunity. *Curr Opin Immunol* **9**, 863–871.

Kraan, M. C., Versendaal, H., Jonker, M. *et al.* (1998). Asymptomatic synovitis precedes clinically manifest arthritis. *Arthritis Rheum* **41**, 1481–1488.

Laman, J. D., van Meurs, M., Schellekens, M. M. *et al.* (1998). Expression of accessory molecules and cytokines in acute EAE in marmoset monkeys (*Callithrix jacchus*). *J Neuroimmunol* **86**, 30–45.

Lawrence, R. C., Helmick, C. G., Arnett, F. C. *et al.* (1998). Estimates of the prevalence of arthritis and selected musculoskeletal disorders in the United States. *Arthritis Rheum* **41**, 778–799.

Ludlage, E. and Mansfield, K. (2003). Clinical care and diseases of the common marmoset (*Callithrix jacchus*). *Comp Med* **53**, 369–382.

Mansfield, K. (2003). Marmoset models commonly used in biomedical research. *Comp Med* **53**, 383–392.

Mansfield, K. G., Lin, K. C., Xia, D. *et al.* (2001). Enteropathogenic *Escherichia coli* and ulcerative colitis in cotton-top tamarins (*Saguinus oedipus*). *J Infect Dis* **184**, 803–807.

Massacesi, L., Genain, C. P., Lee-Parritz, D., Letvin, N. L., Canfield, D., and Hauser, S. L. (1995). Active and passively induced experimental autoimmune encephalomyelitis in common marmosets: a new model for multiple sclerosis. *Ann Neurol* **37**, 519–530.

McClure, H. M., Anderson, D. C., Fultz, P. N., Ansari, A. A., Lockwood, E., and Brodie, A. (1989). Spectrum of disease in macaque monkeys chronically infected with SIV/SMM. *Vet Immunol Immunopathol* **21**, 13–24.

Meinl, E., Hoch, R. M., Dornmair, K. *et al.* (1997). Encephalitogenic potential of myelin basic protein-specific T cells isolated from normal rhesus macaques. *Am J Pathol* **150**, 445–453.

Muchmore, E. A. (2001). Chimpanzee models for human disease and immunobiology. **183**, 86–93.

Myers, L. K., Higgins, G. C., Finkel, T. H. *et al.* (2001). Juvenile arthritis and autoimmunity to type II collagen. *Arthritis Rheum* **44**, 1775–1781.

Nandy, K. (1981). Brain-reactive antibodies in sera of aging non-human primates. *Mech Ageing Dev* **16**, 141–147.

Nielen, M. M., van Schaardenburg, D., Reesink, H. W. *et al.* (2004). Increased levels of C-reactive protein in serum from blood donors before the onset of rheumatoid arthritis. *Arthritis Rheum* **50**, 2423–2427.

Otting, N., Heijmans, C. M., Noort, R. C. *et al.* (2005). Unparalleled complexity of the MHC class I region in rhesus macaques. *Proc Natl Acad Sci USA* **102**, 1626–1631.

Ou, L. S., See, L. C., Wu, C. J., Kao, C. C., Lin, Y. L., and Huang, J. L. (2002). Association between serum inflammatory cytokines and disease activity in juvenile idiopathic arthritis. *Clin Rheumatol* **21**, 52–56.

Pachner, A. R., Gelderblom, H., and Cadavid, D. (2001). The rhesus model of Lyme neuroborreliosis. *Immunol Rev* **183**, 186–204.

Parkin, J. and Cohen, B. (2001). An overview of the immune system. *Lancet* **357**, 1777–1789.

Patel, D. D., Zachariah, J. P., and Whichard, L. P. (2001). CXCR3 and CCR5 ligands in rheumatoid arthritis synovium. *Clin Immunol* **98**, 39–45.

Penn, I. (2000). Post-transplant malignancy: the role of immunosuppression. *Drug Saf* **23**, 101–113.

Peterson, J. W., Bo, L., Mork, S., Chang, A., and Trapp, B. D. (2001). Transected neurites, apoptotic neurons, and reduced inflammation in cortical multiple sclerosis lesions. *Ann Neurol* **50**, 389–400.

Pettit, A. R., Ji, H., von Stechow, D., Muller, R. *et al.* (2001). TRANCE/RANKL knockout mice are protected from bone erosion in a serum transfer model of arthritis. *Am J Pathol* **159**, 1689–1699.

Poliani, P. L., Brok, H., Furlan, R. *et al.* (2001). Delivery to the central nervous system of a nonreplicative herpes simplex type 1 vector engineered with the interleukin 4 gene protects rhesus monkeys from hyperacute autoimmune encephalomyelitis. *Hum Gene Ther* **12**, 905–920.

Pomeroy, I. M., Matthews, P. M., Frank, J. A., Jordan, E. K., and Esiri, M. M. (2005). Demyelinated neocortical lesions in marmoset autoimmune encephalomyelitis mimic those in multiple sclerosis. *Brain* **128**, 2713–2721.

Price, W. S., Mendz, G. L., and Martenson, R. E. (1988). Conformation of a heptadecapeptide comprising the segment encephalitogenic in rhesus monkey. *Biochemistry* **27**, 8990–8999.

Quarta, L., Corrado, A., Melillo, N., and Cantatore, F. P. (2005). Juvenile idiopathic arthritis: an update on clinical and therapeutic approaches. *Ann Ital Med Int* **20**, 211–217.

Raine, C. S., Cannella, B., Hauser, S. L., and Genain, C. P. (1999). Demyelination in primate autoimmune encephalomyelitis and acute multiple sclerosis lesions: a case for antigen-specific antibody mediation. *Ann Neurol* **46**, 144–160.

Ravkina, L., Harib, I., Manovitch, Z., Deconenko, E., Letchinskaja, E., and Papilova, E. (1979). Hyperacute experimental allergic encephalomyelitis in rhesus monkeys as a model of acute necrotizing hemorrhagic encephalomyelitis. *J Neurol* **221**, 113–125.

Rivers, T. M. and Schwenkter, F. F. (1935). Encephalomyelitis accompanied by myelin destruction experimentally produced in monkeys. *J Exp Med* **61**, 698–703.

Rivers, T. M., Sprunt, D. H., and Berry, G. P. (1933). Observations on the attempts to produce acute disseminated allergic encephalomyelitis in primates. *J Exp Med* **58**, 39–53.

Rooney, M., David, J., Symons, J., Di Giovine, F., Varsani, H., and Woo, P. (1995). Inflammatory cytokine responses in juvenile chronic arthritis. *Br J Rheumatol* **34**, 454–460.

Rose, L. M., Richards, T., and Alvord, E. C., Jr. (1994). Experimental allergic encephalomyelitis (EAE) in nonhuman primates: a model of multiple sclerosis. *Lab Anim Sci* **44**, 508–512.

Rose, M. L. (1998). Endothelial cells as antigen-presenting cells: role in human transplant rejection. *Cell Mol Life Sci* **54**, 965–978.

Rose, N. R. and Bona, C. (1993). Defining criteria for autoimmune diseases (Witebsky's postulates revisited). *Immunol Today* **14**, 426–430.

Roses, A. D., Burns, D. K., Chissoe, S., Middleton, L., and St Jean, P. (2005). Disease-specific target selection: a critical first step down the right road. *Drug Discov Today* **10**, 177–189.

Roth, G. S., Mattison, J. A., Ottinger, M. A., Chachich, M. E., Lane, M. A., and Ingram, D. K. (2004). Aging in rhesus monkeys: relevance to human health interventions. *Science* **305**, 1423–1426.

Rothschild, B. M. (1994). Naturally occurring arthritis in monkeys. *Clin Exp Rheumatol* **12**, 347.

Rothschild, B. M. and Woods, R. J. (1989). Spondyloarthropathy in gorillas. *Semin Arthritis Rheum* **18**, 267–276.

Rothschild, B. M. and Woods, R. J. (1991). Reactive erosive arthritis in chimpanzees. *Am J Primatol* **25**, 49–56.

Sachs, D. H. (2003). Tolerance: Of mice and men. *J Clin Invest* **111**, 1819–1821.

Shadidi, K. R., Aarvak, T., Henriksen, J. E., Natvig, J. B., and Thompson, K. M. (2003). The Chemokines CCL5, CCL2 and CXCL12 play significant roles in the migration of Th1 cells into rheumatoid synovial tissue. *Scand J Immunol* **57**, 192–198.

Sigal, L. H. (1993). Cross-reactivity between *Borrelia burgdorferi* flagellin and a human axonal 64,000 molecular weight protein. *J Infect Dis* **167**, 1372–1378.

Sigal, L. H. and Tatum, A. H. (1988). Lyme disease patients' serum contains IgM antibodies to *Borrelia burgdorferi* that cross-react with neuronal antigens. *Neurology* **38**, 1439–1442.

Slierendregt, B. L., Hall, M., 't Hart, B. *et al.* (1995). Identification of an MHC-DPB1 allele involved in susceptibility to experimental autoimmune encephalomyelitis in rhesus macaques. *Int Immunol* **7**, 1671–1679.

Sumpter, T. L. and Wilkes, D. S. (2004). Role of autoimmunity in organ allograft rejection: a focus on immunity to type V collagen in the pathogenesis of lung transplant rejection. *Am J Physiol Lung Cell Mol Physiol* **286**, L1129–1139.

't Hart, B. A. and van Kooyk, Y. (2004). Yin-Yang regulation of autoimmunity by DCs. *Trends Immunol* **25**, 353–359.

't Hart, B. A., Bakker, N. P., Jonker, M., and Bontrop, R. E. (1993). Resistance to collagen-induced arthritis in rats and rhesus monkeys after immunization with attenuated type II collagen. *Eur J Immunol* **23**, 1588–1594.

't Hart, B. A., Bank, R. A., De Roos, J. A. *et al.* (1998a). Collagen-induced arthritis in rhesus monkeys: evaluation of markers for inflammation and joint degradation. *Br J Rheumatol* **37**, 314–323.

't Hart, B. A., Bauer, J., Muller, H. J. *et al.* (1998b). Histopathological characterization of magnetic resonance imaging-detectable brain white matter lesions in a primate model of multiple sclerosis: a correlative study in the experimental autoimmune encephalomyelitis model in common marmosets (Callithrix jacchus). *Am J Pathol* **153**, 649–663.

't Hart, B. A., van Meurs, M., Brok, H. P. *et al.* (2000). A new primate model for multiple sclerosis in the common marmoset. *Immunol Today* **21**, 290–297.

't Hart, B. A., Vervoordeldonk, M., Heeney, J. L., and Tak, P. P. (2003). Gene therapy in nonhuman primate models of human autoimmune disease. *Gene Ther* **10**, 890–901.

't Hart, B., Amor, S., and Jonker, M. (2004a). Evaluating the validity of animal models for research into therapies for immune-based disorders. *Drug Discov Today* **9**, 517–524.

't Hart, B. A., Laman, J. D., Bauer, J., Blezer, E. D., van Kooyk, Y., and Hintzen, R. Q. (2004b). Modelling of multiple sclerosis: lessons learned in a non-human primate. *The Lancet Neurol* **3**, 589–597.

't Hart, B. A., Vogels, J. T., Bauer, J., Brok, H. P. M., and Blezer, E. (2004c). Non-invasive measurement of brain damage in a primate model of multiple sclerosis. *Trends Mol Med* **10**, 85–91.

't Hart, B. A., Amor, S., and Bajramovic, J. J. (2005a). Modeling CNS inflammatory diseases in primates. *Screening Trends Drug Discovery* **206**, 36–38.

't Hart, B. A., Bauer, J., Brok, H. P., and Amor, S. (2005b). Nonhuman primate models of experimental autoimmune encephalomyelitis: variations on a theme. *J Neuroimmunol* **168**, 1–12.

't Hart, B. A., Blezer, E. L., Brok, H. P. *et al.* (2005c). Treatment with chimeric anti-human CD40 antibody suppresses MRI-detectable inflammation and enlargement of pre-existing brain lesions in common marmosets affected by MOG-induced EAE. *J Neuroimmunol* **163**, 31–39.

't Hart, B. A., Brok, H. P., Remarque, E. *et al.* (2005d). Suppression of ongoing disease in a nonhuman primate model of multiple sclerosis by a human-anti-human IL-12p40 antibody. *J Immunol* **175**, 4761–4768.

't Hart, B. A., Losen, M., Brok, H. P. M., and de Baets, M. H. (2005e). Chronic Diseases. In Wolfe-Coote, S. P. ed. *The Laboratory Primate*. Amsterdam: Elsevier Science, pp. 417–433.

't Hart, B. A., Smith, P., Amor, S., Strijkers, G. J., and Blezer, E. L. A. (2005f). MRI-guided immunotherapy development for multiple sclerosis in a primate. *Drug Discov Today* **11**, 58–66.

Tak, P. P., Hart, B. A., Kraan, M. C., Jonker, M., Smeets, T. J., and Breedveld, F. C. (1999). The effects of interferon beta treatment on arthritis. *Rheumatology (Oxford)* **38**, 362–369.

Terato, K., Arai, H., Shimozuru, Y. *et al.* (1989). Sex-linked differences in susceptibility of cynomolgus monkeys to type II collagen-induced arthritis. Evidence that epitope-specific immune suppression is involved in the regulation of type II collagen autoantibody formation. *Arthritis Rheum* **32**, 748–758.

Town, T., Nikolic, V., and Tan, J. (2005). The microglial "activation" continuum: from innate to adaptive responses. *J Neuroinflammation* **2**, 24.

van Beek, J., van Meurs, M., t Hart, B. A. *et al.* (2005). Decay-accelerating factor (CD55) is expressed by neurons in response to chronic but not acute autoimmune central nervous system inflammation associated with complement activation. *J Immunol* **174**, 2353–2365.

van den Berg, W. B. (1991). Impact of NSAID and steroids on cartilage destruction in murine antigen induced arthritis. *J Rheumatol Suppl* **27**, 122–123.

van Holten, J., Pavelka, K., Vencovsky, J. *et al.* (2005). A multicentre, randomised, double blind, placebo controlled phase II study of subcutaneous interferon beta-1a in the treatment of patients with active rheumatoid arthritis. *Ann Rheum Dis* **64**, 64–69.

Van Lambalgen, R. and Jonker, M. (1987). Experimental allergic encephalomyelitis in rhesus monkeys: II. Treatment of EAE with anti-T lymphocyte subset monoclonal antibodies. *Clin Exp Immunol* **68**, 305–312.

Vierboom, M. P., Jonker, M., Bontrop, R. E., and t Hart, B. (2005a). Modeling human arthritic diseases in nonhuman primates. *Arthritis Res Ther* **7**, 145–154.

Vierboom, M. P., Zavodny, P. J., Chou, C. C. *et al.* (2005b). Inhibition of the development of collagen-induced arthritis in rhesus monkeys by a small molecular weight antagonist of CCR5. *Arthritis Rheum* **52**, 627–636.

Villoslada, P., Abel, K., Heald, N., Goertsches, R., Hauser, S. L., and Genain, C. P. (2001). Frequency, heterogeneity and encephalitogenicity of T cells specific for myelin oligodendrocyte glycoprotein in naive outbred primates. *Eur J Immunol* **31**, 2942–2950.

Wedderburn, L. R., Robinson, N., Patel, A., Varsani, H., and Woo, P. (2000). Selective recruitment of polarized T cells expressing CCR5 and CXCR3 to the inflamed joints of children with juvenile idiopathic arthritis. *Arthritis Rheum* **43**, 765–774.

Whitton, J. L. and Fujinami, R. S. (1999). Viruses as triggers of autoimmunity: facts and fantasies. *Curr Opin Microbiol* **2**, 392–397.

Wierda, D., Smith, H. W., and Zwickl, C. M. (2001). Immunogenicity of biopharmaceuticals in laboratory animals. *Toxicology* **158**, 71–74.

Wilkin, T. (1989). Autoimmunity: attack, or defence? (The case for a primary lesion theory). *Autoimmunity* **3**, 57–73.

Wilkin, T. J. (1990). The primary lesion theory of autoimmunity: a speculative hypothesis. *Autoimmunity* **7**, 225–235.

Wollheim, F. A. (2000). Markers of disease in rheumatoid arthritis. *Curr Opin Rheumatol* **12**, 200–204.

Wroblewska, Z., Gilden, D., Devlin, M. *et al.* (1979). Cytomegalovirus isolation from a chimpanzee with acute demyelinating disease after inoculation of multiple sclerosis brain cells. *Infect Immun* **25**, 1008–1015.

Yoon, J. W., Eun, H. M., Essani, K., Roncari, D. A., and Bryan, L. E. (1987). Possible mechanisms in the pathogenesis of virus-induced diabetes mellitus. *Clin Invest Med* **10**, 450–456.

Yu, D. and Kuipers, J. G. (2003). Role of bacteria and HLA-B27 in the pathogenesis of reactive arthritis. *Rheum Dis Clin North Am* **29**, 21–36, v–vi.

Zandman-Goddard, G. and Shoenfeld, Y. (2002). HIV and autoimmunity. *Autoimmun Rev* **1**, 329–337.

Zerhouni, E. (2005). Progress in autoimmune disease research. In *Report to Congress NIH*. Bethesda: NIH, pp. 1–146.

CHAPTER 5

Self-injurious Behavior: Nonhuman Primate Models for the Human Condition

Corrine K. Lutz and Jerrold S. Meyer

EXPRESSION OF SELF-INJURIOUS BEHAVIOR

Self-injurious behavior (SIB) is a serious disorder defined as potential or actual physical damage directed towards one's own body without suicidal intent (Favazza, 1989). SIB is often impulsive (individuals may contemplate self-mutilation for just a few minutes or less before performing the act) (Nock and Prinstein, 2005), and it is also diverse with respect to the forms of the behavior as well as the physical and environmental factors involved. Types of injurious behavior can range from head-banging (Coman and Houghton, 1991; Iwata *et al.*, 1994; Beckett *et al.*, 2002), self-hitting (Coman and Houghton, 1991; Iwata *et al.*, 1994; Dykens and Smith, 1998) and self-biting (Ando and Yoshimura, 1978; Iwata *et al.*, 1994; Dykens and Smith, 1998) to self-burning and cutting (Jones, 1986; Kemperman *et al.*, 1997). Severity can range from little or no tissue damage to extreme mutilation such as eye enucleation (Favazza, 1998) or digit amputation (Nyhan, 1976).

Self-injurious behavior in people

Self-injurious behavior has been associated with a wide range of disorders that include mental retardation or learning disabilities (Griffin *et al.*, 1987; Collacott *et al.*, 1998; Saloviita, 2000; Deb *et al.*, 2001), personality disorders (Schaffer *et al.*, 1982; Gardner and Cowdry, 1985; Kemperman *et al.*, 1997; Bohus *et al.*, 2000), schizophrenia (Green, 1967), autism (Mace *et al.*, 1998), Tourette syndrome (Robertson *et al.*, 1989; Robertson, 1992), and certain rare genetic disorders (Lesch and Nyhan, 1964;

Primate Models of Children's Health and Developmental Disabilities

Sansom *et al.*, 1993; Dykens and Smith, 1998; Symons *et al.*, 1999; Finucane *et al.*, 2001). Although SIB is often associated with institutionalized (Beckett *et al.*, 2002) and prison populations (Jones, 1986; Coid *et al.*, 1992; Fulwiler *et al.*, 1997; Boiko and Lester, 2000; Matsumoto *et al.*, 2005), it also occurs in the general population (Briere and Gil, 1998; Ross and Heath, 2002; Klonsky *et al.*, 2003).

Because of the diverse conditions under which SIB occurs, several authors have proposed classification systems for this disorder. For example, Villalba and Harrington (2000) argue that SIB may be considered as a primary disturbance of either action or thought, and they further subdivide each of these general categories into several subcategories. Simeon and Favazza (2001) propose a somewhat different classification system composed of four categories: (1) stereotypic SIB, (2) major SIB, (3) compulsive SIB, and (4) impulsive SIB. Stereotypic SIB is found in individuals with profound intellectual deficits (e.g. in mental retardation, autism, and genetic defects). In these populations, the expression of SIB is highly repetitive and appears to be largely independent of emotion or social context. Major SIB refers to acts of extreme self-directed violence (e.g. eye enucleation, limb amputation, or castration) that might be associated with a psychotic break. The category of compulsive SIB includes ritualized patterns of self-inflicted wounding (e.g. hair pulling, scratching, or nail biting) that occur repetitively many times a day and are thought to be driven by a compulsive urge to perform the behavior. Finally, impulsive SIB occurs in response to emotional stress or anxiety, is associated with tension reduction and mood elevation, and can be manifested in relatively severe forms of self-injury such as cutting and burning. This form of SIB may occur in certain personality disorders (e.g. borderline or antisocial personality disorder), anxiety disorders (e.g. post-traumatic stress disorder), and other psychiatric conditions, but it also appears to be on the rise among teenagers and young adults in the general population. Having a history of early childhood trauma appears to be an important risk factor for impulsive SIB. As discussed below, the classification scheme of Simeon and Favazza seems to have some usefulness for categorizing SIB in monkeys.

Depending on the population examined, prevalence rates can vary greatly. For example, the extent of SIB in populations with learning disabilities is 1.7% to 23.8% for non-institutionalized individuals (Rojahn, 1986; Griffin *et al.*, 1987; Deb *et al.*, 2001), while the incidence can range from 13.6% to 40.6% for institutionalized populations (Griffin *et al.*, 1986; Saloviita, 2000). The percentages are higher for individuals with schizophrenia (40% based on Green, 1967) as well as those with several genetic disorders that cause a predisposition towards SIB (48.6% to virtually 100% of patients with Smith–Magenis syndrome, Lesch–Nyhan syndrome, Rett syndrome, or Prader–Willi syndrome; Nyhan, 1976; Sansom *et al.*, 1993; Symons *et al.*, 1999; Finucane *et al.*, 2001). The prevalence of SIB is approximately 4% in the general population (Briere and Gil, 1998; Klonsky *et al.*, 2003), but the reported prevalence among adolescents is over three times as high (Ross and Heath, 2002).

Self-injurious behavior in nonhuman species

Self-injurious behavior is not limited to humans. This behavior has been observed in a variety of species including rats and mice (Jinnah *et al.*, 1999; Breese *et al.*, 2005), New World monkeys (McGrogan and King, 1982), Old World monkeys (Bayne *et al.*, 1995; Baker, 2002; Bellanca and Crockett, 2002), and chimpanzees (Walsh *et al.*, 1982; Fritz *et al.*, 1992). As in the human population, the type and extent of self-injury varies and includes such behaviors as self-biting (Fittinghoff *et al.*, 1974; Anderson and Chamove, 1980; see Figure 5.1), self-slapping (Fittinghoff *et al.*, 1974; Anderson and Chamove, 1980), and head-banging (Levison, 1970; Schaefer, 1970).

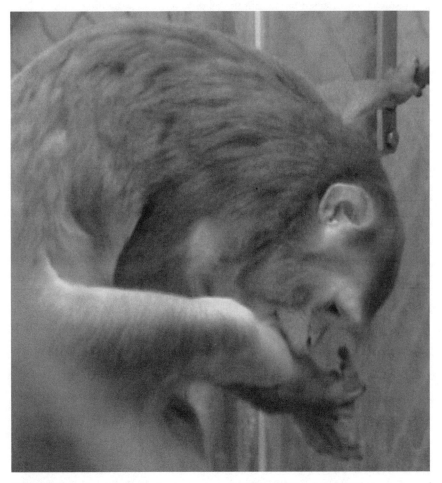

FIGURE 5.1   An adult female rhesus macaque exhibiting self-biting behavior. Photo courtesy of Ernie Davis. (See Plate 3 for the color version of this figure.)

In many laboratory studies, SIB has been experimentally induced through procedures such as brain lesioning (Breese *et al.*, 2005), administration of various drugs (Peffer-Smith *et al.*, 1983; Cromwell *et al.*, 1999; Jinnah *et al.*, 1999), or restrictive rearing practices (e.g. isolation rearing) (Cross and Harlow, 1965; Suomi *et al.*, 1971; Gluck and Sackett, 1974). However, SIB can also occur spontaneously in captive primates (see references in above paragraph). In fact, we and others have noted that a consistent percentage of laboratory-housed macaque monkeys exhibit some form of SIB. These animals are typically reared in social conditions but later housed individually. Retrospective studies of colony records at two different primate facilities found that 11% to 15.8% of individually housed macaque monkeys had a record of self-inflicted injury (Bayne *et al.*, 1995; Lutz *et al.*, 2003b). Self-injury often occurs as a result of self-directed biting, but not all bites result in wounding. Indeed, Lutz and co-workers (2003b) found that wounding was actually infrequent, with a median lifetime incidence of 2 in animals that did wound. Furthermore, over half of the animals with a record of self-biting had not wounded themselves at all. Self-biting often goes unnoticed or untreated, because it usually does not break the skin. Therefore, it is not clear whether self-biting is a precursor to wounding, or whether self-inflicted wounding and non-injurious self-biting are two separate pathologies.

We believe that spontaneously occurring SIB in nonhuman primates is a promising model for the human condition. Unlike previous animal models of self-injury that utilize brain lesions, drug administration, or impoverished rearing conditions, this model does not require special procedures for inducing the behavioral pathology. M. A. Novak has proposed that monkeys that develop a pattern of self-biting and self-injury despite being reared socially are suffering from "reactive SIB" (personal communication). Reactive SIB in monkeys is similar to Simeon and Favazza's category of impulsive SIB in humans. In this form the disorder is hypothesized to result from heightened anxiety and to serve the function of tension reduction and mood elevation. Research from our laboratory not only supports this classification but has also given rise to a novel hypothesis of SIB that is presented in the next section. Later sections will present current findings on the factors that give rise to SIB as well as the treatments for this disorder. Where possible, we will compare the human SIB literature with that of nonhuman primates, focusing particularly on macaque monkeys.

DEVELOPMENT AND MAINTENANCE OF SELF-INJURIOUS BEHAVIOR

Several hypotheses have been proposed to explain the initiation and continuation of SIB in both human and nonhuman primates. According to these hypotheses, self-injury may be initiated or maintained through genetic abnormalities (Cataldo and Harris, 1982; Belfiore and Dattilio, 1990; Symons, 1995), neurochemical abnormalities (Belfiore and Dattilio, 1990; Winchel and Stanley, 1991; King, 1993; Symons, 1995), anxiety reduction/mood regulation (Bennun, 1984; Brain *et al.*, 1998;

Kemperman *et al.*, 1997), self-stimulation (Belfiore and Dattilio, 1990; King, 1993; Symons, 1995), redirected aggression (Bennun, 1984; Simeon *et al.*, 1992), positive and/or negative reinforcement (Belfiore and Dattilio, 1990; King, 1993; Iwata *et al.*, 1994; Symons, 1995; Nock and Prinstein, 2004), social reinforcement (Bennun, 1984), or through a group epidemic (Bennun, 1984). More than one of these hypotheses may be correct, not only because they encompass different levels of analysis (i.e. molecular to behavioral and social) but also because of the diverse categories of SIB as noted earlier. The possibility of multiple etiologic and mechanistic factors in SIB greatly increases the difficulties inherent in formulating effective assessment and treatment strategies.

Our studies of spontaneously occurring SIB in macaque monkeys have led to the conclusion that this disorder arises and is maintained through a combination of developmental, behavioral, and physiological factors. Specifically, our integrated developmental–neurochemical hypothesis proposes that adverse early experiences followed by later stressful events can result in heightened anxiety and a dysregulation of various neurochemical and neuroendocrine systems involved in emotionality and stress. In vulnerable individuals (possibly determined genetically), this increased anxiety and neurochemical/neuroendocrine dysregulation is manifested as SIB, one function of which is to alleviate arousal and stress in the organism (Tiefenbacher *et al.*, 2005c). Evidence in support of this hypothesis will be presented as we discuss the various factors believed to be responsible for the onset and maintenance of SIB.

Adverse early experience

Effects of abuse and neglect in people

In individuals without genetic or developmental disorders, there is a strong association between childhood trauma (e.g. physical or emotional neglect and/or sexual or physical abuse) and SIB (van der Kolk *et al.*, 1991; Briere and Gil, 1998; Lipschitz *et al.*, 1999; Bierer *et al.*, 2003; Yates, 2004). Several studies found that the frequency of childhood abuse was greater in subjects who self-mutilated than in those who did not (Coid *et al.*, 1992; Zweig-Frank *et al.*, 1994); well over half of self-injurers retrospectively reported a history of child abuse or neglect (Favazza and Conteiro, 1989; van der Kolk *et al.*, 1991; Briere and Gil, 1998). In a study of 240 female habitual self-mutilators, 62% of the subjects reported childhood abuse, and the average age of onset was 6–7 years (Favazza and Conterio, 1989). Similar results were obtained in a study of psychiatric inpatients. Those who self-mutilated reported more traumatic childhood experiences than those who did not self-mutilate (Nijman *et al.*, 1999). Conversely, subjects with a history of abuse are more likely to self-injure. In a study of adult women, 20% of those with a history of physical abuse exhibited SIB, while only 9% of subjects with no history of abuse engaged in self-injury (Carlin *et al.*, 1994). Similarly, in a study of institutionally reared orphaned children in Romania, 24% exhibited some form of SIB after joining adoptive families (Beckett et al., 2002). The age at which abuse occurred also plays a role in both the expression and the severity of SIB. In subjects who self-injured by cutting, the earlier the trauma, the more frequently they cut themselves (van der Kolk et al., 1991).

Rearing condition effects in nonhuman primates

As with humans, research on nonhuman primates has demonstrated that maternal separation, isolation, and/or neglect can have devastating effects on the animal's later behavior. Isolation rearing is an extreme form of deprivation for infant monkeys that was studied many years ago but is no longer used in research. In this condition, infant monkeys were separated from their mothers and reared for up to 1 year in chambers in which they could not see, hear, or touch other animals (Harlow and Harlow, 1962a). While isolated, the animals exhibited a number of self-directed behaviors including self-manipulation, grasping, and rubbing (Baysinger et al., 1972). When removed from isolation, the subjects displayed a pattern of isolate disturbance behaviors which included rocking, self-mouthing and self-clasping (Harlow and Harlow, 1962a, 1962b). Moreover, these behaviors tended to decrease over time and be replaced with other kinds of stereotypies and, in some cases, SIB (reviewed by Jones and Barraclough, 1978). Self-injurious behavior in isolate-reared monkeys was also most likely to be observed in male subjects (Gluck and Sackett, 1974).

In the partial isolation condition, infant monkeys are raised in individual wire cages from which they can see and hear, but not touch, conspecifics. This condition has been used for both experimental as well as husbandry situations such as cases of maternal rejection or health problems (Mason and Sponholz, 1963; Bayne and Novak, 1998). Although partial isolation is less extreme than total isolation, animals reared in this condition also exhibited behavioral problems including self-clasping and self-biting to the point of injury (Harlow and Harlow, 1962a). When exposed to a novel environment, partial isolates reacted with clasping, crouching, and stereotyped behavior. In contrast, wild-caught subjects displayed none of these self-directed behaviors and instead, spent more time locomoting (Mason and Green, 1962). In another study in which an experimenter rapped on the subject's cage with a metal dowel, partial isolates exhibited SIB (repeated self-biting and/or self-slapping), whereas this behavior was not observed in the wild-born controls (Fittinghoff et al., 1974). Similarly, self-biting was exclusively demonstrated by subjects raised in partial isolation in comparison to those wild-caught and subsequently individually housed at approximately 2 years of age (Suomi et al., 1971).

Younger animals appear to be more adversely affected by isolation than older ones. The absence of social contact early in life, such as during the first two months of age, is a significant risk factor for SIB (Anderson and Chamove, 1985). For example, rhesus monkeys isolated for six weeks before 90 days of age exhibited many self-directed behaviors, whereas older monkeys (3 years of age) isolated for a longer period of time (80 days) did not display these types of behaviors (McKinney *et al.*, 1973). In general, SIB is less likely to occur in monkeys raised socially, whether in captivity or in the wild (Fittinghoff *et al.*, 1974; Anderson and Chamove, 1980, 1985). However, even when animals are socially reared, the age at which an animal is removed from the social environment and individually housed is important. The earlier that social separation and individual housing occur, the greater the risk of developing SIB at a later time (Lutz *et al.*, 2003b).

Alterations in neurochemical and neuroendocrine systems

In addition to extrinsic factors such as rearing and housing conditions, a variety of neurochemical and neuroendocrine systems also seem to play a role in the development and expression of SIB. Two different approaches have been used to investigate the putative involvement of these systems: (1) comparisons of individuals with and without SIB, and (2) assessments of the therapeutic efficacy of different pharmacologic agents to reduce the incidence of SIB. The majority of this work in humans and/or in nonhuman primates has focused on the serotonergic, dopaminergic, and opioid systems, as well as the hypothalamic-pituitary-adrenal (HPA) axis.

Serotonin

Serotonin (5-HT) is one of the neurotransmitters most frequently implicated in SIB. One common finding has been an association between SIB and a blunting of neuroendocrine (i.e. prolactin and/or cortisol) responses to a serotonergic agonist such as d-fenfluramine or meta-chlorophenylpiperazine (m-CPP). Results of this kind have been reported for patients with personality disorders (Herpertz *et al.*, 1997; New *et al.*, 1997; Dolan *et al.*, 2001) and for women with bulimia nervosa (Steiger *et al.*, 2001) (however, see also Mulder and Joyce, 2002, who found no relationship between SIB and the prolactin response to fenfluramine in depressed men). Moreover, a number of studies have found that treatment with a selective serotonin reuptake inhibitor (SSRI) such as fluoxetine (Prozac), sertraline (Zoloft), or paroxetine (Paxil) reduced the incidence of SIB in patients with mental retardation/developmental disabilities, borderline personality disorder, and Lesch–Nyhan syndrome (Mizuno and Yugari, 1975; Markovitz *et al.*, 1991; Garber *et al.*, 1992; Markowitz, 1992; Ricketts *et al.*, 1993; Jawed *et al.*, 1994; Hellings *et al.*, 1996; Lewis *et al.*, 1996; Davanzo *et al.*, 1998; Singh *et al.*, 1998). Similar findings were obtained using the 5-HT_{1A} receptor agonist buspirone (Verhoeven and Tuinier, 1996).

The findings described above support the possibility that SIB in various human clinical disorders might stem, at least in part, from low activity of the serotonergic system. Yet there is relatively little direct evidence for this hypothesis. For example, SIB has not been reliably associated with low cerebrospinal fluid (CSF) levels of the 5-HT metabolite 5-hydroxyindoleacetic acid (5-HIAA) in patients with personality disorders (Gardner *et al.*, 1990; Simeon *et al.*, 1992), mental retardation (Verhoeven *et al.*, 1999), or Lesch–Nyhan syndrome (Saito and Takashima, 2000). From these findings we can conclude that SIB in humans is unlikely to be caused by reduced 5-HT synthesis or turnover.

Mixed results relating SIB to 5-HT have also been obtained in nonhuman primates (specifically rhesus monkeys). Early work by Kraemer and Clarke (1990) found that SIB in monkeys that had experienced early social deprivation was associated with changes in serotonergic function; however, these changes were complex and varied as a function of the age of the animals. Moreover, later studies from our laboratory that investigated socially reared monkeys with a record of self-inflicted wounding found no difference between these subjects and control (non-wounding) monkeys either in baseline levels of CSF 5-HIAA or hormonal responses to a fenfluramine challenge (Tiefenbacher *et al.*, 2000, 2003). On the other hand, self-directed biting is reportedly reduced by treatment of monkeys with serotonergic agonists such as fluoxetine, buspirone, or the 5-HT precursor L-tryptophan (Weld *et al.*, 1998; Fontenot *et al.*, 2005).

In summary, both the human and nonhuman primate literature provide evidence that SIB can be ameliorated, at least partially, by administration of serotonergic agents. There are also several reports of blunted responses to serotonergic challenge drugs in patients with SIB. Yet these findings are not supported by evidence for differences in serotonergic activity as determined by 5-HIAA levels in the CSF. There are at least two possible reasons for this apparent discrepancy. First, it may be the case that serotonergic dysfunction in SIB occurs postsynaptically, at the level of 5-HT receptor expression and/or signaling, rather than presynaptically. This hypothesis can be tested directly by postmortem studies or (in the case of receptor expression) by appropriate brain imaging studies. Second, we cannot exclude the possibility that 5-HT-based treatments reduce SIB by acting through a mechanism distinct from the neurochemical mechanism that has given rise to the disorder itself. It is also important to note that both aggressive and impulsive behaviors are commonly linked to SIB (Simeon *et al.*, 1992; Herpertz *et al.*, 1997), and thus low serotonergic activity (and its reversal by serotonergic agonists) may be more closely related to those behaviors than specifically to SIB (Brown *et al.*, 1982; Linnoila *et al.*, 1983; Lopez-Ibor *et al.*, 1985; Higley *et al.*, 1992; Mehlman *et al.*, 1994). Therefore, it is critical that future studies separate more carefully the potential involvement of 5-HT in SIB from its role in aggression and impulsivity.

Dopamine

There is also an extensive literature linking SIB to alterations in the dopamine (DA) system. Much of this work has centered around Lesch–Nyhan syndrome, a genetic disorder of purine metabolism that appears to cause a secondary disturbance in the development of the ascending DA pathways innervating the forebrain. This syndrome has a number of behavioral consequences, including severe mental retardation, motor dysfunction, and repetitive SIB that is often manifested as self-biting behavior (Baumeister and Frye, 1985). An early postmortem study comparing small numbers of Lesch–Nyhan patients with age-matched controls found significant reductions in the concentrations of both DA and the DA metabolite homovanillic acid (HVA) in the caudate nucleus, putamen, external pallidum, and nucleus accumbens (Lloyd *et al.*, 1981). No such decreases were observed for either 5-HT or 5-HIAA in these same brain regions. Subsequent studies confirmed this selective dopaminergic deficit by demonstrating reduced CSF levels of HVA but no decreases in 5-HIAA in Lesch–Nyhan patients (Silverstein *et al.*, 1985; Jankovic *et al.*, 1988). Most recently, brain-imaging studies found evidence for a reduced density of DA nerve terminals in the caudate nucleus and frontal cortex (Ernst *et al.*, 1996; Wong *et al.*, 1996), suggesting a deficit in the dopaminergic innervation of these areas. Of course, the mere presence of DA abnormalities does not prove that these abnormalities are responsible for SIB in Lesch–Nyhan patients. However, such a relationship is suggested by research showing that when dopaminergic fibers are destroyed in neonatal rats by administration of the DA neurotoxin 6-hydroxydopamine (6-OHDA), later administration of a DA agonist elicits severe self-biting and self-mutilation (Breese *et al.*, 2005). Denervation-related supersensitivity of D_1 receptors is thought to underlie SIB in the neonatal 6-OHDA-lesioned rat model (Breese *et al.*, 2005), but in Lesch–Nyhan patients there is more evidence for D_2 receptor upregulation (Saito and Takashima, 2000).

If SIB can potentially be produced by stimulation of supersensitive or upregulated DA receptors, then it stands to reason that DA receptor antagonists should be able to attenuate if not block the occurrence of this behavioral pathology. While there is little evidence at present for such an effect of DA antagonists in Lesch–Nyhan syndrome (Nyhan, 2000; Saito and Takashima, 2000), there is a considerable literature on the responses of mentally retarded/developmentally disabled individuals to neuroleptic (antipsychotic) drugs, which generally block D_2 and sometimes also D_1 receptors. Overall, these studies have found mixed results, with positive responses (i.e. reduced incidence or severity of SIB) in some cases but not others (Baumeister *et al.*, 1993; Schroeder *et al.*, 1995; Clarke, 1998). Despite these inconclusive findings, however, there is a continuing interest in the possible therapeutic benefits of DA antagonists, especially atypical neuroleptics such as risperidone, olanzapine, or quetiapine that interact with additional molecular targets such as 5-HT_2 receptors (see later section on drug treatments for SIB).

Several studies have also examined the possible involvement of DA in SIB in non-human primates. When young green monkeys were subjected to unilateral ventromedial tegmental lesions that destroyed most of the DA neurons in this area, administration of mixed D_1/D_2 agonists 10–14 years later elicited significant digit biting contralateral to the lesioned side (Goldstein *et al.*, 1986; Goldstein, 1989). These findings are reminiscent of the effects of DA agonists in adult rats given neonatal 6-OHDA lesions. Other studies have investigated the role of DA in SIB without prior lesioning. For example, the DA-releasing drug amphetamine was demonstrated to increase SIB in stumptailed macaque monkeys that already exhibited the behavior, but not in animals that did not previously exhibit SIB (Peffer-Smith *et al.*, 1983). The mixed DA receptor agonist apomorphine tended to increase the occurrence of SIB in isolate-reared and (to a lesser extent) socially reared rhesus monkeys, although the effect did not quite reach statistical significance (Lewis *et al.*, 1990). Moreover, Taylor and co-workers (2005) reported a case study in which a female monkey suffering from SIB directed towards one of her cheeks was helped by treatment with a low dose of the typical neuroleptic drug chlorpromazine along with environmental enrichment. On the other hand, research from our laboratory found that the levels of HVA in the CSF of rhesus monkeys with a history of self-inflicted wounding did not differ from the levels found in control animals with no such record. In addition, the levels of HVA were not related to the rates of self-directed biting in these animals (Tiefenbacher *et al.*, 2000). Thus, while it may be possible to elicit SIB in nonhuman primates with certain dopaminergic drug treatments, it remains to be shown that spontaneously occurring SIB (such as in the cohort we have studied) is associated with abnormalities in this neurotransmitter system.

Opioid system

A third neurotransmitter/neuromodulator system that is frequently implicated in the expression of SIB is the endogenous opioid system (Herman, 1990). This work began with the publication over 20 years ago of two case studies in which naloxone, a short-acting antagonist of opioid receptors, significantly reduced the occurrence of SIB (Richardson and Zaleski, 1983; Sandman *et al.*, 1983). In the report by Sandman and co-workers, the subjects were suffering from mental retardation, and the majority of subsequent research on the therapeutic efficacy of opioid receptor antagonists has focused on this population. In addition, naloxone was later replaced with naltrexone, another opioid antagonist that is longer acting than naloxone and that can be taken orally. A number of studies have reported that at least some mentally retarded patients with SIB respond positively to naltrexone treatment, although the percentage of responders varies widely as a function of dose, gender, and other factors that have yet to be elucidated (see review by Symons *et al.*, 2004).

The ability of opioid receptor antagonists to reduce SIB raises the possibility of abnormalities in opioid receptors and/or in the synthesis and release of endogenous opioid peptides in people with this behavioral pathology. In support of this idea, elevated baseline levels of plasma β-endorphin have been found in mentally retarded subjects exhibiting SIB compared to control subjects (Sandman, 1988; however, see also Verhoeven *et al.*, 1999 for conflicting results). β-Endorphin and adrenocorticotropic hormone (ACTH) are among several biologically active peptides that are liberated from the same protein precursor (proopiomelanocortin, or POMC), and thus these substances are thought to be co-released (coupled) under normal circumstances. Therefore, it is of interest that Sandman's group has reported that after an episode of SIB, there appears to be an uncoupling of β-endorphin and ACTH such that their respective plasma levels are not significantly correlated as they are under baseline conditions (Sandman *et al.*, 1997, 2003). The cellular mechanism underlying this dissociation remains to be determined.

Acupuncture- or acupressure-analgesia in people has been associated with the release of endogenous opioids (Ulett *et al.*, 1998). In a study of 29 students with intellectual disabilities, 32% of self-injurious behaviors such as biting, slapping, scratching, and rubbing were directed to acupuncture-analgesia body sites, even though only 8% of the body's surface area is covered by these sites (Symons and Thompson, 1997). This result suggests that acts of self-injury may be reinforced by opioid peptide release. Other indirect evidence that SIB may cause the release of endogenous opioids comes from reports of mood enhancement (Kemperman *et al.*, 1997) as well as altered pain sensitivity (Russ *et al.*, 1999; Bohus *et al.*, 2000) following episodes of self-injury.

Two hypotheses relating the opioid system with SIB have been proposed. Although both of these hypotheses have been criticized (see for example, the commentary by King *et al.*, 1991, and the response by DeMet and Sandman, 1991), they continue to inform our thinking about the possible role of endogenous opioids in SIB. The "addiction" hypothesis maintains that individuals can become dependent on endogenous opioids that are released during episodes of SIB (Sandman *et al.*, 1990; Thompson *et al.*, 1995). For example, in patients with moderate to profound mental retardation and with a history of SIB, plasma β-endorphin was elevated after episodes of self-injury, and those with the greatest increase after such episodes showed the greatest reduction in SIB after treatment with naltrexone (Sandman *et al.*, 1997). It is also worth noting that opioid antagonist treatment sometimes causes an initial increase rather than a decrease in SIB (Baumeister *et al.*, 1993). This seemingly paradoxical effect could be interpreted as an extinction burst brought about by removal of the SIB-induced opioid reinforcement.

Alternatively, the "analgesia" hypothesis proposes that individuals who exhibit SIB have an elevated pain threshold brought about by a congenitally hyperactive opioid system (Cataldo and Harris, 1982; Herman, 1990). For example, subjects diagnosed with borderline personality disorder who self-injured reported that they tended not to feel pain when injuring themselves, suggesting that they were experiencing analgesia (Leibenluft *et al.*, 1987; Coid *et al.*, 1992). Subjects with bipolar disorder and a history of SIB also showed a reduction in pain during a cold-pressor test in comparison to control subjects (Russ *et al.*, 1999; Bohus *et al.*, 2000). When naloxone was administered to subjects who reported no pain during bouts of self-injury, the pain intensity ratings increased during the cold-pressor test (Russ *et al.*, 1994). Although both the addiction and the analgesia hypotheses may explain why SIB is maintained in certain subject populations, they do not explain how or why the behavior is initiated in the first place (Carr, 1977).

Much less research has been done to examine the possible role of endogenous opioids in the expression of SIB in nonhuman primates. Nevertheless, a few relevant studies can be mentioned. Rhesus monkeys with a history of self-biting preferentially direct this biting behavior towards areas that can be associated with acupressure analgesia (Marinus *et al.*, 2000), and nonhuman primates have demonstrated acupuncture analgesia (Vierck *et al.*, 1974) that can be reversed with an injection of naloxone (Ha *et al.*, 1981). In one study of rhesus monkeys with a history of self-inflicted wounding, those with a wounding record had lower CSF levels of the opioid peptide metenkephalin than those without such a record. In addition, these levels were positively correlated with the proportion of bites directed towards acupressure sites (Tiefenbacher *et al.*, 2003). These findings suggest that self-directed biting in some cases may be used to release endogenous opioids, which is consistent with the addiction hypothesis of opioid involvement in human SIB.

Hypothalamic-pituitary-adrenal axis

Some investigators have hypothesized that heightened stress, tension, or other types of negative affect could precipitate episodes of SIB, particularly impulsive SIB as described by Simeon and Favazza (2001). Several studies have investigated the relationship between stress and SIB by examining the functioning of the HPA axis, one of the major physiological stress systems. For example, adult mentally retarded subjects rated as having primarily self-injurious aberrant behaviors had a tendency towards lower levels of plasma cortisol and corticosteroid-binding globulin in comparison with a retarded control group (Verhoeven *et al.*, 1999). In contrast, a case study of a patient with borderline personality disorder who exhibited SIB found that night-time urinary cortisol excretion peaked prior to a self-injurious act and then returned to baseline levels afterwards (Sachsse *et al.*, 2002). There was also a significant positive correlation between SIB severity and salivary cortisol in adults with developmental disabilities (Symons *et al.*, 2003). On the other hand, in studies by Sandman and colleagues of developmentally disabled subjects housed in a residential treatment center, there were no significant differences in plasma levels of either cortisol or ACTH measured after a subject exhibited an episode of SIB when compared to control samples taken when no SIB occurred (Sandman *et al.*, 1997, 2003). These latter findings suggest either that SIB is not associated with stress in this clinical population, or that acts of self-injury prevent or alleviate tension/stress so as to prevent stimulation of the HPA axis.

There is also a complex relationship between SIB and HPA axis activity in nonhuman primates. An early study by Faucheux *et al.* (1976) found that stumptail macaques (*Macaca arctoides*) with a history of autoaggression had lower urinary cortisol excretion than non-autoaggressive controls. There was also a negative correlation between the intensity of the autoaggressive behavior and levels of cortisol in the former group. In another study of stumptail macaques, the amount of SIB was inversely related to cortisol secretion (Chamove *et al.*, 1985). More recent studies in our laboratory found that socially reared but individually housed rhesus monkeys with a history of self-wounding showed a blunted plasma cortisol response to the mild stress of restraint and venipuncture (Tiefenbacher *et al.*, 2000). Similar to the findings of Faucheux *et al.*, plasma cortisol levels were negatively correlated with rates of self-biting. In a later study, monkeys that were self-wounders did not differ from non-wounders either with respect to the suppressive effect of a low-dose dex-amethasone challenge on urinary free cortisol excretion or with respect to plasma cortisol concentrations following ACTH stimulation (Tiefenbacher *et al.*, 2004). Interestingly, however, when the same data were analyzed according to rates of self-biting, high-frequency biters showed a decreased negative feedback response to the dexamethasone challenge compared with low frequency biters, and they also exhib-ited a trend towards a reduced plasma cortisol response to ACTH. These results sug-gest that HPA axis dysregulation in rhesus monkeys with SIB can be related either to wounding history or to the behavioral manifestation of the pathology (i.e. self-biting), depending on the circumstances. As a final point, although major environ-mental stressors are capable of eliciting increases in abnormal behavior (including SIB) in monkeys (Davenport, personal communication), we have no evidence at this time for elevated HPA activity during episodes of self-biting. Indeed, samples of salivary cortisol collected shortly after a bout of self-biting in rhesus monkeys were not significantly different from those collected on control days when the monkeys did not bite (Lutz *et al.*, 2002).

Role of anxiety

Humans

Anxiety and stress are two common factors that surround and frequently precede SIB, and the degree of self-injury is often correlated with anxiety (Simeon *et al.*, 1992). Individuals with a history of SIB generally report higher levels of anxiety than control subjects (Penn *et al.*, 2003; Ross and Heath, 2003), and they often use the self-injurious act as a means to counteract their anxiety or enhance their mood (Kemperman *et al.*, 1997). Those who self-injure report engaging in this behavior more for regulating their own emotions than for influencing the behavior of others (Nock and Prinstein, 2004). In a study of female self-injurers by Favazza and Conterio (1989), 72% of the subjects reported that they used self-injury to control their mind when it was racing, and 65% used it to feel relaxed. In a similar study with male prisoners who self-injured, 56% reported that they performed such acts to relieve anxiety or tension. Instead of pain, a sense of well-being often accompanied the injurious act (Fulwiler *et al.*, 1997). In subjects with borderline personality disor-der, SIB was often precipitated by events that were associated with issues of separa-tion, loss, or failure (Leibenluft *et al.*, 1987). Self-cutters reported mounting anxiety, tension, irritability, anger, depression, dysphoria, or emptiness prior to an episode of self-cutting, which then relieved these symptoms (Rada and James, 1982; Coid *et al.*, 1992; Nixon *et al.*, 2002). Even in the general population, 2.5% of men and 2.4% of women endorse the item "When I get very tense, hurting myself physically somehow calms me down" (Klonsky *et al.*, 2003). Although those who self-injured reported an improvement in mood, often they felt worse hours or days later, suggest-ing that the behavior was impulsive (Favazza and Conterio, 1989).

Although the above information is mostly obtained from self-report, studies have also shown physiological responses associated with self-injury that are consistent with a reduction in anxiety. In a study utilizing imaged scripts of self-injury, physiological arousal measured by finger pulse amplitude, heart rate, respiration, and skin conductance level decreased at the stage where actual self-injury was imaged. This pattern differed significantly from arousal patterns elicited from control scripts containing scenes of an accidental injury, an angry interaction, or a neutral event (Haines et al., 1995; Brain et al., 1998).

Nonhuman primates

As in humans, some forms of SIB in nonhuman primates have also been associated with heightened arousal or anxiety. Increased arousal or anxiety in these animals commonly involves stressful conditions brought about by social separation, frustration, aggressive interactions, or specific experimental manipulations. For example, an experimenter can directly induce a stressful situation by rapping on the subject's cage (Fittinghoff et al., 1974), staring at the animal, eliciting threat vocalizations and rattling the cage (Pond and Rush, 1983), or running a catch glove over the cage (Cross and Harlow, 1965). Other means of inducing stress may involve separation from a group (Chamove et al., 1984), from a cage-mate (Erwin et al., 1973), or simply from an artificial cloth surrogate in the case of young animals (McGrogan and King, 1982). As a result of these overtly stressful situations, the subjects showed an increase in SIB.

Frustration can also give rise to stress- or anxiety-related SIB. For example, the incidence of SIB increased when adult stumptail macaques observed companions receiving treats when they themselves did not receive any, or when the subjects observed a companion being tested on a memory task (compared with when they, themselves, were tested) (de Monte et al., 1992). Moreover, providing a single bottle of milk to a group of stumptail macaques increased competition and presumably frustration as well, thereby resulting in increased levels of SIB. Other examples with a similar outcome include placing an orange segment just out of reach of the animal (Chamove et al., 1984), and withdrawing reinforcement (i.e. invoking extinction) in isolation-reared monkeys that had been trained in a lever-pressing task (Gluck and Sackett, 1974).

Self-injurious behavior has sometimes been associated with aggressive behavior and even considered to be social aggression that has been thwarted due to physical (e.g. separate caging) or social (e.g. subordinate status) constraints. According to this view, aggression that would normally be directed towards another individual is redirected to the animal's own body, thus leading to SIB being labeled as "self-fighting" (Allyn et al., 1976) or "self-aggression" (de Monte et al., 1992). Early studies provided some evidence in support of this hypothesis. For example, when an experimenter vocally threatened a male stumptail macaque housed individually in a cage, the animal showed an increase in self-biting behavior (Allyn et al., 1976). Similarly, SIB has occurred in response to receiving social aggression, being displaced by other animals, or simply in response to sudden, unexpected movements by other animals (Anderson and Chamove, 1980). However, Anderson and Chamove (1985) failed to observe a significant correlation between SIB and play-fighting, and recent research suggests that SIB is not due to aggression *per se*, but to the stress and anxiety brought about by the aggression (Rulf Fountain *et al.*, 1997; Lutz *et al.*, 2003a).

Because self-report is not an option in nonhuman primate studies, less information is available concerning the potential stress-reducing effects of SIB. We mentioned earlier that episodes of SIB in rhesus monkeys do not seem to be associated with short-term changes in salivary cortisol levels. On the other hand, other studies on the same cohort of subjects found that when the animals were placed individually in a testing room and videotaped while their heart rate was monitored using radiotelemetry, heart rate significantly increased during a 30-second period prior to a self-biting episode and decreased significantly during the same interval of time after the episode. This heart rate pattern was not observed when animals bit the vest covering the recording electrodes instead of their own body (Marinus *et al.*, 1999). This result raises the possibility that as in the case of some humans who self-injure, SIB may serve the function of reducing stress or anxiety.

TREATMENT

Self-injurious behavior can be difficult to treat because it appears to occur impulsively, giving little time for intervention. In addition, many human subjects who suffer from SIB report a lack of physical pain (Leibenluft *et al.*, 1987; Coid *et al.*, 1992), resulting in a relative insensitivity to the aversive consequences of their behavior. With the possible release of endogenous reinforcing chemicals such as endorphins (Sandman *et al.*, 1990; Thompson *et al.*, 1995), acts of self-injury may instead be reinforcing. These circumstances, along with the severity of self-mutilation that occurs in some cases, underscore the importance of developing effective treatments for SIB. Two general therapeutic approaches have been implemented in this area: behavioral and pharmacological. In human subjects, the behavioral focus has been on training utilizing operant conditioning techniques. In nonhuman primates, the behavioral focus has been on environmental enrichment. Drug therapy has been implemented in both human and nonhuman primates. However, no single procedure has been deemed completely effective in eliminating SIB from either human or primate populations.

Behavioral treatments

Humans

Behavioral training has been utilized as a common method for controlling SIB in human clinical populations, although physical restraint may also be needed in more extreme cases of self-mutilation (Freeman *et al.*, 2002). The behavioral methods utilized are often designed for a particular individual, and what is considered to be a baseline measurement can vary greatly between studies, thus making comparisons difficult. Baselines can range from little to no interaction with a trainer (Carr *et al.*, 1976; Azrin *et al.*, 1988; Roscoe *et al.*, 1998) to presentation of demands or statements by the trainer (Carr *et al.*, 1976; Zarcone *et al.*, 1993). In addition, the sample size in most studies of behavioral intervention is small. For example, in one review of behavioral treatment for self-injury over a period from 1964 to 2000, the number of participants averaged only 1.8 per study (Kahng *et al.*, 2002). Therefore, a general overview will be presented here rather than detailed results. General categories of behavioral intervention may include reinforcement, punishment, extinction, or some combination thereof (Altmeyer *et al.*, 1987; Roscoe *et al.*, 1998; Kahng *et al.*, 2002).

Reinforcement

Several techniques employed in the treatment of SIB utilize the principle of reinforcement. In general, behaviors that are followed by a positive experience or the avoidance of a negative experience will increase in frequency or duration. One type of reinforcement used is the differential reinforcement of other behavior (DRO). In this procedure, reinforcement is provided to the subject following periods in which no SIB occurs. The interval length is increased or decreased as necessary (Favell *et al.*, 1982). A similar procedure is the differential reinforcement of incompatible behavior (DRI) in which the subject receives reinforcement and prompting of behaviors that are incompatible with SIB along with reinforcement for the absence of SIB. Examples of incompatible behavior may include toy play, social behavior, and compliance with requests (Favell *et al.*, 1982). When these procedures were utilized with nine retarded or autistic individuals, the rate of SIB occurrence dropped from 55% of observation intervals during baseline to 34% of intervals during the DRO procedure and only 28% of intervals during the DRI procedures (Azrin *et al.*, 1988).

Non-contingent reinforcement (NCR) is a procedure in which reinforcers are delivered on a fixed time (FT) schedule and occurrences of problem behaviors are ignored. Examples of reinforcement may include food items, toys, or social attention. The intervals between reinforcement are then increased as behavior improves. Utilizing this procedure, SIB was decreased when toys (Roscoe *et al.*, 1998; Kahng *et al.*, 2000) or social attention (Vollmer *et al.*, 1998) were provided to subjects.

The type of reinforcement and reinforcement schedule can vary greatly by subject. For example, in one subject, reinforcement was given once per week on the condition that he had fewer self-inflicted sores than the week before (Carr and McDowell, 1980). Negative reinforcement was also utilized in two subjects who used self-injury as a means to get out of grooming activities. When they were given a button to press for a brief timeout from the grooming, the incidence of SIB was reduced (Steege *et al.*, 1990).

Punishment

Punishment is an alternative behavioral method for the treatment of SIB. Treatment methods involving punishment can include overcorrection, timeout, and demands (Kahng et al., 2002). Overcorrection is a procedure in which subjects are reinforced for appropriate behaviors and for keeping their hands away from sites of self-inflicted injury. If a self-injurious act occurs, the subject receives a verbal reprimand and is then required to practice alternative uses with the head or hands, depending on how the injury was initiated. For example, for a bout of self-hitting, the experimenter would guide the subject's arms to the front and side for 30 seconds (Durand, 1982). Similarly, the procedure for head-banging would be holding the subject's head in specific positions for a period of time (Measel and Alfieri, 1976). These procedures reduced SIB in some, but not all, subjects (Measel and Alfieri, 1976; Durand, 1982), and head-banging actually increased in one subject (Measel and Alfieri, 1976).

Timeout, or interruption, is a procedure that occurs after the subject exhibits a self-injurious act. The experimenter interrupts what the subject is doing and gives the subject a timeout. Examples can include placing the subject in another room for a period of time (Carr and McDowell, 1980) or guiding the subject's hands to the lap where they must remain for a period of time (Azrin et al., 1988). These procedures also reduced the levels of SIB.

Extinction

Extinction involves the elimination of reinforcement that previously followed SIB. For example, if the reinforcement consisted of attention from caretakers, the caretakers would be instructed to ignore the self-injurious act and continue as if the behavior did not occur. In some situations, the reinforcement may be a result of the behavior itself, such as producing sensory stimulation. In this case, extinction may be brought about by placing equipment such as gloves on the subject to reduce the sensory experience gained by this type of SIB (Roscoe et al., 1998). In general, extinction has been found to reduce the incidence of SIB (Repp et al., 1988). However, one problem with extinction is the occurrence of extinction bursts, an immediate but transient increase in the unwanted behavior (Zarcone et al., 1993; Vollmer et al., 1998; Lerman et al., 1999).

Nonhuman primates

Enriching the environment has been proposed as one means of reducing abnormal behavior in nonhuman primates (Bayne et al., 1991; Baker, 1997). Although this approach may be useful for reducing certain abnormal behaviors, there is less evidence supporting the efficacy of environmental enrichment in treating more severe behavioral pathologies such as SIB. For example, despite the fact that enrichment devices such as toys or foraging apparatuses may be used and manipulated by the monkeys, such devices are not consistently effective at reducing rates of self-biting (Kinsey *et al.*, 1997; Novak *et al.*, 1998). In one study testing the effects of puzzle feeders on SIB, two subjects actually bit themselves while manipulating the feeder (Novak *et al.*, 1998). Similarly, when nylon balls were presented to macaque monkeys, one animal incorporated the ball into a pattern of self-biting behavior, alternating biting his leg with biting the nylon ball (Bayne, 1989). However, the presence of simple toys can be beneficial to some animals. One individually housed female baboon ceased self-directed biting around the same time that she developed aggressive biting of a Kong toy. It appeared that she redirected the biting from her knee to the toy (Crockett and Gough, 2002). Similarly, self-aggression decreased in three of four female stumptail macaques when given sticks or a tennis ball to redirect their behavior (Anderson and Stoppa, 1991).

Other behavioral approaches that have been tested include increasing the cage size and housing animals socially instead of individually. Intuitively, it might seem like smaller cages would produce more stress in captive animals, and therefore increasing cage size might reduce this stress and concomitantly result in less SIB. However, actual studies in which we attempted to relate changes in cage size to SIB failed to find a major effect of this manipulation (Jorgensen *et al.*, 1997; Kaufman *et al.*, 2004). In contrast, the social aspects of the housing situation appear to play an important role in the development of SIB in monkeys. Individual housing of both infant (Harlow and Harlow, 1962b; Cross and Harlow, 1965) and adult monkeys (Reinhardt, 1999; Lutz *et al.*, 2003b) increases the likelihood of SIB occurring. Moreover, placing these animals in compatible pairs can reduce, or even eliminate, the expression of SIB after it has developed (Reinhardt, 1999; Weed *et al.*, 2003).

Drug therapies

The development of effective pharmacotherapies for SIB serves two important functions. First and most importantly, drugs can help manage the symptoms of SIB, thereby reducing the amount of tissue damage incurred by patients or laboratory animals. This approach to symptom management is quite common, as shown by one survey of state residential facilities in which 38.8% of the population had received psychoactive drugs to reduce their SIB (Altmeyer *et al.*, 1987). Second, as seen in earlier sections, the ability of specific chemical agents to decrease the incidence or severity of SIB sheds light on the possible neurochemical or neuroendocrine underpinnings of the disorder. We shall discuss several different categories of drugs that have been used to treat SIB either in human clinical populations or in nonhuman primates.

Selective serotonin reuptake inhibitors and other serotonergic agents

As summarized above, SSRIs have been widely used in the treatment of SIB, particularly in patients with developmental disabilities or personality disorders. Because these compounds produce an acute increase in synaptic 5-HT by blocking its reuptake, other pharmacologic approaches to enhancing serotonergic transmission might also be expected to reduce SIB. Two early case studies of Lesch–Nyhan patients examined the effects of 5-hydroxytryptophan, the immediate precursor of 5-HT. The administration of this compound suppressed self-mutilation in one subject, but the efficacy of the drug decreased with time (Castells *et al.*, 1979), and furthermore in another subject, treatment did not reduce levels of self-mutilation (Frith *et al.*, 1976).

Two studies have investigated the effects of serotonergic agents on self-biting in rhesus monkeys with a history of self-wounding. In the first, treatment with the dietary 5-HT precursor L-tryptophan resulted in significant reductions in self-biting that were associated with increased 5-HIAA concentrations in the CSF (Weld *et al.*, 1998). More recently, Fontenot and co-workers (2005) reported that repeated administration of either the SSRI fluoxetine or the 5-HT$_{1A}$ agonist buspirone significantly reduced rates of self-biting in 15 monkeys that had experienced at least one episode of SIB during the previous 5 years. Unfortunately, self-biting returned to previous (or even higher) levels upon cessation of treatment. Further work is needed to determine whether a treatment regimen with SSRIs or any other serotonergic compound can be found that would maintain a long-lasting reduction in SIB without continued drug administration.

Neuroleptic drugs

Neuroleptics, which are DA receptor antagonists used clinically as antipsychotic agents, have also been tested for their ability to control SIB. The results of these trials have been mixed, with some subjects showing benefit but others not. For example, when the classical neuroleptic fluphenazine was given to 15 severely retarded subjects, 11 out of the 15 showed at least some degree of positive response whereas the remaining subjects were unaffected (Gualtieri and Schroeder, 1990). As mentioned earlier, other studies have been conducted with atypical neuroleptics that have fewer extrapyramidal side-effects and that differ in their neurochemical profile from the classical neuroleptics. Thus, an initial case study with risperidone found that it reduced self-mutilation in a Lesch–Nyhan patient (Allen and Rice, 1996), and two subsequent studies with developmentally disabled patients reported efficacy of risperidone in reducing self-injury in at least some of the subjects (Khan, 1997; Cohen *et al.*, 1998). Treatment with olanzapine, a somewhat newer neuroleptic drug, also resulted in decreased SIB in some patients with either learning disabilities (McDonough *et al.*, 2000), autism (Potenza *et al.*, 1999), or anxiety disorders (Garnis-Jones *et al.*, 2000). Finally, there are also reports of successful treatment of SIB using the atypical neuroleptics sulpiride (Rothenberger, 1993) and quetiapine (Hilger *et al.*, 2003). It is interesting to note that in many of the above cited studies, patients had previously received treatment with classical neuroleptic drugs with little or no improvement in their patterns of self-injury.

Unfortunately, little is known about the potential effectiveness of neuroleptic drugs in treating SIB in nonhuman primates. Taylor and co-workers (2005) reported successful elimination of SIB (manifested as repeated chewing of the inside of the cheek) in an adult female rhesus monkey by administration of the classical neuroleptic chlorpromazine in conjunction with environmental enrichment. To our knowledge, atypical neuroleptics have not yet been studied in monkeys with SIB, although the human literature suggests that these compounds could prove beneficial and therefore deserve consideration in future testing.

Opioid antagonists

We mentioned earlier that opioid receptor antagonists such as naltrexone and naloxone have resulted in a reduction of SIB in some studies. In one large study of 56 mentally retarded individuals with SIB, 57% of the subjects treated with naltrexone responded positively to the drug, and 25% of the subjects showed a 50% or more decrease in SIB (Casner et al., 1996). However, other studies showed mixed results and the effect may be dose-dependent (Sandman, 1988; Barrera et al., 1994; Thompson et al., 1994; Garcia and Smith, 1999). Patients with increased plasma levels of β-endorphin after an episode of SIB had the most positive response to naltrexone (Sandman et al., 1997), suggesting that the efficacy of the drug is at least partly dependent on the effects of the behavior itself. In some instances, naloxone actually increased the expression of SIB (Barrett et al., 1989), which may be related in part to the half-life of the drug. Naloxone has a half-life of 81 minutes, while naltrexone has a half-life of 36 hours. Consequently, the increased SIB after treatment with naloxone may be due to an extinction burst that is not observed with the longer acting drug naltrexone (Barrett et al., 1989).

Opioid antagonists have not yet been examined as treatments for SIB in nonhuman primates. However, as with atypical neuroleptics, these agents should be tested to determine whether they are as efficacious in primates as they seem to be in at least some humans who exhibit SIB.

Other pharmacotherapeutic agents

Three additional classes of drugs have been used to treat SIB in nonhuman primates. One is guanfacine, an α_2-adrenergic agonist, which was administered to two rhesus monkeys and one baboon that had been engaging in severe SIB (Macy et al., 2000). At a sufficient dose, this compound successfully reduced self-biting behavior in all three animals, although relapse occurred when treatment was stopped and two of the subjects (one monkey and one baboon) eventually had to be euthanized. The authors hypothesized that guanfacine's beneficial effects were due to enhancement of prefrontal cortical function by activation of postsynaptic α_2 receptors in that brain area.

A second drug that has been tested is the benzodiazepine diazepam, a well-known anti-anxiety agent. At the New England Primate Center, our research group along with the veterinary staff developed a diazepam treatment protocol for monkeys that were referred to the staff for reasons of self-injury. We recently reported on the outcome of eight adult male rhesus monkeys that were enrolled in this protocol (Tiefenbacher *et al.*, 2005a). Four of the monkeys showed a positive response to treatment consisting of a significant reduction in the incidence of self-wounding. Surprisingly, however, the other four subjects showed the opposite effect in which they tended to increase their rate of self-injury. Further analysis indicated that the positive responders differed from the negative responders in their history of individual cage housing and number of minor veterinary procedures, both of which have previously been identified as risk factors for the development of SIB (Novak, 2003). These findings are important for showing that as in humans, there may be multiple categories of SIB in nonhuman primates. In addition, the efficacy of diazepam in reducing self-wounding in one subgroup of monkeys supports the hypothesis that anxiety plays a significant role in maintaining SIB within this subgroup.

The third agent that has been reported to successfully treat SIB in monkeys is cyproterone acetate, a synthetic steroid previously used to manage hyperaggressiveness in men. Eaton and colleagues (1999) found that administration of this compound to adult male rhesus monkeys with SIB significantly reduced the rate of self-biting during the period of treatment. There were concomitant decreases in plasma testosterone and in CSF levels of the neurotransmitter metabolites 5-HIAA and HVA. The authors hypothesized that the beneficial effects of cyproterone acetate on SIB may derive from its antigonadal action. Decreased 5-HIAA and HVA levels were presumed to reflect an inhibition of monoamine oxidase (MAO) activity, thereby enhancing 5-HT and DA availability which could also contribute to the effects of the drug.

CONCLUSIONS

There are some important parallels between SIB in monkeys and SIB in humans who suffer either from developmental disabilities or other disorders with which SIB has been associated. Similarities between monkey and human SIB can be seen with respect to the form of the behavior, the physiological correlates of the behavior, the role of early experience in SIB development, and the beneficial effects of certain pharmacotherapeutic agents. In monkeys, SIB typically establishes itself as self-biting (Lutz *et al.*, 2003b), which also occurs in some humans with SIB (Buitelaar, 1993). However, SIB can take many other forms, such as head-banging and self-hitting, which can be observed in both developmentally disabled individuals as well as nonhuman primates (Levison, 1970; Buitelaar, 1993; Beckett *et al.*, 2002). Humans may also injure themselves by cutting or burning (Favazza and Conterio, 1989), methods that are not available to captive animals. Regardless of this variability in the exact manifestation of the behavior, the end result is the same – bodily injury or at least the potential for injury.

SIB often persists in spite of its pain-inducing potential, suggesting that there is some benefit to the individual such as tension reduction (Brain *et al.*, 1998). In both human and nonhuman primates, SIB often occurs in situations that cause stress or frustration (Chamove *et al.*, 1984; de Monte *et al.*, 1992), and the self-injurious act has been reported to help reduce that stress (Haines *et al.*, 1995; Marinus *et al.*, 1999). Developmentally disabled children have also used SIB as a means to avoid unwanted demands placed on them (Steege *et al.*, 1990). Because there is some benefit of this behavior to the individuals and because many human subjects report a lack of pain during self-injury (Leibenluft *et al.*, 1987; Coid *et al.*, 1992), treatment of SIB can be difficult.

The onset and maintenance of SIB are also influenced strongly by environmental and experiential factors. One such factor involves adverse early experience. For example, monkeys that are either reared in social isolation or separated from conspecifics at an early age are predisposed to exhibit SIB (Cross and Harlow, 1965; Lutz *et al.*, 2003b). Similarly in humans, individuals who experienced neglect (e.g. in an orphanage; Beckett *et al.*, 2002) or abuse during childhood (Briere and Gil, 1998; Bierer *et al.*, 2003) show enhanced vulnerability to developing SIB when older. However, not all individuals who experienced impoverished rearing conditions exhibit SIB, suggesting that such experiences are not sufficient by themselves to result in this kind of behavioral pathology.

Biochemical and physiological studies can play a key role in elucidating the neurobiological and neuroendocrine mechanisms that underlie SIB, and they can also direct the search for more effective therapeutic interventions. In this regard, there are some promising leads showing that several neurotransmitter/neuropeptide systems may be dysfunctional in both humans and monkeys with SIB, and also revealing abnormalities in the HPA stress response system. Furthermore, a number of pharmacologic agents, including SSRIs, neuroleptics, and opioid antagonists, reportedly reduce the incidence and/or severity of SIB in human patients. Unfortunately, many of these studies are open-label (i.e. the researchers and subjects are aware of the drug being administered as opposed to a "double-blind" procedure) or are otherwise poorly controlled, which diminishes the strength of their results. While properly controlled primate studies could be very beneficial in this regard, even those tend to involve small sample sizes and other experimental limitations. In addition, we recently found that pharmacologic treatment of SIB can have greatly different outcomes depending on the monkey's rearing history (Tiefenbacher *et al.*, 2005a).

The existence of significant problems with both the human and nonhuman primate literature underscores the difficulties inherent in studying SIB. Like many kinds of behavioral disorders, SIB is heterogeneous in its etiology and probably also in its mechanistic underpinnings. Therefore, while it can be tempting to bring research on developmentally disabled populations together with findings from Lesch–Nyhan patients and individuals suffering from borderline personality disorder, this approach may ultimately yield more confusion than enlightenment. It is similarly important to identify potential species differences in SIB in nonhuman primates (e.g. macaques versus apes), and also to recognize that SIB which is brought about by certain experimental manipulations such as isolation rearing or DA lesions may not be identical to SIB that develops spontaneously in socially reared animals.

It is not enough to point out the weaknesses in the existing research on SIB; we must also offer a prescription for moving the field forward. In our view, this can best be accomplished in the following way. (1) There must be more attempts to develop testable, biologically based theories of SIB that can help define the research agenda. In the human SIB literature, the dominant biological theory has been the opioid hypothesis in its various forms (Thompson *et al.*, 1995; Sandman and Touchette, 2002). Although this theory has promoted a number of studies on the use of opioid antagonists to treat SIB, many subjects respond either weakly or not at all to these compounds, suggesting that other factors must also be involved in the maintenance of SIB. With respect to nonhuman primates, Kraemer and Clarke (1990) offered some early ideas about the possible role of 5-HT in SIB, and we have proposed a more elaborate "integrated developmental-neurochemical hypothesis" to account for the onset and maintenance of SIB in socially reared rhesus monkeys (Tiefenbacher *et al.* 2005c). Studies are currently underway to test some of the predictions that stem from our model, and more such hypothesis-driven research needs to be carried out by both human and nonhuman primate researchers. (2) Modern research techniques should be brought to bear on the problem of SIB. Schizophrenia can be cited as a good example in this regard. Just as genotyping (e.g. identifying genetic polymorphisms that confer heightened risk), brain imaging, and other powerful techniques are being employed to unravel the complex factors underlying schizophrenia, it is likely that the biological bases of SIB will not be understood until the same approaches are used to study that disorder. For example, we have reported preliminary results suggesting involvement of an MAO-A gene polymorphism in vulnerability for SIB in rhesus monkeys (Tiefenbacher *et al.*, 2005b), but obviously much more work needs to be done to confirm and expand these findings to other candidate genes. (3) There must be an increase in well-controlled studies testing the efficacy of drug treatments in alleviating SIB in nonhuman primates. Furthermore, these trials should make use of medications that have reportedly resulted in positive therapeutic outcomes in human patients (e.g. atypical neuroleptics and opioid antagonists). If we are able to achieve more concordance between the clinical and preclinical literature, then our confidence in the value of particular pharmacotherapeutic agents will be greatly enhanced.

In conclusion, nonhuman primate models can play a central role in the ongoing search for the causes and treatment of SIB. We hope that the literature review and prescriptions for future research presented in this chapter will promote greater development and appreciation for such models. Nonetheless, because no animal model is perfect in all respects, it is important to further explore the similarities and differences between humans and nonhuman primates in the development and maintenance of SIB, as well as their responses to various treatment approaches.

REFERENCES

Allen, S. M. and Rice, S. N. (1996). Risperidone antagonism of self-mutilation in a Lesch–Nyhan patient. *Prog Neuropsychopharmacol Biol Psychiatry* **20**, 793–800.

Allyn, G., Deyme, A., and Begue, I. (1976). Self-fighting syndrome in macaques: I. A representative case study. *Primates* **17**, 1–22.

Altmeyer, B. K., Locke, B. J., Griffin, J. C. *et al.* (1987). Treatment strategies for self-injurious behavior in a large service-delivery network. *Am J Ment Defic* **91**, 333–340.

Anderson, J. R. and Chamove, A. S. (1980). Self-aggression and social aggression in laboratory-reared macaques. *J Abnorm Psychol* **89**, 539–550.

Anderson, J. R. and Chamove, A. S. (1985). Early social experience and the development of self-aggression in monkeys. *Biol Behav* **10**, 147–157.

Anderson, J. R. and Stoppa, F. (1991). Incorporating objects into sequences of aggression and self-aggression by *Macaca arctoides*: An unusual form of tool use? *Lab Primate Newsl* **30**, 1–3.

Ando, H. and Yoshimura, I. (1978). Prevalence of maladaptive behavior in retarded children as a function of IQ and age. *J Abnorm Child Psychol* **6**, 345–349.

Azrin, N. H., Besalel, V. A., Jamner, J. P., and Caputo, J. N. (1988). Comparative study of behavioral methods of treating severe self-injury. *Behav Resid Treat* **3**, 119–152.

Baker, K. (2002). Rearing and housing history of rhesus macaques (*Macaca mulatta*) displaying self-injurious and noninjurious abnormal behaviors. *Am J Primatol* **57**(suppl 1), 82.

Baker, K. C. (1997). Straw and forage material ameliorate abnormal behaviors in adult chimpanzees. *Zoo Biol* **16**, 225–236.

Barrera, F. J., Teodoro, J. M., Selmeci, T., and Madappuli, A. (1994). Self-injury, pain, and the endorphin theory. *J Dev Phys Disabil* **6**, 169–192.

Barrett, R. P., Feinstein, C., and Hole, W. T. 1989. Effects of naloxone and naltrexone on self-injury: a double-blind, placebo-controlled analysis. *Am J Ment Retard* **93**, 644–651.

Baumeister, A. A. and Frye, G. D. (1985). The biochemical basis of the behavioral disorder in the Lesch–Nyhan syndrome. *Neurosci Biobehav Rev* **9**, 169–178.

Baumeister, A. A., Todd, M. E., and Sevin, J. A. (1993). Efficacy and specificity of pharmacological therapies for behavioral disorders in persons with mental retardation. *Clin Neuropharmacol* **16**, 271–294.

Bayne, K. A. L. (1989). Nylon balls re-visited. *Lab Primate Newsl* **28**, 5–6.

Bayne, K. and Novak, M. (1998). Behavioral disorders. In: Bennett, B. T., Abee, C. R., and Henrickson, R. eds. *Nonhuman Primates in Biomedical Research*, Vol. 2: *Diseases*. New York: Academic Press, pp. 485–500.

Bayne, K., Mainzer, H., Dexter, S., Campbell, G., Yamada, F., and Suomi, S. (1991). The reduction of abnormal behaviors in individually housed rhesus-monkeys (Macaca-mulatta) with a foraging grooming board. *Am J Primatol* **23**, 23–35.

Bayne, K., Haines, M., Dexter, S., Woodman, D., and Evans, C. (1995). Nonhuman primate wounding prevalence: A retrospective analysis. *Lab Anim* **24**, 40–44.

Baysinger, C. M., Brandt, E. M., and Mitchell, G. (1972). Development of infant social isolate monkeys (*Macaca mulatta*) in their isolation environments. *Primates* **13**, 257–270.

Beckett, C., Bredenkamp, D., Castle, J., Groothues, C., O'Connor, T. G., Rutter, M., and the English and Romanian Adoptees (E.R.A.) Study Team (2002). Behavior patterns associated with institutional deprivation: a study of children adopted from Romania. *J Dev Behav Pediatr* **23**, 297–303.

Belfiore, P. J. and Dattilio, F. M. (1990). The behavior of self-injury: A brief review and analysis. *Behav Disord* **16**, 23–31.

Bellanca, R. U. and Crockett, C. M. (2002). Factors predicting increased incidence of abnormal behavior in male pigtailed macaques. *Am J Primatol* **58**, 57–69.

Bennun, I. (1984). Psychological models of self-mutilation. *Suicide Life Threat Behav* **14**, 166–186.

Bierer, L. M., Yehuda, R., Schmeidler, J. *et al.* (2003). Abuse and neglect in childhood: relationship to personality disorder diagnoses. *CNS Spectr* **8**, 737–754.

Bohus, M., Limberger, M., Ebner, U. *et al.* (2000). Pain perception during self-reported distress and calmness in patients with borderline personality disorder and self-mutilating behavior. *Psychiatry Res* **95**, 251–260.

Boiko, I. and Lester, D. (2000). Deliberate self-injury in female Russian inmates. *Psychol Rep* **87**, 789–790.

Brain, K. L., Haines, J., and Williams, C. L. (1998). The psychophysiology of self-mutilation: Evidence of tension reduction. *Arch Suicide Res* **4**, 227–242.

Breese, G. R., Knapp, D. J., Criswell, H. E., Moy, S. S., Papadeas, S. T., and Blake, B. L. (2005). The neonate-6-hydroxydopamine-lesioned rat: a model for clinical neuroscience and neurobiological principles. *Brain Res Rev* **48**, 57–73.

Briere, J. and Gil, E. (1998). Self-mutilation in clinical and general population samples: prevalence, correlates, and functions. *Am J Orthopsychiatry* **68**, 609–620.

Brown, G. L., Ebert, M. H., Goyer, P. F. *et al.* (1982). Aggression, suicide, and serotonin: relationships to CSF amine metabolites. *Am J Psychiatry* **139**, 741–746.

Buitelaar, J. K. (1993). Self-injurious behaviour in retarded children: clinical phenomena and biological mechanisms. *Acta Paedopsychiatr* **56**, 105–111.

Carlin, A. S., Kemper, K., Ward, N. G., Sowell, H., Gustafson, B., and Stevens, N. (1994). The effect of differences in objective and subjective definitions of childhood physical abuse on estimates of its incidence and relationship to psychopathology. *Child Abuse Negl* **18**, 393–399.

Carr, E. G. (1977). The motivation of self-injurious behavior: a review of some hypotheses. *Psychol Bull* **84**, 800–816.

Carr, E. G. and McDowell, J. J. (1980). Social control of self-injurious behavior of organic etiology. *Behav Ther* **11**, 402–409.

Carr, E. G., Newsom, C. D., and Binkoff, J. A. (1976). Stimulus control of self-destructive behavior in a psychotic child. *J Abnorm Child Psychol* **4**, 139–153.

Casner, J. A., Weinheimer, B., and Gualtieri, C. T. (1996). Naltrexone and self-injurious behavior: a retrospective population study. *J Clin Psychopharmacol* **16**, 389–394.

Castells, S., Chakrabarti, C., Winsberg, B. G., Hurwic, M., Perel, J. M., and Nyhan, W. L. (1979). Effects of L-5-hydroxytryptophan on monoamine and amino acids turnover in the Lesch-Nyhan syndrome. *J Autism Dev Disord* **9**, 95–103.

Cataldo, M. F. and Harris, J. (1982). The biological basis for self-injury in the mentally retarded. *Anal Interv Dev Disabil* **2**, 21–39.

Chamove, A. S., Anderson, J. R., and Nash, V. J. (1984). Social and environmental influences on self-aggression in monkeys. *Primates* **25**, 319–325.

Chamove, A. S., Bayart, F., Nash, V. J., and Anderson, J. R. (1985). Dominance, physiology, and self-aggression in monkeys. *Aggressive Behav* **11**, 17–26.

Clarke, D. J. (1998). Psychopharmacology of severe self-injury associated with learning disabilities. *Br J Psychiatry* **172**, 389–394.

Cohen, S. A., Ihrig, K., Lott, R. S., and Kerrick, J. M. (1998). Risperidone for aggression and self-injurious behavior in adults with mental retardation. *J Autism Dev Disord* **28**, 229–233.

Coid, J., Wilkins, J., Coid, B., and Everitt, B. (1992). Self-mutilation in female remanded prisoners II: A cluster analytic approach towards identification of a behavioural syndrome. *Crim Behav Ment Health* **2**, 1–14.

Collacott, R. A., Cooper, S. A., Branford, D., and McGrother, C. (1998). Epidemiology of self-injurious behaviour in adults with learning disabilities. *Br J Psychiatry* **173**, 428–432.

Coman, P. and Houghton, S. J. (1991). A functional analysis of self injurious behaviour. *Educ Psychol Pract* **7**, 111–116.

Crockett, C. M. and Gough, G. M. (2002). Onset of aggressive toy biting by a laboratory baboon coincides with cessation of self-injurious behavior. *Am J Primatol* **57**(suppl 1), 39.

Cromwell, H. C., Levine, M. S., and King, B. H. (1999). Cortical damage enhances pemoline-induced self-injurious behavior in prepubertal rats. *Pharmacol Biochem Behav* **62**, 223–227.

Cross, H. A. and Harlow, H. F. (1965). Prolonged and progressive effects of partial isolation on the behavior of macaque monkeys. *J Exp Res Pers* **1**, 39–49.

Davanzo, P. A., Belin, T. R., Widawski, M. H., and King, B. H. (1998). Paroxetine treatment of aggression and self-injury in persons with mental retardation. *Am J Ment Retard* **102**, 427–437.

de Monte, M., Anderson, J. R., and Charbonnier, H. (1992). Self-aggression in stumptail macaques: effects of frustration and social partners. *Primates* **33**, 115–120.

Deb, S., Thomas, M., and Bright, C. (2001). Mental disorder in adults with intellectual disability. 2: The rate of behaviour disorders among a community-based population aged between 16 and 64 years. *J Intellect Disabil Res* **45**, 506–514.

DeMet, E. M. and Sandman, C. A. (1991). Models of the opiate system in self-injurious behavior: A reply. *Am J Ment Retard* **95**, 694–696.

Dolan, M., Anderson, I. M., and Deakin, J. F. W. (2001). Relationship between 5-HT function and impulsivity and aggression in male offenders with personality disorders. *Br J Psychiatry* **178**, 352–359.

Durand, V. M. (1982). Analysis and intervention of self-injurious behavior. *TASH J* **7**, 44–53.

Dykens, E. M. and Smith, A. C. M. (1998). Distinctiveness and correlates of maladaptive behaviour in children and adolescents with Smith-Magenis syndrome. *J Intellect Disabil Res* **42**, 481–489.

Eaton, G. G., Worlein, J. M., Kelley, S. T. *et al.* (1999). Self-injurious behavior is decreased by cyproterone acetate in adult male rhesus (*Macaca mulatta*). *Horm Behav* **35**, 195–203.

Ernst, M., Zametkin, A. J., Matochik, J. A. *et al.* (1996). Presynaptic dopaminergic deficits in Lesch-Nyhan disease. *N Engl J Med* **334**, 1568–1572.

Erwin, J., Mitchell, G., and Maple, T. (1973). Abnormal behavior in non-isolate-reared rhesus monkeys. *Psychol Rep* **33**, 515–523.

Faucheux, B., Bourliere, F., and Lemaire, C. (1976). Decreased adrenal reactivity in partially-isolated auto-aggressive macaques. *Biol Behav* **1**, 329–338.

Favazza, A. R. (1989). Why patients mutilate themselves. *Hosp Community Psychiatry* **40**, 137–145.

Favazza, A. R. (1998). The coming of age of self-mutilation. *J Nerv Ment Dis* **186**, 259–268.

Favazza, A. R. and Conterio, K. (1989). Female habitual self-mutilators. *Acta Psychiatr Scand* **79**, 283–289.

Favell, J.E., Azrin, N.H., Baumeister, A.A. *et al.* (1982). The treatment of self-injurious behavior. *Behav Ther* **13**, 529–554.

Finucane, B., Dirrigl, K. H., and Simon, E. W. (2001). Characterization of self-injurious behaviors in children and adults with Smith-Magenis syndrome. *Am J Ment Retard* **106**, 52–58.

Fittinghoff, N. A., Jr., Lindburg, D. G., Gomber, J., and Mitchell, G. (1974). Consistency and variability in the behavior of mature, isolation-reared, male rhesus macaques. *Primates* **15**, 111–139.

Fontenot, M. B., Padgett, E. E., Dupuy, A. M., Lynch, C. R., De Petrillo, P. B., and Higley, J. D. (2005). The effects of fluoxetine and buspirone on self-injurious and stereotypic behavior in adult male rhesus macaques. *Comparative Med* **55**, 67–74.

Freeman, R. L., Horner, R. H., and Reichle, J. (2002). Functional assessment and self-restraint. In Schroeder, S. R., Oster-Granite, M., and Thompson, T. eds. *Self-Injurious Behavior Gene–Brain–Behavior Relationships.* Washington D.C.: American Psychological Association, pp. 105–118.

Frith, C. D., Johnstone, E. C., Joseph, M. H., Powell, R. J., and Watts, R. W. E. (1976). Double-blind clinical trial of 5-hydroxytryptophan in a case of Lesch-Nyhan syndrome. *J Neurol Neurosurg Psychiatry* **39**, 656–662.

Fritz, J., Nash, L. T., Alford, P. L., and Bowen, J. A. (1992). Abnormal behaviors, with a special focus on rocking, and reproductive competence in a large sample of captive chimpanzees (*Pan troglodytes*). *Am J Primatol* **27**, 161–176.

Fulwiler, C., Forbes, C., Santangelo, S. L., and Folstein, M. (1997). Self-mutilation and suicide attempt: distinguishing features in prisoners. *J Am Acad Psychiatry Law* **25**, 69–77.

Garber, H. J., McGonigle, J. J., Slomka, G. T., and Monteverde, E. (1992). Clomipramine treatment of stereotypic behaviors and self-injury in patients with developmental disabilities. *J Am Acad Child Adolesc Psychiatry* **31**, 1157–1160.

Garcia, D. and Smith, R. G. (1999). Using analog baselines to assess the effects of naltrexone on self-injurious behavior. *Res Dev Disabil* **20**, 1–21.

Gardner, D. L. and Cowdry, R. W. (1985). Suicidal and parasuicidal behavior in borderline personality disorder. *Psychiatr Clin North Am* **8**, 389–403.

Gardner, D. L., Lucas, P. B., and Cowdry, R. W. (1990). CSF metabolites in borderline personality disorder compared with normal controls. *Biol Psychiatry* **28**, 247–254.

Garnis-Jones, S., Collins, S., and Rosenthal, D. (2000). Treatment of self-mutilation with olanzapine. *J Cutan Med Surg* **4**, 161–163.

Gluck J. P. and Sackett G. P. (1974). Frustration and self-aggression in social isolate rhesus monkeys. *J Abnorm Psychol* **83**, 331–334.

Goldstein, M. (1989). Dopaminergic mechanisms in self-inflicting biting behavior. *Psychopharmacol Bull* **25**, 349–352.

Goldstein, M., Kuga, S., Kusano, N., Meller, E., Dancis, J., and Schwarcz, R. (1986). Dopamine agonist induced self-mutilative biting behavior in monkeys with unilateral ventromedial tegmental lesions of the brainstem: possible pharmacological model for Lesch-Nyhan syndrome. *Brain Res* **367**, 114–120.

Green, A. H. (1967). Self-mutilation in schizophrenic children. *Arch Gen Psychiatry* **17**, 234–244.

Griffin, J. C., Williams, D. E., Stark, M. T., Altmeyer, B. K., and Mason, M. (1986). Self-injurious behavior: a state-wide prevalence survey of the extent and circumstances. *Appl Res Ment Retard* **7**, 105–116.

Griffin, J. C., Ricketts, R. W., Williams, D. E., Locke, B. J., Altmeyer B. K., and Stark, M. T. (1987). A community survey of self-injurious behavior among developmentally disabled children and adolescents. *Hosp Community Psychiatry* **38**, 959–963.

Gualtieri, C. T. and Schroeder, S. R. (1990). Pharmacotherapy for self-injurious behavior: preliminary tests of the D1 hypothesis. *Prog Neuropsychopharmacol Biol Psychiatry* **14**(suppl), S81–107.

Ha, H., Tan, E. C., Fukunaga, H., and Aochi, O. (1981). Naloxone reversal of acupuncture analgesia in the monkey. *Exp Neurol* **73**, 298–303.

Haines, J., Williams, C. L., Brain, K. L., and Wilson, G. V. (1995). The psychophysiology of self-mutilation. *J Abnorm Psychol* **104**, 471–489.

Harlow, H. F. and Harlow, M. K. (1962a). The effect of rearing conditions on behavior. *Bull Menninger Clin* **26**, 213–224.

Harlow, H. F. and Harlow, M. K. (1962b). Social deprivation in monkeys. *Sci Am* **207**, 136–146.

Hellings, J. A., Kelley, L. A., Gabrielli, W. F., Kilgore, E., and Shah, P. (1996). Sertraline response in adults with mental retardation and autistic disorder. *J Clin Psychiatry* **57**, 333–336.

Herman, B. H. (1990). A possible role of proopiomelanocortin peptides in self-injurious behavior. *Prog Neuropsychopharmacol Biol Psychiatry* **14**(suppl), S109–139.

Herpertz, S., Sass, H., and Favazza, A. (1997). Impulsivity in self-mutilative behavior: psychometric and biological findings. *J Psychiatr Res* **31**, 451–465.

Higley, J. D., Mehlman, P. T., Taub, D. M. *et al.* (1992). Cerebrospinal fluid monoamine and adrenal correlates of aggression in free-ranging rhesus monkeys. *Arch Gen Psychiatry* **49**, 436–441.

Hilger, E., Barnas, C., and Kasper, S. (2003). Quetiapine in the treatment of borderline personality disorder. *World J Biol Psychiatry* **4**, 42–44.

Iwata, B. A., Pace, G. M., Dorsey, M. F. *et al.* (1994). The functions of self-injurious behavior: an experimental-epidemiological analysis. *J Appl Behav Anal* **27**, 215–240.

Jankovic, J., Caskey, T. C., Stout, J. T., and Butler, I. J. (1988). Lesch-Nyhan syndrome: a study of motor behavior and cerebrospinal fluid neurotransmitters. *Ann Neurol* **23**, 466–469.

Jawed, S. H., Krishnan, V. H. R., and Cassidy, G. (1994). Self-injurious behaviour and the serotonin link: two case illustrations and theoretical overview. *Irish J Psychol Med* **11**, 165–168.

Jinnah, H. A., Yitta, S., Drew, T., Kim, B. S., Visser, J. E., and Rothstein, J. D. (1999). Calcium channel activation and self-biting in mice. *Proc Natl Acad Sci USA* **96**, 15228–15232.

Jones, A. (1986). Self-mutilation in prison a comparison of mutilators and nonmutilators. *Crim Justice Behav* **13**, 286–296.

Jones, I. H. and Barraclough, B. M. (1978). Auto-mutilation in animals and its relevance to self-injury in man. *Acta Psychiatr Scand* **58**, 40–47.

Jorgensen, M. J., Kinsey, J., and Novak, M. A. (1997). Effects of cage size on self-injurious and abnormal behavior in macaques. *Am J Primatol* **42**, 120.

Kahng, S. W., Iwata, B. A., Thompson, R. H., and Hanley, G. P. (2000). A method for identifying satiation versus extinction effects under noncontingent reinforcement schedules. *J Appl Behav Anal* **33**, 419–432.

Kahng, S. W., Iwata, B. A., and Lewin, A. B. (2002). Behavioral treatment of self-injury, 1964 to 2000. *Am J Ment Retard* **107**, 212–221.

Kaufman, B. M., Pouliot, A. L., Tiefenbacher, S., and Novak, M. A. (2004). Short and long-term effects of a substantial change in cage size on individually housed, adult male rhesus monkeys (*Macaca mulatta*). *Appl Anim Behav Sci* **88**, 319–330.

Kemperman, I., Russ, M. J., and Shearin, E. (1997). Self-injurious behavior and mood regulation in borderline patients. *J Personal Disord* **11**, 146–157.

Khan, B. U. (1997). Brief report: risperidone for severely disturbed behavior and tardive dyskinesia in developmentally disabled adults. *J Autism Dev Disord* **27**, 479–489.

King, B. H. (1993). Self-injury by people with mental retardation: a compulsive behavior hypothesis. *Am J Ment Retard* **98**, 93–112.

King, B. H., McCracken, J. T., and Poland, R. E. (1991). Deficiency in the opioid hypotheses of self-injurious behavior. *Am J Ment Retard* **95**, 692–694.

Kinsey, J. H., Jorgensen, M., and Novak, M. (1997). The effects of grooming boards on abnormal behavior in rhesus monkeys (*Macaca mulatta*). *Am J Primatol* **42**, 122–123.

Klonsky, E. D., Oltmanns, T. F., and Turkheimer, E. (2003). Deliberate self-harm in a nonclinical population: prevalence and psychological correlates. *Am J Psychiatry* **160**, 1501–1508.

Kraemer, G. W. and Clarke, A. S. (1990). The behavioral neurobiology of self-injurious behavior in rhesus monkeys. *Prog Neuropsychopharmacol Biol Psychiatry* **14**(suppl), S141–S168.

Leibenluft, E., Gardner, D. L., and Cowdry, R. W. (1987). The inner experience of the borderline self-mutilator. *J Pers Disord* **1**, 317–324.

Lerman, D. C., Iwata, B. A., and Wallace, M. D. (1999). Side effects of extinction: prevalence of bursting and aggression during the treatment of self-injurious behavior. *J Appl Behav Anal* **32**, 1–8.

Lesch, M. and Nyhan, W. L. (1964). A familial disorder of uric acid metabolism and central nervous system function. *Am J Med* **36**, 561–570.

Levison, C. A. (1970). The development of head banging in a young rhesus monkey. *Am J Ment Defic* **75**, 323–328.

Lewis, M. H., Gluck, J. P., Beauchamp, A. J., Keresztury, M. F., and Mailman, R. B. (1990). Long-term effects of early social isolation in *Macaca mulatta*: changes in dopamine receptor function following apomorphine challenge. *Brain Res* **513**, 67–73.

Lewis, M. H., Bodfish, J. W., Powell, S. B., Parker, D. E., and Golden, R. N. (1996). Clomipramine treatment for self-injurious behavior of individuals with mental retardation: a double-blind comparison with placebo. *Am J Ment Retard* **100**, 654–665.

Linnoila, M., Virkkunen, M., Scheinin, M., Nuutila, A., Rimon, R., and Goodwin, F. K. (1983). Low cerebrospinal fluid 5-hydroxyindoleacetic acid concentration differentiates impulsive from nonimpulsive violent behavior. *Life Sci* **33**, 2609–2614.

Lipschitz, D. S., Winegar, R. K., Nicolaou, A. L., Hartnick, E., Wolfson, M., and Southwick, S. M. (1999). Perceived abuse and neglect as risk factors for suicidal behavior in adolescent inpatients. *J Nerv Ment Dis* **187**, 32–39.

Lloyd, K. G., Hornykiewicz, O., Davidson, L. *et al.* (1981). Biochemical evidence of dysfunction of brain neurotransmitters in the Lesch-Nyhan syndrome. *N Engl J Med* **305**, 1106–1111.

Lopez-Ibor, J. J., Jr., Saiz-Ruiz, J., and Perez de los Cobos, J. C. (1985). Biological correlations of suicide and aggressivity in major depressions (with melancholia): 5-hydroxyindoleacetic acid and cortisol in cerebral spinal fluid, dexamethasone suppression test and therapeutic response to 5-hydroxytryptophan. *Neuropsychobiology* **14**, 67–74.

Lutz, C. K., Tiefenbacher, S., Pouliot, A. L., Kaufman, B. M., Meyer, J. S., and Novak, M. A. (2002). Spontaneous episodes of self-biting and associated cortisol levels in captive male *Macaca mulatta*. *Am J Primatol* **57**(suppl 1), 43.

Lutz, C., Marinus, L., Chase, W., Meyer, J., and Novak, M. (2003a). Self-injurious behavior in male rhesus macaques does not reflect externally directed aggression. *Physiol Behav* **78**, 33–39.

Lutz, C., Well, A., and Novak, M. (2003b). Stereotypic and self-injurious behavior in rhesus macaques: a survey and retrospective analysis of environment and early experience. *Am J Primatol* **60**, 1–15.

Mace, A. B., Shapiro, E. S., and Mace, F. C. (1998). Effects of warning stimuli for reinforcer withdrawal and task onset on self-injury. *J Appl Behav Anal* **31**, 679–682.

Macy, J. D. Jr., Beattie, T. A., Morgenstern, S. E., and Arnsten, A. F. T. (2000). Use of guanfacine to control self-injurious behavior in two rhesus macaques (*Macaca mulatta*) and one baboon (*Papio anubis*). *Comp Med* **50**, 419–425.

Marinus, L. M., Chase, W. K., Rasmussen, K. L., Jorgensen, M. J., and Novak, M. A. (1999). Reaction of rhesus monkeys with self-injurious behavior to heart rate testing: Is biting a coping strategy? *Am J Primatol* **49**, 79.

Marinus, L. M., Chase, W. K., and Novak, M. A. (2000). Self-biting behavior in rhesus macaques (*Macaca mulatta*) is preferentially directed to body areas associated with acupuncture analgesia. *Am J Primatol* **51**(suppl 1), 71–72.

Markovitz, P. J., Calabrese, J. R., Schulz, S. C., and Meltzer, H. Y. (1991). Fluoxetine in the treatment of borderline and schizotypal personality disorders. *Am J Psychiatry* **148**, 1064–1067.

Markowitz, P. I. (1992). Effect of fluoxetine on self-injurious behavior in the developmentally disabled: a preliminary-study. *J Clin Psychopharm* **12**, 27–31.

Mason, W. A. and Green, P. C. (1962). The effects of social restriction on the behavior of rhesus monkeys: IV. Responses to a novel environment and to an alien species. *J Comp Physiol Psychol* **55**, 363–368.

Mason, W. A. and Sponholz, R. R. (1963). Behavior of rhesus monkeys raised in isolation. *J Psychiatr Res* **1**, 299–306.

Matsumoto, T., Yamaguchi, A., Asami, T., Okada, T., Yoshikawa, K., and Hirayasu, Y. (2005). Characteristics of self-cutters among male inmates: association with bulimia and dissociation. *Psychiatry Clin Neurosci* **59**, 319–326.

McDonough, M., Hillery, J., and Kennedy, N. (2000). Olanzapine for chronic, stereotypic self-injurious behaviour: a pilot study in seven adults with intellectual disability. *J Intellect Disabil Res* **44**, 677–684.

McGrogan, H. J. and King, J. E. (1982). Repeated separations of 2-year-old squirrel monkeys from familiar mother surrogates. *Am J Primatol* **3**, 285–290.

McKinney, W. T., Jr., Kliese, K. A., Suomi, S. J., and Moran, E. C. (1973). Can psychopathology be reinduced in rhesus monkeys? *Arch Gen Psychiatry* **29**, 630–634.

Measel, C. J. and Alfieri, P. A. (1976). Treatment of self-injurious behavior by a combination of reinforcement for incompatible behavior and overcorrection. *Am J Ment Defic* **81**, 147–153.

Mehlman, P. T., Higley, J. D., Faucher, I. et al. (1994). Low CSF 5-HIAA concentrations and severe aggression and impaired impulse control in nonhuman primates. *Am J Psychiatry* **151**, 1485–1491.

Mizuno, T. and Yugari, Y. (1975). Prophylactic effect of L-5-hydroxytryptophan on self-mutilation in the Lesch-Nyhan syndrome. *Neuropadiatrie* **6**, 13–23.

Mulder, R. T. and Joyce, P. R. (2002). Relationship of temperament and behaviour measures to the prolactin response to fenfluramine in depressed men. *Psychiatry Res* **109**, 221–228.

New, A. S., Trestman, R. L., Mitropoulou, V. et al. (1997). Serotonergic function and self-injurious behavior in personality disorder patients. *Psychiatry Res* **69**, 17–26.

Nijman, H. L. I., Dautzenberg, M., Merckelbach, H. L. G. J., Jung, P., Wessel, I., and a Campo, J. (1999). Self-mutilating behaviour of psychiatric inpatients. *Eur Psychiatry* **14**, 4–10.

Nixon, M. K., Cloutier, P. F., and Aggarwal, S. (2002). Affect regulation and addictive aspects of repetitive self-injury in hospitalized adolescents. *J Am Acad Child Adolesc Psychiatry* **41**, 1333–1341.

Nock, M. K. and Prinstein, M. J. (2004). A functional approach to the assessment of self-mutilative behavior. *J Consult Clin Psychol* **72**, 885–890.

Nock, M. K. and Prinstein, M. J. (2005). Contextual features and behavioral functions of self-mutilation among adolescents. *J Abnorm Psychol* **114**, 140–146.

Novak, M. A. (2003). Self-injurious behavior in rhesus monkeys: new insights into its etiology, physiology, and treatment. *Am J Primatol* **59**, 3–19.

Novak, M. A., Kinsey, J. H., Jorgensen, M. J., and Hazen, T. J. (1998). Effects of puzzle feeders on pathological behavior in individually housed rhesus monkeys. *Am J Primatol* **46**, 213–227.

Nyhan, W. L. (1976). Behavior in the Lesch-Nyhan syndrome. *J Autism Child Schizophr* **6**, 235–252.

Nyhan, W. L. (2000). Dopamine function in Lesch-Nyhan disease. *Environ Health Perspect* **108**(suppl 3), 409–411.

Peffer-Smith, P. G., Smith, E. O., and Byrd, L. D. (1983). Effects of d-amphetamine on self-aggression and posturing in stumptail macaques. *J Exp Anal Behav* **40**, 313–320.

Penn, J. V., Esposito, C. L., Schaeffer, L. E., Fritz, G. K., and Spirito, A. (2003). Suicide attempts and self-mutilative behavior in a juvenile correctional facility. *J Am Acad Child Adolesc Psychiatry* **42**, 762–769.

Pond, C. L. and Rush, H. G. (1983). Self-aggression in macaques: Five case studies. *Primates* **24**, 127–134.

Potenza, M. N., Holmes, J. P., Kanes, S. J., and McDougle, C. J. (1999). Olanzapine treatment of children, adolescents, and adults with pervasive developmental disorders: an open-label pilot study. *J Clin Psychopharmacol* **19**, 37–44.

Rada, R. T. and James, W. (1982). Urethral insertion of foreign bodies. A report of contagious self-mutilation in a maximum-security hospital. *Arch Gen Psychiatry* **39**, 423–429.

Reinhardt, V. (1999). Pair-housing overcomes self-biting behavior in macaques. *Lab Primate Newsl* **38**, 4–5.

Repp, A. C., Felce, D., and Barton, L. E. (1988). Basing the treatment of stereotypic and self-injurious behaviors on hypotheses of their causes. *J Appl Behav Anal* **21**, 281–289.

Richardson, J. S. and Zaleski, W. A. (1983). Naloxone and self-mutilation. *Biol Psychiatry* **18**, 99–101.

Ricketts, R. W., Goza, A. B., Ellis, C. R., Singh, Y. N., Singh, N. N., and Cooke, J. C., III (1993). Fluoxetine treatment of severe self-injury in young adults with mental retardation. *J Am Acad Child Adolesc Psychiatry* **32**, 865–869.

Robertson, M. M. (1992). Self-injurious behavior and Tourette syndrome. *Adv Neurol* **58**, 105–114.

Robertson, M. M., Trimble, M. R., and Lees, A. J. (1989). Self-injurious behaviour and the Gilles de la Tourette syndrome: a clinical study and review of the literature. *Psychol Med* **19**, 611–625.

Rojahn, J. (1986). Self-injurious and stereotypic behavior of noninstitutionalized mentally retarded people: prevalence and classification. *Am J Ment Defic* **91**, 268–276.

Roscoe, E. M., Iwata, B. A., and Goh, H. L. (1998). A comparison of noncontingent reinforcement and sensory extinction as treatments for self-injurious behavior. *J Appl Behav Anal* **31**, 635–646.

Ross, S. and Heath, N. (2002). A study of the frequency of self-mutilation in a community sample of adolescents. *J Youth Adolescence* **31**, 67–77.

Ross, S. and Heath, N.L. (2003). Two models of adolescent self-mutilation. *Suicide Life Threat Behav* **33**, 277–287.

Rothenberger, A. (1993). Psychopharmacological treatment of self-injurious behavior in individuals with autism. *Acta Paedopsychiatr* **56**, 99–104.

Rulf Fountain, A., Tiefenbacher, S., Novak, M. A., and Meyer, J. (1997). Is self injurious behavior in rhesus monkeys related to social aggression? *Am J Primatol* **42**, 144.

Russ, M. J., Roth, S. D., Kakuma, T., Harrison, K., and Hull, J. W. (1994). Pain perception in self-injurious borderline patients: naloxone effects. *Biol Psychiatry* **35**, 207–209.

Russ, M. J., Campbell, S. S., Kakuma, T., Harrison, K., and Zanine, E. (1999). EEG theta activity and pain insensitivity in self-injurious borderline patients. *Psychiatry Res* **89**, 201–214.

Sachsse, U., Von der Heyde, S., and Huether, G. (2002). Stress regulation and self-mutilation. *Am J Psychiatry* **159**, 672.

Saito, Y. and Takashima, S. (2000). Neurotransmitter changes in the pathophysiology of Lesch-Nyhan syndrome. *Brain Dev* **22**(suppl 1), S122–S131.

Saloviita, T. (2000). The structure and correlates of self-injurious behavior in an institutional setting. *Res Dev Disabil* **21**, 501–511.

Sandman, C. A., Datta, P. C., Barron, J., Hoehler, F. K., Williams, C., and Swanson, J. M. (1983). Naloxone attenuates self-abusive behavior in developmentally disabled clients. *Appl Res Ment Retard* **4**, 5–11.

Sandman, C. A. (1988). B-endorphin disregulation in autistic and self-injurious behavior: a neurodevelopmental hypothesis. *Synapse* **2**, 193–199.

Sandman, C. A., Barron, J. L., and Colman, H. (1990). An orally administered opiate blocker, naltrexone, attenuates self-injurious behavior. *Am J Ment Retard* **95**, 93–102.

Sandman, C. A., Hetrick, W., Taylor, D. V., and Chicz-DeMet, A. (1997). Dissociation of POMC peptides after self-injury predicts responses to centrally acting opiate blockers. *Am J Ment Retard* **102**, 182–199.

Sandman, C. A. and Touchette, P. (2002). Opioids and the maintenance of self-injurious behavior. In Schroeder, S. R., Oster-Granite, M., and Thompson, T. eds. *Self-Injurious Behavior Gene–Brain–Behavior Relationships.* Washington D.C.: American Psychological Association, pp. 191–204.

Sandman, C. A., Touchette, P., Lenjavi, M., Marion, S., and Chicz-DeMet, A. (2003). beta-Endorphin and ACTH are dissociated after self-injury in adults with developmental disabilities. *Am J Ment Retard* **108**, 414–424.

Sansom, D., Krishnan, V. H. R., Corbett, J., and Kerr, A. (1993). Emotional and behavioural aspects of Rett syndrome. *Dev Med Child Neurol* **35**, 340–345.

Schaefer, H. H. (1970). Self-injurious behavior: shaping "head-banging" in monkeys. *J Appl Behav Anal* **3**, 111–116.

Schaffer, C. B., Carroll, J., and Abramowitz, S. I. (1982). Self-mutilation and the borderline personality. *J Nerv Ment Dis* **170**, 468–473.

Schroeder, S. R., Hammock, R. G., Mulick, J. A. *et al.* (1995). Clinical trials of D_1 and D_2 dopamine modulating drugs and self-injury in mental retardation and developmental disability. *Ment Retard Dev Disabil Res Rev* **1**, 120–129.

Silverstein, F. S., Johnston, M. V., Hutchinson, R. J., and Edwards, N. L. (1985). Lesch-Nyhan syndrome: CSF neurotransmitter abnormalities. *Neurology* **35**, 907–911.

Simeon, D. and Favazza, A. R. (2001). Self-injurious behaviors: Phenomenology and assessment. In Simeon, D. and Hollander, E. eds. *Self-injurious Behaviors: Assessment and Treatment.* Washington, DC: American Psychiatric Publishing, pp. 1–28.

Simeon, D., Stanley, B., Frances, A., Mann, J. J., Winchel, R., and Stanley, M. (1992). Self-mutilation in personality disorders: psychological and biological correlates. *Am J Psychiatry* **149**, 221–226.

Singh, A. N., Kleynhans, D., and Barton, G. (1998). Selective serotonin re-uptake inhibitors in the treatment of self-injurious behaviour in adults with mental retardation. *Hum Psychopharm* **13**, 267–270.

Steege, M. W., Wacker, D. P., Cigrand, K. C. *et al.* (1990). Use of negative reinforcement in the treatment of self-injurious behavior. *J Appl Behav Anal* **23**, 459–467.

Steiger, H., Koerner, N., Engelberg, M. J., Israel, M., Ng Ying Kin, N. M., and Young, S. N. (2001). Self-destructiveness and serotonin function in bulimia nervosa. *Psychiatry Res* **103**, 15–26.

Suomi, S. J., Harlow, H. F., and Kimball, S. D. (1971). Behavioral effects of prolonged partial social isolation in the rhesus monkey. *Psychol Rep* **29**, 1171–1177.

Symons, F. J. (1995). Self-injurious behavior: A brief review of theories and current treatment perspectives. *Dev Disabil Bull* **23**, 90–104.

Symons, F. J. and Thompson, T. (1997). Self-injurious behaviour and body site preference. *J Intellect Disabil Res* **41**, 456–468.

Symons, F. J., Butler, M. G., Sanders, M. D., Feurer, I. D., and Thompson, T. (1999). Self-injurious behavior and Prader-Willi syndrome: behavioral forms and body locations. *Am J Ment Retard* **104**, 260–269.

Symons, F. J., Sutton, K. A., Walker, C., and Bodfish, J. W. (2003). Altered diurnal pattern of salivary substance P in adults with developmental disabilities and chronic self-injury. *Am J Ment Retard* **108**, 13–18.

Symons, F.J., Thompson, A., and Rodriguez, M.C. (2004). Self-injurious behavior and the efficacy of naltrexone treatment: a quantitative synthesis. *Ment Retard Dev Disabil Res Rev* **10**, 193–200.

Taylor, D. K., Bass, T., Flory, G. S., and Hankenson, F. C. (2005). Use of low-dose chlorpromazine in conjunction with environmental enrichment to eliminate self-injurious behavior in a rhesus macaque (*Macaca mulatta*). *Comp Med* **55**, 282–288.

Thompson, T., Hackenberg, T., Cerutti, D., Baker, D., and Axtell, S. (1994). Opioid antagonist effects on self-injury in adults with mental retardation: response form and location as determinants of medication effects. *Am J Ment Retard* **99**, 85–102.

Thompson, T., Symons, F., Delaney, D., and England, C. (1995). Self-injurious behavior as endogenous neurochemical self-administration. *Ment Retard Dev Disabil Res Rev* **1**, 137–148.

Tiefenbacher, S., Novak, M. A., Jorgensen, M. J., and Meyer, J. S. (2000). Physiological correlates of self-injurious behavior in captive, socially-reared rhesus monkeys. *Psychoneuroendocrinology* **25**, 799–817.

Tiefenbacher, S., Marinus, L. M., Davenport, M. D. *et al.* (2003). Evidence for endogenous opioid involvement in the expression of self-injurious behavior in rhesus monkeys. *Am J Primatol* **60**(suppl 1), 103.

Tiefenbacher, S., Novak, M. A., Marinus, L. M., Chase, W. K., Miller, J. A., and Meyer, J. S. (2004). Altered hypothalamic-pituitary-adrenocortical function in rhesus monkeys (*Macaca mulatta*) with self-injurious behavior. *Psychoneuroendocrinology* **29**, 501–515.

Tiefenbacher, S., Fahey, M. A., Rowlett, J. K. *et al.* (2005a). The efficacy of diazepam treatment for the management of acute wounding episodes in captive rhesus macaques. *Comp Med* **55**, 387–392.

Tiefenbacher, S., Newman, T. K., Davenport, M. D., Meyer, J. S., Higley, J. D., and Novak, M. A. (2005b). The role of two serotonin pathway gene polymorphisms in self-injurious behavior in singly housed *Macaca mulatta*. *Am J Primatol* **66**(suppl 1), 91.

Tiefenbacher, S., Novak, M. A., Lutz, C. K., and Meyer, J. S. (2005c). The physiology and neurochemistry of self-injurious behavior: a nonhuman primate model. *Front Biosci* **10**, 1–11.

Ulett, G. A., Han, S., and Han, J. (1998). Electroacupuncture: mechanisms and clinical application. *Biol Psychiatry* **44**, 129–138.

van der Kolk B. A., Perry J. C., and Herman J. L. (1991). Childhood origins of self-destructive behavior. *Am J Psychiatry* **148**, 1665–1671.

Verhoeven, W. M. A. and Tuinier, S. (1996). The effect of buspirone on challenging behaviour in mentally retarded patients: an open prospective multiple-case study. *J Intellect Disabil Res* **40**, 502–508.

Verhoeven, W. M. A., Tuinier, S., van den Berg, Y. W. M. M. *et al.* (1999). Stress and self-injurious behavior; hormonal and serotonergic parameters in mentally retarded subjects. *Pharmacopsychiatry* **32**, 13–20.

Vierck, C. J., Jr., Lineberry, C. G., Lee, P. K., and Calderwood, H. W. (1974). Prolonged hypalgesia following "acupuncture" in monkeys. *Life Sci* **15**, 1277–1289.

Villalba, R. and Harrington, C. J. (2000). Repetitive self-injurious behavior: a neuropsychiatric perspective and review of pharmacologic treatments. *Semin Clin Neuropsychiatry* **5**, 215–226.

Vollmer, T. R., Progar, P. R., Lalli, J. S. *et al.* (1998). Fixed-time schedules attenuate extinction-induced phenomena in the treatment of severe aberrant behavior. *J Appl Behav Anal* **31**, 529–542.

Walsh, S., Bramblett, C. A., and Alford, P. L. (1982). A vocabulary of abnormal behaviors in restrictively reared chimpanzees. *Am J Primatol* **3**, 315–319.

Weed, J. L., Wagner, P. O., Byrum, R., Parrish, S., Knezevich, M., and Powell, D. A. (2003). Treatment of persistent self-injurious behavior in rhesus monkeys through socialization: a preliminary report. *Contemp Top Lab Anim Sci* **42**, 21–23.

Weld, K. P., Mench, J. A., Woodward, R. A., Bolesta, M. S., Suomi, S. J., and Higley, J. D. (1998). Effect of tryptophan treatment on self-biting and central nervous system serotonin metabolism in rhesus monkeys (*Macaca mulatta*). *Neuropsychopharmacology* **19**, 314–321.

Winchel, R. M. and Stanley, M. (1991). Self-injurious behavior: a review of the behavior and biology of self-mutilation. *Am J Psychiatry* **148**, 306–317.

Wong, D. F., Harris, J. C., Naidu, S. *et al.* (1996). Dopamine transporters are markedly reduced in Lesch-Nyhan disease in vivo. *Proc Natl Acad Sci USA* **93**, 5539–5543.

Yates, T. M. (2004). The developmental psychopathology of self-injurious behavior: compensatory regulation in posttraumatic adaptation. *Clin Psychol Rev* **24**, 35–74.

Zarcone, J. R., Iwata, B. A., Vollmer, T. R., Jagtiani, S., Smith, R. G., and Mazaleski, J. L. (1993). Extinction of self-injurious escape behavior with and without instructional fading. *J Appl Behav Anal* **26**, 353–360.

Zweig-Frank, H., Paris, J., and Guzder, J. (1994). Psychological risk factors for dissociation and self-mutilation in female patients with borderline personality disorder. *Can J Psychiatry* **39**, 259–264.

matrilines consisting of females and their female offspring (Lindburg, 1971; Teas *et al.*, 1980; Berman, 1983; Melnick *et al.*, 1984). This emphasis on females is related to a sex bias in dispersal, in that females remain in their natal troop generally throughout their life whereas males typically emigrate and join new troops (Berard, 1989). Macaques have complex social repertoires that run the gamut from prolonged affiliative responses, as seen in grooming behavior, to highly volatile aggressive altercations that can result in serious injury and even death (e.g. Southwick *et al.*, 1965; Teas *et al.*, 1982). Each troop is essentially a closed society, and troop members typically react to strangers with high levels of aggression (Southwick *et al.*, 1974). Because of their highly complex social nature and their ability to adapt to diverse environments (traits characteristic of humans), macaques may be an ideal model for understanding causes and circumstances surrounding the development of abnormal behavior.

Stereotypic patterns of behavior

Abnormal behavior in nonhuman primates often takes the form of stereotypic behavior, defined as iterative, highly ritualized motor actions which appear to have no identifiable biological function (Berkson, 1968). The word "appear" is important in the definition because it acknowledges that research may ultimately reveal a purpose for various types of stereotypies. Some kinds of abnormal behavior can lead to serious injury (e.g. self-mutilation or head banging). These latter activities are considered in a separate category of pathological behavior because of their potential for self-harm (Bayne and Novak, 1998). Because they are the topic of another chapter in this volume (Chapter 5), they will not be discussed any further here.

In primates, stereotypic behavior is often idiosyncratic (Berkson, 1968; Ridley and Baker, 1982; Bayne and Novak, 1998) and can take many different forms both across and within species of monkeys and apes (Walsh *et al.*, 1982; Bayne *et al.*, 1992). At least two classification schemes have been developed to characterize this variability across primates (Bayne and Novak, 1998). The first scheme emphasizes the form of the motor act, differentiating whole-body, gross motor actions from fine motor movements. Whole-body stereotypies involve repetitive movements through space and time that include pacing, somersaulting, rocking, and bouncing. Fine motor stereotypies consist of activities directed to the animal's own body and include digit sucking, eye saluting, ear covering, clasping, and hair pulling (Berkson, 1968; Bayne *et al.*, 1992).

Because the severity of abnormal behavior can vary substantially across individuals, a second classification scheme is based on the frequency of stereotypic behavior and its potential to disrupt normal activities (Bayne and Novak, 1998). In this scheme stereotypic behavior is divided into two general categories, termed mild and severe. Mild stereotypies can include all of the whole-body and fine motor movements as long as they do not disrupt essential biological processes. However,

Abnormal Behavior in Nonhun Primates and Models of Developm

Melinda A. Novak and Stephen J.

INTRODUCTION

Nonhuman primates raised in captivity can develop a dizzying array of bi unusual patterns of behavior (Bayne and Novak, 1998). These range fron typic activities such as pacing, rocking, self-mouthing, eye covering, and self-grooming to more serious behaviors such as self-inflicted wounding. I captive primates may also display species typical behavior in inappropriate or at levels that are either too high or too low and compromise well-being. discussion of abnormal behavior and its relevance for the human conditic consider both kinds of abnormality. The goals of this chapter are first to d characterize abnormal behavior in nonhuman primates, primarily using as an example; second to identify factors that may contribute to the develc abnormal behavior; and third to explore a functional approach to abnorm ior in primates and identify parallels between human and nonhuman prin respect to these phenomena.

TYPES OF ABNORMAL BEHAVIOR IN MACAQUES

Background

Macaques are a genus of Old World monkeys that can be found in a wid different environments, including remote forests, agricultural areas, sm and even large cities. Rhesus monkeys show arguably the widest range earning the term "weed macaques" because of their ability to thrive in are; estation and human habitation (Teas et al., 1980; Richard et al., 1989). M; highly social and live in large troops that are structured around multig any of these patterns can become severe if its frequency of occurrence disrupts basic processes involved in exploration, feeding, reproduction, or parental behavior or if it replaces other species-typical behavior such as grooming or play. A separate category termed "serious or pathological" is reserved for a suite of behavior patterns that can result in tissue damage, such as self-directed biting, head banging, and hair plucking.

Abnormal forms of species-typical behavior

Discussions of abnormal behavior in captive primates should not be limited to stereotypic patterns of behavior but should also include unusual variation in the expression and/or level of species-typical behavior. However, unlike the presence of bizarre behavior which can be recognized with ease, unusual alterations in species-typical behavior may be much more difficult to identify. Here we focus exclusively on two general temperaments or dispositional styles that when expressed in extreme forms may result in unusual variations in species-typical behavior. These two temperaments have been termed high reactivity and impulsive aggressiveness, respectively, and they have clear-cut human counterparts (Suomi, 2000).

Reactivity

It is now well established that there are marked individual differences in reactivity among nonhuman primates when animals are exposed to novel situations or to relatively minor changes in their social or physical environment. Some rhesus monkeys ($\sim$20%) respond to relatively mild environmental stressors with unusual behavioral disruption and physiological arousal including prolonged activation of the hypothalamic-pituitary-adrenal (HPA) axis as assessed by plasma cortisol and ACTH, increased cerebrospinal fluid (CSF) levels of the norepinephrine metabolite 3-methoxy-4-hydroxyphenylglycol (MHPG), heightened sympathetic nervous system activity as reflected in altered heart rate rhythms, and abnormal immune system response (Coe et al., 1989; Higley et al., 1992b; Suomi, 2000). The same stressors elicit only minor behavioral reactions and transient physiological responses in the remainder of the population (Suomi, 1991; see Kagan and Snidman, 1991, for analogous findings in children). Thus, some monkeys can be characterized as highly reactive – having an anxious or fearful temperament – whereas the majority of monkeys show low–moderate reactivity in response to environmental challenges. These differences have proven to be stable and enduring and are thus characteristic of the individual.

Differences in reactivity become even more pronounced with more severe challenges. For example, separation from the mother or from peers elicits a more profound behavioral and physiological response in highly reactive infant and juvenile monkeys. These individuals consistently exhibit marked distress immediately following separation and are more likely to become withdrawn or depressed if the separation is prolonged or permanent compared to normally reactive monkeys. These patterns are observed in infant monkeys not only under controlled laboratory conditions but also in the wild during times of social disturbance. For example, six-month-old infants frequently experience mother-enforced separations during the breeding season when their mothers form consort relationships with males. Some infants (about 20%) show marked distress responses while the majority of infants show only brief agitation and then seek out their peers and older siblings (Berman et al., 1994). Furthermore, early differences among infants in reactivity are predictive of the timing of later life events, for example the age at which adolescent males emigrate from their troops (Rasmussen and Suomi, 1989).

Impulsive aggression

Another example of unusual variation in species-typical behavior is the presence of impulsive or explosive aggression in a small percentage (5–10%) of the rhesus monkey population, particularly in males. Some male rhesus monkeys living in social groups in the wild or in captivity show heightened levels of aggression in response to relatively innocuous social situations. This aggression is inappropriate not only in terms of its intensity but also with respect to its target (Higley et al., 1990). Furthermore, males with this syndrome often take more risks such as jumping out of trees from a height that sometimes results in injury, show atypical sleep–wakefulness cycles, and have chronically low levels of serotonergic activity as measured by CSF concentrations of the primary central serotonin (5-HT) metabolite 5-hydroxyindoleacetic acid (5-HIAA) (Higley et al., 1992a; Higley et al., 1996b; Zajicek et al., 1997).

FACTORS CONTRIBUTING TO THE DEVELOPMENT OF ABNORMAL BEHAVIOR

Over the last 50 years a variety of factors have been proposed to account for the development of abnormal behavior in monkeys. These factors range from specific environmental situations to neurochemical/cytoarchitectural abnormalities in the brain. A long-standing view is that abnormal behavior in macaques emerges as a result of socially inadequate early rearing experiences (e.g. rearing infants without mothers) or later social separation (e.g. removing animals from social groups and placing them in individual cages). However, abnormal behavior can also be linked to many other factors such as brain damage (Bielefeldt-Ohmann, et al., 2004), painful disorders such as arthritis, and brain neurotransmitter dysfunction (Higley, et al., 1996c). Moreover, some of the behavioral and biological components that characterize both high-reactive and impulsively aggressive monkeys appear to be highly heritable (Higley et al., 1993; Williamson et al., 2003). Recent findings clearly emphasize the need for an integrative model in which abnormal behavior is viewed as the outcome of environmental exposure, physiological changes, and genetic risk factors (Suomi, 2007).

Early rearing environments

The notion that an animal develops stereotypic behavior because of exposure to adverse housing or inadequate environmental conditions first emerged from the early rearing experience work of Harlow (Harlow and Harlow, 1962, 1965) and subsequently was reinforced with studies of social restriction during different stages of the lifespan. The effects of social restriction were found to vary across the stages of development and by the degree of deprivation. Harlow and his colleagues examined several different kinds of early rearing experiences, each of which produced different amounts and types of abnormal behavior.

In most cases, animals reared in these altered conditions were compared with monkeys that were reared with their mothers in social groups consisting minimally of other adult females and offspring. This form of rearing is variously termed normal rearing or mother-peer rearing.

Isolation rearing from birth

Abnormal behavior

Rhesus monkeys reared alone from birth developed a suite of behavioral characteristics that we now refer to as the "isolation syndrome" (Harlow and Harlow, 1962, 1965; Cross and Harlow, 1965; Sackett, 1968; Capitanio, 1986). Isolate reared monkeys showed high levels of abnormal behavior, excessive emotional responses, and little in the way of normal species typical social behavior (Mason, 1968). At six months of age, most of the isolated monkeys exhibited multiple kinds of stereotypic behavior that included both motor stereotypies and self-directed stereotypies, with the three most common patterns being rocking, huddling, and self-clasping. The time allocated to stereotypic behavior was very high, ranging from 35 to 60% of an observation session, and thus severe in nature. The effects described above could not be traced solely to sensory deprivation inasmuch as isolates reared in sensory-rich environments containing toys and manipulanda and exposed to static pictures and movies fared no better in terms of outcome at six months of age (Sackett et al., 1982).

Some forms of abnormal behavior may have represented normal species-typical behavior that the isolates redirected to themselves (e.g. self-clasping instead of clasping a mother). This hypothesis was tested and confirmed by giving infants access to a warm, terry-cloth mother during the period of isolation. When given inanimate surrogate mothers, infants not only clasped their surrogates rather than themselves, they also developed an attachment to these inanimate mothers, using them as a base of operations when exploring novel stimuli (Harlow, 1958; Harlow and Zimmermann, 1959; Harlow and Suomi, 1970). A subsequent study revealed that rocking behavior was reduced by adding motion to the surrogate mother (Mason and Berkson, 1975). Despite the reduction in some forms of stereotypic behavior, the addition of an inanimate surrogate mother did not lead to any marked improvements in later social behavior.

Despite the presence of normal developmental milestones with respect to weight gain and hormonal changes associated with puberty, major isolate deficits in social behavior persisted along with high levels of stereotypic behavior. Some developmental changes in stereotypic behavior were noted in that digit sucking and self-clasping decreased with age, whereas other kinds of stereotypies such as somersaults, head bobs, unusual limb manipulations (e.g. leg behind neck, floating limb), and in some cases, self-injurious behavior (SIB) increased (Mitchell et al., 1966; Sackett, 1967; Mitchell, 1968; Fittinghoff et al., 1974).

Considerable interest was focused on reproductive outcomes and maternal behavior in isolate reared monkeys. Males showed deficits in the motor postures associated with copulation, being unable to perform the double foot clasp mount characteristic of normally reared monkeys. Furthermore, most isolate-reared females were indifferent or abusive to their first-born infants. Surprisingly, some isolate-reared mothers showed substantial improvements in their maternal behavior with the birth of a second infant (Ruppenthal et al., 1976).

Physiological effects

Associated with the pronounced behavioral disruption produced by isolation rearing were major changes in central nervous system (CNS) function. As juveniles, isolate-reared monkeys showed significantly higher levels of central serotonin, as measured by CSF concentrations of 5-HIAA, than socially reared controls (Kraemer et al., 1989). Consistent with disruption of the serotonergic system, abnormal behavior was significantly reduced in juvenile isolates by treatment with the 5-HT$_{1A}$ receptor partial agonist buspirone (Kraemer and Clarke, 1990). However, disruption of the serotonergic system could not be detected in adult isolates, who failed to respond to a number of drugs that either enhanced or suppressed serotonergic activity in socially reared animals (Kraemer et al., 1997). These findings suggest that alterations in serotonin may be related to the presence of abnormal behavior in juvenile monkeys, an effect that apparently disappears prior to reaching adulthood.

Catecholaminergic function also appeared to be altered by isolation rearing. For example, isolates showed unusual responses to amphetamine exposure as juveniles. Amphetamine is well known to provoke stereotypic behaviors in normal animals. However, in a comparison of juvenile isolates and socially reared controls, only the controls showed amphetamine induced stereotypy. The isolates, in contrast, displayed high levels of agonistic behavior with occasional wounding of one another (Kraemer et al., 1984). In a later study by Lewis and co-workers (1990), old adult isolates and old social control monkeys displayed a dose-dependent increase in apomorphine-induced stereotypies, but the isolates showed significantly more whole-body stereotypy than the controls at a dose of 0.3 mg/kg. Together, these studies suggest that early isolation rearing leads to a long-lasting enhancement of catecholaminergic function that is particularly evident following a pharmacologic challenge. This hypothesis is consistent with other studies reporting significant neuroanatomical and physiological changes in the basal ganglia of social isolates (Martin *et al.*, 1991) and reductions in abnormal behavior following treatment of isolates with the dopamine antagonist chlorpromazine (McKinney *et al.*, 1973).

Of considerable interest were possible effects of isolation on stress responsiveness. Juvenile isolate-reared monkeys showed elevated baseline cortisol levels compared to controls (Sackett *et al.* 1973). However, there was no discernable effect of isolation rearing on plasma cortisol levels in adults using a restraint-stress paradigm (Meyer and Bowman, 1972). These results, in combination with the above-reported monamine results, suggest that the differences from controls may be reduced in adults compared to juveniles. This may have resulted from increased vulnerability during the juvenile period and/or because the long period of time since the isolation period resulted in more nonphysical social exposure to other monkeys.

The studies discussed above suggest that isolation rearing influences some of the major monoamine systems as well as possibly yielding differences in cortisol levels. Although these changes may contribute to the abnormal behavior observed in isolate-reared monkeys, several limitations must be noted. First, relatively few monkeys were actually subjected to the isolation rearing condition, and these animals exhibited wide individual differences in the expression of abnormal behavior. This variation has made it difficult to determine any possible connection of particular abnormal behaviors (e.g. stereotypies) to disruptions in normal species-typical behavior patterns such as maternal behavior. Furthermore, existing data do not permit clear causal explanations to be formulated. For example, although it may be tempting to conclude that the monoaminergic abnormalities discussed above underlie the abnormal behaviors exhibited by social isolates, this relationship is almost entirely correlational.

Peer rearing from birth

The isolation research described above revealed that some kind of social experience was necessary for normal development in rhesus monkey infants. A series of studies were conducted to determine if exposure to young naïve infants was sufficient to induce normal development. This rearing condition was called peer rearing and in all the studies mentioned below, infants were removed from their mothers shortly after birth, reared in a nursery for several weeks or more, and then placed in social groups consisting of other like-reared infants. Although these general procedures were followed, some differences existed across research programs that ultimately may explain some of the inconsistent results reported for some measures. Facilities varied with respect to how long the infants were maintained in the nursery, whether they received any social contact during this period, and the size of the social group into which they were ultimately placed. For example, at the Wisconsin

Primate Center (see Clarke *et al.*, 1996), infants were removed from their mothers at birth, placed in single cages in the nursery for six weeks of life during which they received 30 minutes of contact per day with another infant, and at the end of this period were placed into peer groups of three infants. At the California Primate Center (see Capitanio *et al.*, 2005), infants were removed from their mothers at birth, housed individually in incubators for 30 days during which they had access to a stuffed toy and towels, and at the end of this period, were placed in dyads. At the Laboratory of Comparative Ethology (see Higley *et al.*, 1991; Fahlke *et al.*, 2000; Roma *et al.*, 2006), infants were removed from their mothers at birth, placed in individual cages in a nursery for five weeks where they had access to a surrogate mother. At the end of this period, they were placed in social groups of 4–6 infants. Yet another variant of these procedures was followed at the Yerkes Primate Center (see Winslow *et al.*, 2003). In this facility, infants were separated from their mothers at birth, individually housed in a nursery for the first 45–60 days of life. Each infant was then pair housed most of each day except for a separation period of 4–6 hours per day for feeding and bottle training.

Behavioral effects

In marked contrast to early isolation rearing, infants separated from their mothers at birth and reared in peer groups displayed nearly normal social behavior and showed substantially lower levels of stereotypic behavior (Chamove, 1973). Peer-reared monkeys displayed stereotypic behavior about 4–20% of the time and the more common stereotypic patterns included digit sucking and rocking. However, the development of appropriate social behavior was somewhat delayed in comparison to normally reared monkeys (Chamove *et al.*, 1973).

Despite the appearance of many normal patterns of social behavior, peer-reared monkeys also showed heightened fearfulness. They reacted to minor changes in the environment by vocalizing and clutching other members of their peer group for a prolonged period of time, even to the point where they would continue to cling to one another and move around as a train of monkeys (Harlow and Harlow, 1965). Peer-reared monkeys appeared to have very strong attachments to their peer group as seen by their more prolonged and intense reactions to social separation than normally reared monkeys (Higley *et al.*, 1991). However, despite the appearance of a strong attachment bond in infancy, this bond did not provide much social buffering later in development. For example, Winslow and colleagues (2003) reported that juvenile peer-reared males had lower levels of affiliation (e.g. grooming) and were less likely to have their stress levels alleviated by a companion than mother-peer-reared males. Peer-reared monkeys were much more likely to develop impulsively aggressive patterns of response during their juvenile years than their mother-reared counterparts (Higley *et al.*, 1996c). In addition, peer-reared juvenile monkeys also exhibited greater vulnerability to excessive alcohol consumption than normally reared monkeys (Higley *et al.*, 1991; Fahlke *et al.*, 2000).

Subsequent studies have shown that the effects of early peer rearing can extend into adulthood. Considerable attention has been focused on females to determine whether monkeys reared without a mother but with naïve peers can function as normal mothers. A recent study suggests that peer-reared mothers maintained in stable social groups display appropriate maternal behavior and produce infants whose behavior is indistinguishable from the infants of normally reared mothers (Roma *et al.*, 2006).

Physiological effects

As with isolation, the effects of peer rearing extended to various physiological systems, particularly the monoaminergic and neuropeptide systems. Peer-reared infant monkeys showed increased turnover (activity) of the noradrenergic system as indicated by higher CSF levels of the norepinephrine metabolite MHPG compared with normally reared monkeys (Higley *et al.*, 1992b). A subsequent report by Clarke *et al.* (1996) confirmed the increased noradrenergic activity in peer-reared monkey infants. The involvement of the serotonergic system was demonstrated in a comparison of 256 differentially reared infant rhesus monkeys (Shannon *et al.*, 2005). In contrast to isolate-reared monkeys, peer-reared monkeys showed lower central levels of 5-HT across the first year of life than normally reared monkeys as measured by the CSF metabolite 5-HIAA.

A neuroimaging study using positron emission tomography (PET) revealed significantly less serotonin-binding potential and lower rates of cerebral blood flow in many brain regions of juvenile peer-reared monkeys relative to that of mother/peer-reared counterparts (Ichise *et al.*, 2006). Research also suggests that the neuropeptide oxytocin may play a role in peer rearing. Peer-reared juveniles had lower CSF concentrations of oxytocin than normally reared juveniles, and the levels of oxytocin were positively correlated with affiliative social behavior (Winslow *et al.*, 2003). At present, the relationship between these neurotransmitter and neuropeptide alterations and the possible direct effects on stereotypic or other kinds of abnormal behavior remain largely unknown.

Because heightened fearfulness is a key characteristic of peer rearing, the HPA axis has been the focus of a number of studies examining stress responsiveness. Initial studies of cortisol levels were inconclusive in that peer-reared monkeys were reported to have higher concentrations of cortisol (Higley *et al.*, 1992) or lower concentrations of cortisol (Clarke, 1993) compared with mother/peer-reared controls. Peer-reared monkeys also responded to stress with smaller increases in ACTH and cortisol than mother-reared monkeys (Clarke, 1993). A subsequent study was designed to examine infants longitudinally under several different conditions. Mother-reared infants displayed higher concentrations of cortisol than peer-reared monkeys during the first two months of life but showed no difference in their response to 30-minute separation periods (Shannon *et al.*, 1998). In yet another study, neither baseline levels of cortisol or stress levels varied by rearing condition (Winslow *et al.*, 2003). However, a study of 778 infant monkeys provides strong evidence that peer rearing results in a reduced cortisol set-point for the HPA axis (Capitanio *et al.*, 2005). Peer-reared infants showed lower cortisol levels in the afternoon, lower cortisol rises in response to social separation, and were less responsive to both a dexamethasone suppression test and an ACTH challenge test. It should be noted, however, that these differential findings might in part be the result of differences in peer rearing procedures used at the different facilities.

Peer rearing can also result in long-lasting changes in the immune system. Peer-reared monkeys showed greater lymphocyte proliferation responses than mother-reared monkeys (Coe *et al.*, 1989). This vulnerability was associated with lower proportions of CD8 cells and lower natural killer cell activity (Lubach *et al.*, 1995), and a substantially increased risk of diarrhea (Elmore *et al.*, 1992).

Several general conclusions can be drawn from the work on peer rearing. Peer rearing had less of an impact on behavior than isolation rearing in that normal social behavior was present and abnormal behavior was substantially reduced. However, peer-reared monkeys were unable to regulate or modulate both their fearfulness and their aggressiveness, perhaps a failure of social buffering. These behavioral differences have been associated with alterations in monoamine, neuroendocrine, and immune function. However, as in the case of isolate-reared animals, it is difficult at this time to make direct connections between any of these physiological systems and the abnormal behavior patterns seen in peer-reared monkeys.

Finally, research has indicated that many of the above-reported behavioral and biological consequences of peer-rearing are in part mediated by genetic factors, reflecting gene–environment (G × E) interactions. For example, the behavioral and physiological consequences of functional allelic variation in the serotonin transporter gene (*5-HTT*) are far more pronounced for peer-reared rhesus monkeys than for their mother-reared counterparts. Specifically, peer-reared monkeys carrying the "short" (less transcriptionally efficient) allele of the *5-HTT* gene exhibit significantly more aberrant patterns of early neurobehavioral functioning than peer-reared monkeys carrying the "long" (more transcriptionally efficient) allele (Champoux *et al.*, 2002). This includes higher levels of aggression (Barr *et al.*, 2003), lower CSF concentrations of 5-HIAA (Bennett *et al.*, 2002), greater HPA activation following social separation (Barr *et al.*, 2004a), and higher rates of alcohol consumption (Barr *et al.*, 2004b). Of great importance, there were no significant differences attributable to *5-HTT* allelic variation in any of these behavioral and physiological measures among mother-reared monkeys of comparable age and sex. A comparable pattern of G × E interaction involving allelic variation in the MAO-A gene and peer versus mother-peer rearing has been reported for various measures of aggressive behavior in rhesus monkey males (Newman *et al.*, 2005).

Surrogate with limited peer rearing from birth

Nursery rearing of infant monkeys occurs for many reasons, including illness of the mother, prematurity or illness of the infant, rejection by the mother, and research protocol. For many years, peer rearing was the primary way in which nursery-reared monkeys were maintained. In recent years, a second rearing procedure has been examined. The surrogate/peer-rearing condition was instituted in part to overcome the problem of infants serving in the dual role as a mother figure and as playmate. Surrogate/peer-reared monkeys were reared with continuous exposure to an inanimate "terry cloth"-covered mother and were given brief daily exposure to similarly reared peers. Depending on the study, the exposure to peers ranged from 30 minutes to 2 hours a day (Rosenblum, 1961; Hansen, 1966; Meyer *et al.*, 1975). The brief exposure to peers was designed to mimic naturalistic early mother–infant interaction in which infants spend most of their time with their mothers and only interact with other infants for brief periods. The brief exposure was also expected to facilitate play behavior with peers and reduce the risk of developing a primary attachment to peers.

Behavioral effects

In contrast to peer rearing, the surrogate/peer-rearing regimen resulted in the development of normal social behavior without the intense fearful reactions noted in peer-reared monkeys (Hansen, 1966; Ruppenthal *et al.*, 1991). Furthermore, minor differences in vocalization such as geckering and cooing between surrogate/peer-reared and normally reared monkeys disappeared after the first few months of life. Some forms of stereotypic behavior were observed (mostly digit sucking and some rocking against the surrogate surface), occurring about 5–10% of the time. But these patterns declined across age such that surrogate/peer-reared monkeys behaved like normally reared monkeys at one year of age (Hansen, 1966). Surrogate/peer-reared animals continued to develop socially showing adequate skills in grooming, reproduction, and parental care (Novak *et al.*, 1992; Sackett *et al.*, 2002). However, other research has further delineated the differences between the two nursery-rearing regimes, In mixed rearing groups, where monkeys from all three rearing conditions described above were placed together at one year of age, surrogate/peer-reared monkeys were much more likely than peer-reared monkeys to interact with the normally reared monkeys (Strand, 2006). However, a possible emotional deficit was also identified in that surrogate/peer-reared monkeys showed the highest levels of aggression and appeared not to respond readily to the submissive responses of others (Strand and Novak, 2005).

Physiological effects

There are only a few studies of the effect of surrogate/peer rearing on CNS function. To date, the emphasis has been on the HPA axis. Converging evidence suggests that infant surrogate/peer-reared monkeys have significantly lower concentrations of circulating cortisol than mother/peer-reared monkeys (Shannon *et al.*, 2005; Capitanio *et al.*, 2005) and respond significantly less to the stress of brief social separation (Shannon *et al.*, 1998). This difference persisted even after the surrogate/peer-reared monkeys were housed in a large mixed rearing group containing mother/peer-reared and peer-reared monkeys (Davenport *et al.*, 2003).

The information derived from this rearing condition suggests that infants acquire all species-typical social behaviors and show relatively low levels of abnormal behavior when provided with an inanimate surrogate mother and given brief daily peer interaction. Apart from the HPA system findings, we know little about how surrogate/peer rearing influences neurotransmitter activity. However, in considering both types of peer rearing, it is clear that surrogate/peer rearing generally results in better outcome than continuous peer rearing. Obviously, a number of factors may contribute to this difference but key among these is the excessive clinging behavior observed in peer-only reared monkeys. Infants normally cling to mothers; however, mothers control this activity pushing infants away and encouraging independence. Infants reared continuously with each other develop clinging responses that cannot be easily broken. In turn, clinging behavior suppresses exploration of the environment and promotes emotional responses. In contrast, surrogate/peer-reared infants are free to move away from their surrogate and explore their environment. The brief daily contact with other infants facilitates playful interactions rather than clinging behavior. In essence, peer-reared monkeys have to serve as attachment objects and as playmates at the same time and they end up doing a rather poor job of both (Novak and Sackett, 2006).

Later housing environments

Stereotypic behavior is not limited to animals reared in impoverished circumstances during infancy. It can also arise in monkeys at some later point in development. For example, monkeys placed into individual cages can develop a wide range of whole-body and self-directed stereotypies even if normally reared prior to that time (Lutz *et al.*, 2003; Novak, 2003). Unlike the rearing conditions described above, there is considerable variability both in the age at which monkeys are first placed into individual cage housing and the length of exposure to this environment. This makes it difficult to discern general relationships between the development of stereotypies and alterations in neurotransmitter function, HPA axis, or normal behavior. However, it is clear that the earlier the onset of individual cage housing (15 months compared with 28 months) the greater the risk of developing severely abnormal behavior (Lutz *et al.*, 2003; Novak, 2003).

Environmental/social effects

There are at least three features of the individual cage environment which might be implicated in the development of stereotypies: (1) reductions in cage space leading to restrictions on species-typical patterns of locomotion, (2) the abrupt loss of physical contact with other monkeys after a lengthy period of social housing, and (3) the lack of access to other monkeys, thereby depriving the animal of an appropriate target for some of its behavioral repertoire. Cage size may play a role in the development of whole-body motor stereotypies such as backflipping and pacing (Draper and Bernstein, 1963; Paulk et al., 1977). However, once such stereotypies become established in individual cages, they are not always reduced. Monkeys showed no reductions in abnormal behavior when their cage size was doubled (Crockett et al., 1993) or increased sixfold (Kaufman et al., 2004). Only large outdoor housing environments reduced motor stereotypies in monkeys (Draper and Bernstein, 1963). Furthermore, exposure to outdoor environments also appeared to reduce self-directed stereotypies in monkeys even though they remained "individually housed" while outdoors (Fontenot et al., 2006).

The loss of companionship and/or the lack thereof may also be relevant determinants of stereotypy in individually housed monkeys. Monkeys that are placed in individual cages after being reared in social groups for varying periods of time face the loss of familiar companions. Social separation is known to have profound effects on infant monkeys, inducing affective changes that can include depression (Suomi, 1991). Whether social loss plays a significant role in the onset of stereotypy is not clear at this time, particularly because the loss of companionship is generally confounded with exposure to a novel situation and unfamiliar animals. However, it should be noted that the reinstatement of social housing appears to mitigate some forms of abnormal behavior (Bayne et al., 1991; Weed et al., 2003).

The lack of an animal with which to interact may also affect the development of stereotypies (Novak et al., 2006). Monkeys spend considerable time in close physical proximity to other monkeys, engaged in contact, grooming, sex, play, and aggression. Monkeys housed in an individual cage are essentially deprived of a target for many of their social activities. Under these conditions, monkeys may direct certain types of social behavior toward themselves, thus becoming the object of their own social motivation. For example, increases in self-grooming and self-sex in individually housed monkeys may represent an accommodation to the lack of social grooming and sexual activity. Similarly, monkeys may direct play gestures to their own limbs and, when provoked, may focus their aggressive responses on the only convenient target, themselves. This hypothesis is also consistent with the early rearing studies of isolate-reared monkeys in that some forms of abnormal behavior were normal behavior patterns that monkeys redirected to themselves (e.g. self-clasping).

Physiological effects

Less is known about the physiological underpinnings of abnormal behavior in monkeys housed alone after infancy because of considerable individual variability in the age of onset and length of individual cage housing. However, an emerging literature on drug exposure and on drug treatment suggests a role for the dopaminergic and serotonergic systems respectively. Administration of amphetamine, a dopamine releasing agent, produced a decrease in whole-body motor movements (Schlemmer et al., 1996), an increased incidence in floating limb (Levin et al., 1990) and prolonged staring (Ellison *et al.*, 1981). Furthermore, monkeys given repeated low doses of amphetamine showed hallucinatory behavior (complex responses independent of external stimuli) and increases in self-directed stereotypies and other abnormal activities (e.g. mesh weaving) that persisted beyond drug exposure (Castner and Goldman-Rakic, 1999).

Recent research has focused on the role of drugs in alleviating stereotypic behavior. Administration of fluoxetine, a serotonin (5-HT) reuptake inhibitor, markedly reduced self-directed stereotypies in rhesus monkeys (Fontenot *et al.*, 2005) and reduced both whole-body motor stereotypies and self-directed stereotypies in vervet monkeys (Hugo *et al.*, 2003). The use of other drugs such as diazepam has yielded mixed results, working in some monkeys and not others depending on their early history (Tiefenbacher *et al.*, 2005).

THE FUNCTIONS OF ABNORMAL BEHAVIOR IN PRIMATES AND RELATIONSHIP TO MODELS

Considerable effort has been spent characterizing abnormal behavior in monkeys and relating it to early rearing environments. In this regard, monkeys show an amazing array of different kinds of abnormal behavior, much of which can be attributed to impoverished early rearing experiences or later exposure to socially restricted environments. However, less is known about the significance of these behaviors and how they relate to the development of primate models of human health. Are different stereotypies (e.g. pacing, eye poking) indicative of different disorders, do certain stereotypies co-occur with sufficient frequency to form a suite of traits associated with particular disorders, or is the incidence of any stereotypy regardless of its form indicative of the same or similar disorders? There are no clear-cut answers to these questions, and these may be the wrong questions inasmuch as they are focused on form and not function. Increasingly, it may be more important to determine the possible functions of stereotypies rather than to assume that they are functionless. A number of possible functions have actually been proposed ranging from the notion that stereotypies represent maladaptive behavior indicating distress, to the notion that stereotypies represent effective coping strategies, the loss of which might lead to distress. Studies on rodents and farm animals have led to the development of several functional hypotheses for why animals engage in stereotypic behavior (Frith and Done, 1990; Lawrence and Rushen, 1993; Mason and Latham, 2004). Below, we discuss four possible explanations for why animals engage in stereotypic behavior including hypotheses that suggest that stereotypies are beneficial or aversive to well-being.

On the plus side of the equation is the suggestion that stereotypic behavior may be a form of "do it yourself enrichment" (Mason and Latham, 2004). In this context, stereotypies may increase sensory motor stimulation and allow animals to express species-typical behavior in impoverished environments. Are animals that pace or somersault in small cages merely expressing species-typical locomotor activity? If so, it should be possible to show that pacers and somersaulters are more likely to run and to run for longer periods of time in large outdoor environments than non-pacers. This finding would not fully address the hypothesis proposed above but it would be a starting point.

Another possibility is that stereotypies function to reduce arousal and stress. Indeed, there is evidence that self-directed stereotypies such as self-biting in monkeys may reduce heart rate and raise beta-endorphin levels (Novak, 2003; Tiefenbacher et al., 2005; see also Chapter 5). If stereotypies are adaptive coping responses to anxiety-provoking situations, devising strategies to eliminate them without removing the stressor might actually decrease animal well-being (Mason, 1991). The optimal strategy then is to identify potential stressors and eliminate them from the environment. However, if this strategy is impossible to achieve, then pharmacotherapy with serotonin reuptake inhibitors or with anxiolytic drugs might reduce stereotypic behavior. If stereotypies actually function to reduce arousal in particular environments, it raises two possibilities for the animals that do not show stereotypic behavior in the same environment. Either they are less reactive to stressors (e.g. the low reactivity monkeys described earlier) or intriguingly they may be more distressed because they lack effective coping mechanisms.

A third possible explanation (the habit hypothesis) is that stereotypic behavior initially arose in a stressful context which no longer exists but the stereotypic behavior persists as an ingrained habit (Mason and Turner, 1993; Toates, 2000). Such stereotypies might be considered neutral with respect to animal well-being. However, a corollary of the habit hypothesis is that the stereotypic behavior might eventually be elicited by a greater range of stimuli and performed in more diverse situations. Thus, in terms of time and energy expenditure and potential disruption with other species-typical activities, these habits might come to have a negative impact on well-being. Indeed, there may be interesting parallels between this hypothesis and the development and maintenance of obsessive compulsive disorders in humans.

Finally, stereotypies may be maladaptive responses reflecting underlying states of distress and of poor psychological and/or physical well-being. For this latter interpretation, it is important first to determine any physical causes of stereotypic behavior that might include pain or movement disorders such as arthritis (Bayne and Novak, 1998). Once physical causes have been ruled out, then a variety of psychological disorders can be considered. Currently, there is no well-established link between nonhuman primate stereotypies and models of psychological disease. However, it is reasonable to hypothesize that the presence of stereotypic patterns of behavior may reflect several underlying psychological dysfunctions including anxiety (see the role of anxiety in self-injurious behavior in Chapter 5) and impulse control disorders that are most likely elicited in genetically vulnerable individuals by exposure to stressful environments at crucial periods in development. Further research will be required to understand the significance of stereotypies and determine whether they enable animals to cope better with stressful events or serve as a marker for the presence of psychological distress.

REFERENCES

Barr, C. S., Newman, T. K., Becker, M. L. *et al.* (2003). The utility of the non-human primate model for studying gene by environment interactions in behavioral research. *Genes Brain Behav* **2**, 336–340.

Barr, C. S., Newman, T. K., Shannon, C. *et al.* (2004a). Rearing condition and rh5-HTTLPR interact to influence LHPA-axis response to stress in infant macaques. *Biol Psychiatry* **55**, 731–738.

Barr, C. S., Newman, T. K., Lindell, S. *et al.* (2004b). Interaction between serotonin transporter gene variation and rearing condition in alcohol preference and consumption in female primates. *Arch Gen Psychiatry* **61**, 1146–1152.

Bayne, K. A. L. and Novak, M. A. (1998). Psychological disorders. In: Bennett, B. T., Abee, C. R., and Henrickson, R. eds. *Non-human Primates in Biomedical Research*, Vol. II: *Diseases*. New York: Academic Press, pp. 485–500.

Bayne, K., Dexter, S., and Suomi, S. (1991). Social housing ameliorates behavioral pathology in Cebus apella. *Lab Prim Newsletter* **30**, 9–12.

Bayne, K., Dexter, S., and Suomi, S. (1992). A preliminary survey of the incidence of abnormal behavior in rhesus monkeys (*Macaca mulatta*) relative to housing condition. Source: *Lab Animal*. 21 pp: 38, 40, 42–46.

Bennett, A. J., Lesch, K. P., Heils, A. *et al.* (2002). Early experience and serotonin transporter gene variation interact to influence primate CNS function. *Mol Psychiatry* **7**, 118–122.

Berard J. D. 1989. Life histories of male Cayo Santiago macaques. *Puerto Rico Health Sci J* **8**, 61–64.

Berkson, G. (1968). Development of abnormal stereotyped behaviors. *Dev Psychobiol* **1**, 118–132.

Berman, C. M. (1983). Matriline differences and infant development. In: Hinde, R. A. ed. *Primate Social Relationships: An Integrated Approach*. Sunderland, MA: Sinauer Associates.

Berman, C.M., Rasmussen, K. L. R., and Suomi, S. J. (1994). Responses of free-ranging rhesus monkeys to a natural form of social separation. I. Parallels with mother-infant separation in captivity. *Child Dev* **65**, 1028–1041.

Bielefeldt-Ohmann, H., Bellanca, R. U., Crockett, C. M. *et al.* (2004). Subacute necrotizing encephalopathy in a pig-tailed macaque (*Macaca nemestrina*) that resembles mitochondrial encephalopathy in humans. *Comp Med* **54**, 422–433.

Capitanio, J. P. (1986). Behavioral pathology. In: Mitchell, G. and Erwin, J. eds. *Comparative Primate Biology*, Vol. 2, Part A: *Behavior, Conservation, and Ecology*. New York: Alan R. Liss, pp. 411–454.

Capitanio, J.P., Mendoza, S. P., Mason, W. A., and Maninger, N. (2005). Rearing environment and hypothalamic-pituitary-adrenal regulation in young rhesus monkeys (*Macaca mulatta*). *Dev Psychobiol* **46**, 318–330.

Castner, S. A. and Goldman-Rakic, P. S. (1999). Long-lasting psychotomimetic consequences of repeated low-dose amphetamine exposure in rhesus monkeys. *Neuropsychopharmacology* **20**, 10–28.

Champoux, M., Bennett, A. J., Shannon, C., Higley, J. D., Lesch, K. P., and Suomi, S. J. (2002). Serotonin transporter gene polymorphism, differential early rearing, and behavior in rhesus monkey neonates. *Mol Psychiatry* **7**, 1058–1063.

Clarke, A. S, (1993). Social rearing effects on HPA axis activity over early development and in response to stress in rhesus monkeys. *Dev Psychobiol* **26**, 433–446.

Clarke, A. S., Hedeker, D. R., Ebert, M. H., Schmidt, D. E., McKinney, W. T., and Kraemer, G. W. (1996). Rearing experience and biogenic amine activity in infant rhesus monkeys. *Biol Psychiatry* **40**, 338–352.

Chamove, A. S. (1973). Rearing infant rhesus together. *Behaviour* **47**, 48–66.

Chamove, A. S., Rosenblum, L. A., and Harlow, H. F. (1973). Monkeys (*Macaca mulatta*) raised only with peers. A pilot study. *Anim Behav* **21**, 316–325.

Coe, C. L., Lubach, G. R., Ershler, W. B., and Klopp, R. G. (1989). Influence of early rearing on lymphocyte proliferation responses in juvenile rhesus monkeys. *Brain, Behav Immun* **3**, 47–60.

Crockett, C. M., Bowers, C. L., Sackett, G. P., and Bowden, D. M. (1993). Urinary cortisol responses of longtailed macaques to five cage sizes, tethering, sedation, and room change. *Am J Primatol* **30**, 55–74.

Cross, H. A. and Harlow, H. F. (1965). Prolonged and progressive effects of partial isolation on the behavior of macaque monkeys. *J Exp Res Personal* **1**, 39–49.

Davenport, M. D., Novak, M. A., Meyer, J. S. *et al.* (2003). Continuity and change in emotional reactivity in rhesus monkeys throughout the prepubertal period. *Motiv Emot* **27**, 57–76.

Draper, W. A. and Bernstein, I. S. (1963). Stereotyped behavior and cage size. *Percept Mot Skills* **16**, 231–234.

Ellison, G., Nielsen, E. B., and Lyon, M. (1981). Animal model of psychosis: Hallucinatory behaviors in monkeys during the late stage of continuous amphetamine intoxication. *J Psychiatr Res* **16**, 13–22.

Elmore, D. B., Anderson, J. H., Hird, D. W., Sanders, K. D., and Lerche, N. W. (1992). Diarrhea rates and risk factors for developing chronic diarrhea in infant and juvenile rhesus monkeys. *Lab Anim Sci.* **42**, 356–359.

Fahlke, C., Lorenz, J. G., Long, J., Champoux, M., Suomi, S. J., and Higley, J. D. (2000). Rearing experiences and stress-induced plasma cortisol as early risk factors for excessive alcohol consumption in nonhuman primates. *Alcohol Clin Exp Res* **24**, 644–650.

Fittinghoff, N. A. Jr., Lindburg, D. G., Gomber, J., and Mitchell, G. (1974). Consistency and variability in the behavior of mature, isolation-reared, male rhesus macaques. *Primates* **15**, 111–139.

Fontenot, M. B., Padgett, E. E. III. Dupuy, A. M., Lynch, C. R., De Petrillo, P. B., and Higley, J. D. (2005). The effects of fluoxetine and buspirone on self-injurious and stereotypic behavior in adult male rhesus macaques. *Comp Med* **55**, 67–74.

Fontenot, M. B., Wilkes, M. N., and Lynch, C. S. (2006). Effects of outdoor housing on self-injurious and stereotypic behavior in adult male rhesus macaques (*Macaca mulatta*). *J Am Assoc Lab Anim Sci* **45**, 35–43.

Frith, C. D. and Done, D. J. (1990). Stereotyped behavior in madness and health. In: Cooper, S. J. and Dourish, C. T. eds. *Neurobiology of Stereotyped Behavior.* Oxford: Clarendon Press, pp: 232–259.

Hansen, E. W. (1966). The development of maternal and infant behavior in the rhesus monkey. *Behaviour* **27**, 107–149.

Harlow, H. F. (1958). The nature of love. *Am Psychol* **13**, 673–685.

Harlow, H. F. and Harlow, M. K. (1962). The effect of rearing conditions on behavior. *Bull Menninger Clin* **26**, 213–224.

Harlow, H. F. and Harlow, M. K. (1965). The effect of rearing conditions on behavior. *Int J Psychiatry* **1**, 43–51.

Harlow, H. F. and Suomi, S. J. (1970). Nature of love: Simplified. *Am Psychol* **25**, 161–168.

Harlow, H. F. and Zimmermann, R. R. (1959). Affectional responses in the infant monkey. *Science* **130**, 421–432.

Higley, J. D., Suomi, S. J., and Linnoila, M. (1990). Parallels in aggression and serotonin: Consideration of development, rearing history, and sex differences. In van Praag, H. M., Plutchik, R., and Apter, A. eds. *Violence and Suicidality: Perspectives in Clinical and Psychobiological Research.* New York: Brunner/Mazel, pp. 245–256.

Higley, J. D., Suomi, S. J., and Linnoila, M. (1991). CSF monoamine metabolite concentrations vary according to age, rearing, and sex, and are influenced by the stressor of social separation in rhesus monkeys. *Psychopharmacology* **103**, 551–556.

Higley, J. D., Mehlman, P. T., Taub, D. M. *et al.* (1992a). Cerebrospinal fluid monoamine and adrenal correlates of aggression in free-ranging rhesus monkeys. *Arch Gen Psychiatry* **49**, 436–441.

Higley, J. D., Suomi, S. J., and Linnoila, M. (1992b). A longitudinal assessment of CSF monoamine metabolite and plasma cortisol concentrations in young rhesus monkeys. *Biol Psychiatry* **32**, 127–145.

Higley, J. D., Thompson, W. T., Champoux, M. *et al.* (1993). Paternal and maternal genetic and environmental contributions to CSF monoamine metabolites in rhesus monkeys (*Macaca mulatta*). *Arch Gen Psychiatry* **50**, 615–623.

Higley, J. D., King, S. T., Hasert, M. F., Champoux, M., Suomi, S. J., and Linnoila, M. (1996a). Stability of interindividual differences in serotonin function and its relationship to severe aggression and competent social behavior in rhesus macaque females. *Neuropsychopharmacology* **14**, 67–76.

Higley, J. D., Mehlman, P. T., Higley, S. B. *et al.* (1996b). Excessive mortality in young free-ranging male nonhuman primates with low cerebrospinal fluid 5-hydroxyindoleacetic acid concentrations. *Arch Gen Psychiatry* **53**, 537–543.

Higley, J. D., Suomi, S. J., and Linnoila, M. (1996c). A nonhuman model of Type II alcoholism? (Part 2): Diminished social competence and excessive aggression correlates with low CSF 5-HIAA concentrations. *Alcohol Clin Exp Res* **20**, 643–650.

Hugo, C., Seier, J., Mdhluli, C. *et al.* (2003). Fluoxetine decreases stereotypic behavior in primates. *Prog NeuroPsychopharmacol Biol Psychiatry* **27**, 639–643.

Ichise, M., Vines, D. C., Gura, T. *et al.* (2006). Effects of early life stress on [11C] DABS PET imaging of serotonin transporters in adolescent peer- and mother-reared rhesus monkeys. *J Neurosci* **26**, 4638–4643.

Kagan, J. and Snidman, N. (1991). Temperamental factors in human development. *Am Psychol* **46**, 856–862.

Kaufman, B. M., Pouliot, A. L., Tiefenbacher, S. T., and Novak, M. A. (2004). Short and long-term effects of a substantial change in cage size on rhesus monkeys (*Macaca mulatta*). *Appl Anim Behav Sci* **88**, 319–330.

Kraemer, G. W. and Clarke, A. S. (1990) The behavioral neurobiology of self-injurious behavior in rhesus monkeys. *Prog Neuro-psychopharmacol Biol Psychiatry* **14**(suppl), S141–S168.

Kraemer, G. W., Ebert, M. H., Lake, C. R., and McKinney, W. T. (1984). Hypersensitivity to d-amphetamine several years after early social deprivation in rhesus monkeys. *Psychopharmacology* **82**, 266–271.

Kraemer, G. W., Ebert, M. H., Schmidt, D. E., and McKinney, W. T. (1989). A longitudinal study of the effect of different social rearing conditions on cerebrospinal fluid norepinephrine and biogenic amine metabolites in rhesus monkeys. *Neuropsychopharmacology* **2**, 175–189.

Kraemer, G. W., Schmidt, D. E., and Ebert, M. H. (1997). The behavioral neurobiology of self-injurious behavior in rhesus monkeys – current concepts and relations to impulsive behavior in humans. *Ann NY Acad Sci* **836**, 2–38.

Lawrence, A. and Rushen, J. (1993). *Stereotypic Animal Behavior – Fundamentals and Applications to Welfare*. Wallingford: CAB International.

Levin, E. D., Bushnell, P. J., and Baysinger, C. M. (1990). D-Amphetamine-induced "floating limb" syndrome in young rhesus monkeys. *Psychopharmacology* **101**, 112–117.

Lewis, M. H., Gluck, J. P., Beauchamp, A. J., Keresztury, M.F., and Mailman, R. B. (1990). Long-term effects of early social isolation in *Macaca mulatta*: Changes in dopamine receptor function following apomorphine challenge. *Brain Res* **513**, 67–73.

Lindburg, D. G. (1971). The rhesus monkey in North India: An ecological and behavioral study. In: Rosenblum, L. A. ed. *Primate Behavior Developments in Field and Laboratory Research*. New York: Academic Press, pp. 1–106.

Lubach, G. R., Coe, C. L., and Ershler, W. B. (1995). Effects of early rearing environment on immune responses on infant rhesus monkeys. *Brain Behav Immun* **9**: 31–46.

Lutz, C., Well, A., and Novak, M. A. (2003). Stereotypic and self-injurious behavior in rhesus macaques: a survey and retrospective analysis of environment and early experience. *Am J Primatol* **60**, 1–15.

Martin, L. J., Spicer, D. M., Lewis, M. H., Gluck, J. P., and Cork, L. C. (1991). Social deprivation of infant rhesus monkeys alters the chemoarchitecture of the brain. I. Subcortical regions. *J Neurosci* **11**, 3344–3358.

Mason, G. (1991). Stereotypies: a critical review. *Anim Behav* **41**, 1015–1037.

Mason, G. J. and Latham, N. R. (2004). Can't stop, won't stop: is stereotypy a reliable animal welfare indicator. *Anim Welfare* **13**, 557–569.

Mason, G. and Turner, M. (1993). Mechanisms involved in the development and control of stereotypies. In: Bateson, P. ed. *Perspectives in Ethology*, New York: Plenum Press, pp. 53–85.

Mason, W. A. (1968). Early social deprivation in nonhuman primates: Implications for human behavior. In: Glass, D. C. ed. *Environmental Influences*. New York: Rockefeller University and Russell Sage, pp. 70–100.

Mason, W. A. and Berkson, G. (1975). Effects of maternal mobility on the development of rocking and other behaviors in rhesus monkeys: A study with artificial mothers. *Dev Psychobiol* **8**, 197–211.

McKinney, W. T. Jr., Young, L. D., Suomi, S. J., and Davis, J. M. (1973). Chlorpromazine treatment of disturbed monkeys. *Arch Gen Psychiatry* **29**, 490–494.

Melnick, D. J., Pearl, M. C., and Richard, A. F. (1984). Male migration and inbreeding avoidance in wild rhesus monkeys. *Am J Primatol* **7**, 229–243.

Meyer, J. S. and Bowman, R. E. (1972). Rearing experience, stress and adrenocorticosteroids in the rhesus monkey. *Physiol Behav* **8**, 339–343.

Meyer, J. S., Novak, M. A., Bowman, R. E., and Harlow, H. F. (1975). Behavioral and hormonal effects of attachment object separation in surrogate peer-reared and mother-reared infant monkeys. *Dev Psychobiol* **8**, 425–436.

Mitchell, G. D. (1968). Persistent behavior pathology in rhesus monkeys following early social isolation. *Folia Primatol* **8**, 132–147.

Mitchell, G. D., Raymond, E. J., Ruppenthal, G. C., and Harlow, H. F. (1966). Long-term effects of total social isolation upon behavior of rhesus monkeys. *Psychol Rep* **18**, 567–580.

Newman, T. K., Syagaiol, Y, Barr, C. S. *et al.* (2005). Monoamine oxidase A gene promoter polymorphism and infant rearing experience interact to influence aggression and injuries in rhesus monkeys. *Biol Psychiatry* **57**, 167–172.

Novak, M. A. (2003). Self-injurious behavior in rhesus monkeys: new insights on etiology, physiology, and treatment. *Am J Primatol* **59**, 3–19.

Novak, M. and Sackett, G. P. (2006). The effects of rearing experiences: the early years. In: Sackett, G. P., Ruppenthal, G. C., and Elias, K. eds. *Nursery Rearing of Nonhuman Primates in the 21st Century.* New York: Springer, pp. 5–19.

Novak, M. A., O'Neill, P., and Suomi, S. J. (1992). Adjustments and adaptations to indoor and outdoor environments: continuity and change in young adult rhesus monkeys. *Am J Primatol* **28**, 125–138.

Novak, M. A., Tiefenbacher, S. T., Lutz, C., and Meyer, J. S. (2006). Deprived environments and stereotypies: insights from primatology. In Mason, G. and Rushen, J. eds. *Stereotypic Animal Behaviour: Fundamentals and Applications to Welfare*, 2nd edn. Wallingford: CABI, pp. 153–189.

Paulk, H. H., Dienske, H., and Ribbens, L. G. (1977). Abnormal behavior in relation to cage size in rhesus monkeys. *J Abnorm Psychol* **86**, 87–92.

Rasmussen, K. L. R. and Suomi, S. J. (1989). Heart rate and endocrine responses to stress in adolescent male rhesus monkeys on Cayo Santiago. *Puerto Rico Health Sci J* **8**, 65–71.

Richard, A. F., Goldstein, S. J., and Dewar, R. E. (1989). Weed macaques: The evolutionary implications of macaque feeding ecology. *Int J Primatol* **10**, 569–594.

Ridley, R. M. and Baker, H. F. (1982). Stereotypy in monkeys and humans. *Psychol Med* **12**, 61–72.

Roma, P. G., Champoux, M., and Suomi, S. J. (2006). Environmental control, social context, and individual differences in behavioral and cortisol responses to novelty in infant rhesus monkeys. *Child Dev* **77**, 118–131.

Rosenblum, L. A. (1961). The development of social behavior in the rhesus monkey. *Dissertation Abstr* **22**, 926–927.

Ruppenthal, G. C., Arling, G. L., Harlow, H. F., Sackett, G. P., and Suomi, J. S. (1976). A 10-year perspective of motherless-mother monkey behavior. *J Abnorm Psychol* **85**, 341–349.

Ruppenthal, G. C., Walker, C. G., and Sackett, G. P. (1991). Rearing infant monkeys (*Macaca nemestrina*) in pairs produces deficient social development compared with rearing in single cages. *Am J Primatol* **25**, 103–113.

Sackett, G. P. (1967). Some persistent effects of different rearing conditions on preadult social behavior of monkeys. *J Comp Physiol Psychol* **64**, 363–365.

Sackett, G. P. (1968). Abnormal behavior in laboratory-reared rhesus monkeys. In: Fox, M. W. ed. *Abnormal Behavior in Animals.* Philadelphia: Saunders, pp. 293–331.

Sackett, G. P., Bowman, R. E., Meyer, J. S., Tripp, R. L., and Grady, S. S. (1973). Adrenocortical and behavioral reactions by differentially raised rhesus monkeys. *Physiol Psychol* **1**, 209–212.

Sackett, G. P., Tripp, R., and Grady, S. (1982). Rhesus monkeys reared in isolation with added social, nonsocial and electrical brain stimulation. *Annali Dell Istituto Superiore Di Sanita* **18**, 203–213.

Sackett, G. P., Ruppenthal, G. C., and Davis, A. E. (2002). Survival, growth, health, and reproduction following nursery rearing compared with mother rearing in pigtailed monkeys (*Macaca nemestrina*). *Am J Primatol* **56**, 165–183.

Schlemmer, R. F. Jr., Young, J. E., and Davis, J. M. (1996). Stimulant-induced disruption of non-human primate social behavior and the psychopharmacology of schizophrenia. *J Psychopharmacol* **10**, 64–76.

Shannon, C., Champoux, M., and Suomi, S. J. (1998). Rearing condition and plasma cortisol in rhesus monkey infants. *Am J Primatol* **46**, 311–321.

Shannon, C., Schwandt, M. L., Champoux, M. *et al.* (2005). Maternal absence and stability of individual differences in CSF 5-HIAA concentrations in rhesus monkey infants. *Am J Psychiatry* **162**, 1658–1664.

Southwick, C. H., Beg, M. A., and Siddiqi, M. R. (1965). Rhesus monkeys in north India. In Devore, I. ed. *Primate Behavior. Field Studies in Monkeys and Apes*. New York: Holt, Rinehart & Winston, pp. 111–159.

Southwick, C. H., Siddiqi, M. F., Farooqui, M. Y., and Pal, B. C. (1974). Xenophobia among free-ranging rhesus groups in India. In: Holloway, R. ed. *Primate Aggression, Territoriality, and Xenophobia*. New York: Academic Press, pp. 185–209.

Strand, S. C. (2006). Impact of early rearing environment on the behavior and physiology of juvenile and adolescent mother-peer, surrogate-peer, and peer-only reared rhesus monkeys (*Macaca mulatta*). Dissertation. *Abstr Int* **B67(11)**, 134.

Strand, S. C. and Novak, M. A. (2005). Examination of behavior in differently reared monkeys housed together. *Am J Primatol* **66**(suppl 1), 120–121.

Suomi, S. J. (1991). Up-tight and laid-back monkeys: individual differences in the response to social challenges. In: Brauth, S., Hall, W., and Dooling, R. eds. *Plasticity of Development*. Cambridge, MA: MIT Press, pp. 27–56.

Suomi, S. J. (2000). Behavioral inhibition and impulsive aggressiveness: Insights from studies with rhesus monkeys. In: Balter, L. and Tamis-Lamode, C. eds. *Child Psychology: A Handbook of Contemporary Issues*. New York: Taylor and Francis, pp. 510–525.

Suomi, S. J. (2007). Risk, resilience, and gene X environment interactions in rhesus monkeys. *Proc Natl Acad Sci* **1094**, 52–61.

Teas, J., Feldman, H. A., Richie, T. L., Taylor, H. G., and Southwick, C. H. (1982). Aggressive behavior in the free-ranging rhesus monkeys of Kathmandu, Nepal. *Aggress Behav* **8**, 63–77.

Teas, J., Richie, T., Taylor, H., and Southwick, C. (1980). Population patterns and behavioral ecology of rhesus monkeys (*Macaca mulatta*) in Nepal. In: Lindburg, D. ed. *The Macaques Studies in Ecology, Behavior and Evolution*. New York: Van Nostrand Reinhold Company, pp. 247–262.

Tiefenbacher, S. T., Fahey, M. A., Rowlett, J. K. *et al.* (2005). The efficacy of diazepam treatment for the management of acute wounding episodes in captive rhesus macaques. *Comp Med* **55**, 387–392.

Toates, F. (2000). Multiple factors controlling behavior: implications for stress and welfare. In: Moberg, G. and Mench, J. eds. *The Biology of Animal Stress*. Wallingford, UK: CAB International, pp. 199–226.

Walsh, S., Bramblett, C. A., and Alford, P. L. (1982). A vocabulary of abnormal behaviors in restrictively reared chimpanzees. *Am J Primatol* **3**, 315–319.

Weed, J. L., Wagner, P. O., Byrum, R., Parrish, S., Knezevich, M., and Powell, D. A. (2003). Treatment of persistent self-injurious behavior in rhesus monkeys through socialization: A preliminary report. *Cont Top Lab Anim Sci* **42**, 21–23.

Williamson, D. E. *et al.* (2003). Heritability of fearful-anxious endophenotypes in infant rhesus macaques: a preliminary report. *Biol Psychiatry* **53**, 284–291.

Winslow, J. T., Noble, P. L., Lyons, C. K., Sterk, S. M., and Insel, T. R. (2003). Rearing effects on cerebrospinal fluid oxytocin concentration and social buffering in rhesus monkeys. *Neuropsychopharmacology* **28**, 910–918.

Zajicek, K., Higley, J. D., Suomi, S. J., and Linnoila, M. (1997). Rhesus macaques with low CSF 5-HIAA concentrations are unlikely to fall asleep early. *Psychiatr Res* **77**. 15–25.

CHAPTER 7

Neurochemistry and Behavior: Nonhuman Primate Studies

J. Dee Higley and Christina S. Barr

INTRODUCTION

Nonhuman primates are our closest phylogenetic relatives and as a result we share a large percentage of their DNA. These similarities in DNA produce physiological, neuroanatomical, and behavioral homologies that allow researchers to generalize to the human condition more readily than with other, less closely related animal species. For example, unlike rodents who spend a good deal of their existence as solitary nocturnal individuals, nonhuman primates such as macaques are by their nature social (Lindburg, 1980; Thierry *et al.*, 2004). Because of their physical and behavioral likeness, they are particularly good research subjects to model many aspects of human development. Historically, nonhuman primates have been used to study stress, social behaviors, development, and psychopathology. An additional reason to use nonhuman primates in developmental studies is that, like humans, nonhuman primates are highly altricial with a good deal of cortical development occurring outside the womb. As infants and juveniles they need considerable care but develop at a more rapid pace than humans. This allows longitudinal studies to be performed in less time than studies using human subjects.

Another reason that primates are used in developmental studies is that the same behavioral measurements taken on humans can be taken on monkeys and linked to central nervous system (CNS) functioning. For example, Harlow's groundbreaking behavioral studies investigating parental effects, social separation, and psychopathology were linked to group and individual variation in CNS and hypothalamic-pituitary-adrenal (HPA) axis functioning. These early studies of CNS functioning measured biochemicals in the cerebrospinal fluid (CSF), looking at high or low concentrations of neurotransmitters and their metabolites to index specific neurotransmitter activity. In humans, lumbar CSF concentrations of neurotransmitters and/or their metabolites have been shown to change during development and to vary with psychiatric diagnoses. Different concentrations have also been found between men and women and when comparing infants, children, and adults (Andersson and Roos, 1969; Cohen et al., 1974; Langlais et al., 1985; Rogers and Dubowitz, 1970; Seifert et al., 1980; Leckman et al., 1980; Silverstein et al., 1985). Concentrations different from controls have also been reported in patients with mood disorders, aggression, suicide, and alcoholism (e.g. see Asberg et al., 1987; Eichelman, 1987; Linnoila, 1988; Mann and Stanley, 1986; Meltzer and Lowy, 1987; Siever, 1987).

Nonhuman primates have been used to model many of these human disorders (McKinney, 1988; Kalin, 1993; Anderson et al., 2002; Bennett et al., 2002). Studies of CSF monoamine (MAO) concentrations in nonhuman primates allow measurement of neurotransmitter turnover using procedures that are not possible to use regularly with humans. For example, CSF can be routinely obtained from the cisterna magna, which is thought to be a better approximation of neurotransmitter release and turnover in the brain than CSF sampled from the lumbar level of the spine. A recent study illustrates the utility of a primate model for assessment of CNS functioning. This study measured how selective serotonin reuptake inhibitors (SSRIs) function in the brain. While the serotonin metabolite 5-hydroxyindoleacetic acid (5-HIAA) has been widely used to index CNS serotonin functioning, in this study serotonin levels were quantified in the CSF for the first time (Anderson et al., 2002, 2005), This allowed for direct measurement of both short- and long-term action of SSRIs on the CNS serotonin system. Immediately following administration of the SSRI sertraline, CSF concentrations of serotonin rose about 300%, at which level it remained throughout short- and long-term treatment. CSF 5-HIAA concentrations, on the other hand, declined rapidly and remained at similarly reduced levels during long-term treatment. Levels returned to baseline 7 days following sertraline treatment, indicating no lasting effect of SSRI administration. These findings allowed researchers to conclude that SSRIs increase serotonin release rapidly and substantially and the effect is relatively constant during prolonged administration, with values returning to baseline shortly after discontinuation.

This illustration using nonhuman primates to study CNS functioning is important. It showed that a 2–3 week response latency for SSRIs in depression is not due to gradually increasing brain serotonin levels. It also did not support theories that posit SSRI response latency being due to autoreceptor desensitization, transporter downregulation, or drug accumulation. The results also indicate that the reason why previously depressed individuals do not immediately relapse following the termination of SSRI treatment is not because the SSRIs permanently alter serotonin release and uptake (Anderson et al., 2002, 2005).

Many of the early studies investigating CNS and behavior in nonhuman primates were performed by McKinney and Kraemer at the University of Wisconsin. Their studies using CSF measures of monoamines in nonhuman primates were focused on models of depression and psychopathology (McKinney, 1988). These investigations were instrumental in developing the monoamine hypothesis of depression. It had been widely held that depression was a monolithic disorder triggered by stressful events (McKinney, 1988). The Wisconsin work, however, showed that identical stressors failed to produce depression in all individuals.

A number of studies in humans have shown that administration of high doses of reserpine or alpha-methyl-para-tyrosine, drugs designed to deplete monoamines or catecholamines respectively, induced depression in humans who had had a previous episode of depression. Primate work also demonstrated that pharmacologically depleting the monoamines using reserpine or alpha-methyl-para-tyrosine produced severe despair (McKinney *et al.*, 1971; Redmond *et al.*, 1971b). Initially the work was criticized because some of the behaviors could be explained as the sedative effects that result from depleted levels of neurotransmitters. Moreover, some argued that it was unlikely that this could explain human depression because the differences in neurotransmitter levels seen in depressed humans were only a small per cent lower than normal controls but the neurotransmitters were much lower in the animals who had received the selective inhibitors (Kraemer and McKinney, 1979). In response, Kraemer and McKinney (1979) performed an elegant study, which has been largely neglected. They administered a much lower dose of the catecholamine-depleting agent alpha-methyl-para-tyrosine, a dose that under baseline conditions produced no discernable behavioral differences and only minimal monoamine decrements. However, when monkeys receiving alpha-methyl-para-tyrosine were stressed using social separation, they exhibited a profound despair response not seen in controls (Kraemer and McKinney, 1979). Subsequent studies showed that low levels of norepinephrine predicted depression-like behavior during social separation stress (Kraemer *et al.*, 1984a).

These nonhuman primate investigations provided support for the stress–diathesis hypothesis of depression (Akiskal and McKinney, 1975; Akiskal, 1985; McKinney, 1988). The results were also instrumental in demonstrating that the effects of social separation-induced depression in monkeys was reversed using the common anti-depressant treatments of the day, tricyclic antidepressants and electroconvulsive therapy (Lewis and McKinney, 1976; Suomi *et al.*, 1978; McKinney, 1984; Suomi, 1991b).

In these studies only a subset of animals showed the depression-like despair seen in some young primates undergoing social separation (Suomi *et al.*, 1981). More recently, studies have focused on these individual differences. In one study, monkeys were assigned levels of reactiveness during home-cage interactions, based on time spent behaviorally freezing. Subjects were then observed during social separations. Most animals showed reductions in HPA axis response and monoamine turnover during repeated separations. However, highly withdrawn animals, those with high levels of freezing, showed less reduction in serotonin metabolite concentrations over repeated separations than the more bold, outgoing animals. Highly withdrawn subjects also failed to show attenuations in plasma cortisol concentrations across separation weeks (Erickson *et al.*, 2005).

Subsequent studies focused on discovering factors that lead to these differences, examining the role of early experience (Higley and Suomi, 1989). One of the most frequent uses of nonhuman primates is the study of early rearing experiences, particularly those that lead to affective dysregulation. Social separation is a highly stressful event for most primates. Acutely, there is a profound activation of the sympathetic nervous system, resulting in increased heart rate and body temperature (Reite et al., 1974, 1978, 1981). Concomitantly, the adrenal cortex is stimulated, resulting in a sizable elevation of plasma cortisol (Gunnar et al., 1981; Fahlke et al., 2000; Ayala et al., 2004; Barr et al., 2004c, 2004d). Within the central nervous system, catecholamines and serotonin are released, resulting in increased CSF monoamine metabolite concentrations (Wiener et al., 1988; Bayart et al., 1990; Ayala et al., 2004). While social separation induces profound activation of the monoamine and HPA systems, there are wide individual differences in how much it is increased. One of the most replicated findings from these studies is that individual differences in the CSF monoamine metabolites 5-HIAA, 3-methoxy-4-hydroxyphenylglycol (MHPG), and homovanillic acid (HVA) are present early in life and remain relatively stable thereafter (Kraemer et al., 1989; Higley et al., 1996a, 1992c, 1996d, 1996e; Heinz et al., 2003b; Shannon et al., 2005; Howell et al., 2007).

These findings, which show large between-subjects individual differences, provide important clues as to risk and protective CNS factors in depression and other forms of psychopathology. For example, the severity of despair or stress response to separation is directly related to preexisting CSF norepinephrine levels (Kraemer et al., 1984a; Kraemer, 1992). The probability of violent aggression is also predicted by preexisting CSF 5-HIAA concentrations (Higley and Bennett, 1999). This suggests that levels of biochemicals, such as monoamines or corticotropin releasing hormone (CRH) in the CSF, may reflect underlying life-long risk for certain forms of psychopathology or adjustment to challenges.

As Harlow's work showing the psychological effects of early parental absence was coming to a close, Kraemer and McKinney's work was instrumental because it extended Harlow's studies on maternal influence and showed that the basis of environmentally induced psychopathology lay in the brain. Thus, parental input early in life was seen to be critical for normal CNS development. Given the widely held belief that repeated stress affects the organism's capacity to respond to future stress, these assessments that unlocked the black box of the brain showed how early life events sensitize the CNS to respond to subsequent stress and how parental absence leads to brain dysfunction.

THE ROLE OF PARENTS IN CNS DEVELOPMENT

Because primates are born altricial, with only limited cortical processes complete at birth, proper nurturing is of critical importance for further CNS maturation. Warmth and nutrition are of primary importance for all altricial mammals. Parents, particularly in primates, play another critical role. Classic studies by Levine (1970), since replicated and expanded by others (Meaney and Szyf, 2005; Roman et al., 2005;

Roman *et al.*, 2006) show that even in rodents, maternal contact and nurturance lead to a healthy CNS response to stress. In the absence of maternal influence the response of the HPA axis is blunted. Subsequent studies have shown that this is true centrally as well, with a variety of CNS systems dysregulated when mother is absent (van Oers *et al.*, 1998a, 1998b; Vazquez *et al.*, 2000, 2002; Levine, 2005). Given the critical importance of appropriate CNS input for synaptic pruning and dendritic branching, it is likely that evolutionary selective pressures have played an important role in assuring that appropriate input is present as CNS systems are developing. It is likely that parents are primary in that role, particularly in primates whose cortical and limbic development occur in the context of social environments.

Among macaques and most Old World primates, mothers play the principle nurturing role, providing early developmental input. As the limbic system develops and synaptic connections are made with the prefrontal cortex and other regions important to down-modulating emotionality, mothers provide limbic input, reducing fear, over-arousal, and providing security, allowing the infant to eventually become self-reliant as it uses its mother as a secure base from which to explore (Harlow and Harlow, 1965; Harlow, 1969). Later, at a time that the frontal areas are undergoing synaptic pruning, mothers provide the appropriate CNS input necessary for the development of frontal inhibitory functioning by punishing inappropriate behaviors and reinforcing appropriate social behaviors with contact and grooming (Harlow and Harlow, 1965; Harlow, 1969).

Nature appears to have a genetic plan for how the CNS is to be laid down. Within that plan, however, there is considerable variability. Studies show a partial genetic origin for individual differences in monoamine functioning (Higley *et al.*, 1993; Clarke *et al.*, 1995). There are also important environmental effects on the development of the monoamine and other systems. In the absence of parental input, pathological CNS development results (Barr *et al.*, 2004e). For example, as adolescents, monkeys reared in isolation during the first year of life exhibit alterations in the reward system, showing CNS hyperresponsivity to amphetamines (Kraemer *et al.*, 1984b). Mother-reared monkeys exhibit month-to-month interindividual stability in the response of the monoamine system and modest individual correlations between the functioning of the different monoamine systems, serotonin, dopamine, and norepinephrine. In the absence of early maternal influence the within-individual positive correlation between the separate systems disappears. This shows the importance of parental input in "wiring" monoamine systems and ensuring their proper interaction (Kraemer *et al.*, 1989). On the other hand, a larger data set found interindividual stability across time regardless of early experience (Shannon *et al.*, 2005).

ATTACHMENT

Today we know that the central task of developmental psychiatry is to study the endless interaction of the internal and external and how the one is constantly influencing the

other, not only during childhood but during adolescence and adult life as well. John
Bowlby, *American Journal of Psychiatry* **145**, 1.

A fundamental aspect of the infant's psychological development is its native curiosity. As the curious infant leaves the safety of its mother's grasp to explore its environment, the mother serves as a secure base from which the infant can derive security.
This serves to reduce arousal and anxiety (Harlow and Harlow, 1965; Harlow, 1969)
as the mother employs contact comfort and other methods to reduce her infant's
anxiety and fear. As Bowlby and Ainsworth both illustrate, for a sense of security and
a secure attachment to form, the mother must adjust her behavior to reliably provide such a secure base.

While this psychological hypothesis is observable and can be measured using
behavior, what is not readily apparent are the changes that occur centrally. As Bowlby
stated, central systems that underlie attachment are activated which dictate the
behaviors that will be expressed and their intensity. High arousal induces proximity,
and with arousal reduced, systems that underlie exploration are activated. In the
absence of its mother or an attachment source to serve as a secure base, an infant's
exploration is severely reduced and behaviors that increase the probability of maternal
contact increase (Harlow and Harlow, 1965).

Centrally, when the infant is separated from its mother, CNS stress responsive systems are vigorously activated. Plasma epinephrine and norepinephrine (Ayala *et al.*,
2004), as well as central serotonin and dopamine release are markedly increased (Bayart
et al., 1990; Ayala *et al.*, 2004). The HPA axis shows robust activation with increased
plasma ACTH and cortisol (Champoux *et al.*, 1989; Bayart *et al.*, 1990; Higley *et al.*,
1991a, 1992c, 1996d, 1996e; Fahlke *et al.*, 2000; Ayala *et al.*, 2004). There are quite
marked individual differences in this acute response to separation, with some infants
showing high rates of vocalizations and agitation in response to maternal separation.
High rates of distress calls are positively correlated with plasma cortisol (Becker *et al.*,
2004). With prolonged separation from their attachment source, a subset of monkeys
fall into a depression–like despair. High levels of despair early in life during separation
are predictive of future bouts of despair later in life following stress (Higley, 1985).
Monkeys with low CSF norepinephrine are particularly vulnerable to the effects of
separation from their attachment source, showing high rates of despair during a social
separation stressor (Kraemer *et al.*, 1984a). Antidepressants reverse such despair and prevent its reoccurrence during subsequent stress (Suomi *et al.*, 1978; Higley *et al.*, 1992a).

To the extent that monoamines underlie such affective disorders in monkeys,
long–term individual differences in the response to separation and the risk for subsequent stress-mediated affective pathology may be related to individual differences
in the response of the monoamine systems. One of the most replicated findings in
our laboratory is that individual differences in the responsiveness of the
monoamines is trait–like. Thus, monoamine turnover, as measured by concentrations of their metabolites in the CSF, are highly stable across time and situation
(Raleigh *et al.*, 1986, 1992; Kraemer *et al.*, 1989; Higley *et al.*, 1992c, 1996a,

1996e; Insel, 1992; Carter *et al.*, 1995; Anderson *et al.*, 2002; Kendrick, 2004; Shannon *et al.*, 2005).

A number of other biochemical systems are also important in attachment behaviors. Rodent and ungulate studies show that oxytocin is a primary central neurochemical involved in mother–infant bonding (Keverne and Kendrick, 1992). In species such as voles, for example, oxytocin plays an important role in adult long-term pair bonding and maternal care (Insel, 1992; Carter *et al.*, 1995; Kendrick, 2004). However, cross-species generalizations have not been forthcoming in primates. Some primate studies have shown oxytocin to be stress sensitive (Kalin *et al.*, 1985), and higher in the CSF of lactating females (Amico *et al.*, 1990).

In Old World species such as macaques we are unaware of any studies showing that oxytocin plays a primary function in mother–infant attachment bonds. Moreover, in several studies in our laboratory, CSF oxytocin concentrations were not correlated with mother–infant behavior. We attempted to induce maternal care in females which had rejected their own infants by injecting oxytocin, but this failed to induced maternal care. On the other hand, oxytocin is found in brain areas responsible for the control of social behavior in the cynomolgus monkey (Boccia *et al.*, 2001) and it is higher in the CSF of the more gregarious and affiliative bonnet macaques than in the less social pigtail macaques (Rosenblum *et al.*, 2002). Recent studies of rhesus monkeys by Winslow and colleagues are some of the first to show that CSF oxytocin in young adults and adolescents is positively related to affiliative behaviors. Also, males reared without their mothers show impaired sociality and low CSF oxytocin later in life (Winslow, 2005; Winslow *et al.*, 2003). Ziegler suggested that if investigations focused on New World monogamous species rather than on the more promiscuous Old World monkeys, such oxytocin-bonding biobehavioral relationships might be detected (Ziegler, 2000). It would be interesting to assess oxytocin levels in caregivers in these long-term bonded species, be they fathers, siblings, or mothers.

Research in both rodent and nonhuman primates shows that the endogenous opioid system is important in modulating mother–infant attachment and other types of bonding behavior. Pharmacological and gene knockout studies of rodents were instrumental in suggesting that μ-opioid receptor activation may be primary in the establishment and maintenance of social bonding (Nelson and Panksepp, 1998; Depue and Morrone-Strupinsky, 2005). During rodent mother–infant separation, for example, endogenous opioids are important in modulating separation distress (Kehoe and Blass, 1986; Moles *et al.*, 2004). In a series of studies, Kalin and his group showed that this is true in primates as well (Kalin *et al.*, 1988, 1995; Kalin and Shelton, 1989). These studies show that once the mother and infant are reunited, attachment behaviors are activated at high levels, with mothers grooming and cradling, and when the infant is not in contact it is kept within arms length.

All of these behaviors activate the endogenous opioid system and reinforce attachment (Panksepp *et al.*, 1994). As evidence of this, infant macaques administered low doses of morphine decrease contact with their mothers, while infants given the nonspecific opioid receptor antagonist naltrexone increase contact with their mother (Kalin *et al.*, 1995) (but see Martel *et al.*, 1993). During separation from the mother, contact-eliciting coos were reduced by morphine and augmented by the endogenous opioid antagonist naltrexone (Kalin and Shelton, 1989). Although this could be due to reduction of the general fear and anxiety resulting from mother–infant separation, primate studies have been particularly revealing by showing that the opioid system may be specific in modulating attachment systems. For example, proximity-eliciting coos were not affected by other anxiolytic compounds such as the benzodiazepines, but are reduced by administration of low doses of morphine. This shows the specificity of the opioid system in attachment and bonding regulation (Kalin and Shelton, 1989).

Following the discovery that CRH plays a primary role in modulating fear- and anxiety-like behaviors in rodents (Smith *et al.*, 1989), Kalin began a series of studies showing that CRH plays a major role in fear and anxiety and in having a reactive or timid temperament among primates (Kalin *et al.*, 1989). Social separation is a potent activator of the CRH system in monkeys (Kalin *et al.*, 1989; Ayala *et al.*, 2004). One well-replicated finding is that among both humans and nonhuman primates, right frontal cortex activation is more likely during fear-provoking situations (Davidson *et al.*, 1992, 1993).

There are notable individual differences, however, in the response of infants to identical fear-provoking stimuli. Infants who are temperamentally more fearful show increased right frontal activation when compared with less fearful animals (Buss *et al.*, 2003). These findings also showed that the degree of fear and right frontal cortex activation were both correlated with CSF CRH concentrations (Buss *et al.*, 2003). The response of the CRH system is trait-like, showing interindividual stability across time, beginning in infancy and persisting at least into adolescence (Kalin *et al.*, 1998, 2000).

Other studies have shown that during mother–infant separation, the CRH system shows a substantial activation that is augmented with repeated exposure to separations (Gerald *et al.*, 2000). Administration of the recently discovered CRH1 antagonist antalarmin reduced anxiety and increased environmental exploration during social separation (Ayala *et al.*, 2004). The role of CRH in anxiety is not limited to infants. For example, intruder stress increases anxiety and CRH in adult nonhuman primates and blocking the CRH1 receptor using a recently discovered CRH1 antagonist reduces both stress-provoked anxiety and CSF CRH (Habib *et al.*, 2000).

One rearing condition known to affect the response to a wide variety of stressors, including social separation, is chronic peer rearing in the absence of adults. This is a particularly interesting rearing paradigm because monkeys reared in this particular environment do not lack for social contact; indeed, they have social partners 24 hours a day. Only adults are missing, which allows researchers to tease out the effects of parental absence versus isolation. Moreover, unlike isolates, they show a full range of social behaviors, including grooming, dominance relationships, and ultimately parental care. There are variations in the peer-rearing methods used such as 24-hour peer access versus access limited to only a few hours a day in a playroom (Meyer et al., 1975; Ruppenthal et al., 1991; Champoux et al., 1999) and there are also species differences (Laudenslager et al., 1990; Ruppenthal et al., 1991). The condition most often studied in neurobiological studies is the 24-hour, chronic-access condition first described by Harlow and Harlow (1965) (hereafter referred to as peer reared or peer rearing in this paper).

Peer rearing is associated, however, with patterns of behavior denoting increased anxiety and fearfulness (Harlow, 1969; Chamove et al., 1973; Higley and Suomi, 1989). During social separation challenge peer-reared monkeys are more likely than mother-reared to show depression-like behaviors and despair (Mineka and Suomi, 1978). As infants, peer-reared monkeys show chronic hypercortisolism, high stress-induced plasma ACTH, and high CSF CRH (Champoux et al., 1989; Higley et al., 1991a, 1992c, 1996d, 1996e; Fahlke et al., 2000; Ayala et al., 2004; Barr et al., 2004a, 2004d), although Clarke (1993) and Barr et al. (2004) found higher ACTH, but not cortisol. Decrements in norepinephrine and serotonin, as measured by low CSF NE, MHPG, and 5-HIAA concentrations, have also been found (Kraemer and McKinney, 1979; Kraemer et al., 1989, 1991; Higley et al., 1991b, 1992c, 1996d, 1996e; Clarke et al., 1996; Bennett et al., 2002; Shannon et al., 2005). Post infancy, between 1 and 3 years old, is a period roughly corresponding to early childhood in human children. During this age range, peer-reared monkeys are more sensitive than older animals to the effects of pharmacological challenges, showing diminished norepinephrine in response to social separation (Kraemer and McKinney, 1979).

Given the biochemical differences, it is not surprising that several studies have shown neuroanatomical deficits in peer-reared monkeys. Parental absence and social isolation, for example, result in deficits in the basal ganglia and dentate gyrus of the hippocampus (Lewis et al., 1990, 2000), which may in part explain some of the learning deficits seen in these subjects (Bennett et al., 1999). Parental absence, even in the presence of other social companions, leads to impaired 5-HT$_{1A}$ receptor binding in addition to altered levels of mineralcorticoid and glucocorticoid receptor mRNAs (Lopez et al., 2001).

In a series of studies, the accessibility and reliability of mother as a secure base was manipulated by varying the mother's daily foraging demands. This rearing environment forced mothers to either spend a good deal of their time looking for food or varied the requirements for foraging from sparse to plenty on a random daily basis. This gave the infant no sense of her availability as a secure base, ultimately resulting in impaired attachment relations (Andrews and Rosenblum, 1991a, 1991b; Andrews and Rosenblum, 1992; Coplan et al., 1992; Rosenblum et al., 1994).

In discussing foraging rearing condition variations it is important to note that adequate calories were available even on days when foraging was a predominant part of the day. In fact, mothers in the sparse condition, who always spent a large percentage of their time each day foraging, produced infants who differed little from mothers who always foraged for a short daily period. The important variable was the predictability of the mother's availability. Under conditions where foraging demands were unpredictable there were a number of behavioral deficits. This suggests that unpredictable experience was even more stressful than the demands that daily high maternal foraging imposed on the infant. Under the variable foraging condition a number of the infant's central neurochemical systems appeared to be chronically activated, as measured by high CSF concentrations of CRH, 5-HIAA, HVA, and somatostatin (Coplan *et al.*, 1998). However. there may be some species differences in this response. Similar studies in more metabolically active squirrel monkeys show that infants having mothers with high foraging demands exhibited high levels of cortisol (Lyons *et al.*, 1998).

These studies are important because they suggest that the biochemical differences seen in the monkeys reared without adults are not simply a result of chronic early stress. There is also something fundamental about the availability and presence of an adult caregiver for the monoamine systems to adequately develop. On the other hand, findings from the Old World species studied suggest that the infant's attachment figure must be predictably and reliably available (a fundamental aspect of secure attachment) for normal CNS development to occur.

AGGRESSION

Aggression is experienced by infant primates very early in life as a result of challenges and attacks on its mother as well as during mother–infant interchanges. One of the principal functions of the adult caregiver is to restrain and inhibit their infant's inappropriate social behaviors such as stealing food or hurting the mothers when nursing, and unrestrained threatening acts towards other members of the group. This is typically done through punishment or the threat of punishment. This seems to function in a stimulus-response fashion to modify inappropriate behaviors. It probably also provides stimulation for proper cortical growth and development of inhibitory cortical connections. Monkeys reared without parents in semi-isolation show inappropriate aggression such as attacking animals two or three times their size, make poor social companions, and are not preferred as social partners (Sackett, 1968, 1970). They are generally shunned by other monkeys (Sackett, 1968, 1970; Capitanio, 1986), and end up low in social dominance rank (Bastian *et al.*, 2003).

The infant learns behavioral restraint during a major period of development of the frontal and prefrontal cortex. Functioning frontal, prefrontal, and orbitofrontal cortex are of critical importance for controlling impulsive behavior. For example, monkeys with orbitofrontal damage exhibit inappropriate aggression and impaired social competence. As a result they may be ostracized by other group members (Raleigh *et al.*, 1979; Raleigh and Steklis, 1981). A positron emission tomography (PET) study of monkeys predisposed to aggression found that low CSF 5-HIAA concentrations – a risk factor for violence – were strongly correlated with cortical glucose uptake in a variety of areas in the cortex, but particularly the orbital frontal cortex (Doudet *et al.*, 1995). This is important because, as noted above, orbital frontal damage often leads to violent behavior and indicates a possible dysregulation in the orbital frontal cortex of animals with low CSF 5-HIAA concentrations.

As they develop, both peer-reared and semi-isolate subjects are more likely than parentally reared subjects to exhibit impulse control deficits resulting in violence and self-aggression, particularly in the rhesus macaque (Mitchell, 1970; Ruppenthal *et al.*, 1976; Suomi and Ripp, 1983; Capitanio, 1986; Kraemer *et al.*, 1991; Suomi, 1991a; Higley *et al.*, 1994, 1996d, 1996e). For example, when they are provoked, nursery-reared rhesus are likely to express aggression at inappropriate targets or in unexpected settings, and they are particularly prone to violently aggressive behaviors (Mitchell, 1970; Suomi and Ripp, 1983; Capitanio, 1986; Kraemer *et al.*, 1991; Suomi, 1991a; Higley *et al.*, 1994, 1996d, 1996e). Moreover, peer-reared monkeys during adolescence are more likely to show deficits in CNS inhibitory systems (Higley and Linnoila, 1997) of the frontal and prefrontal cortex regions (Doudet *et al.*, 1995; Heinz *et al.*, 1998).

Lopez and colleagues found a number of cortical parallels between the frontal cortical regions of peer-only reared macaques and humans who complete suicide (Lopez *et al.*, 2001). Brain injuries in these areas often result in impulse control deficits and impulsive aggression (Davidson *et al.*, 2000). Studies suggest that parental input is of critical importance for developing CNS inhibitory controls functioning to restrain aggression (Doudet *et al.*, 1995). Mothers are particularly well-suited to inculcate such inhibitions. As the inhibitory influences of the frontal cortex are maturing and making connections, mothers punish inappropriate aggression, probably inducing cortical growth in the inhibitory control centers. Without such input, monkeys often develop into hyperaggressive adults who act violently toward infants and even older monkeys (Suomi, 1982).

A second period of qualitative change in brain activity occurs at puberty. In human adolescence this may be a time of substantial change in sensation seeking and behavior dysregulation in some individuals (Steinberg, 2004). On average, high-risk behaviors in both humans and nonhuman primates increase during the adolescent period. Among many nonhuman primate species this is a period when males migrate from their troop of origin. In rhesus as many as 20–25% of the male population die during the period of migration (Drickamer, 1974; Dittus, 1979; Meikle and Vessey, 1988). One could postulate that a loosening of behavior control and dependency in the young male at this time may serve some adaptive functions. An overregulation of impulses may make it difficult for the young male to leave his natal environment, remaining dependent on his family and without opportunities to seek breeding partners. On the other hand, excessive impulsivity can lead to premature migration and other risky behaviors such as violence.

CSF 5-HIAA, a major neurotransmitter that modulates impulsive behavior (Higley *et al.*, 1996c; Soubrié, 1986), shows a substantial fall at adolescence (Higley *et al.*, 1996d, 1996e). Males with low CSF 5-HIAA concentrations migrate at an early age, often at a time when they lack the sophistication to defend themselves.

As a consequence they may be more likely to die than monkeys with high CSF 5-HIAA concentrations that migrate at an older age (Higley *et al.*, 1996b). This may in large part be because they are impulsively violent, showing significantly higher rates of aggression than males with higher CSF 5-HIAA concentrations (Higley *et al.*, 1996b, 1996c; Howell *et al.*, 2007).

BIOLOGICAL SUBSTRATES OF AGGRESSION

Serotonin

> Recent pharmacological and genetic studies have dramatically expanded the list of neurotransmitters, hormones cytokines, enzymes, growth factors, and signaling molecules that influence aggression. In spite of this expansion, serotonin remains the primary molecule determinant of inter-male aggression, whereas other molecules appear to act indirectly through serotonin signaling. J. Grafman, 2003, *Molecular Psychiatry* **8**, 131

The neurochemistry of aggression and violence continues to be a major research area among a wide variety of disciplines. Of all the biochemicals investigated, perhaps the most replicated relationship between a biological measure and aggression is that between serotonin and aggression. Studies show that impaired or low CNS serotonin functioning, whether naturally occurring or pharmacologically induced, is related to violence and impulsive aggression. In his classic comprehensive review of serotonin and impulse control, Soubrié (1986) summarizes the research in rodents and humans showing that aggression is higher in subjects with impaired or compromised central serotonin functions. Across a wide variety of subprimate species (e.g. dogs, cats, fish, lobsters, rodents, foxes, horses) pharmacological agents that increase serotonin activity decrease aggression, while agents that decrease serotonin activity or block its action increase aggression (Siegel and Pott, 1988; Miczek and Donat, 1990; Olivier and Mos, 1990; Olivier *et al.*, 1990; Nikulina *et al.*, 1992). For example, aggressive dogs that severely bite their owners or others without warning are more likely than nonbiters to show diminished CNS serotonin activity (Reisner *et al.*, 1996).

In humans and nonhuman primates, the principal method used to assess naturally occurring individual differences in serotonin and aggression is to measure the serotonin metabolite 5-HIAA in the CSF. Perhaps the most replicated finding in psychiatry is that men with low lumbar CSF 5-HIAA concentrations exhibit increased unplanned aggression and impulsive violence (Brown *et al.*, 1979, 1982; Linnoila *et al.*, 1983; Lidberg *et al.*, 1985; Roy *et al.*, 1985; Limson *et al.*, 1991; Virkkunen *et al.*, 1994a, 1994b). Studies using male nonhuman primates show that, like humans, low cisternal CSF 5-HIAA concentrations are correlated with high rates of wounding, unprovoked and unrestrained violence, and violent deaths (Higley *et al.*, 1992b, 1996a, 1996b, 1996c, 1996d, 1996e; Mehlman *et al.*, 1992, 1995). But see Yodyingyuad *et al.* (1985) for an exception to this frequently replicated finding.

Low concentrations of CSF 5-HIAA identify an underactive or impaired central serotonin system. Studies using CSF 5-HIAA concentrations have been widely used in humans, typically measuring lumbar CSF 5-HIAA concentrations. One major advantage of nonhuman primates for such studies is that CSF can be directly obtained from the cisterna magna at the base of the brain, probably reflecting a more accurate assessment of central functioning than lumbar measures. Measuring these monoamine metabolites in CSF to index central neurotransmitter activity is based on investigations in animals and postmortem studies in humans showing that concentrations of CSF monoamine metabolites, particularly in the cisternal magna, are correlated with both regional and whole-brain metabolite concentrations (Wilk and Stanley, 1978; Banki, 1981; Stanley et al., 1985; Elsworth et al., 1987; Knott et al., 1989). Studies using CSF to index CNS monoamine activity cannot pinpoint the relative contributions of CSF monoamine concentrations in specific brain areas. However, the method can assess whether a specific CNS neurotransmitter system is activated and its degree of involvement in the behavioral activity under study without compromising the CNS (Wood, 1980; Stone and McCarty, 1983; Anisman and Zacharko, 1990). This is important because when lumbar CSF is obtained from humans, there is always a question of peripheral origin of the serotonin measures. This is not a question in studies of nonhuman primates, where CSF is obtained from the cistern magna.

In the initial study of correlation between CSF 5-HIAA concentration and rates of aggression in nonhuman primates, Higley and colleagues (1992) blind-rated adolescent male macaques for aggressiveness based on the number and location of wounds. Males with low CSF 5-HIAA had more frontal wounds, indicating they were not fleeing when they were wounded, and were rated as more aggressive (Higley et al., 1992b). This was followed by a study in which radio collars were used to facilitate locating monkeys for direct behavioral observations. In this study there was no correlation between CSF 5-HIAA and overall aggression, but there was a strong correlation between high rates of impulsive or violent aggression and low CSF 5-HIAA concentrations (Mehlman et al., 1994). A number of studies of other species in the same and other laboratories replicated these findings, showing that males with low CSF 5-HIAA exhibit violent behavior (Higley et al., 1996b, 1996c; Reisner et al., 1996; Champoux et al., 1997; Fairbanks et al., 2001). Low CSF 5-HIAA concentrations may be modulated by individual differences in MAO activity. Rhesus monkeys with low platelet MAO consumed alcohol to excess, exhibited low CSF 5-HIAA concentrations, were less competent socially, and exhibited higher rates of aggression (Fahlke et al., 2002).

In a lifespan longitudinal research – the first of its kind – male juvenile, 2.5-year-old rhesus monkeys with low CSF 5-HIAA concentrations were studied for nearly a decade into their middle-aged period. The results showed that subjects with low CSF 5-HIAA concentrations exhibit a life-long pattern of antisocial behavior and violence. CSF 5-HIAA taken when the subjects were juveniles, still dependent on their mothers for much of their psychological needs and protection, predicted both

CSF 5-HIAA concentrations and violent behavior nearly a decade later (Howell *et al.*, 2007).

Consistent with earlier findings from monkeys who die as adolescents and young adults during their first migration (Higley *et al.*, 1996b), males with low CSF 5-HIAA concentrations were less likely to survive into middle adulthood (Howell *et al.*, 2007). They were loners not only as juveniles, but throughout life (Mehlman *et al.*, 1997; Howell *et al.*, 2007). At night, they slept on the edge of the group and awoke frequently. During the breeding season, they were less likely to be selected by adult females for consort relationships that led to breeding. While the males with high CSF 5-HIAA concentrations were observed to frequently produce sperm plugs in the females, there were no observed inseminations by males with low CSF 5-HIAA concentrations (Mehlman *et al.*, 1997).

Within the laboratory, where males lived in pairs and paternities could be accurately assessed, the male of the pair who had the highest CSF 5-HIAA concentration was most likely to sire offspring (Gerald *et al.*, 2002). However, among younger males, those with the lowest CSF 5-HIAA concentrations were more likely to produce offspring. This suggests that a "live-fast-die-young" strategy may be present for males with low CSF 5-HIAA concentrations (Gerald *et al.*, 2002). These differences in reproductive rates were not simply a product of physiological differences such as sperm quality (Roudebush *et al.*, 2002).

In a series of interesting studies investigating silver foxes, researchers employed a selective breeding program to produce a calm, placid, and increasingly docile temperament. As selective breeding produced animals with less and less aggressive temperaments, there was a concomitant increase in CNS concentrations of serotonin and its breakdown product 5-HIAA (Namboodiri *et al.*, 1985; Popova *et al.*, 1991a, 1991b). As each generation showed an increasingly placid and docile temperament, there was a parallel increase in the enzyme tryptophan hydroxylase, which converts the amino acid tryptophan into serotonin. There was also a corresponding decrease in monoamine oxidase type A, an enzyme that breaks down serotonin (Popova *et al.*, 1997).

Such parallel CNS serotonin strain and species differences may also be present in nonhuman primates. Westergaard and colleagues (1999b), investigating species differences in CNS serotonin functioning, found that CSF 5-HIAA concentrations were lower in the highly aggressive rhesus macaque than in the more gregarious and less aggressive pigtail macaques (Westergaard *et al.*, 1999b). Champoux and colleagues (1997) found that when comparing rhesus macaque stains, the more aggressive Chinese rhesus macaques possessed lower CSF 5-HIAA concentrations than their more peaceable Indian-derived rhesus cousins. Paralleling these findings, hamadryas baboons, which show less inter-male aggression than anubis baboons, exhibited higher CSF 5-HIAA than the anubis species (Kaplan *et al.*, 1999).

Other procedures have been used to assess CNS serotonin–aggression relationships. One of the principal methods widely used in humans is prolactin challenge. This involves administration of a serotonin-enhancing drug, such as fenfluramine hydrochloride or another serotonin reuptake inhibitor, then measuring blood prolactin. High levels of prolactin are taken as evidence of an active serotonin system, low levels as evidence of impaired serotonin activity. Numerous challenge studies have found evidence for impaired central serotonin functioning in aggressive men and violent patients (Newman *et al.*, 1998). Similarly, adult male cynomolgus monkeys who were given fenfluramine and responded with low prolactin were more likely to exhibit aggressive responses to pictures of humans making threatening gestures (Kyes *et al.*, 1995) than were males with high prolactin.

Serotonin and aggression: The female story

The relationship between low or impaired CNS serotonin and aggression has not been systematically studied in human females, but nonhuman primate studies suggest that this relationship may extend to females as well as males. In female cynomolgus monkeys, low blood plasma levels of prolactin following fenfluramine administration are associated with high rates of aggression (Botchin *et al.*, 1993; Shively *et al.*, 1995). In laboratory, studies, unrelated adolescent and adult female macaques who were removed from their group for excessive aggression or those that exhibited high rates of impulsive aggression and violence had lower CSF 5-HIAA concentrations than females not involved in aggression (Higley *et al.*, 1996a, 1996d, 1996e; Westergaard *et al.*, 1999b). A low CSF 5-HIAA-high aggression relationship in unrelated females is not limited to rhesus, but is also seen in female pigtail macaques (Westergaard *et al.*, 1999b).

When females were observed longitudinally, antisocial behaviors were seen that paralleled findings in males. For example, they showed reproductive deficits. Nulliparous females who did not give birth during their first breeding season had lower CSF 5-HIAA than females who gave birth during their first breeding season (Cleveland *et al.*, 2004). Among rhesus females with low CSF 5-HIAA who give birth, first-born infants were more likely to die during the infant's first postnatal year (Westergaard *et al.*, 2003a). Also paralleling male findings, females with low CSF 5-HIAA concentrations were more likely to show spontaneous, dangerous, long leaps, spend long periods alone, and seldom interacted socially (Westergaard *et al.*, 2003b).

On the other hand, the story may be different for females living in a natural family setting of extended matrilineal family members consisting of mother, grandmothers, sisters, aunts, and their offspring. For females living with close female kin, high CNS serotonin functioning is not correlated with violent aggression. It is correlated with the overall level of milder forms of aggression, and the females with mild aggression have higher plasma cortisol, indicating chronic stress (Westergaard *et al.*, 2003b). In the natural setting family squabbles and kin disagreements are the leading cause of interfemale aggression. But in family disagreement, aggression may be less likely to escalate than in unrelated laboratory groups. That is not to say that such aggression is meaningless, as these females exhibited increased signs of stress such as high cortisol.

Females with low CSF 5-HIAA living in their natural family setting were also more likely to require clinical treatments for illnesses than those with high CSF 5-HIAA

(Westergaard *et al.*, 2003a). Like males with low CSF 5-HIAA, low-concentration females were also more likely to suffer from premature mortality. But unlike males with low CSF 5-HIAA concentrations, these females did not die disproportionately of violence. They died for a variety of causes including illnesses such as wasting and diarrhea, although there were some cases of premature death following violence (Westergaard *et al.*, 2003a). This again may reflect a difference between males and females in life history, with feral females living in family groups not likely to engage in severe violence leading to death.

Child abuse

Some female monkeys seriously abuse their infants. The most intensely studied female abusers and their infants come from work by Maestripieri. His research group acquired a relatively large number of rhesus macaque females that abused their infants and followed them and their offspring longitudinally for over a decade.

Biochemically, there were a number of differences between nonabusing controls and abusing females. An initial study showed that abusing females had higher CSF CRH and 5-HIAA concentrations (Maestripieri *et al.*, 2005). Unlike earlier studies in which high rates of aggression were correlated with low CSF 5-HIAA, for both abusers and controls aggression levels were correlated with higher 5-HIAA, as well as higher CRH and MHPG concentrations. When the females who abused their infants were compared with the nonabusing controls, the abusing females had higher CSF 5-HIAA concentrations (Maestripieri *et al.*, 2005).

Higher CSF 5-HIAA, MHPG, and CRH concentrations in these abusing females may reflect high, chronic stress. In subsequent studies of the infants, however, the picture was more consistent with earlier studies, yielding a negative correlation between CSF 5-HIAA concentrations and aggression. For example, infants that underwent high rates of rejection by their mothers during the first six months engaged in solitary but not in social play and subsequently demonstrated low CSF 5-HIAA concentrations (Maestripieri *et al.*, 2006b). Not surprisingly, abused infants that were rejected most often developed lower CSF 5-HIAA and HVA than infants that were rejected least often.

Only a subset of abused infants went on to become mothers who abused their own infants. However, females that did abuse their infants had been rejected by their mothers more often and demonstrated lower CSF 5-HIAA than those who did not abuse their offspring (Maestripieri *et al.*, 2006a, 2007). According to the arguments presented next, this suggests that low central serotonin may cause the high maternal rejection leading abused females to abuse their own infants when they become adults.

Correlation and causation

Finding correlations between CSF 5-HIAA and behavior leaves open the question of causation. When central serotonin is enhanced via pharmacological agents rates of aggression decrease and when CNS serotonin is diminished via pharmacological agents aggression increases. For example, vervet monkeys that consume experimental diets high in the serotonin precursor tryptophan exhibit decreased aggression, whereas individuals placed on diets low in tryptophan exhibit increased aggression. However, these effects may be stronger for males than for females (Raleigh et al., 1985, 1986, 1991; Chamberlain et al., 1987). Similarly, treatments which augment CNS serotonin, such as short-term administration of SSRIs, decrease aggression (Chamberlain et al., 1987; Raleigh et al., 1980, 1985, 1986, 1991; Higley et al., 1998). On the other hand, long-term treatment with the SSRI fenfluramine, which decreases CNS serotonin turnover, increases aggression in nonhuman primates (Raleigh et al., 1983, 1986). Aggression also shows marked increases following the administration of the serotonin synthesis inhibitor p-chlorophenylalanine, which acts to diminish serotonin production (Raleigh et al., 1980; Raleigh and McGuire, 1986).

Impaired serotonin and an impulsive temperament

Soubrié (1986) suggested that the reason aggression is higher in animals with impaired CNS serotonin functioning is because their impulse-control capabilities are defective. In reviewing this research, Ferrari and colleagues (2005) concluded that the relationship between serotonin, impulsivity, and aggression in primates is a different form of aggression than that which is seen in rodents. In rodents aggression often leads to some form of reinforcement. In primates, they argue, serotonin-mediated aggression serves little biological function. They conclude that in most of the nonhuman and human primate studies aggression and impulsivity are so closely linked that the two terms could be used interchangeably. While aggression can take many forms and often serves biological functions, serotonin-mediated aggression in nonhuman primates often appears on the surface to be maladaptive. In support of this, low CSF 5-HIAA is not correlated with the overall levels of aggression used to maintain status or obtain resources. Instead, it is only seemingly unprovoked, impulsive, aggression that escalates out of control, and only this type shows the negative correlation with CSF 5-HIAA (Higley et al., 1996a, 1996b, 1996c; Mehlman et al., 1992, 1994). Indeed, high levels of impulsive or escalated aggression were even predictive of premature death (Howell et al., 2007), suggesting that Ferrari's analysis of the nonhuman primate serotonin–aggression story may be close to the mark.

One reason why serotonin-mediated primate aggression may be seen as maladaptive is because the original studies were designed to model impulsive violence in humans. A large number of studies have investigated the diminished serotonin-increased aggression and violence relationship. The results suggest that monkeys with impaired CNS serotonin functioning show a cluster of closely related behaviors and traits centering around impaired impulse control (Apter et al., 1990). Cloninger's biosocial theory of personality posits that personality disorders related to dysfunctional social relationships, aggression, and diminished social bonding are neurobiologically based on diminished serotonin and possibly reduced dopamine (Cloninger, 1988).

Clarke and colleagues (1999) assessed CSF 5-HIAA taken from febrile human neonates. Three years later, as toddlers, the subjects with low CSF 5-HIAA concentrations as neonates exhibited high scores on externalizing behavior (Clarke et al., 1999). Other studies of human children (Kruesi et al., 1990), as well as nonhuman primates (Mehlman et al., 1995; Higley et al., 1996a, 1996e; Higley and Suomi, 1996), showed that individuals high in social deviancy or who exhibit less competent social behavior exhibit relatively low CSF 5-HIAA. These low CSF 5-HIAA concentrations early in life predict later externalizing behavior, conduct disorder, and other antisocial outcomes (Kruesi, 1989; Kruesi et al., 1990; Kruesi et al., 1992; Howell et al., 2007).

Soubrié's (1986) review of serotonin and impulsivity in animals and other studies that have since followed, show that serotonin plays a role in controlling impulses other than aggression. For example, serotonin-enhancing pharmacological treatments decrease alcohol consumption in both rodents and nonhuman primates (Gill and Amit, 1989; McBride et al., 1989; Higley et al., 1992a). Conversely, in rodents, pharmacologically reducing CNS serotonin activity increases the frequency of performing a response despite the threat of punishment for responding (Soubrié, 1986; Gleeson et al., 1989; Miczek et al., 1989). Additionally, among humans, men with low CSF 5-HIAA concentrations exhibit evidence of impaired impulse control such as increased unplanned fire setting (Virkkunen et al., 1987), and increased violent criminal recidivism (Virkkunen et al., 1989).

Consistent with Soubrié's (1986) review, nonhuman primates with low CSF 5-HIAA concentrations are more likely to exhibit impulse control deficits such as spontaneous, unprovoked long leaps between trees at dangerous heights, approach of a potentially dangerous stranger, and repeated re-entry into baited traps in which they had been captured previously (Mehlman et al., 1994; Higley et al., 1996c; Fairbanks et al., 1999, 2004; Fairbanks, 2001). In the laboratory setting, when monkeys are allowed access to a novel baited black box, all monkeys show interest, but monkeys with low CSF 5-HIAA concentrations approach the box rapidly and spend more time in close proximity than do monkeys with high CSF 5-HIAA (Bennett et al., 1998). Rhesus macaques with impaired CNS serotonin or low CSF 5-HIAA concentrations are also dysregulated in their patterns of alcohol intake, showing a high likelihood to consume especially large amounts of alcohol once drinking begins (Higley et al., 1994, 1996d, 1996e; Heinz et al., 2003a; Barr et al., 2004b).

Other laboratories have also found a relationship between low CSF 5-HIAA and impaired impulse control. Fairbanks and colleagues used a standardized test of impulse control to measure the relationship between impulsivity and CNS serotonin. They measure the latency to approach an unfamiliar similar aged monkey. Monkeys with low CSF 5-HIAA were more likely to approach the potentially dangerous intruder and did so more rapidly (Fairbanks et al., 2001). Similar results were found using the fenfluramine test. Monkeys that moved within close proximity of the potentially dangerous intruder had lower prolactin responses compared to animals that failed to approach the intruder (Manuck et al., 2003).

This relationship between low or impaired CNS serotonin impulsivity and aggression may be a causal one. The monkey intruder method was also used to study central serotonin using the SSRI fluoxetine. Following administration, monkeys were slower to approach the unfamiliar adult male than those dosed with placebo (Fairbanks *et al.*, 2001). If excessive aggression is a result of an impulse control deficit, it would be predicted that rates of impulsivity would also be positively correlated with rates of escalated aggression or violence. Given the negative correlation between CSF 5-HIAA and the two serotonin-mediated behaviors violence and impulsivity, it is not surprising that there is a strong correlation between violent aggression and impulsivity. Thus, in separate studies, rates of apparently unprovoked dangerous long leaps between trees at very high heights were positively correlated with rates of violent behavior (Mehlman *et al.*, 1994; Higley *et al.*, 1996c). Similarly, Fairbanks and colleagues found that monkeys who quickly approached an unfamiliar male were more likely to act aggressively toward the male intruder (Fairbanks *et al.*, 2001). These results all suggest that high levels of escalated aggression and violence in individuals with impaired central serotonin functioning is a result of deficient impulse control regulation.

Low CSF 5-HIAA concentrations, high aggression and social alienation

Aggressive males are not sought as often as companions and seldom affiliate with adult females (Chapais, 1986; Mehlman *et al.*, 1995; Mehlman *et al.*, 1997). Because monkeys with low CSF 5-HIAA are more aggressive and exhibit impulse control deficits, it seems reasonable to hypothesize that males with low CSF 5-HIAA concentrations will also show impairments in sociality. Like humans, individual primates vary in sociality, some exhibiting gregariousness and others introversion. Chamove and colleagues identified sociality as one of three core personality traits in rhesus monkeys (Chamove *et al.*, 1972). Sociality in monkeys is a trait similar to the personality trait extroversion that Eysenck identified in humans (Eysenck and Eysenck, 1971). As in humans, sociality is an enduring trait in monkeys (Stevenson-Hinde and Simpson, 1980; McGuire *et al.*, 1994).

Several nonhuman primate studies demonstrate that sociality is positively correlated with CNS serotonin function. In a sample of free-ranging adolescent male rhesus monkeys, aggressive subjects with low CSF 5-HIAA exhibited reduced levels of four measures of sociality: time spent grooming other monkeys; time spent in close proximity to others; time spent in general affiliative social behaviors; and mean number of companions within a 5-meter radius (Mehlman *et al.*, 1995). In laboratory studies of juveniles, low rates of positive social interactions were correlated with low CSF 5-HIAA in both sexes (Mehlman *et al.*, 1995, 1997; Higley *et al.*, 1996a, 1996d, 1996e; Higley and Suomi, 1996). Also, serotonin-stimulated plasma prolactin was lower in monkeys described as loners (Botchin *et al.*, 1993).

This relationship between CNS serotonin and sociality may also be a casual one. For example, across repeated studies of captive vervet monkeys, Raleigh and colleagues found that enhancing serotonin by administering tryptophan, fluoxetine, or quipazine decreased aggression while increasing positive social behaviors such as approaching and grooming other monkeys (Raleigh et al., 1983, 1985, 1980). When investigators reduced serotonin functioning by administering low doses of the tryptophan hydroxylase enzyme inhibitor p-chlorophenylalanine, opposite effects were seen. The monkeys withdrew, and avoided social proximity and affiliative social interactions (Raleigh et al., 1980, 1985; Raleigh and McGuire, 1990).

Studies of both aggressive humans (Brown et al., 1982) and nonhuman primates (Raleigh et al., 1989; McGuire et al., 1994) have shown that individuals high in social deviancy or who are rated as low in competent social behaviors (Kruesi et al., 1990), have low CSF 5-HIAA. In some primate species, social dominance is acquired and maintained through the formation of affiliative bonds with other troop members, who then support the dominant male during hostile and challenging social encounters (Packer and Pusey, 1979; Raleigh and Steklis, 1981; Smuts, 1987; Walters and Seyfarth, 1987). As noted previously, building coalitions and maintaining social support is crucial to acquire and maintain a high social dominance rank (Chapais, 1986; Raleigh and McGuire, 1986; Chapais, 1988; Raleigh et al., 1991; Higley and Suomi, 1996). Thus it is reasonable to predict that monkeys low in CSF 5-HIAA would be more likely to be low in social dominance. Indeed, in a series of studies within our laboratory and others, a frequently replicated finding is that naturally occurring low CNS serotonin functioning, measured by low CSF 5-HIAA (Raleigh et al., 1986; Higley et al., 1992b, 1996a, 1996b, 1996c, 1996d, 1996e; Raleigh and McGuire, 1994; Mehlman et al., 1994; Westergaard et al., 1999a, 1999b; Fairbanks et al., 2001) or pharmacologically reducing CNS serotonin functioning (Raleigh et al., 1983, 1986) is linked to low social dominance ranking. This finding may not be true for all species, as studies of cynomolgus monkeys have not always found a positive correlation between low rank and impaired CNS serotonin (Botchin et al., 1993; Shively et al., 1995).

Serotonin and other deficits

Primates with low CSF 5-HIAA concentrations also show other forms of behavior pathology. In what has been interpreted as an aspect of irritable temperament, they also exhibit high levels of stereotyped motor behaviors (Erickson et al., 2001). Other studies show that they are dysregulated in daily activity patterns and circadian sleep–activity cycles. When compared with subjects with high CSF 5-HIAA, juvenile monkeys with low CSF 5-HIAA take longer to fall asleep at night and exhibit more overall motor activity during the day. This is unlikely to be an aspect of captivity, because in this unique field study aggressive macaques with low CSF 5-HIAA woke up more often during the night, spent more time active at night, and napped more often during the daytime than controls (Zajicek et al., 1997; Mehlman et al., 2000).

Testosterone

Investigations of the relationship between testosterone and aggression have a long history, with many animal studies suggesting that it is the primary hormone modulating violent aggression (Archer, 1991). This is largely because when testosterone is blocked or animals are castrated they are unlikely to engage in aggression, but when testosterone is replaced they again engage in agonistic behavior (Archer, 1991). More recently, however, it has become clear that testosterone is probably not the major cause of violent aggression, particularly in primates. Those studies suggest that testosterone probably functions more to modulate competitiveness or an overall aggressive motivation than to induce violence or aggression (Olweus, 1984, 1986; Christiansen and Knussmann, 1987; Archer, 1991; Buchanan et al., 1992). When aggression and testosterone are measured directly, studies showing a positive correlation between the two often fail to replicate (Olweus, 1986; Archer, 1991). Interestingly, when testosterone and aggression correlations are found, they are detected most often when both are measured during competition or during social status challenges (Scaramella and Brown, 1978; Mazur, 1983) or during provocation or threat (Olweus et al., 1980, 1988; Olweus, 1986). Among humans, a correlation between testosterone and aggression is found among violent criminals (Olweus, 1986; Archer, 1991). This may be because they also possess other personality deficits that center around impulse control.

Individually, most men and women with high circulating testosterone are not violent, they are restrained in their use of aggression. They express aggression in settings that are socially acceptable. This may be expression of a function for which testosterone-mediated aggression was selected; namely, maintenance of social status and defense of competitive challenges. Moreover, correlations between testosterone and behavior are not limited to aggression. Testosterone also shows correlations with seemingly positive traits such as toughness (Dabbs et al., 1987), social dominance (Ehrenkranz et al., 1974; Christiansen and Knussmann, 1987; Lindman et al., 1987; Booth et al., 1989), social assertiveness (Lindman et al., 1987), and competitiveness and physical vigor (Mattsson et al., 1980; Booth et al., 1989).

Among male rhesus macaques, which are seasonal breeders, aggression and testosterone show similar seasonal peaks, reaching their apex during the breeding season (Kaufman, 1967; Gordon et al., 1976; Bernstein et al., 1977; Gordon et al., 1978; Rose et al., 1978; Paul, 1989; Kuester and Paul, 1992; Wickings and Dixson, 1992). Paralleling studies in humans, a number of nonhuman primate investigations have found no relationship between aggression and testosterone (Rose et al., 1972, 1975; Eaton and Resko, 1974; Gordon et al., 1976). When testosterone was increased in male talapoin monkeys, neither aggression nor social dominance rank changed (Keverne et al., 1983). In a separate study of male macaques, subjects received injections of chorionic gonadotropin twice a week to stimulate testosterone production, but they showed no change in aggression (Gordon et al., 1979). On the other hand, when cynomolgus macaques were injected with testosterone propionate, rates of aggression increased in dominant subjects, but not in subordinates (Rejeski *et al.*, 1988). This suggests that testosterone's effect on aggression is mediated by social dominance rank. Consistent with this interpretation, in a follow-up study of the monkeys that were injected with testosterone, rates of aggression increased in dominant monkeys, but decreased in the subordinates.

Separate roles for serotonin and testosterone

These findings, as well as others in animals and humans (e.g. Olweus *et al.*, 1980, 1988; Soubrié, 1986; Archer, 1991), suggest that testosterone modulates aggressive motives and competitiveness rather than violence and physical aggression. Consistent with this interpretation, testosterone and noncontact aggressive challenges were both found to peak during the breeding season, while violent aggression showed no seasonal variability (Gordon *et al.*, 1976). Moreover, testosterone was positively correlated with day-to-day lower level aggression, but not with violent aggression (Gordon *et al.*, 1976). While testosterone may modulate competition and agonism to challenge, impaired impulse control could determine the onset and intensity of the expression of such agonism. Serotonin, as discussed previously, functions to inhibit a variety of impulses. One might hypothesize that CNS serotonin determines the initiation of aggression, limiting aggression to proper times, settings, and intensity. As a direct test of the testosterone-competition/serotonin impulse control hypothesis, we took both CSF testosterone and 5-HIAA from a group of free-ranging young adult male rhesus monkeys and measured rates of impulsivity, restrained competitive aggression, and violent aggression (Higley *et al.*, 1996c). Consistent with testosterone and serotonin performing different roles in modulating aggression, three findings emerged. First, CNS testosterone, indexed by CSF free testosterone concentration, was positively correlated with overall aggressiveness and aggression used to compete for status and resources, but not with measures of impulsivity such as spontaneous long leaps nor rates of capture. Second, CSF 5-HIAA was negatively correlated with the impulsive behaviors above and severe violent aggression, but not with competitive overall rates of aggression. Moreover, high rates of impulsive behavior were positively correlated with severe, unrestrained aggression, but not overall rates of aggression. Third, there was an interaction between serotonin and testosterone. Subjects with low CSF 5-HIAA exhibited high rates of aggression. High CSF testosterone further augmented rates and intensity of aggression in subjects with low CSF 5-HIAA. However, the most severe forms of aggression were unaffected by high testosterone. Such findings suggest that high central testosterone is associated with competitive aggression, while low impaired serotonin is associated with severe aggression resulting from impaired impulse control and perseverative behavior (Higley *et al.*, 1996c).

One possible interpretation of these data is that testosterone and serotonin may contribute differentially to the expression of aggressive behavior. We hypothesize that testosterone influences aggressive motivation and serotonin regulates the threshold, intensity, and frequency of aggressive expression. Thus, individuals with low testosterone would be unmotivated to compete or to engage in any form of aggression, regardless of their serotonin levels. But when they have impaired central serotonin functioning they might act impulsively in other behaviors. On the other hand, individuals with above average testosterone level but normal serotonin may express aggression in a variety of settings, but generally would not express violence or unrestrained aggression. They would also be expected to exhibit more assertive behaviors that characterize social dominance such as threats, displacements, or mounting of other male monkeys. Individuals with lower than average serotonin functioning would be expected to exhibit impaired impulse control, resulting in a low threshold to display aggression and difficulties inhibiting aggression once they begin an agonistic exchange. Ultimately they would engaging in more frequent and higher intensity of violence.

Due to increased aggressive motivation, high testosterone would further augment the propensity to engage in aggression in subjects with low CSF 5-HIAA. Once an aggressive act had begun, high testosterone subjects with low CSF 5-HIAA would exhibit deficits in stopping the aggression before it escalated into violence with a high probability of injury. Put simply, these interpretations say that testosterone provides the push to act competitively and serotonin provides the brakes that determine the timing and intensity.

ETIOLOGICAL INVESTIGATIONS OF INDIVIDUAL DIFFERENCES

Individual nonhuman primates differ considerably under baseline and stressful conditions. It is possible to test etiological hypotheses concerning individual differences in ways not possible in humans. Parents can be selected to study genetic and environmental influences and to assess how genetic and environmental influences interact. Studies can be planned with controlled rearing conditions to study their effects on development. For example, as discussed above, in infant nonhuman primates parental absence leads to long-term, possibly permanent, monoamine functioning deficits (Kraemer, 1986; Kraemer et al., 1989; Higley et al., 1990, 1991a, 1991b, 1996d, 1996e; Clarke et al., 1996; Shannon et al., 1998, 2005; Fahlke et al., 2000; Bennett et al., 2002; Champoux et al., 2002; Bastian et al., 2003; Barr et al., 2004a, 2004d; Lorenz et al., 2006). Thus, adult influence, particularly maternal input, is critical for development of the CNS serotonin system.

In the absence of adult input early in life, the development of CNS serotonin functioning is impaired. CSF 5-HIAA was obtained from neonatal and infant peer-only-reared and mother-reared monkeys on postnatal days 14, 30, 60, 90, 120, and 150. Parentally absent peer-reared subjects exhibited lower CSF 5-HIAA concentrations than mother-reared subjects (Shannon et al., 2005). Another study with a limited sample size suggested that the effect of early rearing experiences on CSF 5-HIAA may disappear by adolescence (Higley *et al.*, 1991b), but subsequent studies suggest that early parental absence in infancy, when input is necessary to guide and assure synaptic survival, leads to long-term serotonin and catecholamine deficits. Since this study, several others have involved peer- and mother-reared rhesus subjects measured longitudinally from infancy into adulthood. Results show that rhesus peer-reared subjects possess lower CSF 5-HIAA concentrations than mother-reared subjects both in infancy and young adulthood (five-year-olds) (Higley *et al.*, 1996d, 1996e; Shannon *et al.*, 2005). It would be of interest to test this effect in other species, such a pigtail macaques, to see if a species that shows less behavioral deficits to peer rearing also shows low CSF 5-HIAA concentrations when they are reared in peer-only groups.

The difference in activity of the serotonin system between peer- and mother-reared subjects was particularly evident in a recent PET study using a newly discovered serotonin transporter ligand. In the young adult male peer-reared monkeys, binding was reduced in virtually every area measured that is rich in serotonin, with specific reductions of 10–23% across a range of brain areas including the raphe, thalamus, hypothalamus, caudate and putamen, globus pallidum, anterior cingulate gyrus, and medial temporal regions, amygdale, and hippocampus (Ichise *et al.*, 2006).

GENETIC CONTRIBUTIONS

Parents also contribute genes to their offspring, which can influence individual differences in offspring neurobiology. Additive genetic influences on CSF monoamine metabolite concentrations have been investigated using nonhuman primate infants reared with or apart from their parents. Paternal genetic influence was tested by rearing infants apart from their fathers, which allowed a paternal genetic half-sibling analysis. Maternal genetic influences were studied by rearing infants with either their biological mothers, adopted unrelated lactating females, or without adults in peer-only groups.

When the subjects were six months of age, CSF was obtained prior to and during the stress of social separation. The results showed that CSF 5-HIAA was a significantly heritable effect ($h^2 > 0.5$) with no differences between the sexes. In addition, there were substantial maternal genetic influences on 5-HIAA ($h^2 > 0.5$). Although lower additive genetic effects were found for catecholamines, there was substantial heritability for the catecholamine metabolites MHPG and HVA. Paternal additive genetic contributions to CSF monoamine concentrations were independently replicated by another group studying nonhuman primates (Clarke *et al.*, 1994). Together these findings suggest that a significant portion of the variance in the turnover of CNS serotonin is determined by genetic mechanisms. These discoveries led researchers to begin studies looking for genetic variation that may be associated with this trait in nonhuman primates.

GENE–ENVIRONMENT INTERACTION

The study of candidate gene effects in nonhuman primates has resulted in several advances in understanding primate neurochemistry and behavior. One of the most exciting discoveries is that phenotypic outcome may not be an additive genetic–environment effect, but instead may be a quantitative or qualitative gene–environment interaction. In studies of humans and nonhuman primates one of the most widely studied candidates is a variant linked to the serotonin transporter gene called the serotonin transporter linked polymorphic region (*5-HTTLPR*). Initial human studies indicated that there are two major alleles, the long and short varieties. People with the short allele have a decrease in transcriptional efficiency, resulting in a variety of serotonin deficits (Collier *et al.*, 1996; Hranilovic *et al.*, 1996; Lesch *et al.*, 1996; Little *et al.*, 2006; Reist *et al.*, 2001).

In the first primate study of its kind, the orthologous region was screened for variation in rhesus macaques. The results revealed variation similar to humans. As predicted, subjects with the short, less-efficient variant, had low CSF 5-HIAA concentrations (Bennett *et al.*, 2002). The more interesting discovery came when Bennett and colleagues grouped the subjects by rearing and genotype. If the subjects were reared by their parents in a social group, there was no association of the *5-HTTLPRs* allele with differences in CSF 5-HIAA concentrations. The effect was quite different when peer-reared subjects were considered. There was substantial genetic influence in the subjects reared without adults in peer-only groups. They had low CSF 5-HIAA, but only if they were carriers of the short allele (Bennett *et al.*, 2002). Peer-reared subjects homozygous for the long allele did not differ from mother-reared subjects. This finding that genetic influence is rearing-dependent was an important breakthrough in many ways, changing the common thinking of how genes are expressed phenotypically.

Since this discovery, many studies have found similar gene × environment interactions at both the behavioral and CNS levels. Barr and colleagues demonstrated *HTTLPR* by rearing interactions on other phenotypes. One example is level of intoxication following a standardized alcohol dose (Barr *et al.*, 2003). Champoux and colleagues, studying rhesus neonates, performed a standardized battery of neonatal biobehavioral tests. These included assessments of state, temperament, motor maturity, and orienting to interesting novel objects. For orientation there was no effect of genotype if the subjects were reared by their mothers, but for the peer-reared subjects there was a substantial genetic contributions. Peer-reared subjects showed impaired performance, but only if they had the less efficient short allele. While there were trends for the other tests showing the same interaction, genetic effects were statistically significant only for orientation. (Champoux *et al.*, 2002).

Rearing by allele interactions may also affect CNS functions such as HPA axis activation (Barr *et al.*, 2004d). As noted earlier, during a social separation stressor plasma levels of cortisol and ACTH rise, but there are substantial group differences. Peer-reared infants that carried the *5-HTTLPRs* allele had higher ACTH levels than those without the *5-HTTLPRs* allele. Mother-reared subjects, on the other hand, were undifferentiated by genotype. In a more detailed analysis, it became evident that this interaction was limited to females. This later finding is important because it suggests that the gene × environment interactions are not monolithic but instead may at times be limited to only one sex (Barr *et al.*, 2004a). Other extrinsic factors, such as stress, must also be taken into account when considering gene × environment interactions.

While this review of candidate genes is selective (a number of other genes have been screened for variation including MAO-A, the mu-opioid receptor, TPH-2, NPY, and CRH) these studies illustrate the utility of the nonhuman primate model for examining interactions between functional genetic variants and early stress exposure. Not all studies have shown interacting gene × environment effects. In some cases only rearing effects have been detected and others detected only genotype effects.

Since there is a growing trend to genotype animals and to include genotype data in the analyses, a caution is in order. Most CNS and behavior phenotypes are polygenic in origin. In most studies candidate gene effects are small, accounting for less than 10–15% of the genetic variance. This means that to detect statistical significance, a large number of animals must be phenotyped under identical conditions. Sample sizes of 30 have been the standard for human clinical research and many primate studies, but these are underpowered for detecting many main effects or most gene × environment effects.

CONCLUSIONS

The studies reviewed in this chapter presented a great deal of evidence that nonhuman primates offer a powerful research tool to assess CNS function and its role in behavior. Because of their similarity to humans, many primate species are particularly useful for modeling human brain–behavior relationships and neurotransmitter psychopathology. We now have a complete rhesus genome. Thus, many new gene variants will emerge. These can be used to assess not only gene × environment interactions, but even how different genes themselves interact to produce phenotypes.

REFERENCES

Akiskal, H. S. (1985). Interaction of biologic and psychologic factors in the origin of depressive disorders. *Acta Psychiatr Scand* **319**, 131–139.

Akiskal, H. S. and McKinney, W. T. (1975). Overview of recent research in depression. *Arch Gen Psychiatry* **32**, 285–305.

Amico, J. A., Challinor, S. M., and Cameron, J. L. (1990). Pattern of oxytocin concentrations in the plasma and cerebrospinal fluid of lactating rhesus monkeys (Macaca mulatta), evidence for functionally independent oxytocinergic pathways in primates. *J Clin Endocrinol Metab* **71**, 1531–1535.

Anderson, G. M., Bennett, A. J., Weld, K. P., Pushkas, J. G., Ocame, D. M., and Higley, J. D. (2002). Serotonin in cisternal cerebrospinal fluid of rhesus monkeys, basal levels and effects of sertraline administration. *Psychopharmacology (Berl)* **161**, 95–99.

Anderson, G. M., Barr, C. S., Lindell, S., Durham, A. C., Shifrovich I., and Higley, J. D. (2005). Time course of the effects of the serotonin-selective reuptake inhibitor sertraline on central and peripheral serotonin neurochemistry in the rhesus monkey. *Psychopharmacology (Berl)* **178**, 339–346.

Andersson, H. and Roos B. E. (1969). "5-hydroxyindoleacetic acid in cerebrospinal fluid of hydrocephalic children." *Acta Paediatrica Scandinavica* **58**: 601–608.

Andrews, M. W. and Rosenblum, L. A. (1991). Attachment in monkey infants raised in variable- and low-demand environments. *Child Dev* **62**, 686–693.

Andrews, M. W. and Rosenblum, L. A. (1991). Dominance and social competence in differentially reared bonnet macaques. In: Ehara, A., Kimura, T., Takenaka, O., and Iwamoto, M. eds. *Primatology Today*. New York: Elsevier Science Publishers, pp. 347–350.

Andrews, M. W. and Rosenblum, L. A. (1992). Response of bonnet macaque dyads to an acute foraging task under different motivational conditions. *Dev Psychobiol* **25**, 559–566.

Anisman, H. and Zacharko, R. M. (1990). Multiple neurochemical and behavioral consequences of stressors: Implications for depression. *Pharmacol Ther* **46**, 119–136.

Apter, A., van Praag, H. M., Plutchik, R., Sevy, S., Korn, M., and Brown, S. L. (1990). Interrelationships among anxiety, aggression, impulsivity, and mood, A serotonergically linked cluster? *Psychiatry Res* **32**, 191–199.

Archer, J. (1991). The influence of testosterone on human aggression. *Br J Psychol* **82**, 1–28.

Ayala, A. R., Pushkas, J., Higley, J. D. *et al.* (2004). Behavioral, adrenal, and sympathetic responses to long-term administration of an oral corticotropin-releasing hormone receptor antagonist in a primate stress paradigm. *J Clin Endocrinol Metab* **89**, 5729–5737.

Banki, C. M. (1981). Factors influencing monoamine metabolites and tryptophan in patients with alcohol dependence. *J Neural Transm* **50**, 89–101.

Barr, C. S., Newman, T. K., Becker, M. L. *et al.* (2003). Serotonin transporter gene variation is associated with alcohol sensitivity in rhesus macaques exposed to early-life stress. *Alcohol Clin Exp Res* **27**, 812–817.

Barr, C. S., Newman, T. K., Lindell, S. *et al.* (2004a). Early experience and sex interact to influence limbic-hypothalamic-pituitary-adrenal-axis function after acute alcohol administration in rhesus macaques (*Macaca mulatta*). *Alcohol Clin Exp Res* **28**, 1114–1119.

Barr, C. S., Newman, T. K., Lindell, S *et al.* (2004b). Interaction between serotonin transporter gene variation and rearing condition in alcohol preference and consumption in female primates. *Arch Gen Psychiatry* **61**, 1146–1152.

Barr, C. S., Newman, T. K., Schwandt, M. *et al.* (2004c). Sexual dichotomy of an interaction between early adversity and the serotonin transporter gene promoter variant in rhesus macaques. *Proc Natl Acad Sci USA* **101**, 12358–12363.

Barr, C. S., Newman, T. K., Shannon, C. *et al.* (2004d). Rearing condition and rh5-HTTLPR interact to influence limbic-hypothalamic-pituitary-adrenal axis response to stress in infant macaques. *Biol Psychiatry* **55**, 733–738.

Barr, C. S., Schwandt, M. L., Newman, T. K., and Higley, J. D. (2004e). The use of adolescent nonhuman primates to model human alcohol intake, neurobiological, genetic, and psychological variables. *Ann N Y Acad Sci* **1021**, 221–233.

Bastian, M. L., Sponberg, A. C., Suomi, S. J., and Higley, J. D. (2003). Long-term effects of infant rearing condition on the acquisition of dominance rank in juvenile and adult rhesus macaques (*Macaca mulatta*). *Dev Psychobiol* **42**, 44–51.

Bayart, F., Hayashi, K. T., Faull, K. F., Barchas, J. D., and Levine, S. (1990). Influence of maternal proximity on behavioral and physiological responses to separation in infant rhesus monkeys (*Macaca mulatta*). *Behav Neurosci* **104**, 98–107.

Becker, M. L., Bernhards, D. E., Chisholm, K. L. *et al.* (2004). Calling rate as a measure of stress reactivity in mother- and nursery-reared rhesus infants (*Macaca mulatta*). *Am J Primatol* **62**, 60.

Bennett, A. J., Tsai, T., Pierre, P. J. *et al.* (1998). Behavioral response to novel objects varies with CSF monoamine concentrations in rhesus monkeys. *Soc Neurosci Abstr* **24**, 954.

Bennett, A. J., Tsai, T., Hopkins, W. D. *et al.* (1999). Early social rearing environment influences acquisition of a computerized joystick task in rhesus monkeys (*Macaca mulatta*). *Am J Primatol* **49**, 33–34.

Bennett, A. J., Lesch, K. P., Heils, A. *et al.* (2002). Early experience and serotonin transporter gene variation interact to influence primate CNS function. *Mol Psychiatry* **7**, 118–122.

Bernstein, I. S., Rose, R. M., and Gordon, T. P. (1977). Behavioural and hormonal responses of male rhesus monkeys introduced to females in the breeding and non-breeding seasons. *Anim Behav* **25**, 609–614.

Boccia, M. L., Panicker, A. K., Pedersen, C., and Petrusz, P. (2001). Oxytocin receptors in non-human primate brain visualized with monoclonal antibody. *Neuroreport* **12**, 1723–1726.

Booth, A., Shelley, G., Mazur, A., Tharp, G., and Kittok, R. (1989). Testosterone, and winning and losing in human competition. *Horm Behav* **23**, 556–571.

Botchin, M. B., Kaplan, J. R., Manuck, S. B., and Mann, J. J. (1993). Low versus high prolactin responders to fenfluramine challenge, Marker of behavioral differences in adult male cynomolgus macaques. *Neuropsychopharmacology* **9**, 93–99.

Brown, G. L., Goodwin, F. K., Ballenger, J. C., Goyer, P. F., and Major, L. F. (1979). Aggression in humans correlates with cerebrospinal fluid amine metabolites. *Psychiatry Res* **1**, 131–139.

Brown, G. L., Ebert, M. H., Goyer, P. F. *et al.* (1982). Aggression, suicide, and serotonin, Relationships to CSF amine metabolites. *Am J Psychiatry* **139**, 741–746.

Buchanan, C. M., Eccles, J. S., and Becker, J. B. (1992). Are adolescents the victims of raging hormones, Evidence for activational effects of hormones on moods and behavior at adolescence. *Psychol Bull* **111**, 62–107.

Buss, K. A., Schumacher, J. R., Dolski, I., Kalin, N. H., Goldsmith, H. H., and Davidson, R. J. (2003). Right frontal brain activity, cortisol, and withdrawal behavior in 6-month-old infants. *Behav Neurosci* **117**, 11–20.

Capitanio, J. P. (1986). Behavioral pathology. In: Mitchell, G., and Erwin, J. eds. *Comparative Primate Biology, Behavior, Conservation and Ecology*, Vol 2. New York: Alan R. Liss, pp. 411–454.

Carter, C. S., DeVries, A. C., and Getz, L. L. (1995). Physiological substrates of mammalian monogamy, the prairie vole model. *Neurosci Biobehav Rev* **19**, 303–314.

Chamberlain, B., Ervin, F. R., Pihl, R. O., and Young, S. N. (1987). The effect of raising or lowering tryptophan levels on aggression in vervet monkeys. *Pharmacol Biochem Behav* **28**, 503–510.

Chamove, A. S., Eysenck, H. J., and Harlow, H. F. (1972). Personality in monkeys, Factor analysis of rhesus social behavior. *Q J Exp Psychol* **24**, 496–504.

Chamove, A. S., Rosenblum, L. A., and Harlow, H. F. (1973). Monkeys (*Macaca mulatta*) raised with only peers. A pilot study. *Anim Behav* **21**, 316–325.

Champoux, M., Coe, C. L., Schanberg, S., Kuhn, C., and Suomi, S. J. (1989). Hormonal effects of early rearing conditions in the infant rhesus monkey. *Am J Primatol* **19**, 111–117.

Champoux, M., Higley, J. D., and Suomi, S. J. (1997). Behavioral and physiological-characteristics of Indian and Chinese-Indian hybrid rhesus macaque infants. *Dev Psychobiol* **31**, 49–63.

Champoux, M., Shannon, C., Airoso, W. D., and Suomi, S. (1999). Play and attachment behavior of peer-only reared, and surrogate/peer-reared rhesus monkey infants in their social groups. In: Riefel, S. ed. *Play and Culture Studies, Play Context Revisited*, Vol 2. Stamford, CA: Ablex, pp. 209–217.

Champoux, M., Bennett, A., Shannon, C., Higley, J. D., Lesch, K. P., and Suomi, S. J. (2002). Serotonin transporter gene polymorphism, differential early rearing, and behavior in rhesus monkey neonates. *Mol Psychiatry* **7**, 1058–1063.

Chapais, B. (1986). Why do male and female rhesus monkeys affiliate during the birth season? In: Rawlins, R. G. and Kessler, M. *The Cayo Santiago Macaques.* Chicago: SUNY Press, pp. 173–200.

Chapais, B. (1988). Rank maintenance in female Japanese macaques, Experimental evidence for social dependency. *Behaviour* **102**, 41–59.

Christiansen, K. and Knussmann, R. (1987). Androgen levels and components of aggressive behavior in men. *Horm Behav* **21**, 170–180.

Clarke, A. S. (1993). Social rearing effects on HPA axis activity over early development and in response to stress in rhesus monkeys. *Dev Psychobiol* **26**, 433–446.

Clarke, A. S., Wittwer, D. J., Abbott, D. H., and Schneider, M. L. (1994). Long-term effects of prenatal stress on HPA axis activity in juvenile rhesus monkeys. *Dev Psychobiol* **27**, 257–269.

Clarke, A. S., Kammerer, C. M., George, K. P., Kupfer, D. J., McKinney, W. T., and Spence, M. A. (1995). Evidence for heritability of biogenic amine levels in the cerebrospinal fluid of rhesus monkeys. *Biol Psychiatry* **38**, 572–578.

Clarke, A. S., Hedeker, D. R., Ebert, M. H., Schmidt, D. E., McKinney, W. T., and Kraemer, G. W. (1996). Rearing experience and biogenic amine activity in infant rhesus monkeys. *Biol Psychiatry* **40**, 338–352.

Clarke, R. A., Murphy, D. L., and Constantino, J. N. (1999). Serotonin and externalizing behavior in young children. *Psychiatry Res* **86**, 29–40.

Cleveland, A., Westergaard, G. C., Trenkle, M. K., and Higley, J. D. (2004). Physiological predictors of reproductive outcome and mother-infant behaviors in captive rhesus macaque females (*Macaca mulatta*). *Neuropsychopharmacology* **29**, 901–910.

Cloninger, C. R. (1988). A unified biosocial theory of personality and its role in the development of anxiety states, A reply to commentaries. *Psychiatr Dev* **6**, 83–120.

Collier, D. A., Stober, G., Li, T. *et al.* (1996). A novel functional polymorphism within the promoter of the serotonin transporter gene, Possible role in susceptibility to affective disorders *Mol Psychiatry* **1**, 453–460.

Cohen, D. J., Shaywitz, B. A., Johnson W. T., and Bowers M. D. (1974). "Biogenic amines in autistic and atypical children." *Archives of General Psychiatry* **31**: 845–853.

Coplan, J. D., Rosenblum, L. A., Friedman, S., Bassoff, T. B., and Gorman, J. M. (1992). Behavioral effects of oral yohimbine in differentially reared nonhuman primates. *Neuropsychopharmacology* **6**, 31–37.

Coplan, J. D., Trost, R. C., Owens, M. J. *et al.* (1998). Cerebrospinal fluid concentrations of somatostatin and biogenic amines in grown primates reared by mothers exposed to manipulated foraging conditions. *Arch Gen Psychiatry* **55**, 473–477.

Dabbs, J. M. J., Frady, R. L., Carr, T. S., and Besch, N. F. (1987). Saliva testosterone and criminal violence in young adult prison inmates. *Psychosom Med* **49**, 174–182.

Davidson, R. J., Kalin, N. H., and Shelton, S. E. (1992). Lateralized effects of diazepam on frontal brain electrical asymmetries in rhesus monkeys. *Biol Psychiatry* **32**, 438–451.

Davidson, R. J., Kalin, N. H., and Shelton, S. E. (1993). Lateralized response to diazepam predicts temperamental style in rhesus monkeys. *Behav Neurosci* **107**, 1106–1110.

Davidson, R. J., Putnam, K. M., and Larson, C. L. (2000). Dysfunction in the neural circuitry of emotion regulation – a possible prelude to violence. *Science* **289**, 591–594.

Depue, R. A. and Morrone-Strupinsky, J. V. (2005). A neurobehavioral model of affiliative bonding, implications for conceptualizing a human trait of affiliation. *Behav Brain Sci* **28**, 313–350; discussion 350–395.

Dittus, W. P. J. (1979). The evolution of behaviors regulating density and age-specific sex ratios in primate population. *Behaviour* **69**, 265–302.

Doudet, D., Hommer, D., Higley, J. D. *et al.* (1995). Cerebral glucose metabolism, CSF 5-HIAA levels, and aggressive behavior in rhesus monkeys. *Am J Psychiatry* **152**, 1782–1787.

Drickamer, L. C. (1974). A ten-year summary of reproductive data for free-ranging *Macaca mulatta*. *Folia Primatol* **21**, 61–80.

Eaton, G. G. and Resko, J. A. (1974). Plasma testosterone and male dominance in a Japanese macaque (*Macaca fuscata*) troop compared with repeated measures of testosterone in laboratory males. *Horm Behav* **5**, 251–259.

Ehrenkranz, J., Bliss, E., and Sheard, M. H. (1974). Plasma testosterone, Correlation with aggressive behavior and social dominance in man. *Psychosom Med* **36**, 469–475.

Eichelman, B. (1987). Neurochemical and psychopharmacologic aspects of aggressive behavior. In: Meltzer, H. Y. ed. *Psychopharmacology: The Third Generation of Progress.* New York, Raven Press: 697–704.

Elsworth, J. D., Leahy, D. J., Roth, R. H., and Redmond, D. E. (1987). Homovanillic acid concentrations in brain, CSF and plasma as indicators of central dopamine function in primates. *J Neural Transm* **68**, 51–62.

Erickson, K., Lindell, S., Champoux, M. *et al.* (2001). Relationships between behavior and neurochemical changes in rhesus macaques during a separation paradigm. *Soc Neurosci Abstr* **27**, program 572, 14.

Erickson, K., Gabry, K. E., Lindell, S. *et al.* (2005). Social withdrawal behaviors in nonhuman primates and changes in neuroendocrine and monoamine concentrations during a separation paradigm. *Dev Psychobiol* **46**, 331–339.

Eysenck, S. B. and Eysenck, H. J. (1971). A comparative study of criminals and matched controls on three dimensions of personality. *Br J Soc Clin Psychol* **10**, 362–366.

Fahlke, C., Lorenz, J. G., Long, J., Champoux, M., Suomi, S. J., and Higley, J. D. (2000). Rearing experiences and stress-induced plasma cortisol as early risk factors for excessive alcohol consumption in nonhuman primates. *Alcohol Clin Exp Res* **24**, 644–650.

Fahlke, C., Garpenstrand, H., Oreland, L., Suomi, S. J., and Higley, J. D. (2002). Platelet monoamine oxidase activity in a nonhuman primate model of type 2 excessive alcohol consumption. *Am J Psychiatry* **159**, 2107–2109.

Fairbanks, L. A. (2001). Individual differences in response to a stranger, social impulsivity as a dimension of temperament in vervet monkeys (*Cercopithecus aethiops sabaeus*). *J Comp Psychol* **115**, 22–28.

Fairbanks, L. A., Fontenot, M. B., Phillips-Conroy, J. E., Jolly, C. J., Kaplan, J. R., and Mann, J. J. (1999). CSF monoamines, age and impulsivity in wild grivet monkeys (*Cercopithecus aethiops aethiops*). *Brain Behav Evol* **53**, 305–312.

Fairbanks, L. A., Melega, W. P., Jorgensen, M. J., Kaplan, J. R., and McGuire, M. T. (2001). Social impulsivity inversely associated with CSF 5-HIAA and fluoxetine exposure in vervet monkeys. *Neuropsychopharmacology* **24**, 370–378.

Fairbanks, L. A., Jorgensen, M. J., Huff, A., Blau, K., Hung, Y. Y., and Mann, J. J. (2004). Adolescent impulsivity predicts adult dominance attainment in male vervet monkeys. *Am J Primatol* **64**, 1–17.

Ferrari, P. F., Palanza, P., Parmigiani, S., de Almeida, R. M., and Miczek, K. A. (2005). Serotonin and aggressive behavior in rodents and nonhuman primates, predispositions and plasticity. *Eur J Pharmacol* **526**, 259–273.

Gerald, M., Habib, K. E., Weld, K. P. *et al.* (2000). Effects of acute and chronic social stress on levels of CSF corticotropin-releasing hormone. *Biol Psychiatry* **47**(suppl 1), S71.

Gerald, M. S., Higley, S., Lussier, I. D., Westergaard, G. C., Suomi, S. J., and Higley, J. D. (2002). Variation in reproductive outcomes for captive male rhesus macaques (macaca mulatta) differing in CSF 5-hydroxyindoleacetic acid concentrations. *Brain Behav Evol* **60**, 117–124.

Gill, K. and Amit, Z. (1989). Serotonin uptake blockers and voluntary alcohol consumption. A review of recent studies. *Recent Dev Alcohol* **7**, 225–248.

Gleeson, S., Ahlers, S. T., Mansbach, R. S., Foust, J. M., and Barrett, J. E. (1989). Behavioral studies with anxiolytic drugs. VI. Effects on punished responding of drugs interacting with serotonin receptor subtypes. *J Pharmacol Exp Ther* **250**, 809–817.

Gordon, T. P., Rose, R. M., and Bernstein, I. S. (1976). Seasonal rhythm in plasma testosterone levels in the rhesus monkey (*Macaca mulatta*), A three year study. *Horm Behav* **7**, 229–243.

Gordon, T. P., Bernstein, I. S., and Rose, R. M. (1978). Social and seasonal influences on testosterone secretion in the male rhesus monkey. *Physiol Behav* **21**, 623–637.

Gordon, T. P., Rose, R. M., Grady, C. L., and Bernstein, I. S. (1979). Effects of increased testosterone secretion on the behavior of adult male rhesus living in a social group. *Folia Primatol* **32**, 149–160.

Gunnar, M. R., Gonzalez, C. A., Goodlin, B. L., and Levine, S. (1981). Behavioral and pituitary–adrenal responses during a prolonged separation period in infant rhesus macaques. *Psychoneuroendocrinology* **6**, 65–75.

Habib, K. E., Weld, K. P., Rice, K. C. *et al.* (2000). Oral administration of a corticotropin-releasing hormone receptor antagonist significantly attenuates behavioral, neuroendocrine, and autonomic responses to stress in primates. *Proc Natl Acad Sci USA* **97**, 6079–6084.

Harlow, H. F. (1969). Age-mate or peer affectional system. *Adv Study Behav* **2**, 333–383.

Harlow, H. F. and Harlow, M. K. (1965). The affectional systems. In: Schrier, A. M., Harlow, H. F., and Stollinitz, F. eds. *Behavior of Nonhuman Primates*, Vol 2. New York: Academic Press, pp. 287–334.

Heinz, A., Higley, J. D., Gorey, J. G. *et al.* (1998). In vivo association between alcohol intoxication, aggression, and serotonin transporter availability in nonhuman primates. *Am J Psychiatry* **155**, 1023–1028.

Heinz, A., D. W. Jones, Gorey, J. G. *et al.* (2003). Serotonin transporter availability correlates with alcohol intake in non-human primates. *Mol Psychiatry* **8**, 231–324.

Higley, J. D. (1985). Continuity of social separation behaviors in rhesus monkeys from infancy to adolescence, University of Wisconsin, Madison.

Higley, J. D. and Bennett, A. J. (1999). Central nervous system serotonin and personality as variables contributing to excessive alcohol consumption in non-human primates. *Alcohol Alcohol* **34**, 402–418.

Higley, J. D. and Linnoila, M. (1997). A nonhuman primate model of excessive alcohol intake, Personality and neurobiological parallels of Type I- and Type II-like alcoholism. *Recent Dev Alcohol* **13**, 192–219.

Higley, J. D. and Suomi, S. J. (1989). Temperamental reactivity in non-human primates. In: Kohnstamm, G. A., Bates, J. E., and Rothbart, M. K. eds. *Temperament in Childhood*. New York: John Wiley & Sons, pp. 153–167.

Higley, J. D. and Suomi, S. J. (1996). Effect of reactivity and social competence on individual responses to severe stress in children, Investigations using nonhuman primates. In: Pfeffer, C. R. ed. *Intense Stress and Mental Disturbance in Children*. Washington, D.C.: American Psychiatric Press, pp. 1–69.

Higley, J. D., Suomi, S. J., and Linnoila, M. (1990). Parallels in aggression and serotonin, Consideration of development, rearing history, and sex differences. In: van Praag, H. M., Plutchik, R., and Apter, A. eds. *Violence and Suicidality, Perspectives in Clinical and Psychobiological Research*. New York: Brunner/Mazel, pp. 245–256.

Higley, J. D., Suomi, S. J., and Linnoila, M. (1991). CSF monoamine metabolite concentrations vary according to age, rearing, and sex, and are influenced by the stressor of social separation in rhesus monkeys. *Psychopharmacology (Berl)* **103**, 551–556.

Higley, J. D., Hasert, M. F., Suomi, S. J., and Linnoila, M. (1991). Nonhuman primate model of alcohol abuse, effects of early experience, personality, and stress on alcohol consumption. *Proc Natl Acad Sci USA* **88**, 7261–7265.

Higley, J. D., Hasert, M. F., Dodson, A., Linnoila, M., and Suomi, S. J. (1992a). *Treatment of Excessive Alcohol Consumption Using the Serotonin Reuptake Inhibitor Sertraline in a Nonhuman Primate Model of Alcohol Abuse*. San Diego, CA: Research Society on Alcoholism.

Higley, J. D., Mehlman, P., Taub, D. *et al.* (1992b). Cerebrospinal fluid monoamine and adrenal correlates of aggression in free-ranging rhesus monkeys. *Arch Gen Psychiatry* **49**, 436–441.

Higley, J. D., Suomi, S. J., and Linnoila, M. (1992c). A longitudinal assessment of CSF monoamine metabolite and plasma cortisol concentrations in young rhesus monkeys. *Biol Psychiatry* **32**, 127–145.

Higley, J. D., Thompson, W. W., Champoux, M. *et al.* (1993). Paternal and maternal genetic and environmental contributions to cerebrospinal fluid monoamine metabolites in rhesus monkeys (*Macaca mulatta*). *Arch Gen Psychiatry* **50**, 615–623.

Higley, J. D., Linnoila, M., and Suomi, S. J. (1994). Ethological contributions, Experiential and genetic contributions to the expression and inhibition of aggression in primates. In: Hersen, M., Ammerman, R. T., and Sisson, L. eds. *Handbook of Aggressive and Destructive Behavior in Psychiatric Patients*. New York: Plenum Press, pp. 17–32.

Higley, J. D., King, S. T., Hasert, M. F., Champoux, M., Suomi, S. J., and Linnoila, M. (1996a). Stability of interindividual differences in serotonin function and its relationship to severe aggression and competent social behavior in rhesus macaque females. *Neuropsychopharmacology* **14**, 67–76.

Higley, J. D., Mehlman, P. T., Higley, S. B. *et al.* (1996b). Excessive mortality in young free-ranging male nonhuman primates with low cerebrospinal fluid 5-hydroxyindoleacetic acid. *Arch Gen Psychiatry* **53**, 537–543.

Higley, J. D., Mehlman, P. T., Poland, R. E. *et al.* (1996c). CSF testosterone and 5-HIAA correlate with different types of aggressive behaviors. *Biol Psychiatry* **40**, 1067–1082.

Higley, J. D., Suomi, S. J., and Linnoila, M. (1996d). A nonhuman primate model of type II alcoholism? Part 2. Diminished social competence and excessive aggression correlates with low cerebrospinal fluid 5-hydroxyindoleacetic acid concentrations. *Alcohol Clin Exp Res* **20**, 643–650.

Higley, J. D., Suomi, S. J., and Linnoila, M. (1996e). A nonhuman primate model of type II excessive alcohol consumption? Part 1. Low cerebrospinal fluid 5-hydroxyindoleacetic acid concentrations and diminished social competence correlate with excessive alcohol consumption. *Alcohol Clin Exp Res* **20**, 629–642.

Higley, J. D., Hasert, M. F., Suomi, S. J., and Linnoila, M. (1998). The serotonin reuptake inhibitor sertraline reduces excessive alcohol consumption in nonhuman primates, Effect of stress. *Neuropsychopharmacology* **18**, 431–443.

Howell, S., Westergaard, G. C., Hoos, B. *et al.* (2007). Serotonergic influences on life history outcomes in free-ranging male primates. *American Journal of Primatology* **69**, 1–15.

Hranilovic, D., Lesch, K. P., Ugarkovic, D., Cicin-Sain, L., and Jernej, B. (1996). Identification of serotonin transporter mRNA in rat platelets. *Journal of Neural Transm* **103**, 957–965.

Ichise, M., Vines, D. C., Gura, T. *et al.* (2006). Effects of early life stress on [11C]DASB positron emission tomography imaging of serotonin transporters in adolescent peer- and mother-reared rhesus monkeys. *J Neurosci* **26**, 4638–4643.

Insel, T. R. (1992). Oxytocin – a neuropeptide for affiliation, evidence from behavioral, receptor autoradiographic, and comparative studies. *Psychoneuroendocrinology* **17**, 3–35.

Kalin, N. H. (1993). The neurobiology of fear. *Scientific American* **268**, 94–101.

Kalin, N. H. and Shelton, S. E. (1989). Defensive behaviors in infant rhesus monkeys, Environmental cues and neurochemical regulation. *Science* **243**, 1718–1721.

Kalin, N. H., Gibbs, D. M., Barksdale, C. M., Shelton, S. E., and Carnes, M. (1985). Behavioral stress decreases plasma oxytocin concentrations in primates. *Life Sci* **36**, 1275–1280.

Kalin, N. H., Shelton, S. E., and Barksdale, C. M. (1988). Opiate modulation of separation-induced distress in non-human primates. *Brain Res* **440**, 285–292.

Kalin, N. H., Shelton, S. E., and Barksdale, C. M. (1989). Behavioral and physiologic effects of CRH administered to infant primates undergoing maternal separation. *Neuropsychopharmacology* **2**, 97–104.

Kalin, N. H., Shelton, S. E., and Lynn, D. E. (1995). Opiate systems in mother and infant primates coordinate intimate contact during reunion. *Psychoneuroendocrinology* **20**, 735–742.

Kalin, N. H., Larson, C., Shelton, S. E., and Davidson, R. J. (1998). Asymmetric frontal brain activity, cortisol, and behavior associated with fearful temperament in rhesus monkeys. *Behav Neurosci* **112**, 286–292.

Kalin, N. H., Shelton, S. E., and Davidson, R. J. (2000). Cerebrospinal fluid corticotropin-releasing hormone levels are elevated in monkeys with patterns of brain activity associated with fearful temperament. *Biol Psychiatry* **47**, 579–585.

Kaplan, J. R., Phillips-Conroy, J., Fontenot, M. B., Jolly, C. J., Fairbanks, L. A., and Mann, J. J. (1999). Cerebrospinal fluid monoaminergic metabolites differ in wild anubis and hybrid (*Anubis hamadryas*) baboons, possible relationships to life history and behavior. *Neuropsychopharmacology* **20**, 517–524.

Kaufman, J. H. (1967). Social relations of adult males in a free-ranging band of rhesus monkeys. In: Altmann, S. A. ed. *Social Communication Among Primates.* Chicago: University of Chicago Press, pp. 73–98.

Kehoe, P. and Blass, E. M. (1986). Opioid-mediation of separation distress in 10-day-old rats, reversal of stress with maternal stimuli. *Dev Psychobiol* **19**, 385–398.

Kendrick, K. M. (2004). The neurobiology of social bonds. *J Neuroendocrinol* **16**, 1007–1008.

Keverne, E. B. and Kendrick, K. M. (1992). Oxytocin facilitation of maternal behavior in sheep. *Ann N Y Acad Sci* **652**, 83–101.

Keverne, E. B., Eberhart, J. A., and Meller, R. E. (1983). Plasma testosterone, sexual and aggressive behavior in social groups of talapoin monkeys. In: Steklis, H. D. and King A. S. eds. *Hormones, Drugs and Social Behavior in Primates.* New York: Spectrum, pp. 33–55.

Klinteberg, B., Schalling, D., Edman, G., Oreland L., and Asberg M. (1987). "Personality correlates of platelet monoamine oxidase (MAO) activity in female and male subjects." *Neuropsychobiology* **18**: 89–96.

Knott, P., Haroutunian, V., Bierer, L. *et al.* (1989). Correlations post-mortem between ventricular CSF and cortical tissue concentrations of MHPG, 5-HIAA, and HVA in Alzheimer's disease. *Biol Psychiatry* **25**, 112A.

Kraemer, G. W. (1986). Causes of changes in brain noradrenaline systems and later effects on responses to social stressors in rhesus monkeys, The cascade hypothesis. *CIBA Found Symp* **123**, 216–233.

Kraemer, G. W. (1992). A psychobiological theory of attachment. *Behav Brain Sci* **15**, 493–541.

Kraemer, G. W. and McKinney, W. T. (1979). Interactions of pharmacological agents which alter biogenic amine metabolism and depression – An analysis of contributing factors within a primate model of depression. *J Affect Disord* **1**, 33–54.

Kraemer, G. W., Ebert, M. H., Lake, C. R., and McKinney, W. T. (1984a). Cerebrospinal fluid measures of neurotransmitter changes associated with pharmacological alteration of the despair response to social separation in rhesus monkeys. *Psychiatry Res* **11**, 303–315.

Kraemer, G. W., Ebert, M. H., Lake, C. R., and McKinney, W. T. (1984b). Hypersensitivity to d-amphetamine several years after early social deprivation in rhesus monkeys. *Psychopharmacology (Berlin)* **82**, 266–271.

Kraemer, G. W., Ebert, M. H., Schmidt, D. E., and McKinney, W. T. (1989). A longitudinal study of the effect of different social rearing conditions on cerebrospinal fluid norepinephrine and biogenic amine metabolites in rhesus monkeys. *Neuropsychopharmacology* **2**, 175–189.

Kraemer, G. W., Ebert, M. H., Schmidt, D. E., and McKinney, W. T. (1991). Strangers in a strange land, A psychobiological study of infant monkeys before and after separation from real or inanimate mothers. *Child Dev* **62**, 548–566.

Kruesi, M. J. (1989). Cruelty to animals and CSF 5HIAA [letter]. *Psychiatry Res* **28**, 115–116.

Kruesi, M. J., Rapoport, J. L., Hamburger, S. *et al.* (1990). Cerebrospinal fluid monoamine metabolites, aggression, and impulsivity in disruptive behavior disorders of children and adolescents. *Arch Gen Psychiatry* **47**, 419–426.

Kruesi, M. J., Hibbs, E. D., Zahn, T. P. *et al.* (1992). A 2-year prospective follow-up study of children and adolescents with disruptive behavior disorders. Prediction by cerebrospinal fluid 5-hydroxyindoleacetic acid, homovanillic acid, and autonomic measures? *Arch Gen Psychiatry* **49**, 429–435.

Kuester, J. and Paul, A. (1992). Influence of male competition and female mate choice on male mating success in Barbary macaques (*Macaca sylvanus*). *Behaviour* **120**, 192–217.

Kyes, R. C., Botchin, M. B., Kaplan, J. R., Manuck, S. B., and Mann, J. J. (1995). Aggression and brain serotonergic responsivity, Response to slides in male macaques. *Physiol Behav* **57**, 205–208.

Laudenslager, M. L., Held, P. E., Boccia, M. L., Reite, M. L., and Cohen, J. J. (1990). Behavioral and immunological consequences of brief mother-infant separation, A species comparison. *Dev Psychobiol* **23**, 247–264.

Leckman, J. F., Cohen, D. J., Shaywitz, B. A., Caparulo, B. K., Heninger, G. R., and Bowers, M. B. (1980). "CSF monoamine metabolites in child and adult psychiatric patients. A developmental perspective." *Archives of General Psychiatry* **37**: 677-681.

Lesch, K. P., Bengel, D., Heils, A. *et al.* (1996). Association of anxiety-related traits with a polymorphism in the serotonin transporter gene regulatory region. *Science* **274**, 1527–1531.

Levine, S. (1970). The pituitary-adrenal system and the developing brain. *Progr Brain Res* **32**, 79–85.

Levine, S. (2005). Developmental determinants of sensitivity and resistance to stress. *Psychoneuroendocrinology* **30**, 939–946.

Lewis, J. K. and McKinney, W. T. (1976). The effect of electrically induced convulsions on the behavior of normal and abnormal rhesus monkeys. *Dis Nerv Syst* **37**, 687–693.

Lewis, M. H., Gluck, J. P., Beauchamp, A. J., Keresztury, M. F., and Mailman, R. B. (1990). Long-term effects of early social isolation in Macaca mulatta, changes in dopamine receptor function following apomorphine challenge. *Brain Res* **513**, 67–73.

Lewis, M. H., Gluck, J. P., Petitto, J. M., Hensley, L. L., and Ozer, H. (2000). Early social deprivation in nonhuman primates, long-term effects on survival and cell-mediated immunity. *Biol Psychiatry* **47**, 119–126.

Lidberg, L., Tuck, J. R., Åsberg, M., Scalia-Tomba, G. P., and Bertilsson, L. (1985). Homicide, suicide and CSF 5-HIAA. *Acta Psychiatr Scand* **71**, 230–236.

Limson, R., Goldman, D., Roy, A. *et al.* (1991). Personality and cerebrospinal fluid monoamine metabolites in alcoholics and controls. *Arch Gen Psychiatry* **48**, 437–441.

Lindburg, D. G. (1980). *The Macaques: Studies in Ecology, Behavior, and Evolution.* New York: Van Nostrand Reinhold Co.

Lindman, R., Järvinen, P., and Vidjeskog, J. (1987). Verbal interactions of aggressively and nonaggressively predisposed males in a drinking situation. *Aggressive Behav* **13**, 187–196.

Linnoila, M., Virkkunen, M., Scheinin, M., Nuutila, A., Rimon, R., and Goodwin, F. K. (1983). Low cerebrospinal fluid 5-hydroxyindoleacetic acid concentration differentiates impulsive from nonimpulsive violent behavior. *Life Sci* **33**, 2609–2614.

Linnoila, M. (1988). Monoamines and impulse control. *Depression, anxiety, and aggression.* Swinkels, J. A. and Blijleven, W. Houten, Medidact b.v.i.o. Peppelkade 2C: 167–172.

Little, K. Y., Zhang, L., and Cook, E. (2006). Fluoxetine-induced alterations in human platelet serotonin transporter expression, serotonin transporter polymorphism effects. *J Psychiatry Neurosci* **31**, 333–339.

Lopez, J. F., Vazquez, D. M., Zimmer, C. A., Little, K. Y., and Watson, S. J. (2001). Chronic unpredictable stress and antidepressant modulation of mineralocorticoid, and glucocorticoid receptors. *Soc Neurosci Abstr* **27**, program 352.

Lorenz, J. G., Long, J. C., Linnoila, M. , Goldman, D., Suomi, S. J. and Higley, J. D. (2006). Genetic and other contributions to alcohol intake in rhesus macaques (*Macaca mulatta*). *Alcohol Clin Exp Res* **30**, 389–398.

Lyons, D. M., Kim, S., Schatzberg, A. F., and Levine, S. (1998). Postnatal foraging demands alter adrenocortical activity and psychosocial development. *Dev Psychobiol* **32**, 285–291.

Maestripieri, D., Lindell, S. G., Ayala, A., Gold, P. W., and Higley, J. D. (2005). Neurobiological characteristics of rhesus macaque abusive mothers and their relation to social and maternal behavior. *Neurosci Biobehav Rev* **29**, 51–57.

Maestripieri, D., Higley, J. D., Lindell, S. G., Newman, T. K., McCormack, K. M., and Sanchez, M. M. (2006a). Early maternal rejection affects the development of monoaminergic systems and adult abusive parenting in rhesus macaques (*Macaca mulatta*). *Behav Neurosci* **120**, 1017–1024.

Maestripieri, D., McCormack, K., Lindell, S. G., Higley, J. D., and Sanchez, M. M. (2006b). Influence of parenting style on the offspring's behaviour and CSF monoamine metabolite levels in crossfostered and noncrossfostered female rhesus macaques. *Behav Brain Res* **175**, 90–95.

Maestripieri, D., Lindell, S. G., and Higley, J. D. (2007). Intergenerational transmission of maternal behavior in rhesus macaques and its underlying mechanisms. *Dev Psychobiol* **49**, 165–171.

Mann, J. J. and Stanley, M. Eds. (1986). *Psychobiology of Suicidal Behavior.* Annals of the New York Academy of Sciences. New York, New York Academy of Sciences.

Manuck, S. B., Kaplan, J. R., Rymeski, B. A., Fairbanks, L. A., and Wilson, M. E. (2003). Approach to a social stranger is associated with low central nervous system serotonergic responsivity in female cynomolgus monkeys (*Macaca fascicularis*). *Am J Primatol* **61**, 187–194.

Martel, F. L., Nevison, C. M., Rayment, F. D., Simpson, M. J., and Keverne, E. B. (1993). Opioid receptor blockade reduces maternal affect and social grooming in rhesus monkeys. *Psychoneuroendocrinology* **18**, 307–321.

Mattsson, A., Schalling, D., Olweus, D., Löw, H., and Svensson, J. (1980). Plasma testosterone, aggressive behavior, and personality dimensions in young male delinquents. *J Am Acad Child Psychiatry* **19**, 476–490.

Mazur, A. (1983). Hormones, aggression, and dominance in humans. In: Svare, B. B. ed. *Hormones and Aggressive Behavior.* New York: Plenum Press, pp. 563–576.

McBride, W. J., Murphy, J. M., Lumeng, L., and Li, T. K. (1989). Serotonin and ethanol preference. *Recent Dev Alcohol* **7**, 187–209.

McGuire, M. T., Raleigh, M. J., and Pollack, D. B. (1994). Personality factors in vervet monkeys, The effects of sex, age, social status, and group composition. *Am J Primatol* **33**, 1–13.

McKinney, W. T. (1984). Animal models of depression, An overveiw. *Psychiatr Dev* **2**, 77–96.

McKinney, W. T. (1988). *Models of Mental Disorders, A New Comparative Psychiatry.* New York: Plenum Medical.

McKinney, W. T., Jr., Suomi, S. J., and Harlow, H. F. (1971). Depression in primates. *Am J Psychiatry* **127**, 1313–1320.

Meaney, M. J. and Szyf, M. (2005). Environmental programming of stress responses through DNA methylation, life at the interface between a dynamic environment and a fixed genome. *Dialogues Clin Neurosci* **7**, 103–123.

Mehlman, P. T., Higley, J. D., Faucher, I. *et al.* (1992). CNS 5-HIAA and aggression in free-ranging adolescent rhesus males. *Am J Primatol* **27**, 46–47.

Mehlman, P. T., Higley, J. D., Faucher, I. *et al.* (1994). Low CSF 5-HIAA concentrations and severe aggression and impaired impulse control in nonhuman primates. *Am J Psychiatry* **151**, 1485–1491.

Mehlman, P., Higley, J. D., Faucher, I. *et al.* (1995). Correlation of CSF 5-HIAA concentration with sociality and the timing of emigration in free-ranging primates. *Am J Psychiatry* **152**, 907–913.

Mehlman, P. T., Higley, J. D., Fernald, B. J., Sallee, F. R., Suomi, S. J., and Linnoila, M. (1997). CSF 5-HIAA, testosterone, and sociosexual behaviors in free-ranging male rhesus macaques in the mating season. *Psychiatry Res* **72**, 89–102.

Mehlman, P. T., Westergaard, G. C., Hoos, B. J. *et al.* (2000). CSF 5-HIAA and nighttime activity in free-ranging primates. *Neuropsychopharmacology* **22**, 210–218.

Meikle, B. B. and Vessey, S. H. (1988). Maternal dominance rank and lifetime survivorship if male and female rhesus monkeys. *Behav Ecol Sociobiol* **23**, 379–383.

Meltzer, H. Y. and Lowy, M. Y. (1987). The serotonin hypothesis of depression. *Psychopharmacology: The third generation of progress.* Meltzer, H. Y. New York, Raven Press: 513–526.

Meyer, J. S., Novak, M. A., Bowman, R. E., and Harlow, H. F. (1975). Behavioral and hormonal effects of attachment object separation in surrogate-peer-reared and mother-reared infant rhesus monkeys. *Dev Psychobiol* **8**, 425–435.

Miczek, K. A. and Donat, P. (1990). Brain 5-HT system and inhibition of aggressive behavior. In: Archer, T., Bevan, P., and Cools, A. eds. *Behavioral Pharmacology of 5-HT.* Hillsdale, NJ: Lawrence Erlbaum Associates, pp. 117–144.

Miczek, K. A., Mos, J., and Olivier, B. (1989). Brain 5-HT and inhibition of aggressive behavior in animals, 5-HIAA and receptor subtypes. *Psychopharmacol Bull* **25**, 399–403.

Mineka, S. and Suomi, S. J. (1978). Social separation in monkeys. *Psychol Bull* **85**, 1376–1400.

Mitchell, G. (1970). Abnormal behavior in primates. In: Rosenblum, R. A. ed. *Primate Behavior, Developments in Field and Laboratory Research*, Vol 1. New York: Academic Press, pp. 195–249.

Moles, A., Kieffer, B. L., and D'Amato, F. R. (2004). Deficit in attachment behavior in mice lacking the mu-opioid receptor gene. *Science* **304**, 1983–1986.

Namboodiri, M. A., Sugden, D., Klein, D. C., Tamarkin, L., and Mefford, I. N. (1985). Serum melatonin and pineal indoleamine metabolism in a species with a small day/night N-acetyltransferase rhythm. *Comp Biochem Physiol B* **80**, 731–736.

Nelson, E. E. and Panksepp, J. (1998). Brain substrates of infant-mother attachment, contributions of opioids, oxytocin, and norepinephrine. *Neurosci Biobehav Rev* **22**, 437–452.

Newman, M. E., Shapira, B., and Lerer, B. (1998). Evaluation of central serotonergic function in affective and related disorders by the fenfluramine challenge test, A critical review. *Int J Neuropsychopharmacol* **1**, 49–69.

Nikulina, E. M., Avgustinovich, D. F., and Popova, N. K. (1992). Role of 5HT1A receptors in a variety of kinds of aggressive behavior in wild rats and counterparts selected for low defensiveness to man. *Aggressive Behav* **18**, 357–364.

Olivier, B. and Mos, J. (1990). Serenics, serotonin and aggression. *Progr Clin Biol Res* **361**, 203–230.

Olivier, B., Mos, J., Tulp, M., Schipper, J., and Bevan, P. (1990). Modulatory action of serotonin in aggressive behavior. In: Archer, T., Bevan, P., and Cools, A. eds. *Behavioral Pharmacology of 5-HT.* Hillsdale, NJ: Lawrence Erlbaum Associates, pp. 89–116.

Olweus, D. (1984). Development of stable aggressive reaction patterns in males. *Adv Study Aggression* **1**, 103–137.

Olweus, D. (1986). Aggression and hormones, Behavioral relationship with testosterone and adrenaline. In: Olweus, D., Block, J., and Radke-Yarrow, M. eds. *Development of Antisocial and Prosocial Behavior.* New York: Academic Press, pp. 51–72.

Olweus, D., Mattsson, A., Schalling, D., and Löw, H. (1980). Testosterone, aggression, physical, and personality dimensions in normal adolescent males. *Psychosom Med* **42**, 253–269.

Olweus, D., Mattsson, A., Schalling, D., and Löw, H. (1988). Circulating testosterone levels and aggression in adolescent males, A causal analysis. *Psychosom Med* **50**, 261–272.

Packer, C. and Pusey, A. E. (1979). Female aggression and male membership in troops of Japanese macaques and olive baboons. *Folia Primatol* **31**, 212–218.

Panksepp, J., Nelson, E., and Siviy, S. (1994). Brain opioids and mother-infant social motivation. *Acta Paediatr Suppl* **397**, 40–46.

Paul, A. (1989). Determinants of male mating success in a large group of Barbary macaques (*Macaca sylvanus*) at Affenberg Salem. *Primates* **30**, 344–349.

Popova, N. K., Kulikov, A. V., Nikulina, E. M., Kozlachkova, E. Y., and Maslova, G. B. (1991a). Serotonin metabolism and serotonergic receptors in Norway rats selected for low aggressiveness towards man. *Aggressive Behav* **17**, 207–213.

Popova, N. K., Voitenko, N. N., Kulikov, A. V., and Avgustinovich, D. F. (1991b). Evidence for the involvement of central serotonin in mechanism of domestication of silver foxes. *Pharmacol Biochem Behav* **40**, 751–756.

Popova, N. K., Kulikov, A. V., Avgustinovich, D. F., Voitenko, N. N., and Trut, L. N. (1997). Effect of domestication of the silver fox on the main enzymes of serotonin metabolism and serotonin receptors. *Genetika* **33**, 370–374.

Raleigh, M. J. and McGuire, M. T. (1986). Animal analogues of ostracism, Biological mechanisms and social consequences. *Ethol Sociobiol* **7**, 53–66.

Raleigh, M. J. and McGuire, M. T. (1990). Social influences on endocrine function in male vervet monkeys. In: Ziegler, T. E. and Bercovitch, F. B. eds. *Socioendocrinology of Primate Reproduction*. New York: Wiley-Liss, pp. 95–111.

Raleigh, M. J. and McGuire, M. T. (1994). Serotonin, aggression, and violence in vervet monkeys. In: Masters, R. D. and McGuire, M. T. eds. *The Neurotransmitter Revolution*. Carbondale, Southern Illinois University Press, pp. 129–145.

Raleigh, M. J. and Steklis, H. D. (1981). Effect of orbitofrontal and temporal neocortical lesion on the affiliative behavior of vervet monkeys (*Cercopithecus aethiops sabaeus*). *Exp Neurol* **73**, 378–379.

Raleigh, M. J., Steklis, H. D., Ervin, F. R., Kling, A. S., and McGuire, M. T. (1979). The effects of orbitofrontal lesions on the aggressive behavior of vervet monkeys (*Cercopithecus aethiops sabaeus*). *Exp Neurol* **66**, 158–168.

Raleigh, M. J., Brammer, G. L., Yuwiler, A., Flannery, J. W., and McGuire, M. T. (1980). Serotonergic influences on the social behavior of vervet monkeys (*Cercopithecus aethiops sabaeus*). *Exp Neurol* **68**, 322–334.

Raleigh, M. J., Brammer, G. L., and McGuire, M. T. (1983). Male dominance, serotonergic systems, and the behavioral and physiological effects of drugs in vervet monkeys (*Cercopithecus aethiops sabaeus*). In: Miczek, K. A. ed. *Ethopharmacology, Primate Models of Neuropsychiatric Disorders*. New York: Alan R. Liss, pp. 185–197.

Raleigh, M. J., Brammer, G. L., McGuire, M. T., and Yuwiler, A. (1985). Dominant social status facilitates the behavioral effects of serotonergic agonists. *Brain Res* **348**, 274–282.

Raleigh, M. J., Brammer, G. L., Ritvo, E. R., Geller, E., McGuire, M. T., and Yuwiler, A. (1986). Effects of chronic fenfluramine on blood serotonin, cerebrospinal fluid metabolites, and behavior in monkeys. *Psychopharmacology* **90**, 503–508.

Raleigh, M. J., McGuire, M. T., and Brammer, G. L. (1989). Subjective assessment of behavioral style, Links to overt behavior and physiology in vervet monkeys. *Am J Primatol* **18**, 161–162.

Raleigh, M. J., McGuire, M. T., Brammer, G. L., Pollack, D. B., and Yuwiler, A. (1991). Serotonergic mechanisms promote dominance acquisition in adult male vervet monkeys. *Brain Res* **559**, 181–190.

Raleigh, M. J., Brammer, G. L., McGuire, M. T., Pollack, D. B., and Yuwiler, A. (1992). Individual differences in basal cisternal cerebrospinal fluid 5-HIAA and HVA in monkeys. The effects of gender, age, physical characteristics, and matrilineal influences. *Neuropsychopharmacology* **7**, 295–304.

Redmond, D. E. J., Maas, J. W., Kling, A., and Dekirmenjian, H. (1971a). Changes in primate social behavior after treatment with alpha-methyl-para-tyrosine. *Psychosom Med* **33**, 97–113.

Redmond, D. E. J., Maas, J. W., Kling, A., Graham, C. W., and Dekirmenjian, H. (1971b). Social behavior of monkeys selectively depleted of monoamines. *Science* **174**, 428–431.

Reisner, I. R., Mann, J. J., Stanley, M., Huang, Y. Y., and Houpt, K. A. (1996). Comparison of cerebrospinal fluid monoamine metabolite levels in dominant-aggressive and non-aggressive dogs. *Brain Res* **714**, 57–64.

Reist, C., Mazzanti, C., Vu, R., Tran, D., and Goldman, D. (2001). Serotonin transporter promoter polymorphism is associated with attenuated prolactin response to fenfluramine. *Am J Med Genet* **105**, 363–368.

Reite, M., Kaufman, I. C., Pauley, J. D., and Stynes, A. J. (1974). Depression in infant monkeys: Physiological correlates. *Psychosom Med* **36**, 363–367.

Reite, M., Short, R., and Seiler, C. (1978). Loss of your mother is more than loss of a mother. *Am J Psychiatry* **135**, 370–371.

Reite, M., Short, R., Seiler, C., and Pauley, J. D. (1981). Attachment, loss, and depression. *J Child Psychol Psychiatry* **22**, 141–169.

Rejeski, W. J., Brubaker, P. H., Herb, R. A., Kaplan, J. R., and Koritnik, D. (1988). Anabolic steroids and aggressive behavior in cynomolgus monkeys. *J Behav Med* **11**, 95–105.

Rogers, J. J. and Dubowitz, V. (1970). "5-hydroxyindoles in hydrocephalus: A comparative study of cerebrospinal fluid and blood levels." *Developmental Medicine and Child Neurology* **12**: 461–466.

Roman, E., Gustafsson, L., Hyytia, P., and Nylander, I. (2005). Short and prolonged periods of maternal separation and voluntary ethanol intake in male and female ethanol-preferring AA and ethanol-avoiding ANA rats. *Alcohol Clin Exp Res* **29**, 591–601.

Roman, E., Gustafsson, L., Berg, M., and Nylander, I. (2006). Behavioral profiles and stress-induced corticosteroid secretion in male Wistar rats subjected to short and prolonged periods of maternal separation. *Horm Behav* **50**, 736–747.

Rose, R. M., Gordon, T. P., and Bernstein, I. S. (1972). Plasma testosterone levels in the male rhesus, Influences of sexual and social stimuli. *Science* **178**, 643–645.

Rose, R. M., Bernstein, I. S., and Gordon, T. P. (1975). Consequences of social conflict on plasma testosterone levels in rhesus monkeys. *Psychosom Med* **37**, 50–61.

Rose, R. M., Gordon, T. P., and Bernstein, I. S. (1978). Diurnal variation in plasma testosterone and cortisol in rhesus monkeys living in social groups. *J Endocrinol* **76**, 67–74.

Rosenblum, L. A., Coplan, J. D., Friedman, S., Bassoff, T., Gorman, J. M., and Andrews, M. W. (1994). Adverse early experiences affect noradrenergic and serotonergic functioning in adult primates. *Biol Psychiatry* **35**, 221–227.

Rosenblum, L. A., Smith, E. L., Altemus, M. *et al.* (2002). Differing concentrations of corticotropin-releasing factor and oxytocin in the cerebrospinal fluid of bonnet and pigtail macaques. *Psychoneuroendocrinology* **27**, 651–660.

Roudebush, W. E., Gerald, M. S., Cano, J. A., Lussier, I. D., Westergaard, G., and Higley, J. D. (2002). Relationship between platelet-activating factor concentration in rhesus monkey (*Macaca mulatta*) spermatozoa and sperm motility. *Am J Primatol* **56**, 1–7.

Roy, A., Pickar, D., Linnoila, M., Doran, A. R., Ninan, P., and Paul, S. M. (1985). Cerebrospinal fluid monoamine and monoamine metabolite concentrations in melancholia. *Psychiatry Res* **15**, 281–292.

Ruppenthal, G. C., Arling, G.L., Harlow, H. F., Sackett, G. P., and Suomi, S. J. (1976). A 10-year perspective of motherless-mother monkey behavior. *J Abnorm Psychol* **85**, 341–349.

Ruppenthal, G. C., Caffery, S. A., Goodlin, B. L., Sackett, G. P., Vigfusson, N. V., and Peterson, V. G. (1991). Rearing infant monkeys (*Macaca nemestrina*) in pairs produces deficient social development compared with rearing in single cages. *Am J Primatol* **25**, 103–113.

Sackett, G. P. (1968). Abnormal behavior in laboratory-reared monkeys. In: Fox, M. W. ed. *Abnormal Behavior in Animals*. St. Louis, MO: W.B Saunders Company, pp. 293–331.

Sackett, G. P. (1970). Unlearned responses, differential rearing experiences, and the development of social attachments by rhesus monkeys. In: Rosenblum, R. A. ed. *Primate Behavior, Developments in Field and Laboratory Research*, Vol 1. New York: Academic Press, pp. 111–140.

Scaramella, T. J. and Brown, W. A. (1978). Serum testosterone and aggressiveness in hockey players. *Psychosom Med* **40**, 262–265.

Schalling, D., Åsberg, M., Edman, G., and Oreland, L. (1987). "Markers for vulnerability to psychopathology: Temperament traits associated with platelet MAO activity." *Acta Psychiatrica Scandinavica* **76**: 172-182.

Seifert, W. E. J., Foxx, J. L., and Butler, I. J. (1980). "Age effect on dopamine and serotonin metabolite levels in cerebrospinal fluid." *Annals of Neurology* **8**: 38–42.

Shannon, C., Champoux, M., and Suomi, S. J. (1998). Rearing condition and plasma cortisol in rhesus monkey infants. *Am J Primatol* **46**, 311–321.

Shannon, C., Schwandt, M. L., Champoux, M. *et al.* (2005). Maternal absence and stability of individual differences in CSF 5-HIAA concentrations in rhesus monkey infants. *Am J Psychiatry* **162**, 1658–1664.

Shively, C. A., Fontenot, M. B., and Kaplan, J. R. (1995). Social status, behavior, and central serotonergic responsivity in female cynomolgus monkeys. *Am J Primatol* **37**, 333–340.

Siegel, A. and Pott, C. B. (1988). Neural substrates of aggression and flight in the cat. *Progr Neurobiol* **31**, 261–283.

Siever, L. J. (1987). Role of noradrenergic mechanisms in the etiology of the affective disorders. *Psychopharmacology: The Third Generation of Progress.* Meltzer, H. Y. New York, Raven Press: 493–504.

Silverstein, F. S., Johnston, M. V., Hutchinson, R. J., and Edwards, N. L. (1985). "Lesch-Nyhan syndrome: CSF neurotransmitter abnormalities." *Neurology* **35**: 907–911.

Smith, M. A., Kling, M. A., Whitfield, H. J. *et al.* (1989). Corticotropin-releasing hormone, From endocrinology to psychobiology. *Horm Res* **31**, 66–71.

Smuts, B. B. (1987). Gender, aggression and influence. In: Smuts, B. B.,Cheney, D. L., Seyfarth, R. M., Wrangham, R. W., and Struhsaker, T. T. *Primate Societies.* Chicago: University of Chicago Press, pp. 400–412.

Soubrié, P. (1986). Reconciling the role of central serotonin neurons in human and animal behavior. *Behav Brain Sci* **9**, 319–364.

Stanley, M., Traskman-Bendz, L., and Dorovini-Zis, K. (1985). Correlations between aminergic metabolites simultaneously obtained from human CSF and brain. *Life Sci* **37**, 1279–1286.

Steinberg, L. (2004). Risk taking in adolescence, What changes, and why? *Ann N Y Acad Sci* **1021**, 51–58.

Stevenson-Hinde, J. and Simpson, M. J. A. (1980). Subjective assessment of rhesus monkeys over four successive years. *Primates* **21**, 66–82.

Stone, E. A. and McCarty, R. (1983). Adaptation to stress, Tyrosine hydroxylase activity and catecholamine release. *Neurosci Biobehav Rev* **7**, 29–34.

Suomi, S. J. (1982). Abnormal behavior and primate models of psychopathology. In: Fobes, J. L. and King, J. E. eds. *Primate Behavior.* New York: Academic Press, pp. 171–215.

Suomi, S. J. (1991a). Early stress and adult emotional reactivity in rhesus monkeys. *CIBA Found Symp* **156**, 171–183.

Suomi, S. J. (1991b). Primate separation models of affective disorders. In: Madden, J. I. ed. *Neurobiology of Learning, Emotion and Affect.* New York: Raven Press, pp. 195–214.

Suomi, S. J. and Ripp, C. (1983). A history of mother-less mother monkey mothering at the University of Wisconsin Primate Laboratory. In: Reite, M. and Caine, N. eds. *Child Abuse, The Nonhuman Primate Data.* New York: Alan R. Liss, pp. 50–78.

Suomi, S. J., Seaman, S. F., Lewis, J. K., DeLizio, R. D., and McKinney, W. T. (1978). Effects of imipramine treatment of separation-induced social disorders in rhesus monkeys. *Arch Gen Psychiatry* **35**, 321–325.

Suomi, S. J., Kraemer, G. W., Baysinger, C. M., and DeLizio, R. D. (1981). Inherited and experiential factors associated with individual differences in anxious behavior displayed by rhesus monkeys. In: Klein, D. F. and Rabkin, J. eds. *Anxiety, New Research and Changing Concepts.* New York: Raven Press, pp. 179–199.

Thierry, B., Mewa, S., and Kaumanns, W. (2004). *Macaque Societies: A Model for the Study of Social Organization.* Cambridge and New York: Cambridge University Press.

van Oers, H. J., de Kloet, E. R., and Levine, S. (1998a). Early vs. late maternal deprivation differentially alters the endocrine and hypothalamic responses to stress. *Brain Res Dev Brain Res* **111**, 245–252.

van Oers, H. J., de Kloet, E. R., Whelan, T., and Levine, S. (1998b). Maternal deprivation effect on the infant's neural stress markers is reversed by tactile stimulation and feeding but not by suppressing corticosterone. *J Neurosci* **18**, 10171–10179.

Vazquez, D. M., Lopez, J. F., Van Hoers, H., Watson, S. J., and Levine, S. (2000). Maternal deprivation regulates serotonin 1A and 2A receptors in the infant rat. *Brain Res* **855**, 76–82.

Vazquez, D. M., Eskandari, R., Zimmer, C. A., Levine, S., and Lopez, J. F. (2002). Brain 5-HT receptor system in the stressed infant rat, implications for vulnerability to substance abuse. *Psychoneuroendocrinology* **27**, 245–272.

Virkkunen, M., Nuutila, A., Goodwin, F. K., and Linnoila, M. (1987). Cerebrospinal fluid monoamine metabolite levels in male arsonists. *Arch Gen Psychiatry* **44**, 241–217.

Virkkunen, M., De Jong, J., Bartko, J., Goodwin, F. K., and Linnoila, M. (1989). Relationship of psychobiological variables to recidivism in violent offenders and impulsive fire setters. A follow-up study. *Arch Gen Psychiatry* **46**, 600–603.

Virkkunen, M., Kallio, E., Rawlings, R. *et al.* (1994a). Personality profiles and state aggressiveness in Finnish alcoholic, violent offenders, fire setters, and healthy volunteers. *Arch Gen Psychiatry* **51**, 28–33.

Virkkunen, M., Rawlings, R., Tokola, R. *et al.* (1994b). CSF biochemistries, glucose metabolism, and diurnal activity rhythms in alcoholic, violent offenders, fire setters, and healthy volunteers. *Arch Gen Psychiatry* **51**, 20–27.

Walters, J. R. and Seyfarth, R. M. (1987). Conflict and cooperation. In: Smuts, B. B., Cheney, D. L., Seyfarth, R. M., Wrangham R. W., and Struhsaker, T. T. eds. *Primate Societies.* Chicago: University of Chicago Press, pp. 306–317.

Westergaard, G. C., Izard, M. K., Drake, J. H., Suomi, S. J., and Higley, J. D. (1999a). Rhesus macaque (*Macaca mulatta*) group formation and housing, wounding and reproduction in a specific pathogen free (SPF) colony. *Am J Primatol* **49**, 339–347.

Westergaard, G. C., Mehlman, P. T., Shoaf, S. E., Suomi, S. J., and Higley, J. D. (1999b). CSF 5-HIAA and aggression in female macaque monkeys, Species and interindividual differences. *Psychopharmacology* **146**, 440–446.

Westergaard, G. C., Cleveland, A., Trenkle, M. K., Lussier, I. D., and Higley, J. D. (2003a). CSF 5-HIAA concentration as an early screening tool for predicting significant life history outcomes in female specific-pathogen-free (SPF) rhesus macaques (Macaca mulatta) maintained in captive breeding groups. *J Med Primatol* **32**, 95–104.

Westergaard, G. C., Suomi, S. J., Chavanne, T. J. *et al.* (2003b). Physiological correlates of aggression and impulsivity in free-ranging female primates. *Neuropsychopharmacology* **28**, 1045–1055.

Wickings, E. J. and Dixson, A. F. (1992). Testicular function, secondary sexual development, and social status in male mandrills (*Mandrillus sphinx*). *Physiol Behav* **52**, 909–916.

Wiener, S. G., Coe, C. L., and Levine, S. (1988). Endocrine and neurochemical sequelae of primate vocalizations, 367–394.

Wilk, S. and Stanley, M. (1978). Dopamine metabolites in human brain. *Psychopharmacology* **14**, 77–81.

Winslow, J. T. (2005). Neuropeptides and non-human primate social deficits associated with pathogenic rearing experience. *Int J Dev Neurosci* **23**, 245–251.

Winslow, J. T., Noble, P. L., Lyons, C. K., Sterk, S. M., and Insel, T. R. (2003). Rearing effects on cerebrospinal fluid oxytocin concentration and social buffering in rhesus monkeys. *Neuropsychopharmacology* **28**, 910–918.

Wood, J. H. (1980). Sites of origin and cerebrospinal fluid concentration gradients. In: Wood, J. H. ed. *Neurobiology of Cerebrospinal Fluid*. New York: Plenum Press, pp. 53–62.

Yodyingyuad, U., de la Riva, C., Abbott, D. H., Herbert, J., and Keverne, E. B. (1985). Relationship between dominance hierarchy, cerebrospinal fluid levels of amine transmitter metabolites (5-hydrox-yindole acetic acid and homovanillic acid) and plasma cortisol in monkeys. *Neuroscience* **16**, 851–858.

Zajicek, K. B., Higley, J. D., Suomi, S. J., and Linnoila, M. (1997). Rhesus macaques with high CSF 5-HIAA concentrations exhibit early sleep onset. *Psychiatry Res* **73**, 15–25.

Ziegler, T. E. (2000). Hormones associated with non-maternal infant care, a review of mammalian and avian studies. *Folia Primatol* **71**, 6–21.

CHAPTER 8

Assessing Environmental Complexity for Both Normal and Deviant Development

Matthew F. S. X. Novak

Regardless of the causal mechanism, differences in sensory and perceptual experiences and abilities form a cornerstone of many developmental disabilities. This leads to differences in how an organism experiences complexity in the environment. Attempting to quantify and understand environmental complexity has long defied objective measurement. This chapter explores the components of complexity that are essential to its understanding and offers an heuristic framework from which the interested scientist can explore both the objective aspects and the subjective aspects of complexity phenomena. Historical attempts to characterize organism–environment interactions are briefly reviewed as a foundation for new meaningful progress in this area. Examples are presented from research with nonhuman primates (*Macaca nemestrina*) that attempt to demonstrate the usefulness of biobehavioral signatures for classifying individuals in regards to varying levels of environmental stimulation. Translational uses of the ideas discovered from nonhuman primate studies are then discussed. Translational studies across human and nonhuman primate taxa involving differently reared groups and even closely related species of nonhuman primates are essential to understanding individual differences in the role that organism–environment interactions play in developmental disabilities.

INTRODUCTION

In order to understand adaptive behavior in the developmentally disabled, politicians, scientists, educators, therapists, and family members must walk a mile in the shoes of the disabled. We must come to understand that for many developmental disabilities, both sensory and perceptual processes are altered. This, in turn alters the nature

Primate Models of Children's Health and Developmental Disabilities

and complexity of each and every moment of each and every day. In his seminal paper, "Mice, monkeys, men and motives," Harry Harlow provides both a review for and a challenge to psychologists to come and attack the attackable problems in psychology "without regard to, or fear of, difficulty" (Harlow, 1953, p. 31). He suggested that if we apply contemporary tools to the unsolvable problems that have been left behind, we may find ourselves standing on the edge of a different understanding. One such problem involved predicting the behavior of individuals and understanding complexity within organism–environment interactions.

Great progress in organism–environment interactions has been made on a number of fronts. Studies have shown that the nature–nurture question is more fact than a question. From the organismic point of view, the nature–nurture relationship is more a connection or a statement that the two go hand in hand and cannot or should not be considered independently. The starting point for complex organisms and behaviors is 50:50 in terms of genes relative to the environments. From the standpoint of the idea that there are no main effects in behavioral research (Sackett, 1991; Baumrind, 1993; Rosenzweig, 1996; Gould and Gross, 2002; Curtis and Cicchetti, 2003; Sameroff and Mackenzie, 2003; Suomi, 2003; Fleshner and Laudenslager, 2004; Segerstrom, 2005 as a few examples from a range of developmental fields), it is exceedingly unwise to attempt an understanding of genetic or biological processes and how they interact without being aware that the very processes and interactions which may be functioning are driven by the environment. Likewise, it is also unwise to assume that environments drive behavior independently from biological, physiological, and genetic restraints.

In the nonhuman primate literature, one of the best examples of the powerful relationship between the organism and the environment was demonstrated by Harlow, his students and colleagues in their ground-breaking work on differential rearing of infant macaque monkeys. The research can be best understood in the context of social and health policies in existence at the time. Early in the twentieth century, babies in long-term care in hospitals, institutionalized or reared in foundling homes from under the age of six months suffered from high rates of failing to thrive syndrome and very high death rates approaching 100% in some New York hospitals (Bawkin, 1942). Differential rearing studies with nonhuman primates, in which various forms of altered rearing experiences were used, produced a variety of animals with sensory deficits and altered perceptual abilities. Often overlooked, and not typically understood, even within the world of primatology, is the finding that isolation rearing syndrome, which can be debilitating to a rhesus monkey, is not a main effect (Sackett et al., 1976, 1981a). A thorough review of this literature shows that there are species differences, age differences, and timing differences (Capitanio, 1986; Sackett et al., 1999). One goal of Harlow and his colleagues' work was to uncover the necessary and sufficient sensory and perceptual conditions to produce normative development. This work added to what was then a nascent literature on the importance of "contact comfort," which Harlow himself would later term "love" (Harlow, 1958, 1959; Harlow and Harlow, 1966). One has to look no further than any introductory psychology textbook to recognize that these studies are part of the foundation for social and emotional developmental theory. Collectively, these studies contributed to vast improvements in the early care and survivorship of human infants.

Today the problems associated with deficits in sensation and perception are no less prevalent. It is quite likely that the species differences among closely related macaques in response to differential rearing conditions and even forms of sensory isolation provide an excellent model for understanding individual differences in human children suffering from developmental disabilities including learning disabilities (Wright and Zecker, 2004), mental retardation (Greenfield, 1985), autism spectrum disorder (Dawson and Watling, 2000), and self-injurious behavior (Schmahl et al., 2004), all of which have been associated with sensory deprivation and/or altered sensory processing. In order for a model of this type to succeed, however, we must first address the subjective nature of experience.

Nature and nurture

The realization of an organismic relationship between genes and environments is multifaceted (Rutter, 2002; Moffit et al., 2005). Sameroff has provided a thought-provoking assessment of contextualism that scales generations and cultures on a global level (1975, 1981). Sackett et al. (1981b) furthered these ideas in the developmental context of understanding continuity versus discontinuity. However, it is behavior genetics research that has most keenly lauded the relationship between environments and genes, moving us out of the theoretical into the domain of computational (Plomin, 1994; Plomin and Craig, 1997; Saudino, 2005) and beyond that into molecular genetics (Plomin and Rutter, 1998; Plomin and Kovas, 2005; Rutter et al., 2006). Despite challenges associated with the assumptions and beliefs about phenotypic variance due to shared versus non-shared environments (Dunn and Plomin, 1991; Rutter and Plomin, 1997; Plomin et al., 2001; Dunn, 2005; Turkheimer et al., 2005) this work holds great promise and moves the science of psychology closer to becoming an interval-scale science, rather than the ordinal-scale science it is currently.

A second challenge to using behavioral genetics research as a window on organismic complexity involves the null hypothesis. The question needs to be asked whether a finding of 50% genetic basis for complex traits or a finding of 5% genetic basis for that same trait is more profound. If the expectation is that there is no genetic basis for a behavioral process then the finding of 50% is interesting. However, if the nature and nurture hypothesis is correct, then for any even moderately complex behavior a finding of 50% genetic influence represents a failure to reject the null, and 5%, which may not differ from 0, might be quite profound. Considering the heralded preponderance of genetic contribution estimates near 50%, plus or minus a small 95% confidence interval, a re-evaluation would at the very least be heuristic for the field.

Beyond these considerations, behavioral genetics research has confirmed the important caveat that the relationship among genes, environments and organisms is multidirectional. Not only do genes drive environments (Scarr and McCartney, 1983; Plomin and Bergeman, 1991; Scarr, 1992; Plomin, 1994) but environments drive genes (Bakshi and Kalin, 2000; Anway *et al.*, 2005; Weaver *et al.*, 2006). Furthermore, environmental variation can produce nongenetic intergenerational changes in populations that result in genetic changes over evolutionary time (Gottlieb, 2002).

In nonhuman primates, Suomi and colleagues have accomplished what could be called "experimental behavior genetics" with literal manipulations of environmental rearing conditions relative to the phenotypic expression of the long and short alleles of the serotonin transporter gene (Barr *et al.*, 2003, 2004; Shannon *et al.*, 2005). For rhesus macaques and humans there appear to be associations between the genes for the serotonin system, the functioning of the serotonin system, and behavioral phenotypes that involve impulsivity, aggression, and even propensity for alcohol consumption. However, early rearing environment and enrichment modify the expression of this genetic predisposition such that more species-typical rearing and environmental enrichment can buffer or overcome the genetic vulnerability (Suomi, 2005).

The purpose of this chapter is to both consider and propose methods about how to differentiate the experience of the environment among and within organisms. Specifically, this chapter focuses on the individual and the processes by which experience varies over time and across situations.

An integral part of any nature–nurture discovery is the person–environment relationship, which for our purposes is defined as how the organism experiences its environment. Identical environments will surely be experienced differently by different organisms. However, environments will also be experienced differently by the same organism at different times. And for all the reasons stated thus far, there is no such thing as identical organisms. Even if novelty were not an issue, it is unlikely that an individual organism would always respond the same to the same situation. How then, if the measurable environment has not changed, do scientists find a systematic way to understand the remaining variation in responses that an organism expresses? Can this variation be measured, or, are we forever doomed to send some portion of intra- and interindividual differences to the trash heap of the error term in our analyses?

One possibility is that within-individual variation is random error that defies systematic measurement and prediction. However, it is also possible that measuring single variables to represent biological systems does not provide a robust characterization of the system from which patterns can be discerned. A third possibility is that we measure the wrong variables. This could be due to technological limitations and/or intellectual limitations in our understanding of the process. The challenge here lies in generating a systematic and empirical method to understand the subjective nature of experience. And, as is the case for nonhuman animals, how do we assess the subjective without asking an animal how it feels? How do we go about making the subjective objective?

SENSATION

The issue of environmental complexity starts with the senses. This realization is not new, and the fact that complexity consists of more than just the empirical dimensions of a stimulus has contributed to the consternation of many scientists (Lewis, 2004; Sackett et al., 1999). This chapter attempts to address this issue by integrating sensory experience as the gateway dimension to a more comprehensive organismic response that can be measured systematically. In order to accomplish this task, it is first useful to understand the idea of complexity from a developmental perspective.

While development has been an integral part of complexity research, it is uncommon for the endpoints of the developmental timespan to include prenatal development when the sensory systems are first beginning to function. How an organism experiences its environment must start with the inductive phases of sensory system development during which an organism first begins to interact with the outside world.

There are two theoretical viewpoints about the nature of sensory development to consider. The first argues for an integrationist point of view where sensory systems develop relatively independently and undergo maturational processes which involve an increase in the ability of sensory systems to work together and coordinate parallel and competing stimuli into different systems (Piaget, 1952; Lewkowicz, 2000). The second argues from a differentiationist point of view. First, "generalized sense" is induced. Then as development proceeds, necessity and experience drive differentiation, inducing separate senses to be developed by the organism (Gibson, 1969, 1988). While both viewpoints take a developmental approach, looking at them more sequentially and across both fetal and infant time periods rather than in competition with each other during postnatal development provides a more comprehensive developmental scale from which these two competing ideas can bring synergy to the understanding of the sensory systems.

While both sets of ideas tend to pick up development at birth, all the sensory systems are functional well before birth (Gottlieb, 1971). During embryological/fetal development there is an induction point before which the organism is unable to undergo a sensory experience of the environment; and after which, sensory experience becomes possible. Considerable research has gone into various factors that can and do cause individual variation in the onset and timing of sensory development (Lecanuet et al., 1995; Lickliter, 2000; Ronca, 2003). Given the timing relative to the rest of brain development, it is unlikely that an organism is wired to be aware of the energy form of the stimulus. In addition, it is unlikely that initially the sensation is anything other than white noise. The exception to the white noise is dedicated neurons for specific components of sensory stimulation, such as face neurons in the anterior superior temporal sulcus and the inferior temporal gyrus (Eifuku et al., 2004), mirror neurons in the premotor cortex (Rizzolatti and Craighero, 2004; Ferrari et al., 2005), object-aspect neurons from the inferior temporal cortex or even the visual cortex (Fujita, 2002; Zhou et al., 2000, respectively) and others that may be predisposed to respond to specific types of stimulation. However, whether or not any of these actually work in the neonate, let alone the fetus, needs to be demonstrated. In addition, the levels to which each are experienced independently needs to be investigated.

Lewkowicz's integrationist point of view argues for very early multimodality of sensory systems. At first this may seem antithetical to the developmental differentiation point of view. And, in fact, this is how these two viewpoints are often presented. However, I do not believe this to be the case. Before pattern recognition can occur, sensation must occur. Only with time and the organismic process of maturation will multiple senses come first to function and then to be differentiated. It is likely that the driving force behind this differentiation is the environment. The differentiationist view I am proposing suggests that the environment will only drive differentiation of meaningful differences among sensory stimulation. Within this context, intermodal invariants (Gibson, 1966) or intersensory equivalents (Lewkowicz, 1994) would result from a failure of differentiation. From this perspective then, crossmodal abilities are like blocking in classical conditioning, in which the additional information does not increase the predictability of the association and therefore is not learned (Kamin, 1969). From the standpoint of the senses, this means that the link between the senses is not broken for this type of stimulation and therefore they remain integrated. Certainly with time, more complex brain structures may allow for reintegration, higher level integration and even perhaps other subtler connections to be made later during postnatal development, as is proposed and demonstrated by the integrationist perspective of sensory development.

Postnatally, individual differences in sensory sensitivity and perception are also driven by experiential factors. Musicians come to be able to recognize subtleties in music (Peretz and Zatorre, 2005); mothers may become able to differentiate their own babies crying (Zeskind and Huntington, 1984; LaGasse et al., 2005); blind people come to depend on their other senses more readily than sighted people (Kellogg, 1962; Dufour et al., 2005), and we all learn to pay attention to language sounds that matter while slowly losing the plasticity to perceive those that are not meaningful (Zhang et al., 2005). Similarly, it is likely that a developing fetus will come to differentiate sound from somatosensory stimulation only when such a differentiation increases their ability to adapt or cope with the demands of their environment.

Gottlieb (1971) demonstrated that the sensory systems all develop in the same order across a wide array of species. This is consistent with a pivotal role for maturation processes in sensory differentiation. Nonetheless, these maturational processes are firmly entrenched in the environment in which they develop. As long as there is environmental variation and an organism has the ability to detect these cause–effect variations, both classical and operant conditioning principles are at work in even the simplest developing organisms. Within these somewhat simplistic behaviorist boundaries, what is necessary to the organism at a particular developmental stage will evolve into sensitivity to environmental variation. The evolved sensitivity would then drive how and when the sensory systems mature and what the organism "chooses" to pay attention to. Since the sensory systems are functional prior to birth, the developmental time-course of differentiation must begin during the prenatal period.

In terms of environmental complexity, the order of differentiation of the senses may also inform us when it comes to ranking two equal stimuli of differing modalities. The later the developing system (i.e. vision), the more evolved it is in detecting complexity. Therefore, with a somatosensory stimulus and a visual stimulus that differ only in modality and are equal in every other aspect, the visual stimulus will be more complex than the somatosensory one. This is a hypothesis that I will revisit later in the chapter.

NOVELTY

A second aspect of complexity that is relevant to this discussion is novelty. Novelty preferences (Hughes, 1965; Bevins and Besheer, 2005; Kendal et al., 2005; Stansfield and Kirstein, 2006) and avoidances (Mineka, 1985; Timmermans et al., 1994) have been documented in both nonhuman primates and other species. Berlyne (1950, 1966) offered an excellent behaviorally based account of novelty as it pertains to curiosity, postulating that curiosity is a drive stimulus-producing response. As time of exposure passes, the drive stimulus-producing response, curiosity, diminishes as measured by exploration. According to Berlyne, pattern recognition is the key. Complex organisms have evolved a "generalized habit of learning" in order to increase the probability of survival. Therefore, the parameters and constraints of this learning may also be under evolutionary influence as well. This evolutionary pressure may have pushed curiosity and novelty-seeking processes and/or learning to distinguish patterns into the prenatal period of development. Said another way, we have evolved neural circuits for learning. Once these neural circuits have formed, they will function! If there is variation in the induction of functioning circuits, and there is an advantage to learning early, then evolution would select for this advantage. Alternatively, if early learning increased the vulnerability to risk factors, then the early learning phenomena might not be selected for.

Marks (1978) noted that the only sensory experience that can be reliably detected by all the senses is time. If true, this may give us unique insight into the phenomena and significance of novelty, which is also based in time. Curiosity results from the organism's sensitivity to, or anticipation of, the consequences of environmental change. What is learned is that differentiating the environment increases one's ability to respond adaptively to experience. Over time and successful learning bouts, the propensity or valence of the seeking should increase. In most cases curiosity will most likely increase on a variable ratio scale, which over time leads to more and more responding. However, the exact nature of this learning curve needs to be assessed. The phenomena described here are similar in nature to the conditioning of variability in responding, proposed and documented by Neuringer as the basis for creativity (Neuringer, 2002, 2004).

Curiosity or attraction to novelty would diminish as sensation within a sensory system ultimately approaches an asymptote on the time axis. Therefore, from a sensory point of view, novelty is a search for maximum sensory stimulation across as many sensory systems as possible. As each sensory system documents the stimulus, the number of constants increases and variation decreases, which leads to less attention needed to seek newness in the stimulus. Hence, the stimulus becomes less novel, and more resources become available for curiosity and novelty-seeking elsewhere. By this definition and line of reasoning then, novelty and complexity are thoroughly intertwined. Certainly the first time an organism experiences a specific combination of inputs, a stimulus is more complex than during later exposures to the same stimulus.

Research on the neuronal mechanisms for learning and memory shows permanent alteration of how stimuli are represented in the visual cortex of the adult monkey. Desimone (1996) describes three specific changes to neuronal functioning: repetition suppression, enhancement, and delay. Any or all of these changes may account for how stimuli switch from novel to non-novel in the visual system. Similarly, concomitant changes in the function of neuronal circuits in other CNS sensory areas may also be occurring.

COMPLEXITY

The subjective components of the complexity experience have, to date, yielded an impermeable wall to researchers (Dember and Earl, 1957; Dember, Earl and Paradise, 1957; Berlyne, 1966; Suess and Berlyne, 1978; Kang and Shaver, 2004; Lewis, 2004; Zautra et al., 2005). The idea of objectifying a subjective process is daunting. We offered a developmental version of Complexity Dissonance Theory as a theoretical model to show how rearing environment, psychological complexity of an animal, and development might interact to produce both group differences and developmental change for an individual (Sackett et al., 1999).

Earl (1961) defined complexity, K, computationally as a mediator of within-individual variation in behavior. Although he postulated variables that may account for the role that complexity plays in producing behavior, it was his student, Gene Sackett, who provided experimental tests of complexity in nonhuman primates (Sackett, 1965).

Objective aspects of complexity

Frequency, number, duration

Sackett (1965) studied the psychological maturity of juvenile monkeys (*Macaca mulatta*) who were reared in the differentially complex environments of total social isolation, partial isolation, and the forests of India. The animals were exposed to various manipulanda and the amount of time spent interacting with each object was recorded. The objects varied in complexity from a straight bar, to a moving T-bar, to a hanging chain. The straight bar was stationary and solid, the T-bar was slightly more complex involving the "T" shape and it moved up and down in one dimension. The chain stimulus was the most complex because it could be moved into multiple shapes, made various noises, and could move freely across all three dimensions. The results showed that stimulus complexity preference was directly related to the complexity of the rearing environment.

Objective complexity can also vary according to its frequency or number during an exposure. For example, it would be difficult to argue at the objective level that a social interaction with 11 individuals is less complex than one involving two. This too, however, is not a fixed value. Both maturation and experience will alter the perceptual demands beyond the simply objective count. Duration and intensity are also unique processes in the objective realm of complexity. For duration, longer exposures lead to habituation, which results in reduced complexity. But for highly complex stimuli, increased durations may overwhelm an organism's ability to respond adaptively to the stimulation and therefore the complexity increases relative to the organism's acute adaptive psychological complexity level. The objective components of intensity follow a similar nonlinear relationship to complexity. In most cases increases in intensity are related to increasing objective complexity, number, or even rate.

Other differences in intensity move to the subjective, personal experience side of the equation and are not so clear. In research on language-capable humans, self-report as to the intensity of a given stressor may prove to be an adequate measure. However, in young children and animals this avenue is not available to researchers. Therefore, the challenge is to develop another method of detecting the perception and intensity of stimulation.

Subjective aspects of complexity

The basis for objectifying the subjective nature of sensory experience lies in the sensory systems themselves and in the assumption that necessity drives differentiation. We know from the classical conditioning literature that necessity, also referred to as surprise by Rescorla and Wagner (1972), drives associative learning (Fanselow, 1998). Classical studies on blocking demonstrated that if a conditioned stimulus using one sensory stimulus predicts the unconditioned stimulus with a certain probability, then a newly intended conditioned stimulus paired with it will not come to be learned unless it provides more information than the initial conditioned stimulus (Kamin, 1969). For example, once a dog has been classically conditioned to salivate to a bell, combining the bell with a light such that the light and bell provide the same information to the dog will not come to produce salivation to the light alone. The bell blocks the light stimulus from being learned. For fear conditioning, this

blocking of new but extraneous information is related to the production of endogenous opioids (Fanselow and Bolles, 1979; Bolles and Fanselow, 1980). Why should an
organism devote more resources to learning an association than is necessary? From an
evolutionary point of view, this devotion to wasted resource would not long survive.

Nature, nurture, organismic development

Expanding on his experimental work (1965), Sackett reviewed the status of research
on the effects of differential rearing (Sackett et al., 1999). In the resulting developmental version of Complexity Dissonance Theory, he proposed that every organism starts with a genetic pacer range. A pacer range is a developmentally paced range
of environmental experiences to which an organism will respond adaptively. This
pacer range, although based in genetics, is shaped by the environments to which
the organism is exposed; and the result of this interaction establishes a unique psychological complexity for the organism. Beyond this point developmentally, nature
and nurture continue to inform the organism. However, both now interact epige-
netically with the organismic psychological complexity level.

It is against this organismic background that we need to assess the amount, type,
and intensity of how organisms perceive their environments. To do this we move out
of the cognitive/perceptual region, where one might be biased to look for the
answer, into the physiological/perceptual domain. As the demand requirements of a
stimulus increases, the organism will devote more and more resources to cope with
the demand. Regardless of the objective status of the stimulus, the more resources
(sensory, behavioral, neurophysiological) an organism devotes to a given stimulus, the
more complex that stimulus is. A stimulus that evokes both visual and tactile sensation is more complex than one that evokes only one sensory system. Two different
stimuli with the same objective and sensory complexity could then be differentiated
by the degree of demand they place on an organism's physiological response systems.

A THEORETICAL PROPOSAL

In a review of the effects of early rearing experience, we proposed a definition of
complexity that includes measuring the number of sensory systems activated by a
given experience in order to gain some perspective on how complex an event is to
a given individual (Sackett et al., 1999). In a later paper, I proposed a similar solution
related to intensity of response to stressful or challenging stimuli (Novak, M. F. S. X.
2004). In the updated version, the organismic focus shifted from the breadth of
sensory stimulation to the breadth of response dimensions required to respond
adaptively to an environmental stimulus. Instead of sensory systems, I proposed that
there are response dimensions within the body, and that the sensory systems are just
one of these dimensions. Any environmental event that activates more of these
dimensions is more intense than an event that activates fewer of these dimensions.

Here I reconcile both presentations into a single framework. To accomplish this, I map intensity of responding onto the processes of novelty versus habituation. As discussed, novel objects demand more of an organism's resources than well-learned objects. Objects to which one has habituated require even fewer resources from an individual. Therefore, measuring complexity will involve not only the objective, measurable qualities of a stimulus, but also both the range of sensory stimulation and psychophysiological demand required to adaptively respond to the stimulus. These demands will shift as the object moves from novel, to learned, to habituated.

Dimensions

The responses involved in complexity of a stimulus include sensory, behavioral, cardiovascular, endocrine and immune, metabolic, cognitive and emotional dimensions. However, the primary or gateway dimension through which provocation of the others occurs is the sensory dimension. All of these dimensions are likely to be interrelated, but this may not always be so. For example, Weinberg and Levine (1980) demonstrated that behavioral and physiological dimensions could be disassociated in an avoidance paradigm where rats produced a maladaptive behavioral repertoire but still showed signs of reduction in stress hormones. Hennessy *et al.* (1979) showed a similar dissociation in surrogate-reared squirrel monkeys. Coe and Levine (1981) suggest that behavior and physiology are often correlated, but that the assumption of correlation, "can also lead to serious misinterpretations" (p. 172). The dissociations between physiology and behavior are often discussed as noise. However, an equally likely alternative is that the dissociations are the data. Dissociations across all the response dimensions need further study. The characterization that intensity increases as the number of response dimensions activated increases yields a heuristic model from which testable hypotheses can be generated.

The term dimension is intended to categorize the relative difference and interactions of these arbitrarily defined systems. Therefore, any stimulus that activates more of these dimensions is considered more intense. For example, a challenging environmental stimulus accounted for by an alteration of the thought dimension is less intense than one that alters thought and initiates an emotional response. Likewise, a stimulus that alters both thought and emotion is less intense than one affecting cognition, emotion, and heart rate.

The boundaries between dimensions have become increasingly arbitrary as research gains new levels of understanding. For example, the boundary between what is thought of as the immune system and the endocrine system is not precise and many of the functions of these two systems interact. It is probable that response dimensions, while dissociable, are rarely independent; each overlapping to varying degrees with other dimensions. Some boundaries may be classifications imposed on an organism by those who study it.

In addition, it is likely an oversimplification to place all dimensions on an even par with one another. Hierarchies may exist such that the interaction of two particular response dimensions is not more intense than a particular single dimension. This situation can be tested experimentally. A second oversimplification concerns the time for a dimension to become activated. The cardiovascular/endocrine dimensions may respond very quickly to perceived stressors, whereas other dimensions such as the immune/metabolic may be slower to respond. This temporal variation may be of significance in objectively identifying the subjective intensity of perceived stimuli. Again, this is an issue for empirical studies.

Systems

I used the term dimension carefully in the preceding argument. Here, the term "system" refers to the traditional dependent-variable classifications that have been used to identify functional units in an organism. Historically speaking, many of the advances in physiological understanding of behavior were based on what we were capable of measuring at the time. Rather than a theoretical discussion of what we should measure, we are all too often limited to what we can measure. Fortunately, the drive for advancement within, and to, newer technologies now leaves us in the position of being able to measure the same or similar things in multiple ways. One example is heart rate, which can be assessed both as raw heart rate and as vagal tone (Porges, 2003). Porges argues that vagal tone is better, but he also acknowledges that the two are not completely uncorrelated. To the degree that they are not correlated they are actually different methods to measure the cardiovascular system. A second example might be adrenocorticotropic hormone (ACTH) and cortisol. Again to the degree that they provide us with unique information, they are different measures of the hypothalamic-pituitary-adrenal (HPA) axis system. Within the framework proposed here we refer to each of these dependent variables as systems. Collectively these systems make up the response dimensions.

The ability of any organism to respond to its environment is multifaceted. It can include the sensory dimension within which any or all of the sensory systems may become activated. Likewise it can involve emotion, thought, behavior, immune, cardiovascular, metabolic, and endocrine dimensions. This taxonomy becomes relevant because it creates a testable hierarchy. A stimulus which activates two systems within a dimension is less complex than a stimulus that activates two systems from different dimensions. The more systems within a dimension that something activates, the more complex the subjective experience of the stimulus. Also, the more dimensions a stimulus activates the more complex the stimulus.

Rank, order, importance

The point at which three systems within one dimension becomes more complex than two systems from different dimensions will need to be investigated and empirically determined. For the sensory systems it may be possible to create a hierarchy of significance using information about how the sensory systems develop. Returning to the premise of necessity driving sensory development, the pattern would be the opposite of developmental order, with visual stimuli ranking highest and somatosensory stimuli ranking lowest (Gottlieb, 1971). Again, this proposal can be tested empirically.

AN EXPERIMENTAL MODEL

The model I am proposing can occur both at the systemic and dimensional level. At both levels, acuteness is time-based or transitory. The breadth of response such as a single system responding versus multiple systems is not a measure of acuteness, but is related to the intensity of response, as discussed above.

Research on the experience of various forms of stimulation and environmental challenges can usually be categorized into two separate types of studies. Event studies categorized subjects according to some aspect of the environment. Reaction studies categorized subjects according to extreme values of some characteristic (systems and/or dimensions) of the organism. Within the category of reaction research, subdivisions exist that are consistent with the discussion of dimensions and systems. Organismic responses, for example, can differ depending on whether they are sensory, behavioral, physiological, emotional or metabolic. In addition, each of these organismic responses may have an acute phase, or both acute and chronic phases. Each of these dimensions sheds light on the assessment of experiential phenomena. Only by combining information from both types of research can we begin to understand these complex and transactional phenomena.

Using traditional deductive experimentation, researchers have developed a number of different tools and theoretical perspectives for investigating experiential phenomena. A great deal of literature is devoted to arguing for and against different terminology, different methods of measuring, and different ways of thinking about environmental events and reactions to the environment (Selye, 1980; Lazarus, 1991). Certainly, these discussions have been fruitful and bring the scientific community to its current level of understanding. The next step in our understanding of the individual is to step away from these debates and to use the information provided by each of these systems to look at idiographic patterns of responding.

At the very least, the inter- and intra-individual variability demonstrated in these competing research perspectives is used to weaken both its significance and credibility. In order to move in a more productive direction, the similarities and differences demonstrated by various techniques and perspectives may be able to be combined such that the patterns demonstrated can themselves be used as dependent variables. In essence, what are often thought of as the weaknesses of this research area may actually be strengths.

Each individual to be studied experimentally can be exposed to several types of situations. Each situation can be presented multiple times. The result is data that reveal the effect of a type of stimulation for each presentation. In addition, however, each individual would demonstrate a pattern across the entirety of the manipulations. This pattern of results is a dependent variable in itself. Individuals with different patterns may be more informative for the advancement of theory than the particular effect of a given event. Consistent with this idea, Corneal and Nesselroade (1994) used factor analysis of several personality assessments to evaluate different effects environments could have on emotional experience. In their experiments, the number of factors that the assessments loaded onto was the dependent variable. Shoda (1999) and Shoda and Mischel (2000) propose that patterns demonstrated by individuals across multiple dependent variables and situations reveal a "behavioral signature" for an individual. The same may be true for an individual's biobehavioral pattern of responding to varying levels of stimulation.

The idea of a biobehavioral signature starting from the sensory dimension and then encompassing other response dimensions of an organism is adapted from social psychology research interested in predicting an individual's behavior from environmental and person characteristics of that individual. Correlations across situations are often quite low (Bem and Allen, 1974; Mischel and Peake, 1982), and yet there is considerable belief among both professionals and lay people that individuals are consistent over time. In order to demonstrate consistency in individuals, research has attempted to incorporate context into the assessment of a person's reaction across time and situations (Corneal and Nesselroade, 1994). By incorporating context into the correlations across situations, the percentage of variance explained by personality judgments increases (Shoda et al., 1993). That individuals demonstrate considerable variability in their response to different levels of complexity and even that the complexity level of a stimulus will change for an individual over time, context and experience, is an example of Shoda's behavioral signature expanded to include biobehavioral dimensions. Inductive data from idiographic studies designed to uncover the biobehavioral signature for individual organisms may assist in defining experimental group assignments in later deductive studies on complexity.

A conceptual example of the biobehavioral signature idea will help illustrate its usefulness. This example is drawn from stress theories. Traditionally, stress research has had a number of theoretical perspectives (i.e. Cannon, 1929; Selye, 1975, or Kanner et al., 1981). These perspectives have often been discussed as contradictory to one another rather than complimentary, especially between Lazarus and Selye. Attempting to unite these research ideas creates one example of an organism's biobehavioral signature.

Research on stress and stress phenomena must be able to operationalize both the environmental context of the stress and the response of the individual to stress. Environmental stressors (Selye, 1980) are often objectifiable and could literally be any environmental demand. However, quantifying the event itself is not enough. Consistent with Lazarus's ideas about the perception and appraisal of stress, research must include a measure of the acute stress response (Coyne and Lazarus, 1980). These measures could include self-report, sensation, behavioral, cardiovascular, endocrine and immune, metabolic, and even cognitive and emotional changes. Combining the ideas of stressors and the stress reactions into a single theory generates additional parameters that are not often discussed together in stress research.

Expanding this idea beyond merely stress to environmental challenges and stimulus complexity helps to clarify experimental groups from which data can be generated. In the simplest model, a 2×2 research design, the presence or absence of a stimulus is crossed with the presence or absence of the reaction to a stimulus. Mere activation of systems within the sensory dimension represents the lowest intensity stimulus. However, even at this lowest level, this generates four types of individuals (see Table 8.1). The first type is usually thought to be the traditional subjects of stress studies: people who experience the stimulus and who become stimulated. In the context of the current argument, the type of stimulation (i.e. stress) is irrelevant and in fact will mislead the argument into the domain of "good" versus "bad." Instead, it is more useful to characterize the interaction, which subsequently may or may not be stressful, into those who at the very least experience a sensation in response to stimulation. In Table 8.1, this is the condition occupied by the upper left cell. However, the upper left cell is often not what is actually operationalized by studies of this type in the literature. Traditionally, stressor studies expose individuals to a potentially challenging environment but do not measure whether an acute response has occurred. The entire left column would represent this situation. The subjects that were exposed to a stimulus but exhibited no sensation let alone a response in other dimensions, the lower left, usually would be error variance in traditional studies. This second group might be characterized as a resistant group. In the model being proposed, resistant individuals are characterized as different from the stimulated individuals, and become part of the analysis and no longer part of the error term. The third group, in the lower right, does not experience the stimulation and consequently does not initiate a response to stimulation. This group is the proper control group for many studies. A final group, in the upper right, does not experience the targeted stimulation, and yet exhibits a stimulated response profile. This group can be said to be chaotic, perhaps even psychopathological. In this group, the stimulation response may vary in chronicity, or the organism may be responding to an unmeasured or latent stimulation.

There is added variation at both the stimulation and responsiveness levels just introduced according to whether the event or reaction is acute or both acute and chronic. Acute is the time segment most proximal to a given event. The chronic

TABLE 8.1   Four biobehavioral signatures are created by crossing environmental events and organism response models

	Environmental event	No environmental event
Organismic reaction	Stimulated	Chaotic
No organismic reaction	Resistant	Unstimulated

dimension is more distal. All stimulation, whether an external event or an organismic response, by this definition has an acute phase but not necessarily a chronic phase. Hereafter, the term chronic refers to a process with both an acute and chronic phase. What we are left with then is no longer a 2×2 design in the simplest form, but a 3×3 design. For example, an organism might be exposed to an acute stressor but exhibit both an acute and chronic response. In contrast, an organism might be exposed to an acute and chronic stressor and only exhibit an acute response due to habituation to the stressor.

All nine combinations can and have been previously separated along similar lines (Novak, M. F. S. X. 2006). However, within the context of the discussion in this chapter, the nine-celled characterization model depicted as the learned level (middle level of Figure 8.1) is also overly simplified and not complete. The size of individual cells in this characterization, and the size of the matrix itself will vary as a function of novelty or duration. This increased level of complexity rapidly starts to become a large, unwieldy model. However, this final axis is necessary. As Figure 8.1 suggests, the sizes of the individual cells, which represent the percentage of individuals or the probability of a particular biobehavioral signature, will vary as a function of novelty, between the top, middle and bottom levels. In the example depicted, the cells are larger during early exposures and get smaller as an organism first learns and then habituates to stimulation. In addition, however, as depicted, it is also possible that at some levels of learning more or fewer distinguishable groups exist. These and other possibilities should be considered and tested empirically.

The sensory systems are a single response dimension and make up one portion of complexity. The other response systems discussed previously (Novak, 2002, 2004, 2006) add to complexity along the intensity dimension. For each of these response dimensions, there could be a figure like Figure 8.1. Future research can test which components are meaningful. Both for the sake of this discussion and in practice, working with smaller pieces of a larger model is necessary. As we come to understand each of these pieces, they can be assembled into the larger and more complete biobehavioral signature. When working with these pieces, the goal is to keep the larger interactive multiple response dimension context in perspective. Lobel (1994) suggests this type of approach in her review of prenatal stress literature. Likewise, Sandman et al. (1997) advocate a similar type of approach in their investigation of the relationship between psychosocial stress and HPA axis activity.

RESPONSIVENESS TO THE ENVIRONMENT

Individual consistencies and inconsistencies in responsiveness to environmental demand can be theoretically determined but are all too often limited by what we can measure. In this final section, I offer an example from my own research into the acute maternal and acute fetal responses to maternal psychological challenges in pig-tailed macaque monkeys (*Macaca nemestrina*). I have proposed such a characterization

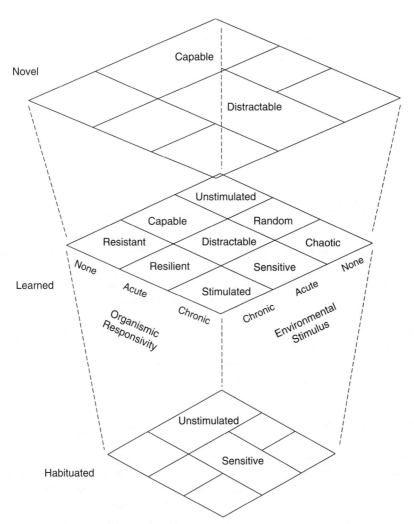

FIGURE 8.1   Complexity as a function of novelty, environmental stimulation, type of reaction, and intensity or breadth of reaction for a given stimulus. Depicts one possibility of how complexity may vary with time. Changes over time across and within individual organismic cells present phenotypic variation to be determined empirically.

for measuring the acute and chronic response of a mother and fetus to psychological experiences of the mother (Table 8.2). In our laboratory, we maintain pregnant pigtailed and rhesus monkeys on chronic indwelling catheters for the last 6–8 weeks of pregnancy in order to study maternal and fetal cardiovascular response and to have chronic access to maternal and fetal blood supply. Access to the blood supply gives us the opportunity to sample hormone, immune, and metabolic constituents of blood

TABLE 8.2   Systems and dimensions assessed as potential stress responders

Organism	Dimension	System
Mother	Behavioral	Postures
		Specific behaviors
	Cardiovascular	Heart rate
		Blood pressure
		Heart rate variability
Fetus	Cardiovascular	Heart rate
		Blood pressure
		Heart rate variability
Mother–fetus	Cardiovascular	Within-system mother–fetus interactions

without restraint or anesthesia, and allows us to administer experimental manipulations to either or both the mother and the fetus. Previously, we have demonstrated the efficacy of our procedures in producing species-typical births (Novak, 2002, 2006). In this case, the focus was on the presence or absence of an immediate response in the mother and the fetus as measured by the acute cardiovascular and behavioral response of mothers and cardiovascular responses of fetuses during a range of maternal environmental events. A second goal was to study the relationship between maternal and fetal cardiovascular responses, and how this relationship changes in response to variation in events in the maternal environment.

The biobehavioral signature

Identifying systems and dimensions to be included for consideration in a more comprehensive biobehavioral signature is an empirical question. Although it is unlikely that two entire systems will respond identically, if two systems are identified that always respond in the same way, or fail to respond at all, then the redundancy is not useful. In this analysis, both postures and behaviors changed in response to the events presented. Sometimes the frequency of posture changes increased, sometimes they decreased. If any change at all in the variable is the metric of interest then these two systems appear redundant. However, if the direction of change is also of interest then there is important information to be gained by including the reaction of both systems in the biobehavioral signature.

Identifying variables within a response system is also an empirical question. Although mean value of heart rate (HR), blood pressure (BP), and heart rate variability (VAR) may characterize the cardiovascular system, the log–linear analysis of these same variables revealed other aspects which may also be important (Novak, 2002). The shape of the distribution may be as important as the mean level. Most likely, a combination of the two would be best. The analyses showed that the maternal

(M)–fetal (F) interaction between cardiovascular variables is another characteristic, in addition to the acute maternal and fetal response to environmental events, that may need to be included in the maternal–fetal biobehavioral signature. In the 2002 study, animals were watched under baseline conditions for four 5-minute time blocks prior to the onset of a 5-minute anticipating-capture challenge. Following the conclusion of the challenge, animals were observed but undisturbed for an additional 45 minutes. The capture manipulation consisted of presenting the subject with all the environmental cues of an imminent capture without actually following through and capturing the subject. During the 5-minute manipulation, the researcher would enter the room, approach the cage, enable, but not actually use, a mechanism on the cage typically used to immobilize subjects and remain at the cage interacting with the subject for the entire 5-minute period. The time-course of the treat-other manipulation was similar. The researcher would enter the room at the end of baseline, this time with fruit food treats in hand. Across the 5-minute period, treats would be offered and given individually to all animals in the room. However, the treats were offered to the subject but not given. Both manipulations were performed twice across a five-week period at the end of gestation. Each manipulation was alternated with baseline days conducted at the same time of day when nothing happened. Data for both baseline and experimental manipulations were collected remotely via closed circuit video. The cardiovascular data were then collapsed into quintiles resulting in categories for which we had frequencies for the number of times that a cardiovascular signal occurred in low, low moderate, moderate, high moderate or high ranges.

Direct, one-to-one comparison was attempted between maternal and fetal cardiovascular variables revealing maternal–fetal interactions for both heart rate and blood pressure. The maternal–fetal interaction for heart rate variability was less clear. Based on this analysis, the maternal–fetal interaction is not a variable to be included to describe heart rate variability in a maternal–fetal model of a biobehavioral signature. Table 8.3 applies the theoretical structure of the stress signature described in Table 8.2 to several of the results from this study. Using a similar format to the conceptual table (Table 8.2), the response pattern of the several potential response variables during the two most stressful events and no-event (baseline day) condition are summarized.

For the subject represented in Table 8.3, several of the variables exhibited consistencies within an event type. These consistencies occurred more often during events than baselines. Four variables exhibited both consistency within event types and differentiation between event types. The occurrence of negative behaviors was similar for both the capture and treat-other events, and both days were different from the baseline days. On the baseline days the negative behaviors did not occur. The mean change in fetal heart rate (FHR) consistently differentiated between the treat-other and baseline events. FHR dropped in response to both treat-other events, but either did not change or increased during the four baselines. It is doubtful that this consistent difference between test and baseline would hold up under repeated testing. Assuming baselines are indeed baselines, the probability of no change, increasing, and decreasing should approach equality over time. Fetal blood pressure

TABLE 8.3   Biobehavioral signature in response to capture, treat-other and baseline events

Systems	Capture	Treat-other	No event
Behavioral dimension			
Postures – different number	+ −	− +	− − n n
Behaviors – different number	+ −	− +	+ n − +
– *negative*	*Y y*	*y y*	*n n n n*
Cardiovascular dimension			
MHR – mean change	+ +	+ +	+ n + +
– extreme value for day	y y	y y	n n n y
– distribution shift	y y	y y	y n y y
– high values elevated	y y	y y	n n n y
– low values suppressed	n n	y n	n n n y
FHR – *mean change*	− +	− −	+ n + n
– extreme value for day	n y	**n n**	**n n n n**
– distribution shift	**y y**	y y	**y y y y**
– high values elevated	n y	y n	n n y n
– low values suppressed	n y	y n	n n y n
MHR–FHR – interaction	n y	y n	**n n n n**
MBP – mean change	+ +	+ +	+ − n−
– extreme value for day	**y y**	**y y**	n y n n
– distribution shift	**y y**	**y y**	y n y y
– high values elevated	**y y**	**y y**	y n n n
– low suppressed	y n	y n	**n n n n**
FBP – mean change	+ +	+ +	+ n n n
– *extreme value for day*	*y y*	**n n**	*n n n n*
– distribution shift	**y y**	y y	**y y y y**
– high values elevated	n y	**y y**	y n n n
– low values suppressed	**n n**	**y y**	y n n n
MBP–FBP – interaction	**y y**	**n n**	y n n y
MVAR – mean change	+ +	+ +	− n n+
– extreme value for day	**y y**	**y y**	n y n n
– *distribution shift*	*y y*	n −	*n n − −*
– high values elevated	**y y**	n −	y n − −
– low values suppressed	**y y**	y −	y n − −
FVAR – mean change	+ +	+ +	+ − + n
– extreme values for day	y n	n y	n n y n
– distribution shift	**y y**	n y	n y y n

(*Continued*)

TABLE 8.3   (*Continued*)

Systems	Capture	Treat-other	No event
– high values elevated	**y y**	n y	n n y n
– low values suppressed	y n	**n n**	n n y y
MVAR–FVAR – interaction	**n n**	**n n**	**n n n n**

Comparisons summarize exposure to stimulus and changes from baseline period to exposure period. **Bold values indicate consistencies across replications of event types.**

Italics indicates consistent replicated differences between baseline and test.

+, increase; −, decrease between baseline and test periods; y, yes; n, no indicates occurrence during test or control time period.

For postures and behaviors, different numbers of unique behaviors are exhibited.

Negative = fear/disturbance, threat/aggression, or stereotypy. Mean change = outside 99.9% confidence interval (CI). Extreme value for day = high or low mean value across 14 5-minute time blocks. Distribution shift = change in significant quintiles from baseline to challenges. High values elevated = values in the highest 20% occurring more often than expected in best-fit model. Low values suppressed = values in lowest 20% occurring less often than expected in best-fit model. Interaction = maternal–fetal interaction term included in model.

values achieved maximum daily values in response to both capture events. This never occurred on the baseline days. Again, random chance should disrupt the consistency of the baselines across repeated testing. The pattern of the maternal VAR quintiles shifted in response to both capture events. During baselines, the maternal VAR term was only included in the best-fit log-linear model on 2 of 4 days, but on both days the pattern of significant quintiles did not shift (Novak, 2002).

Any or all of the variables in Table 8.3 may need to be included in a comprehensive biobehavioral signature for an organism. Table 8.3 is, however, only a partial signature. There are other data from within this distribution that might prove useful. For example, FHR decreased in response to both presentations of the treat-other challenge. In this case it may be more important to observe whether low values are elevated and high values suppressed, as opposed to the opposite which was included in the table. In addition, there are other aspects of both the behavioral and cardiovascular dimensions not covered, as well as other dimensions such as sensory, endocrine, immune, and metabolic which were not measured. In these cases, further empirical research will continue in order to develop the biobehavioral signature that describes an organism's response to various environments.

More replications of each test event are necessary. On most test days the response was consistent. However, on most baseline days, the patterns were variable. Psychological challenges to pregnant females may not result in all-or-none differences between baseline and test days. Instead, the effect may be to alter the probabilities of different patterns appearing in the data. For example, under baseline conditions high maternal heart rate may become elevated in 25% of time blocks. In response to stress, though, that probability may shift to a different value, or even 100% of the time as suggested by Table 8.3. These changes in response probabilities may alter development by restricting the range of responding that can occur. More replication of both baselines and tests would help to illustrate this possibility and is currently underway.

Historically, as analyses have evolved from mean changes, to vagal tone and respiratory sinus arrhythmia, to analyses of the power spectrum, previous types of analyses often get dropped. Unless the two analyses explain the same variance, information is being lost. Often we exchange explanation of one piece of variance for the explanation of another piece. An example of this comes from the analysis of vagal tone rather than mean heart rate. Porges *et al.* (1996, 2003) argue that vagal tone is indicative of vagal influences on the heart and is more informative than simple mean fluctuations in heart rate. He suggests that often when effects on heart rate are expected, changes in vagal tone occur with no change in mean heart rate. This is taken as evidence that vagal tone is a better variable to represent the cardiovascular system. I argue that both measures are important. Future analyses with both variables using multivariate techniques to partial out unique portions of variance may be particularly valuable. In addition, multivariate techniques may help to define how variables cluster into different systems and dimensions.

From the data presented here, it is clear that the prior state of the organism is essential to understanding the reaction of systems and dimensions to environmental events and is particularly important for the formation of the biobehavioral signature. The clearest example of this understanding comes from the postural and behavioral data, which exhibit a floor effect. When the mother exhibited only a single posture or behavior during the time-block prior to the challenge event, the only way the mother could change the number of postures or behaviors being exhibited was to increase them. When the mother exhibited more than one posture or behavior during the block prior to an event test, she can react to the stress with either an increase or a decrease in the number of different behaviors or postures.

This same concept can be applied to the cardiovascular data as well. In terms of mean changes, there are most likely both ceiling and floor effects during normal functioning. In situations where the cardiovascular variable is already at one extreme the only possibility of change is to go in the opposite direction. Therefore, there may be times when the cardiovascular response of an organism to an environmental event is exactly the opposite due to the prior state of the organism. This phenomenon is also true of frequency of particular ranges of values. The occurrence of any given value range cannot be less than zero or greater than the total possible occurrences for a given amount of observation time. Therefore, in order for a fluctuation in cardiovascular signals to occur, there are times that the direction of the change is predetermined by the prior state of the organism. It is also likely that there are times when the prior state of the organism has little to do with the response that occurs. Without these careful considerations of prior state and how we define the variables being studied, consistencies in responding to similar situations often may be mistaken for inconsistencies and visa versa.

Combining systems and dimensions into a single analysis is the eventual goal of the research framework laid out in this proposal. However, testing specific hypotheses within portions of the framework using basic simple experiments is not only important, but essential in building a meaningful framework. As the number of variables, systems, and dimensions in an analysis increases, the analysis and the reporting of the analysis rapidly becomes unwieldy. A balance needs to be achieved between getting work done and including consideration of enough of the environmental and experiential phenomena to produce results that move understanding of the subjective nature of complexity phenomena in a meaningful direction.

Conceptualizing subjectivity in a given individual as untestable is a condition that has plagued this type of research. Perhaps the troubling news from stress and complexity research, namely that there are as many different ideas about both as there are researchers (Rutter, 1988), is not a weakness after all. Perhaps, by incorporating the possibility of variation into our models we can reach a new level of understanding about the concept of complexity.

Translational uses

Testing batteries are needed to produce biobehavioral signatures. An individual's biobehavioral signature would document the range of environments in which adaptive behavior is willingly produced. Practical use of these ideas could allow clinicians to either tailor or document why a strategy that works with one patient would not be expected to work with another. Equally useful would be a demonstration of why two very different strategies might have the same effect with different individuals. For example, an autistic child can be tested and a biobehavioral signature can identify the types of stimulation to which that individual has already habituated, the types of stimulation that are interesting, and the types of stimulation that are too complex to process. No longer is assessment left to a judgment as to which of two stimulations is more challenging to this patient. The biobehavioral signature will allow the therapist or practitioner to systematically assess the types of stimuli that are in the range that will and will not produce adaptive behavior. Then the therapist, educator, or other practitioner can target stimulation that meets the goals of upcoming interactions, rather than rely on objective assessment scales.

As opposed to strategies where children's behavior is assessed and then operant strategies are designed to extinguish unwanted behavior, we can systematically assess the levels of complexity that produce the unwanted behavior so that these levels can be avoided in the future. The levels of complexity to be avoided would be true of both similar and divergent forms of stimulation. Additionally, a biobehavioral signature allows for the targeting of types of stimulation where adaptive behavior is likely to occur and even be willingly produced. The strategies used to keep children concentrated on a computerized learning task can be adapted to each individual's signature. The mode of sensory stimulation can be more visual and tactile to the hearing impaired so as to keep the level of complexity in an acceptable range. Alternatively, auditory information can be augmented for the visually impaired.

More importantly developmentally appropriate tasks can be designed to treat modes of stimulation judged to be necessary or important to adaptive functioning.

In children with auditory deficits, exposure to auditory stimulation can be measured such that it does not overwhelm them. In this case the biobehavioral signature offers insight in two ways. First, it provides background information as to the complexity level to which a child might respond adaptively. This pacer range will, of course, change with development and need to be continually updated as interventions proceed so that the targeted pacer range stays in the stimulating range without becoming excessively complex or too simple (Sackett et al., 1999). Second, further assessment of the biobehavioral signature will allow practitioners to document progress of an intervention in a systematic way. Documenting a patient's reaction to complexity through systems and dimensions allows for comparison of seemingly divergent stimulation from the perspective of the patient himself or herself, thereby going considerably beyond self report which, in many cases of developmental disability, may not be possible.

CONCLUSION

As long as the information provided offers insight on individuals from a developmental perspective, the biobehavioral signature could be used to tailor education programs, therapies, and even home environments. As we increase the amount of time adaptive behavior is willingly produced, we increase access that individuals have to normative developmental processes.

For many developmental disabilities, organism environment interactions involve altered sensory and perceptual processes. The diversity of nonhuman primate species offers opportunities to model biobehavioral signatures in different societies with different biophysical and ecological constraints (Thierry et al., 2004). Furthermore, the species differences themselves between closely related nonhuman primate species are an excellent opportunity to understand individual differences in human populations. However, before developmental disabilities can be studied in either human or nonhuman primate models, we must generate a conceptual structure for interpreting and understanding both the objective and subjective side of sensory and perceptual experience and complexity. By understanding an organism's biobehavioral signature, researchers will come to understand group and individual differences in the bidirectional interactions between structure and function through which complex organisms meet the demands of both typical and atypical development.

Acknowledgments

Data presented in this paper supported by Washington National Primate Research Center Core Grant RR00166 and Center for Human Development and Disability

Core grant NICHD-HD02274. Preparation of the manuscript supported by the Intramural Research Program of the NICHD at the NIH.

REFERENCES

Anway, M. D., Cupp, A. S., Uzumcu, M., and Skinner, M. K. (2005). Epigenetic transgenerational actions of endocrine disruptors and male fertility. *Science* **308**, 1466–1469.

Bakshi, V. P. and Kalin, N. H. (2000). Corticotropin-releasing hormone and animal models of anxiety: Gene-environment interactions. *Biol Psychiatry* **48**, 1175–1198.

Barr, C. S., Newman, T. K., Becker, M. L. *et al.* (2003). The utility of the non-human primate model for studying gene by environment interactions in behavioral research. *Genes Brain Behav* **2**, 336–340.

Barr, C. S., Newman, T. K., Shannon, C. *et al.* (2004). Rearing condition and rh5-HTTLPR interact to influence limbic-hypothalamic-pituitary-adrenal axis response to stress in infant macaques. *Biol Psychiatry* **55**, 733–738.

Baumrind, D. (1993). The average expectable environment is not good enough: a response to Scarr. *Child Dev* **64**, 1299–1317.

Bawkin, H. (1942). Lonliness in infants. *Am J Dis Child* **63**: 30–40.

Bem, D. J. and Allen, A. (1974). On predicting some of the people some of the time: Assessing the personality of situations. *Psychol Rev* **81**, 506–520.

Berlyne, D. E. (1950). Novelty and curiosity as determinants of exploratory behavior. *Br J Psychol* **41**, 68–80.

Berlyne, D. E. (1966). Curiosity and exploration. *Science* **153**, 25–33.

Bevins, R. A. and Besheer, J. (2005). Novelty reward as a measure of anhedonia. *Neurosci Biobehav Rev* **29**, 707–714.

Bolles, R. C. and Fanselow, M. S. (1980). A perceptual-defensive-recuperative model of fear and pain. *Behav Brain Sci* **3**, 291–301.

Cannon, W. B. (1929). Organization for physiological homeostasis. *Psychol Rev* **9**, 399–431.

Capitanio, J. P. (1986). Behavioral pathology. In: Mitchell, G. and Erwin, J. eds. *Comparative Primate Biology*, Vol. 2: *Behavior, Conservation, and Ecology*. New York: A. R. Liss, pp. 411–454.

Coe, C. L. and Levine, S. (1981). Normal responses to mother-infant separation in nonhuman primates. In: Klein, D. F. and Rabkin, J. eds. *Anxiety: New Research and Changing Concepts*. New York: Raven Press, pp. 155–177.

Corneal, S. E. and Nesselroade, J. R. (1994). A stepchild's emotional experience across two households: An investigation of response patterns by p-technique factor analysis. *Multivariate Exp Clin Res* **10**, 167–180.

Coyne, J. C. and Lazarus, R. L. (1980). Cognitive style, stress perception, and coping. In: *Handbook on Stress and Anxiety: Contemporary Knowledge, Theory, and Treatment*. San Francisco: Jossey-Bass Inc., pp. 144–158.

Curtis, W. J. and Cicchetti, D. (2003). Moving research on resilience into the 21st century: Theoretical and methodological considerations in examining the biological contributors to resilience. *Dev Psychopathol* **15**, 773–810.

Dawson, G. and Watling, R. (2000). Interventions to facilitate auditory, visual, and motor integration in autism: a review of the evidence. *J Autism Dev Disord* **30**, 415–421.

Dember, W. N. and Earl, R. W. (1957). Analysis of exploratory, manipulatory, and curiosity behaviors. *Psychol Rev* **50**, 91–96.

Dember, W. N., Earl, R. W., and Paradise, N. (1957). Response by rats to differential stimulus complexity. *J Comp Physiol Psychol* **50**, 514–518.

Desimone, R. (1996). Neural mechanisms for visual memory and their role in attention. *Proc Natl Acad Sci USA* **93**, 13494–13499.

Dufour, A., Despres, O., and Candas, V. (2005). Enhanced sensitivity to echo cues in blind subjects. *Exp Brain Res* **165**, 515–519.

Dunn, J. (2005). Commentary: siblings in their families. *J Fam Psychol* **19**, 654–657.

Dunn, J. and Plomin, R. (1991). Why are siblings so different? The significance of differences in sibling experiences within the family. *Fam Process* **30**, 271–283.

Earl, R. W. (1961). A theory of stimulus selection: Human factors section. *Special Document SD61–132*. Hughes Aircraft Company Ground Systems: Fullerton, CA.

Eifuku, S., De Souza, W. C., Tamura, R., Nishijo, H., and Ono, T. (2004). Neuronal correlates of face identification in the monkey anterior temporal cortical areas. *J Neurophys* **91**, 358–371.

Fanselow, M. S. (1998). Pavlovian conditioning, negative feedback, and blocking: mechanisms that regulate association formation. *Neuron* **20**, 625–627.

Fanselow, M. S. and Bolles, R. C. (1979). Triggering of the endorphin analgesic reaction by a cue previously associated with shock: Reversal by naloxone. *Bull Psychonom Soc* **14**, 88–90.

Ferrari, P. F., Rozzi, S., and Fogassi, L. (2005). Mirror neurons responding to observation of actions made with tools in monkey ventral premotor cortex. *J Cogn Neurosci* **17**, 212–226.

Fleshner, M. and Laudenslager, M. L. (2004). Psychoneuroimmunology: Then and now. *Behav Cogn Neurosci Rev* **3**, 114–130.

Fujita, I. (2002). The inferior temporal cortex: architecture, computation, and representation. *J Neurocytol* **31**, 359–371.

Gibson, E. J. (1969). *Principles of Perceptual Learning and Development*. New York: Appleton.

Gibson, E. J. (1988). Exploratory behavior in the development of perceiving, acting, and the acquiring of knowledge. *Annu Rev Psychol* **39**, 1–41.

Gibson, J. J. (1966). The perceptual systems. In: *The Senses Considered as Perceptual Systems*. Boston: Houghton Mifflin, pp. 47–58.

Gottlieb, G. (1971). Ontogenesis of sensory function in birds and mammals. In: Tobach, E., Aronson, L. A., and Shaw, E. eds. *Biopsychology of Development*. New York: Academic Press, pp. 67–128.

Gottlieb, G. (2002). Developmental-behavioral initiation of evolutionary change. *Psychol Rev* **109**, 211–218.

Gould, E. and Gross, C. G. (2002). Neurogenesis in adult mammals: Some progress and problems. *J Neurosci* **22**, 619–623.

Greenfield, D. B. (1985). Facilitating mentally retarded children's relational learning through novelty-familiarity training. *Am J Ment Defic* **90**, 342–348.

Harlow, H. F. (1953). Mice, monkeys, men, and motives. *Psychol Rev* **60**, 23–32.

Harlow, H. F. (1958). The nature of love. *Am Psychol* **13**, 673–685.

Harlow, H. F. (1959). The development of learning in the rhesus monkey. *Am Sci* **47**, 459–479.

Harlow, H. F. and Harlow, M. (1966). Learning to love. *Am Sci* **54**, 244–277.

Hennessy, M. B., Kaplan, J. N., Mendoza, S. P., Lowe, E. L., and Levine, S. (1979). Separation distress and attachment in surrogate-reared squirrel monkeys. *Physiol Behav* **23**, 1017–1023.

Hughes, R. N. (1965). Food deprivation and locomotor exploration in the white rat. *Anim Behav* **13**, 30–32.

Kamin, L. J. (1969). Predictability, surprise, attention, and conditioning. In: Campbell, B. A. and Church, R. M. eds. *Punishment and Aversive Behavior*. New York: Appleton-Century-Crofts, pp. 279–296.

Kang, S. M. and Shaver, P. R. (2004). Individual differences in emotional complexity: Their psychological implications. *J Person* **72**, 687–726.

Kanner, A. D., Coyne, J. C., Schaefer, C., and Lazarus, R. S. (1981). Comparison of two modes of stress management: Daily hassles and uplifts versus major life events. *J Behav Med* **4**, 1–39.

Kellogg, W. N. (1962). Sonar systems of the blind. *Science* **131**, 399–404.

Kendal, R. L., Coe, R. L., and Laland, R. N. (2005). Age differences in neophilia, exploration, and innovation in family groups of callitichid monkeys. *Am J Primat* **66**, 167–188.

LaGasse, L., Neal, A. R., and Lester, B. M. (2005). Assessment of infant cry: acoustic cry analysis and parental perception. *Ment Retard Dev Disabil Res Rev* **11**, 83–93.

Lazarus, R. S. (1991). *Emotion and Adaptation*. New York: Oxford University Press.

Lecanuet, J. -P., Fifer, W. P., Krasnegor, N. A., and Smotherman, W. P. (eds) (1995). *Fetal Development: A Psychobiological Perspective*. Hillsdale, NJ: Lawrence Erlbaum Associates.

Lewis, M. H. (2004). Environmental complexity and central nervous system development and function. *Ment Retard Dev Disabil Res Rev* **10**, 91–95.

Lewkowicz, D. J. (1994). Reflections on infants' response to temporally based intersensory equivalence: The effect of synchronous sounds on visual preferences for moving stimuli. *Infant Behav Dev* **15**, 297–324.

Lewkowicz, D. J. (2000). The development of intersensory temporal perception: An epigenetic systems/limitations view. *Psychol Bull* **126**, 281–308.

Lickliter, R. (2000). Atypical perinatal sensory stimulation and early perceptual development: Insights from developmental psychobiology. *J Perinat* **20**, s45–s54.

Lobel, M. (1994). Conceptualization, measurement and effects of prenatal maternal stress on birth outcomes. *J Behav Med* **17**, 225–272.

Marks, L. E. (1978). *The Unity of the Senses*. New York: Academic Press.

Mineka, S. (1985). Animal models of anxiety–based disorders: Their usefulness and limitations. In: Tuma, A. H. and Maser, J. eds. *Anxiety and the Anxiety Disorders*. Hillsdale, NJ: Lawrence Erlbaum Associates, pp. 199–244.

Mischel, W. and Peake, P. K. (1982). Beyond deja vu in the search for cross-situational consistency. *Psychol Rev* **89**, 730–755.

Moffit, T. E., Caspi, A., and Rutter, M. (2005). Strategy for investigating interactions between measured genes and measured environments. *Arch Gen Psychiat* **62**, 473–481.

Neuringer, A. (2002). Operant variability: Evidence, functions and theory. *Psychonom Bull Rev* **9**, 672–705.

Neuringer, A. (2004). Reinforced variability in animals and people: implications for adaptive action. *Am Psychol* **59**, 891–906.

Novak, M. S. (2002). A model experimental system for studying prenatal stress in pigtailed macaque monkeys (*Macaca nemestrina*). Doctoral dissertation, University of Washington, Seattle.

Novak, M. F. S. X. (2004). Fetal–maternal interactions: Prenatal psychobiological precursors to adaptive infant development. *Contemp Top Dev Biol* **59**, 37–51.

Novak, M. F. S. X. (2006). Tethering with maternal and fetal catheterization as a model for studying pre- to postnatal continuities. In: Sackett, G. P., Ruppenthal, G. C. and Elias, K. eds. *Nursery Rearing of Infant Monkeys in the 21st Century*. New York: Springer, pp. 513–536.

Peretz, I. and Zatorre, R. J. (2005). Brain organization for music processing. *Annu Rev Psychol* **56**, 89–114.

Piaget, J. (1952). *The Origins of Intelligence in Children*. New York: International Universities Press.

Plomin, R. (1994). *Genetics and Experience: The Interplay between Nature and Nurture*. Thousand Oaks, CA: Sage Publications Inc.

Plomin, R. and Bergeman, C. S. (1991). The nature of nurture: Genetic influences on environmental measures. *Behav Brain Sci* **14**, 373–427.

Plomin, R. and Craig, I. (1997). Human behavioural genetics of cognitive abilities and disabilities. *Bioassays* **19**, 1117–1124.

Plomin, R. and Kovas, Y. (2005). Generalist genes and learning disabilities. *Psychol Bull* **131**, 592–617.

Plomin, R. and Rutter, M. (1998). Child development, molecular genetics and what to do with genes once they are found. *Child Dev* **69**, 1223–1242.

Plomin, R., Asbury, K., and Dunn, J. (2001). Why are children in the same family so different? Nonshared environment a decade later. *Can J Psychiat* **46**, 225–233.

Porges, S. W. (2003). The polyvagal theory: Phylogenetic contributions to social behavior. *Physiol Behav* **79**, 503–513.

Porges, S. W. (2003). The Polyvagal Theory: Phylogenetic contributions to social behavior. *Physiol Behav* **79**, 503–513.

Porges, S. W., Doussard-Roosevelt, J. A., Portales, A. L., and Greenspan, S. I. (1996). Infant regulation of the vagal "brake" predicts child behavior problems: A psychobiological model of social behavior. *Dev Psychobiol* **29**, 697–712.

Rescorla, R. A. and Wagner, A. R. (1972). In: Black, A. H. and Prokasy, W.F. eds. *Classical Conditioning II: Current Theory and Research*. New York: Appleton Century Crofts, pp. 85–99.

Rizzolatti, G. and Craighero, L. (2004). The mirror-neuron system. *Annu Rev Neurosci* **27**, 169–192.

Ronca, A. E. (2003). Studies toward birth and early mammalian development in space. *Adv Space Res* **32**, 1483–1490.

Rosenzweig, M. R. (1996). Psychobiology of plasticity: Effects of training and experience on brain and behavior. *Behav Brain Res* **78**, 57–65.

Rutter, M. (1988). Stress, coping, and development: Some issues and some questions. In: Garmezy, N. and Rutter, M. eds. *Stress Coping and Development in Children*. Baltimore: Johns Hopkins University Press, pp. 1–41.

Rutter, M. (2002). Nature, nurture, and development: From evangelism through science toward policy and practice. *Child Dev* **73**, 1–21.

Rutter, M. and Plomin, R. (1997). Opportunities for psychiatry from genetic findings. *Br J Psychiatry* **171**, 209–219.

Rutter, M., Kim-Cohan, J., and Maughan, B. (2006). Continuities and discontinuities in psychopathology between childhood and adult life. *J Child Psychol Psychiatry* **47**, 276–295.

Sackett, G. P. (1965). Manipulatory behavior in monkeys reared under different levels of early stimulation variation. *Percep Mot Skills* **20**, 985–988.

Sackett, G. P. (1991). Toward a more temporal view of organism-environment interaction. In: Wachs, T. D. and Plomin, R. eds. *Conceptualization and Measurement of Organism Environment Interaction*. Washington D.C.: American Psychological Association, pp. 11–28.

Sackett, G. P., Holm, R. A., and Ruppenthal, G. C. (1976). Social isolation rearing: Species differences in behavior of macaque monkeys. *Dev Psychol* **12**, 283–288.

Sackett, G. P., Ruppenthal, G. C., Fahrenbruch, C. E., Holm, R. A., and Greenough, W. T. (1981a). Social isolation rearing effects in monkeys vary with genotype. *Dev Psychol* **17**, 313–318.

Sackett, G. P., Sameroff, A. J., Cairns, R. B., and Suomi, S. J. (1981b). Continuity in behavioral development: Theoretical and empirical issues. In: Immelmann, K., Barlow, G., Petrinovich, L., and Main, M. eds. *Behavioral Development: The Bielefeld Interdisciplinary Project*. London: Cambridge University Press, pp. 23–67.

Sackett, G. P., Novak, M. F. S. X., and Kroeker, R. (1999). Early experience effects on adaptive behavior: Theory revisited. *Ment Retard Dev Disabil Res Rev* **5**, 30–40.

Sameroff, A. J. (1975). Early influences on development: Fact or fancy? *Merrill-Palmer Q* **21**, 267–294.

Sameroff, A. J. (1981). Development and the dialectic: The need for a systems approach. In: Collins, W. A. ed. *Minnesota Symposium on Child Psychology*, Vol 15. Hillsdale, NJ: Lawrence Erlbaum Associates, pp. 83–103.

Sameroff, A. J. and Mackenzie, M. J. (2003). Research strategies for capturing transactional models of development: the limits of the possible. *Dev Psychopathol* **15**, 613–640.

Sandman, C. A., Wadwha, P. D., Chicz-Demet, A, Dunkel-Schetter, C., and Porto, M. (1997). Maternal stress, HPA activity and fetal/infant outcome. *Ann NY Acad Sci* **814**, 266–275.

Saudino, K. J. (2005). Behavioral genetics and child temperament. *J Dev Behav Pediatr* **26**, 214–223.

Scarr, S. (1992). Developmental theories for the 1990s: development and individual differences. *Child Dev* **63**, 1–19.

Scarr, S. and McCartney, K. (1983). How people make their own environments: A theory of genotype greater than environment effects. *Child Dev* **54**, 424–435.

Schmahl, C., Greffrath, W., Baumgartner, U. *et al.* (2004). Differential nociceptive deficits in patients with borderline personality disorder and self-injurious behavior: laser-evoked potentials, spatial discrimination of noxious stimuli, and pain ratings. *Pain* **110**, 470–479.

Segerstrom, S. C. (2005). Optimism and immunity: do positive thoughts always lead to positive effects? *Brain Behav Immun* **19**, 195–200.

Selye, H. (1975). Confusion and controversy in the stress field. *J Hum Stress* **1**, 37–44.

Selye, H. (1980). The stress concept today. In: *Handbook on Stress and Anxiety: Contemporary Knowledge, Theory, and Treatment*. San Francisco: Jossey-Bass Inc., pp. 127–143.

Shannon, C., Schwandt, M. L., Champoux, M. *et al.* (2005). Maternal absence and stability of individual differences in CSF 5-HIAA concentrations in rhesus monkey infants. *Am J Psychiatry* **162**, 1658–1664.

Shoda, Y. (1999). Behavioral expressions of a personality system: Generation and perception of behavioral signatures. In: Cervone, C. and Shoda, Y. eds. *The Coherence of Personality: Social-cognitive Bases of Personality Consistency, Variability, and Organization*. New York: Guilford, pp. 155–181.

Shoda, Y. and Mischel, W. (2000). Reconciling contextualism with the core assumptions of personality psychology. *Eur J Person* **14**, 407–428.

Shoda, Y., Mischel, W., and Wright, J. C. (1993). The role of situational demands and cognitive competencies in behavior organization and personality coherence. *J Person Soc Psychol* **65**, 1023–1035.

Stansfield, K. H. and Kirstein, C. L. (2006). Effects of novelty on behavior in the adolescent and adult rat. *Dev Psychobiol* **48**, 10–15.

Suess, W. M. and Berlyne, D. E., (1978). Exploratory behavior as a function of hippocampal damage, stimulus complexity, and stimulus novelty in the hooded rat. *Behav Biol* **23**, 487–499.

Suomi, S. J. (2003). Gene-environment interactions and the neurobiology of social conflict. *Ann NY Acad Sci* **1008**, 132–139.

Suomi, S. J. (2005). Aggression and social behaviour in rhesus monkeys. *Novartis Found Symp* **268**, 216–222.

Thierry, B., Singh, M., and Kaumans, W. (eds) (2004). *Macaque Societies: A Model for the Study of Social Organization*. New York: Cambridge University Press.

Timmermans, P. J. A., Vochteloo, J. D., Vossen, J. M. H., Roder, E. L., and Duijghuisen, J. A. H. (1994). Persistent neophobic behaviour in monkeys: A habit or a trait? *Behav Processes* **31**, 177–196.

Turkheimer, E., D'Onofrio, B. M., Maes, H. H., and Eaves, L. J. (2005). Analysis and interpretation of twin studies including measures of the shared environment. *Child Dev* **76**, 1217–1233.

Weaver, I. C., Meaney, M. J., and Szyf, M. (2006). Maternal care effects on the hippocampal transcriptome and anxiety-mediated behaviors in the offspring that are reversible in adulthood. *Proc Natl Acad Sci USA* **103**, 3480–3485.

Weinberg, J. and Levine, S. (1980). Psychobiology of coping in animals: The effects of predictability. In: Levine, S. and Ursin, H. eds. *Coping and Health*. New York: Plenum Press.

Wright, B. A. and Zecker, S. G. (2004). Learning problems, delayed development, and puberty. *Proc Natl Acad Sci USA* **101**, 9942–9946.

Zautra, A. J., Affleck, G. G., Tennen, H., Reich J. W., and Davis, M. C. (2005). Dynamic approaches to emotions and stress in everyday life: Bolger and Zuckerman reloaded with positive as well as negative affects. *J Person* **73**, 1511–1538.

Zeskind, P. S. and Huntington, L. (1984). The effects of within-group and between-group methodologies in the study of perceptions of infant crying. *Child Dev* **54**, 1658–1665.

Zhang, Y., Kuhl, P. K., Imada, T., Kotani, M., and Tohkura, Y. (2005). Effects of language experience: neural commitment to language-specific auditory patterns. *Neuroimage* **26**, 703–720.

Zhou, H., Friedman, H. S., and von der Heydt, R. (2000). Coding of border ownership in monkey visual cortex. *J Neurosci* **20**, 6594–6611.

CHAPTER 9

Prenatal Stress Influences on Neurobehavior, Stress Reactivity, and Dopaminergic Function in Rhesus Macaques

Mary L. Schneider, Colleen F. Moore, Onofre T. DeJesus, and Alexander K. Converse

The notion that the environment in which a fetus develops is critical for long-term health and optimal developmental outcome is well supported by research. Less well recognized is the view that adaptation of the pregnant mother to psychological challenges or threats to homeostasis (i.e. stress) can have adverse effects on the offspring's development. Moreover, the pathways that link prenatal stress to suboptimal development in the offspring remain uncertain. Recent data suggest that stressful experiences in the life of the pregnant mother may be incorporated into the offspring's biology by altering both neural and hormonal processes (Uno *et al.*, 1990; Weinstock, 1997; Roberts *et al.*, 2004). Potential mechanisms that underlie these processes are just beginning to be described.

An important question that arises from this research is whether prenatal stress could contribute to health disparities among the economically less privileged sector of society. In the less privileged sector, individuals are more likely subjected to uncontrollable daily pressures and serious stressors such as frequent relocation and unemployment, along with its cascade of related consequences. Another concern is the clustering of negative events, such that pregnant women of any social class who are under stress are more likely to smoke cigarettes, consume alcohol and engage in other behaviors that can induce adverse developmental outcomes in their offspring. The extent to which we understand how maternal stress may, in part, account for health disparities could yield information which could ultimately be used for the prevention of developmental disabilities.

Primate Models of Children's Health and Developmental Disabilities

This chapter first reviews the evidence establishing a relationship between prenatal stress, birth outcomes, and child behavior problems in humans. Possible mechanisms for these effects are next discussed. Following this, we review the findings from our series of prospective, longitudinal studies with nonhuman primates at the University of Wisconsin-Madison. We describe evidence that prenatal stress compromises birth weight, infant neurobehavior, behavioral/hypothalamic-pituitary-adrenal (HPA) axis reactivity to challenge, response to sensory stimulation, and dopaminergic function in rhesus monkey offspring. Our results, replicated across several primate studies, provide a start at understanding some of the mechanisms underlying the effects of prenatal stress. It is becoming clear that determining the effects of stress during pregnancy on offspring outcome must become a research priority to optimize long-term health and optimal developmental outcome, preventing or minimizing developmental disabilities.

HUMAN STUDIES

The initial human studies of prenatal stress were retrospective. These studies compared the reported prenatal conditions of individuals with various psychiatric diagnoses to those of other individuals without those diagnoses, or compared groups of individuals with different prenatal backgrounds (i.e. war victims or refugees versus those not subjected to these conditions during the prenatal period). These studies are interesting but have methodological problems (see Lobel, 1994, for a review), including that memory is reconstructive and can be biased (Gorin and Stone, 2001), the questionnaires used tended to show skewed distributions (Paarlberg et al., 1995), and alcohol and/or tobacco use, and differential parenting can co-vary with prenatal stress (Cliver et al., 1992).

Researchers in Finland found that an increased risk of schizophrenia and criminality was associated with paternal death during pregnancy compared with paternal death during the first year after birth (Huttunen and Niskanen, 1978). Another retrospective study found that stress during pregnancy was one of four significant predictors of diagnosis (other significant variables were an index of medical risk variables, smoking during pregnancy, and months to term) of attention deficit hyperactivity disorder (ADHD) or undifferentiated attention deficit disorder (UADD) compared with no diagnosis (McIntosh et al., 1995). Meijer (1985) compared a cohort of boys in Israel who were either in gestation or born shortly before the Six Day War of 1967 with a cohort born 2 years later. The war cohort showed delays in developmental milestones such as speech development and independent toileting. Teachers rated children from the war cohort as showing more social withdrawal and less consideration of peers than the comparison cohort.

More recently, work on prenatal stress has been both prospective and longitudinal, and has focused on birth outcomes such as preterm birth and low birth weight (see

Wadhwa and Federenko, 2006). These are important outcomes that are associated with later child functioning. A number of well-controlled, methodologically rigorous, population-based studies involving pregnant women of various racial/ethnic, socioeconomic, and national backgrounds have shown that women under social or psychological stress during pregnancy are at increased risk for shorter gestation/ preterm delivery as well as for reduced fetal growth, low birth weight, and small for gestation age, after statistically controlling for other risk factors (Wadhwa et al., 1993; Hedegaard et al., 1996; Rini et al., 1999; Dole et al., 2003). Because low-income women are at higher risk of having offspring with these same outcomes, it has been hypothesized that the effects of prenatal stress on birth outcomes may be responsible, at least to some extent, for the disparities in health outcomes associated with social disadvantage. This hypothesis is based on the association of economic disadvantage with increased stress and lack of psychosocial resources (Zambrana et al., 1997; Wadhwa and Federenko, 2006).

Prenatal stress and maternal anxiety during pregnancy have also been linked with later child behavior problems. Studies with smaller samples have used direct observational measures and/or standardized testing of infants and children, while studies with large sample sizes have relied on maternal report. Oyemade and colleagues (1994) conducted a prospective study of African American women that included self-report measures of prenatal stress (trait anxiety, stressful life events and "daily hassles") and a standardized test of neonatal neurobehavioral development (Brazelton Neonatal Behavioral Assessment Scale, the BNBAS, see Brazelton, 1984), administered before two weeks of age. Maternal prenatal stress was negatively associated with the attention and habituation measures of the BNBAS. In another one of the first prospective longitudinal studies, Wadhwa (1998) assessed infant temperament with questionnaires as well as with a laboratory-based behavioral assessment and found that higher levels of prenatal stress and maternal stress hormones were associated with a more difficult infant temperament. In addition, maternal anxiety and depression during the prenatal, but *not* the postnatal period, was correlated with infant behavioral reactivity to novelty. In utero measures of fetal arousal and reactivity were also associated with difficult temperament during infancy.

Prospective longitudinal studies also show that the effects of prenatal stress can extend into childhood. The Avon Longitudinal Study on Parents and Children of approximately 7500 children in England found that maternal anxiety, but not depression, during pregnancy predicted child behavior and emotional problems at age 4 (O'Connor et al., 2002a, 2002b). Maternal depression was also associated with child behavior problems, but when prenatal anxiety was entered into the model as a covariate, the association was no longer significant. In a smaller sample of children from this cohort, handedness was assessed by maternal report at 42 months of age from a scale based on six items, including throwing a ball and using a toothbrush. Prenatal stress was associated with mixed handedness at 42 months, independent of parental handedness, prenatal risks, and postnatal anxiety (Glover *et al.*, 2004; Lobel, 2004). Finally, in a sample of 74 10-year-olds from this longitudinal cohort, prenatal anxiety was associated with individual differences in cortisol at awakening after controlling for postnatal maternal anxiety and depression (O'Connor *et al.*, 2005).

Another longitudinal prospective study underway in the Netherlands showed that anxiety during pregnancy averaged across three pregnancy periods predicted decreased attention regulation at three and eight months assessed by observer ratings on the Infant Behavior Rating of the Bayley Scales of Infant Development (Huizink *et al.*, 2002). Moreover, at 27 months of age, anxiety during pregnancy was also related to parental reports of lower temperamental adaptability and higher behavioral problems on the Infant Characteristics Questionnaire and the Achenbach Child Behavior Checklist (Gutteling *et al.*, 2005b). At age 5, children whose mothers had higher morning cortisol during pregnancy and more fear of bearing a child with a handicap, showed higher cortisol on school days (Gutteling *et al.*, 2005a).

Recent longitudinal prospective research has also found that prenatal stress may be related to psychological dysfunction in childhood. In a sample of approximately 72 Belgian children, researchers found that prenatal anxiety predicted attention deficit disorder symptoms and externalizing problems in 8- to 9-year-old children (Van den Bergh and Marcoen, 2004). This study also showed that greater impulsivity during attention tasks at age 15 was associated with prenatal maternal anxiety (Van den Bergh *et al.*, 2005).

One research project has produced the intriguing suggestion that both too little and too much stress might compromise development, while moderate amounts might facilitate neurodevelopment. The sample consisted of low-risk, nonsmoking, financially stable women who were well-educated and who wanted their pregnancies. Prenatal anxiety, nonspecific stress, and depressive symptoms measured during the second half of pregnancy were associated with more *advanced* motor development in children at 24 months of age. Also at 24 months of age, both maternal anxiety and depression were positively correlated with mental development on the Bayley Scales (DiPietro *et al.*, 2006). The authors suggested that mild stress might accelerate growth and development in a fashion similar to the well-characterized inverted U-shaped relationship between arousal and performance. More emotionally reactive mothers might produce more variety in acoustic and somatosensory stimuli in utero. Such stimulation could enhance neural development. Excessive amounts of stimulation, on the other hand, might overwhelm or disturb the capabilities of the fetus (DiPietro *et al.*, 2003; Monk *et al.*, 2003; Novak, 2004). It is important to note that the women in this study did not report traumatic events during pregnancy and they did not show clinical levels of anxiety or depression. Thus these findings may not generalize to women experiencing intense or prolonged stress or clinical populations of anxious or depressed women. Clearly more research is needed to increase our understanding of the effects of different degrees of stressors and the resources available to women.

POSSIBLE MECHANISMS OF PRENATAL STRESS EFFECTS

Recent research evidence also suggests that the effects of prenatal stress on offspring are likely to be produced by complex multifaceted processes. For decades it has been known that stress activates the limbic-hypothalamic-pituitary-adrenal (LHPA) axis. Stressful conditions, physical or psychological challenges that threaten the stability of homeostasis of the organism's internal milieu, result in an elaborate, integrated pattern of behavioral, autonomic, sensorimotor, cognitive, immune, vascular, and neuroendocrine responses including the LHPA axis (Selye, 1936; Sanchez et al., 2001). Information relating to stress or challenges is integrated into the paraventricular nucleus of the hypothalamus by neurons that express corticotropin releasing hormone (CRH) (Swanson et al., 1983). CRH subsequently stimulates the synthesis of proopiomelanocortin, which in turn stimulates the release of stored adrenocorticotropic hormone (ACTH) from the anterior pituitary. Other neuroactive peptides, such as arginine vasopressin, are also expressed by the same neurons that express CRH and act along with CRH to stimulate ACTH release (Plotsky, 1991). ACTH, in turn, causes the release of glucocorticoids from the adrenal gland. Cortisol is the major glucocorticoid in primates, including humans. Glucocorticoids mobilize energy and act as transcriptional regulators for the adrenal cortex. Therefore, cortisol is the major hormonal end product synthesized by the LHPA axis in primates. Glucocorticoids are part of a negative feedback loop that act to prevent further LHPA axis activity at pituitary and central sites mediated by both mineralocorticoid and glucocorticoid receptors in a number of brain regions including the hippocampus (Jacobson and Sapolsky, 1991; de Kloet et al., 1998). Adaptation to a stressful event is regarded as depending in part upon an individual's ability to produce increased levels of cortisol and to reduce the production of cortisol once the stressor has subsided.

A critical issue for explaining the effects of prenatal stress on infant outcome is whether and how activation of the LHPA axis of the *mother* during pregnancy affects the *fetus*. Communication between the mother and fetus occurs through maternal factors acting on placental activity or through exchange of substances carried across the placenta (Wadhwa and Federenko, 2006). Wadhwa and colleagues (2006) suggest that chronic maternal stress may act through a combination of neuroendocrine, immune/inflammatory, and vascular pathways to alter the maternal–placental–fetal (MPF) systems that regulate fetal growth and parturition. Placental CRH is likely to have a critical role in coordinating these effects on fetal growth and parturition. Early or excessive activation of MPF neuroendocrine axis, fetal inflammation from infection, or placental vascular lesions, perhaps acting in concert, may influence birth outcomes (see Wadhwa and Federenko, 2006).

Research has addressed several of the mechanisms that may mediate the effects of prenatal stress on offspring. Several studies suggest that stress-related vascular disorders during pregnancy might contribute to adverse birth outcomes. For example, maternal catecholamines (dopamine, epinephrine, norepinephrine) released during a stressful event could constrict placental blood vessels and cause fetal hypoxia, or reduced fetal oxygenation, which may contribute to alterations in brain development and function. Women who scored as highly anxious on self-report questionnaires had significantly different uterine blood flow velocity waveform patterns than those without high anxiety, suggesting reduced blood flow to the fetus and placenta (Teixeira et al., 1999). High trait anxiety was also associated with altered blood flow in the umbilical artery (Sjostrom et al., 1995).

Effects of maternal stress on fetal oxygenation have also been shown in studies with rhesus monkeys. Meyers (1975) used indwelling catheters placed in the femoral arteries of pregnant monkey mothers and their fetuses and showed that short periods of maternal stress caused fetal heart rate slowing, depression of fetal blood pressure, and impairment in fetal oxygenation. Similarly, Morishima et al. (1978) found that maternal agitation was associated with a decrease in fetal heart rate and arterial oxygenation. Additionally, infusing catecholamines (epinephrine or norepinephrine) into the maternal circulation reduced fetal oxygenation (Adamsons et al., 1971). These studies suggest that stress-induced vascular changes may be a contributing factor for maternal psychosocial stress effects on the offspring.

MATERNAL STRESS HORMONES

Several studies suggest that maternal stress hormones cross the placenta and compromise fetal development and offspring outcome. Human studies show a striking relation between maternal and fetal cortisol levels ($r = 0.58$, Gitau et al., 1998). Experimental studies in rodents support a causal role of maternal stress hormones on the HPA axis of the offspring. For example, repeated exposure to stressful events was found to interfere with the ability of cortisol to return to prestress levels (Takahashi et al., 1998). Moreover, elevated levels of glucocorticoids and beta-endorphins in the rodent dam cross the placental barrier and have been shown to affect areas of the fetal brain that contain glucocorticoid receptors (Maccari et al., 1995; Barbazanges et al., 1996; Weinstock, 1997). When pregnant dams were injected with CRH from day 14 to 21 of gestation, the pups showed effects similar to those observed from prenatally stressed females, including reduced weight of offspring and increased ultrasonic vocalizations during isolation (Williams et al., 1995). Injecting the dams with ACTH during the last third of pregnancy induced higher resting levels of circulating corticosterone in offspring. The offspring also had lower corticosterone levels after a stressful event than controls (Fameli et al., 1994). When glucocorticoid secretion was blocked in rodent dams by adrenalectomy, the effects of prenatal stress on the offspring were also suppressed (Barbazanges et al., 1996). These studies provide compelling evidence for the involvement of the maternal LHPA axis in prenatal stress effects on offspring.

MORPHOLOGICAL AND NEUROTRANSMITTER CHANGES IN PRENATALLY-STRESSED ANIMALS

Because rodent, primate, and human studies all show that glucocorticoids cross the placenta, glucocorticoids are implicated as part of the chain of events by which prenatal stress alters offspring. The question is then how and what aspects of offspring brain morphology and neurotransmitter activity are altered.

Rodent studies show that prenatal stress exposure modifies the levels of biogenic amines in various brain regions (Peters, 1982; Fride and Weinstock, 1988, 1989). Prenatally stressed rodents in comparison to controls exhibit increased dopaminergic activity in the right prefrontal cortex and decreased dopaminergic activity in the right nucleus accumbens. These findings indicate that prenatal stress may alter the cerebral lateralization of dopaminergic activity (Fride et al., 1986). Other studies have found that prenatal stress decreased dopamine activity in striatum at adulthood and increased serotonergic activity in striatum and cerebral cortex (Fameli, et al., 1994). Still others have reported that prenatal stress produced increased concentrations of norepinephrine (NE) and NE metabolites in the rat cerebral cortex and locus coeruleus and reduced dopamine (DA) levels but increased concentration of DA metabolites in the locus coeruleus (Takahashi et al., 1992). Peters (1986, 1988) reported altered development of serotonin neurons in several brain regions in prenatally stressed rats, possibly due to increased levels of plasma tryptophan expressed by the stressed mother (Peters, 1990). Primate studies have shown a substantial reduction in the size of the hippocampus caused by prenatal stress (Coe et al., 2003). Along similar lines, in rodent studies, prenatal stress induced a 50% reduction in brain cell proliferation within the hippocampus at postnatal days 1 and 5 (Van den Hove et al., 2006). Prenatal stress was also found to impair long-term potentiation (LTP) in the hippocampus CA1 region and enhance the adverse effects of acute postnatal stress on the hippocampus in young rat offspring (Yang et al., 2006).

The hippocampal glucocorticoid receptors partially regulate the negative feedback of glucocorticoids on the HPA axis in adult animals (McEwen et al., 1986; de Kloet and Reul, 1987). Studies in rodents found that prenatal stress reduced hippocampal cell proliferation and reduced the number of differentiated new neurons in both young and old prenatally stressed rats. Interestingly, these adverse effects were reversed with neonatal handling (Lemaire et al., 2006). Other rodent studies suggest that permanent change in the expression of corticosteroid receptors in the hippocampus may be responsible for prenatal stress-induced alterations in basal corticosterone levels and LHPA axis responsiveness. Prenatal stress was found to upregulate mineralocorticoid receptor (MR) and glucocorticoid receptor (GR) binding in the hippocampus of adult male rats and to decrease MR binding in the hippocampus of diestrous females and GR binding in the hypothalamus of estrous females (Rimanoczy et al., 2006). Prenatally stressed rats also exhibited increased numbers of FOS proteins in the hippocampus and locus coeruleus, brain regions that regulate feedback control of the HPA axis (Viltart et al., 2006). Alterations in glucocorticoid expression may involve GR promoter DNA methylation patterns, which are important in the complex regulation of gene expression. Thus changes during the prenatal period in promoter demethylation could produce fine-tuning of the promoter and subsequent programming of regulatory events occurring during development. This process could provide a mechanism for control of gene activity by environmental events early in life, which in turn could persist throughout life (Nyirenda *et al.*, 2006).

Prenatal stress also altered an important molecular regulator of development and plasticity, the expression of basic fibroblast growth factor in the prefrontal cortex, entorhinal cortex, and striatum (Fumagalli *et al.*, 2005). This finding provides additional mechanistic evidence of how prenatal stress could induce life-long effects on synaptic function.

Such changes in neurotransmitters and morphology can mediate behavioral effects depending on the parts of the brain in which they occur. For example, alterations in the serotonin system were found to mediate prenatal stress-induced increased pain sensitivity in rats (Butkevich *et al.*, 2005). Also, prenatally stressed rats exhibited a more intense startle response than controls after both groups were treated with a serotonergic agonist. The prenatally stressed group showed reduced binding of the serotonin $5-HT_{1A}$ agonist in the hippocampus (Griffin *et al.*, 2005). The areas of the brain affected (hippocampus, cerebral cortex, locus coeruleus, nucleus accumbens) are those involved in attention, learning, pain, regulation of emotion, regulation of the LHPA axis and stress responsiveness, sensory processing, voluntary control of movement, and complex planning and problem solving, functions found to be adversely impacted by prenatal stress in rodent, primate, and human studies.

ADVANTAGES OF THE NONHUMAN PRIMATE MODEL OF PRENATAL STRESS EFFECTS

Primate studies are important in that they afford the opportunity to use randomized experiments and to establish causal connections between treatments such as prenatal stress and offspring behavior and brain function. Causal inferences are almost always tentative in studies of humans due to uncontrolled confounding factors. Also, the richness of primate social organization and complex cognitive capabilities and the similarity in brain structure to humans make nonhuman primate studies more attractive than rodent models for studying prenatal stress effects on behavior–brain relationships. Due to the shorter lifespan of the nonhuman primate, longitudinal studies are more feasible than with humans, allowing a full assessment of the long-term effects of prenatal stress on offspring outcome through adulthood and even into old age. The normative pattern of rhesus monkey behavioral development is well known so that alterations from norms can be detected (see Suomi, 1997, for a review). A variable of interest can be isolated from other lifestyle factors that may accompany that variable in human studies.

For the study of prenatal stress in particular, the primate model also permits the administration of a standard prenatal stress treatment during a specific period of pregnancy. Also, behavioral, hormonal, and neurotransmitter measurements on the offspring can be standardized and performed under baseline and challenging conditions repeatedly across the lifespan in order to characterize the long-term effects of prenatal stress. Finally, certain nonhuman primates, such as the rhesus monkeys, are quite responsive to mild stress, behaviorally and physiologically, yet they produce viable offspring that are available for prospective longitudinal observations.

NONHUMAN PRIMATE PRENATAL STRESS STUDIES AT THE UNIVERSITY OF WASHINGTON, SEATTLE

There has been a long tradition evaluating the influence of psychosocial stress induced by simple events such as social separation on the physiological and behavioral systems in nonhuman primates (Coe et al., 1978). Studies extending this stress work to prenatal stress are sparse. Newell-Morris and colleagues (1991) reported that exposure to prenatal stress by once-daily capture, five times per week, from day 30 through 130 post conception increased fetal loss in pigtailed macaques that had excellent breeding histories. However, prenatal stress did not affect the abortion rate for females at high risk for a poor pregnancy outcome. Prenatally stressed pigtailed macaque offspring showed higher dermatoglyphic asymmetry (differences in pattern and number of dermal ridges between the left and right hand), a symptom associated with a higher incidence of infant mortality (Newell-Morris et al., 1989). These studies laid the groundwork for a series of prenatal stress studies conducted at the University of Wisconsin Harlow Primate Laboratory.

PRENATAL STRESS EFFECTS IN RHESUS MONKEYS ON NEUROBEHAVIOR, HPA AXIS REGULATION, AND BRAIN FUNCTION AT THE UNIVERSITY OF WISCONSIN

In our primate studies conducted at the University of Wisconsin, the focus is on the developmental course of prenatal stress effects on neurobehavior, stress reactivity, sensory processing, learning, immunity and brain function (Schneider and Moore, 2000; Roberts et al., 2004; Coe and Lubach, 2006). It is important to establish whether small changes during fetal life can persist during postnatal development, as the individual matures and acts on the environment. Moreover, how new experiences can then lead to an increasing divergence in developmental outcomes for certain individuals is a guiding viewpoint of our work (Boyce et al., 1998). Thus, we view prenatal stress as probabilistically increasing the likelihood of certain developmental problems through a sequence of events in which both the fetal and postnatal environments interact dynamically with genetic influences.

Our rhesus monkeys (*Macaca mulatta*) come from a colony of approximately 500 monkeys founded over 50 years ago by Harry Harlow. Approximately 50–100 breedings per year yield infants for developmental studies. The similarity of the physiology of the female monkey to women in terms of the hypothalamic-pituitary axis during pregnancy makes this species an excellent model for examining prenatal stress. All females in our prenatal stress studies were of optimal reproductive age (5–18 years), multiparous and without a history of birth complication or fetal loss.

In all our studies, we randomly assign the breeding females to treatments. In conditions that involve prenatal stress, we expose the pregnant female monkey to a mild daily stressor during specific gestation periods. In the majority of our studies the pregnant female was removed from her home cage, taken in a transport cage to a darkened room, where she heard three noise bursts (115 dB sound at 1 m, 1300 Hz) randomly dispersed over a 10-minute period. She was then returned to her home cage. The stressor was administered five times per week at 1600 hours for females in the stress condition. The stress treatment was chosen as a model of recurrent daily episodic stress. In pilot work we verified that this procedure activates the maternal hypothalamic-pituitary axis, significantly raising plasma cortisol levels (baseline = 25.2 ± 2.2 μg/dL; post stress = 34.8 ± 2.4 μg/dL [mean ± SEM]). Controls were undisturbed during pregnancy, except for normal animal husbandry.

In our first study (Noise stress/nursery rearing) (Schneider, 1992a, 1992b, 1992c), we administered the noise stressor to pregnant females on days 90–145 of a 165-day gestation period. We refer to this timing of the stressor as "middle-to-late gestation" stress. We specifically avoided the very early gestation period in order to minimize the risk of inducing early fetal loss. Similarly, we avoided administering the stressor during late gestation to reduce the chance of inducing early parturition. In the Noise stress/nursery rearing study, the infants were reared in a primate nursery in order to avoid confounding prenatal stress with differential maternal care (see Schneider and Suomi, 1992, for details).

In study 2 (Noise stress/mother rearing) (Schneider et al., 1997, 1999) we compared infants whose mothers received the identical home cage removal and noise stressor (described above) but the gestational timing varied: early gestation (days 45–90 post conception), or middle-to-late gestation (days 90–145 post conception). The monkeys in this study were reared with their mothers for the first six months of life and then placed in mixed-sex peer groups. When they were 24 months old they were removed from their peer groups and housed with same sex peers thereafter.

Because we were interested in the potential role of the pituitary-adrenal hormones in mediating the effects of prenatal stress, we also conducted behavioral assessments of monkeys from a study in which ACTH, a hormone released from the pituitary that stimulates the adrenal gland to release cortisol, was administered to pregnant females from days 120 to 134 post conception (see Schneider et al., 1992, for details) (study 3: ACTH treatment/mother rearing). We also assessed monkeys from a study in which the impact of relocation of the pregnant female, or moving females to a new cage and new social group during pregnancy was assessed (see Schneider and Coe, 1993, for details) (study 4: social relocation/acute versus chronic stress). Previous studies have shown that changes in the composition of monkey social groups does yield changes in behavior, autonomic, and endocrine activity that persist several weeks (Mendoza *et al.*, 1979; Kaplan *et al.*, 1990). Also, naturalistic studies with monkeys have shown that dominance relations during pregnancy influence both reproductive success and infant development (Wasser *et al.*, 1988).

PRENATAL STRESS AND FETAL ALCOHOL EXPOSURE

Because prenatal stress can covary with fetal alcohol exposure in women, how prenatal stress and fetal alcohol exposure together affect development is an issue of concern. Moreover, the issue of whether *moderate* level fetal alcohol exposure, alone or in conjunction with prenatal stress, has adverse effects on development has only recently been studied. Moderate level alcohol exposure is defined as 7–14 drinks per week in humans (Dawson *et al.*, 1995). Rodent studies indicate that moderate alcohol exposure produces deficits in learning and CNS changes including inhibition of cell–cell adhesion, reductions in long-term synaptic potentiation, decreases in hippocampal synaptic plasticity and altered glial development (Savage *et al.*, 1991; Goodlett *et al.*, 1993; Charness *et al.*, 1994; Sutherland *et al.*, 1997).

In study 5 (Noise stress/fetal alcohol exposure), pregnant monkeys voluntarily consumed a moderate alcohol dose once a day. The alcohol was administered alone or in combination with the noise stress treatment described above. All monkeys in this experiment were from mothers screened for their willingness to voluntarily consume 0.6 g/kg in a 6% (v/v) solution sweetened with NutraSweet daily throughout gestation at 4:00 pm (comparable to 1–2 drinks for an average-sized woman). They were randomly assigned to one of four conditions: alcohol, prenatal stress-alone, alcohol with prenatal stress, and no-stress:no-alcohol controls. Alcohol consumption was begun 5 days before breeding and ended at parturition. The control and prenatal stress-alone mothers consumed a sucrose solution that was designed to be approximately equivolemic and equicaloric (8 g/100 mL water) to the alcohol solution. During the remainder of the day, all females were housed under identical conditions, undisturbed except for necessary routine animal husbandry at all times except during the stress exposure.

INFANT OUTCOME VARIABLES

Gestation duration and birth weight

We did not find any significant effects of the relatively mild psychological stressors described above on gestation duration. However, prenatal stress accompanied by prenatal alcohol consumption during gestation resulted in 23% fetal losses (3 of 13 pregnancies aborted or stillborn) (Schneider et al., 1997). Of 51 monkeys born in the noise stress/mother rearing and noise stress/fetal alcohol exposure experiments, the only other fetal loss was to one mother treated with prenatal stress during early gestation. The normal occurrence of fetal loss in our colony is 5% (Schneider et al., 1999) (Table 9.1).

Birth weight was significantly affected by prenatal stress in two of the studies. In study 1 (noise stress/nursery rearing) the mean birth weight of the prenatal-stress group was significantly lower than that in the control group (495 ± 14 and 527 ± 12, respectively) (Schneider, 1992a). In study 2 (noise stress/mother rearing) the early gestation prenatal-stress group had lower birth weights than the middle-to-late gestation prenatal-stress group (476 ± 19 and 544 ± 15, respectively) whereas

TABLE 9.1   Neonatal neurobehavioral effects

Study	Conditions	Prenatal stress findings	Reference
1	Noise stress, rhesus, gestational days 90–145, nursery reared, $n = 12$ per group	↓ Birth weight, motor maturity (tone, response speed, coordination, balance) and motor activity ↑ Distractibility, passivity, and days to independence in self-feeding	Schneider, 1992a
2	Noise stress, rhesus, gestational days 45–90 (early stress), 90–145 (mid–late stress), mother reared, $n = 8$–10 per group	↓ Birth weight, attention, motor activity and postrotary nystagmus (early stress) ↓ Motor maturity and orientation (early and mid–late stress) Early gestation poses the greatest vulnerability to prenatal stress	Schneider et al., 1999
3	ACTH treatment, rhesus, gestational days 120–134, mother reared, $n = 6$ per group	↓ Motor maturity, orientation, state control, and attention ↑ Drowsy state and irritability	Schneider et al., 1992; Roughton et al., 1998
4	Social relocation, squirrel, once mid-gestation vs chronic stress, mother reared, $n = 18$–26 per group	↓ Motor maturity, motor activity, attention, muscle tone, and postrotary nystagmus (chronic)	Schneider and Coe, 1993
5	Noise stress, rhesus, gestational days 90–145 (mid–late stress), mother reared, and alcohol consuming (0.6 g/kg) throughout gestation (alcohol/stress) $n = 10$–12 per group	↓ Birth weight (males) ↓ Coordination and response speed (alcohol/stress) ↓ Motor maturity and orientation	Schneider et al., 1997

↓ and ↑ denote a decrease or increase, respectively, in the dependent variable compared with control animals.

the control group fell in between (498 ± 14) (Schneider *et al.*, 1999). Also, males in study 5 (noise stress/fetal alcohol) in the alcohol/stress condition had reduced birth weights compared with males from the alcohol or control groups (495 ± 18 versus 568 ± 41, and 551 ± 12, respectively) (Schneider *et al.*, 1997). There were no birth weight effects found in the other two studies (ACTH/mother rearing and social relocation/acute versus chronic) (Schneider *et al.*, 1992; Schneider and Coe, 1993). It should be noted, however, that all birth weights were within two standard deviations of what is considered "normal" for rhesus monkeys; therefore none of our subjects would be categorized as having low birth weight analogous to the clinical diagnosis in human infants.

Neonatal neurobehavior

At birth, rhesus macaque infants demonstrate neuromotor capabilities and temperamental characteristics that are remarkably similar to human neonates (Schneider and Suomi, 1992). This facilitates the use of certain tests that can be adapted directly from human tests, such as the Brazelton Newborn Assessment Scale (Brazelton, 1984). The first author of this paper developed the Primate Neonatal Neurobehavioral Assessment (PNNA) as a primate analog of the widely used Brazelton test (Schneider *et al.*, 1991; Schneider and Suomi, 1992). We use four indices of function from the test: Orientation, Motor maturity, Motor activity, and State control.

All infants were tested repeatedly across the first month of life on the PNNA. A pattern of neurobehavioral deficits related to prenatal stress was apparent across studies (see Table 9.1). This profile included shortened attention span (reduced Orientation) and reduced neuromotor performance (reduced Motor maturity). For example, infants from the social relocation/acute versus chronic study whose mothers were relocated repeatedly during pregnancy (i.e. they were moved prior to conception, during early gestation, and during late gestation), had shorter attention spans, poorer motor maturity, and impaired balance compared with monkeys whose mothers experienced a *single* relocation during middle gestation or controls from undisturbed pregnancies. Also, prenatal stress (noise stressor/mother rearing) during an early gestation period was found to produce increased vulnerability for neuromotor deficits compared with prenatal stress during the middle-to-late gestation period (Schneider *et al.*, 1999).

Our overall conclusion is that early gestation stress is linked to more severe motor abnormalities and lower birth weight (Schneider *et al.*, 1999). A question that arises concerns whether this represents a sensitive period. If one considers a sensitive period as a point at which the effects of a teratogen peak, followed by a gradual offset, one could consider that early gestation is a sensitive period for prenatal stress influences on infant functioning (Bornstein, 1989). Moreover, the period during which the early stressor was implemented approximates the period of neuronal migration (gestation days 40 through 70–100). This period represents the time during which fetal cortical brain cells migrate along radial glial fascicles, enter the developing cortical plate, and form ontogenetic columns (Rakic, 1995). Studies have indicated that neuronal cell migration is highly sensitive to various perturbations, such as toxins, viruses and genetic mutations. Further, defective neuronal migration is considered to be a possible cause of both gross and subtle abnormalities in synaptic circuits (Barth, 1987; Rakic, 1988; Caviness *et al.*, 1989), including developmental dyslexia (Galaburuda *et al.*, 1989) and schizophrenia (Kotrla *et al.*, 1997). Correct cell migration is necessary for communication to occur between the early and late forming neurons at critical developmental stages, before they make their synaptic connections (Rakic, 1985).

The alcohol/stress-exposed monkeys in the noise stress/fetal alcohol exposure study differed from controls for neonatal Orientation and Motor maturity. Also, while moderate alcohol consumption alone failed to induce significant impairments in coordination and response speed, exposure to *both* alcohol and prenatal stress produced infants with poorer coordination and slower speeds of responding, suggesting that maternal stress during pregnancy can exacerbate the effects of fetal alcohol exposure in the motor domain (Schneider *et al.*, 1997). This may be because both alcohol and stress activate the maternal LHPA axis. Increased maternal neuroendocrine activity from prenatal stress with fetal alcohol exposure could alter fetal brain development and mediate neurodevelopmental problems. They may act together to enhance or alter the likelihood of adverse consequences beyond that which each variable contributes alone.

Behavioral reactivity from infancy through adolescence

The next question we asked was how the prenatal-stressed infants would respond to a novel, challenging situation and whether the observed patterns of response to stress would persist into adulthood. Over the course of this research program we have conducted a variety of behavior assessments in response to challenges. The behavioral assessments were the most thorough in the noise stress/nursery rearing study. In our other experiments (noise stress/mother rearing and noise stress/fetal alcohol exposure) we assessed behavioral responses to challenge and HPA axis measures at 6 and 18 months (Schneider *et al.*, 2004).

Table 9.2 summarizes the behavioral responses of the monkeys in the noise stress/nursery rearing group and controls to a variety of environmental challenges from six months to adolescence. The first experiment in this series was undertaken when the monkeys were approximately 6 months old (Schneider, 1992c). For this study, the monkeys were tested for 15 minutes each day for three consecutive days in a primate playroom. The playroom consists of a large room containing a variety of movable and non-movable wire mesh climbing and sitting platforms. Testers observed the monkeys through a glass observation window and recorded the duration and frequency of well-defined behaviors using a computer-assisted scoring system.

TABLE 9.2   Novelty challenge results for hand-reared monkeys

Experiment	Novelty challenge test	Behavioral findings	Reference
1	6-month playroom	↓ Exploratory ↑ Self-directed ↑ Sleep ↑ Clinging	Schneider, 1992c
2	8-month separation/reunion	↓ Locomotion, play, climb ↑ Self-grooming ↑ Clinging	Schneider et al., 1998
3	18-month challenge	↓ Proximity, contact ↑ Abnormal (clinging)	Clarke and Schneider, 1993
4	3–4 year playroom	↓ Exploration ↑ Vocalization (at first)	Clarke et al., 1996
5	4-year new group formation	↓ Play and exploration ↑ Stereotypes ↑ General disturbance ↑ Freezing ↑ Self-clasping	Clarke et al., 1996

↓ and ↑ denote a decrease or increase, respectively, in the dependent variable as a function of prenatal stress.

Playroom studies have been employed for decades at the Harlow Primate Laboratory. The typical response for a monkey in this situation is initial wariness followed by eventual exploratory behavior. In fact, this is what we observed in the control monkeys. Controls spent more time than prenatally stressed monkeys in gross motor or exploratory behavior (more locomotion, climbing and exploring the environment). In contrast, the prenatally stressed monkeys showed high levels of disturbance behavior (clinging to each other, and self-directed behaviors). In addition, an unexpected finding was that 50% of the prenatal-stressed monkeys fell asleep, a highly unusual phenomenon (Schneider, 1992c). We speculate that the enhanced disturbance behavior (evidenced by excessive clinging and self-directed behaviors) could have contributed to the prenatal-stressed monkeys lapsing into drowsiness or sleep state. Emde and colleagues (1971) reported that human infants showed an increase in nonrapid eye movement (NREM) sleep following circumcision. Their interpretation was that NREM sleep or quiet sleep served as a coping mechanism after a stressful event, to assist recovery from the perturbation. Similarly, Gunnar and her colleagues found that newborn human infants showed increases in quiet or NREM sleep after circumcision. Moreover, they demonstrated an association between quiet sleep and the re-establishment of baseline adrenocortical hormone levels (Gunnar et al., 1985).

Table 9.2 also presents the behavioral findings when the monkeys were separated from their cage-mates at eight months of age and housed individually for 3 days. During this 3-day period, we scored their behavior three times daily and collected blood samples and CSF samples as well (the physiological measures will be discussed later). Examination of the behavioral data indicated that prenatally stressed monkeys exhibited more self-grooming and more clinging than controls (these are considered abnormal behaviors), and less locomotion, less play and less climbing behaviors (Schneider *et al.*, 1998). Thus, it is evident that the prenatally stressed monkeys exhibited more disturbance behaviors and fewer exploratory behaviors. Interestingly, it is well documented that despair or depression in rhesus monkeys is characterized by sharp decreases in play and increases in passive, self-directed behaviors (Kaufman and Rosenblum, 1967; Suomi *et al.*, 1978). This raises the question of whether prenatal stress might be a risk factor for depression.

When the monkeys were 18 months of age, they were exposed to a sequence of five challenges: baseline, move to a new cage, move to a new cage and exposure to noise stressor, separation from cage-mates, and separation from cage-mates and exposure to noise stressor (the latter four were employed in a random order). There were striking differences across groups in social behaviors, with prenatally stressed monkeys engaging in more clinging to peers (a disturbance behavior for rhesus monkeys) and less species-typical social behavior (i.e. proximity and social contact) (Clarke and Schneider, 1993).

When the monkeys were 3–4 years of age, we observed the prenatally stressed and control monkeys after they were separated from their cage-mates and placed into a new group. New group formation is a challenging event for rhesus monkeys, in that they must negotiate new social structures and relationships (Mendoza *et al.*, 1979). Under these conditions, prenatally stressed monkeys were found to show more stereotyped behavior, self-clasping, and general disturbance behavior compared with controls. They were also observed to spend significantly less time in play behavior, less time in exploratory behavior, and more time in "freezing" behavior or inactivity than controls. Prenatally stressed males showed the greatest amount of clinging to cage-mates (Clarke *et al.*, 1996) (see Table 9.2).

The first study (noise stress/nursery rearing) demonstrates that prenatal stress can have long-lasting effects, extending past infancy into adolescence. Interestingly, the reduction of exploration at six months of age in the playroom, the increased clinging to peers and reduced locomotion during the eight-month social separation and reunion, the increased clinging to peers during the 18 months challenge, and the self-clasping, freezing, and reduced exploration at 4 years of age during new group formation all suggest that a small effect early in life can persist and perhaps even become amplified over the course of maturation.

HYPOTHALAMIC-PITUITARY-ADRENAL AXIS REGULATION

It is well documented in rodents that prenatal stress results in HPA axis dysregulation. Altered HPA axis function might subserve some of the neurobehavioral effects associated with prenatal stress. Thus, we designed manipulations to determine whether our prenatally stressed monkeys would also show alterations in HPA regulation. In the noise stress/nursery rearing study, we examined levels of plasma cortisol in prenatally stressed and control monkeys under baseline and stress (social separation conditions) at eight months of age. Cortisol levels for the entire sample were approximately threefold from an average of 21.5 (1.3)μg/dL at baseline to 73.3 (2.7)μg/dL 2 hours after separation. However, the increase from baseline was significantly larger for the prenatally stressed monkeys. We repeated the social separation a second time in order to obtain test–retest reliability for the cortisol data. The intra-individual consistency from the first to the second separation study was $r = 0.64$, $P < 0.0007$, thus indicating the reliability of our results (Schneider and Moore, 2000).

Our next logical question was to ask whether this apparent increase in HPA reactivity noted in the prenatally stressed monkeys would extend beyond the eight-month period. Therefore, when the monkeys were 18-month-old juveniles, they were exposed to a series of stressors over a six-week period of time (Clarke and Schneider, 1993). Following a baseline period, they experienced the following episodes in a random order: (1) placement in a novel cage; (2) placement in a novel cage and exposure to a noise stressor; (3) separation from peers and placement in an individual cage; and (4) placement in an individual cage and exposure to a noise stressor (Clarke et al., 1994). The prenatal stress group showed higher ACTH values than controls under all four sampling times, indicating that the increased HPA reactivity we had observed in these monkeys at eight months of age persisted into the juvenile period. Cortisol levels were also higher for the prenatally stressed monkeys; however, the effects did not reach significance (see Clarke et al., 1994, for details).

STRIATAL DOPAMINE FUNCTION

A relatively large literature from rodent studies indicates that prenatal stress induces changes in brain neurotransmitter activity (see Weinstock, 2006, for a review). The recent development and availability of neuroimaging techniques has enabled us to conduct noninvasive studies of brain neurotransmitter function associated with prenatal stress in monkeys. Based on rodent findings of alterations in dopamine turnover in the right prefrontal cortex and left striatum and increased density of D_2 receptors in the nucleus accumbens in prenatally stressed rats (Fride and Weinstock 1989; Alonso et al., 1994; Henry et al., 1995), we opted to assess dopamine function in the striatum in our primate studies. We are fortunate to have funding to conduct these studies on monkeys from the noise stress/mother rearing and noise stress/fetal alcohol exposure studies.

In order to assess dopamine system function, we used positron emission tomography (PET). We chose to examine both D_2-binding availability and DA synthesis in the striatum because this brain region is rich in dopaminergic synapses, and therefore should be sensitive to any treatment that alters DA function. The methodology for PET studies of these particular DA system components is well established, resulting from decades of research into neurodegenerative disorders such as Parkinson disease. In addition, we assessed the ratio of PET measures of striatal DA synthesis and D_2 receptor density in each individual animal to assess the balance between the pre- and postsynaptic elements of the striatal dopamine system, given the complementary relationship between DA synthesis and DA receptors. The striatum, which consists of the caudate nucleus and putamen, receives inputs from all cortical areas and the thalamus and projects to frontal lobe areas (prefrontal, premotor, and supplementary motor areas). Those circuits regulate the cortex, play a role in predicting future events, and act in shifting attention sets, movement, and spatial working memory (Herrero et al., 2002).

Striatal DA synthesis was assessed using 6-[^{18}F]-fluoro-m-tyrosine (FMT) as a PET tracer. FMT imaging provides a quantitative measure of dopa decarboxylase activity, reflecting the enzymatic action required to produce DA (Dejesus et al., 2005). The tracer used to assess D_2 receptors was [^{18}F]-fallypride (FAL), an F-18 labeled raclopride analog developed by Mukherjee and colleagues (1997). FAL has a high affinity for D_2 receptors and high brain uptake – almost three times higher than [^{11}C]-raclopride. The details of our methodology are available elsewhere (Roberts et al., 2004). The central goal was to obtain an index of receptor density by assessing FAL binding and an index of dopamine synthesis by using FMT.

Animals were anesthetized with ketamine and maintained on isoflurane. After positioning the animals in the scanner, a transmission scan was first performed for later attenuation correction. Tracer injection of 5 mCi in 1–5 mL normal saline was followed by a dynamic sequence of images over 90 minutes, including a total of 13 frames with duration increasing from 2 to 10 minutes. At the end of scanning the animals were extubated, allowed to awaken, returned to their transport cages, and immediately transported to the animal care facility.

PET images were reconstructed from the raw data using the Ordered Subset Estimation Method (OSEM) (Hudson and Larkin, 1994). Standard regions of interest (ROI) were placed on the occipital cortex (an area known to contain little significant D_2 dopaminergic innervation) in order to produce reference region time–activity curves for use as input functions in graphical analysis. Other ROIs were placed to cover both left and right caudate and putamen in the basal ganglia, and time–activity (TAC) data for these ROIs were generated. The FMT data were analyzed with the graphical approach of Patlak and Blasberg (1985). The FAL data were analyzed using the graphical method of Logan et al. (1996). The Logan method assumes that the unbound components of the tracers are the same in the target regions (e.g. striatum) as in the reference region (occipital cortex).

Monkeys from the prenatally stressed pregnancies (prenatal stress alone and prenatal stress + fetal alcohol exposure) showed upregulated striatal dopamine fallypride binding, indicative of increased dopamine receptor binding (see Roberts et al., 2004, for details). The control mean differed significantly from the prenatally stressed and the alcohol + stress means. This finding is consistent with findings of altered dopamine system function in laboratory rats from prenatally stressed pregnancies (Fride and Weinstock, 1989; Alonso et al., 1994; Henry et al., 1995). We also found an increase in the ratio between D_2 receptor (D_2R) binding and presynaptic DA synthesis in prenatal stress conditions (prenatal stress alone and prenatal stress + fetal alcohol exposure) compared with controls, due mainly to upregulated D_2R binding since no significant difference in dopamine synthesis was observed. Upregulation of D_2R binding may be a feedback response to conditions of lower synaptic dopamine levels due to increased metabolism in the prenatal stress conditions. Either an increase or a decrease in D_2R binding can have repercussions on normal DA functioning.

It has been shown that there is a critical range of DA activity for optimal functioning (Arnsten, 1997). DA is an important neurotransmitter that modulates the activity of many brain regions, promoting both excitatory and inhibitory signals. In particular, DA is a critical regulator of frontal–striatal function, which is identified as a system involved in the modulation of complex cognitive functions, such as attention and executive function, as well as movement, affect, and inhibitory control. DA underlies the response to important or salient events, whether aversive or appetitive (Berridge and Robinson, 1998; Redgrave et al., 1999). If D_2R density is too high, DA function may be more responsive or supersensitive, which could result in heightened sensitivity to novel stimuli and/or unfamiliar situations (Volkow et al., 2002). Higher striatal D_2R binding has been found in unmedicated patients with schizophrenia compared with normal controls (Laruelle, 1998). Higher striatal D_2R density was also found in adolescents with a history of ADHD who had low cerebral blood flow (suggesting low oxygen and/or metabolites) at preterm birth (Lou et al., 2004). Future studies will assess D_1 receptor binding and dopamine transporter binding in this same group of monkeys (noise stress/gestational timing and noise stress/fetal alcohol).

SENSORY PROCESSING

Our most recent assessment of our longitudinal cohort of prenatally stressed monkeys (noise stress/mother rearing and noise stress/fetal alcohol exposure studies) involves a new measure that we developed to assess sensory processing function in monkeys. We were interested in this domain based on a growing literature suggesting that disrupted sensory processing, characterized by over- and underresponsiveness to environmental stimuli, occurs in children with a variety of developmental disabilities (Ayres and Tickle, 1980; Baranek and Berkson, 1994; Miller et al., 1999). The question we posed was whether prenatal stress, alone or in conjunction with moderate level prenatal alcohol exposure, would alter behavioral responses to repeated tactile stimuli. We also explored the relationship of tactile sensitivity to dopamine system function using our PET data described in the previous section. The sensory processing scale we used was adapted from the published sensory processing assessments for children (Baranek and Berkson, 1994; Miller et al., 1999).

When the animals reached 5 to 7 years of age, sensory processing testing was conducted in a 53 × 44 cm testing cage with vertical bars spaced 5.5 cm apart, situated in a dimly lit and sound-shielded room (62 dB) with a masking white noise of 65–70 dB. A human experimenter who stood beside the cage and administered the tactile stimulation items through the bars of the cage tested each monkey individually. A second experimenter videotaped the session for later scoring. Both experimenters were blind to the experimental conditions of the animals. The animals did not know the human experimenters.

The first tactile stimulus consisted of a 12.5 cm feather, which delivered light tactile stimulation. The second stimulus, a 7 cm cotton ball, delivered a soft but slightly firmer tactile stimulation. Finally, the third stimulus, a 15 cm stiff craft brush delivered a scratchy but innocuous tactile stimulation. All stimuli were attached to a 91 cm dowel so the experimenter could maintain a safe distance. Six trials of each stimulus were administered to assess the pattern of responsiveness across trials. On each trial the light feather, soft cotton ball and stiff brush were administered in an invariant order, as listed here, as a swipe to the cheek and neck area. Prior to the first presentation of each stimulus, the stimulus was placed in full view and touching range of the monkey and remained there for approximately 3 seconds. Once the animal looked at the object, the examiner slowly moved the stimulus into the cage and began the series of six trials. Stimuli were applied for approximately 2 seconds per trial, with an inter-trial interval of approximately 2 seconds, and an approximate 4-second pause between each of the textures. The entire testing session lasted for approximately 10 minutes. Following the completion of the testing, the monkey re-entered the transport cage and was immediately returned to the home cage.

Raters blind to the condition and history of the animals scored the videotapes. The total of 18 trials, six trials each with the light feather, soft cotton ball, and stiff brush stimuli were scored for degree of withdrawal from tactile stimuli in 0.25 increments on a 0–3 rating scale with the integers labeled as follows: 0 = no withdrawal; 1 = slight withdrawal, such as turning head away from the stimulation; 2 = moderate withdrawal, such as turning full body away from stimulation; 3 = extreme withdrawal, such as moving body away from stimulation. Inter-rater reliability as percentage agreement within ±0.25 on the rating scale exceeded 99%.

Control monkeys (no prenatal alcohol/no prenatal stress) showed a relatively strong initial withdrawal response to tactile stimuli followed by a decrease in response across trials (the expected pattern of habituation) for feather and cotton textures. Prenatal stress-only monkeys, on the other hand, showed a slightly lower initial response for feather, followed by slightly *increased* magnitude of withdrawal responses across trials (a pattern of *sensitization*). Alcohol/stress monkeys showed a relatively high initial response that remained high compared to controls. Prenatal alcohol-alone monkeys showed relatively high initial response scores that decreased slightly across trials. When we correlated the sensory scores with our PET data described in the previous section, we found reduced habituation to repeated tactile stimulation and higher average withdrawal response was associated with increased striatal D_2R binding and increased ratio of D_2R binding to DA synthesis. This is the first finding to our knowledge linking prenatal stress to behavioral sensitization to repeated non-noxious sensory stimuli. Moreover, we hypothesize that one factor contributing to sensory processing disorders in prenatally stressed offspring may involve alterations in the functioning of basic neural circuits involved in dopaminergic regulatory systems.

SUMMARY

We have reviewed evidence suggesting that maternal stress during pregnancy has important influences on offspring outcome that persist throughout life. While the mechanisms for these effects are not known, they may involve inter-related and possibly overlapping neuroendocrine, immune, vascular, and epigenetic processes. We discussed the effects found in our own primate studies, which include reduced birth weight, altered HPA axis regulation, enhanced sensitization to tactile stimuli, and altered dopaminergic system function. Early gestation appears to be a sensitive period for these effects, and some of the effects seem to be compounded by other factors including exposure to alcohol consumption during pregnancy.

We interpret these findings within the context of probablistic epigenesis, or the view that prenatal perturbations, such as prenatal stress and prenatal alcohol exposure, are not linked in a one-to-one fashion with a particular outcome (Gottlieb and Halpern, 2002). Rather, it is the combination or co-action of environmental factors, genetic factors, neural activity, behavior, and probably timing of their co-action, that leads to certain outcomes. Prenatal stress and prenatal alcohol exposure can be regarded as probabilistically rather than deterministically increasing the likelihood of the expression of developmental disabilities. Further, just as prenatal stress and prenatal alcohol exposure do not necessarily result in the same outcome, more than one developmental pathway can lead to a certain developmental outcome (Cicchetti and Rogosch, 1996).

Further work is needed to increase our understanding of the effects of timing and duration of prenatal stress and interaction with other teratogens, including alcohol, and to explore interventions to optimize long-term outcomes of the offspring. We also need to further explore how prenatal stress influences structure and function of systems that underlie health and disease risk. Moreover, it is important to continue to explore the evolutionary significance of prenatal stress effects. If the HPA axis and/or dopaminergic system of prenatally stressed offspring is permanently altered, does this assist the organism in adapting to the environment into which it will be born? In other words, if the environment is hostile, such as an environment with a potentially high level of predation, is it adaptive for the offspring to be more vigilant than normal? Could this explain the increased dopaminergic receptor density ("super-sensitive" receptors), heightened sensory aversions, and altered HPA axis regulation in prenatally stressed monkeys?

The primate model is useful in that it allows a more detailed and rapid exploration of systems and phenotypic changes and neural pathways affected by prenatal stress than is possible with humans. Further noninvasive neuroimaging studies are planned to explore the effects of prenatal stress on other aspects of the DA system including D_1R binding, DA transporter binding and dynamic studies, including dynamic radioligand displacement studies under challenge. The primate model also allows us to test interventions, including both pharmacologic manipulations and behavioral interventions, such as the behavioral treatments used by occupational therapists to reduce tactile sensitivities (Wilbarger and Wilbarger, 2002). Such interventions are needed to prevent or attenuate the adverse consequences of prenatal stress.

REFERENCES

Adamsons, K., Mueller-Heubach, E., and Meyers, R. E. (1971). Production of fetal asphyxia in the rhesus monkey by administration of catecholamines to the mother. *Am J Obstet Gynecol* **109**, 248–262.

Alonso, S. J., Navarro, E., and Rodriguez, M. (1994). Permanent dopaminergic alterations in the n. accumbens after prenatal stress. *Pharmacol Biochem Behav* **49**, 353–358.

Arnsten, A. F. T. (1997). Catecholamine regulation of the prefrontal cortex. *J Psychopharmacol* **11**, 151–162.

Ayres, A. J. and Tickle, L. S. (1980). Hyper-responsivity to touch and vestibular stimuli as a predictor of positive response to sensory integration procedures by autistic children. *Am J Occup Ther* **34**, 375–381.

Baranek, G. T. and Berkson, G. (1994). Tactile defensiveness in children with developmental disabilities: Responsiveness and habituation. *J Autism Dev Disord* **24**, 457–471.

Barbazanges, A., Piazza, P. V., Le Moal, M., and Maccari, S. (1996). Maternal glucocorticoid secretion mediates long-term effects of prenatal stress. *J Neurosci* **16**, 3943–3949.

Barth, P. G. (1987). Disorders of neuronal migration. *Can J Neurol Sci* **14**, 1–16.

Berridge, K. C. and Robinson, T. E. (1998). What is the role of dopamine in reward: Hedonic impact, reward learning, or incentive salience? *Brain Res Brain Res Rev* **28**, 309–369.

Bornstein, M. H. (1989). Sensitive periods in development: Structural characteristics and causal interpretations. *Psychol Bull* **105**, 179–197.

Boyce, W. T., Frank, E., Jensen, P. S., Kessler, R. C., Nelson, C. A., and Steinberg, L. (1998). Social context in developmental psychopathology: Recommendations for future research from the MacArthur Network on Psychopathology and Development. The MacArthur Foundation Research Network on Psychopathology and Development. *Dev Psychopathol* **10**, 143–164.

Brazelton, T. B. (1984). *Neonatal Behavioral Assessment Scale*, 2nd edn, Vol. 88. Philadelphia and London: Spastics International Medical Publications, J.B. Lippincott.

Butkevich, I. P., Mikhailenko, V. A., and Leont'eva, M. N. (2005). Sequelae of prenatal serotonin depletion and stress on pain sensitivity in rats. *Neurosci Behav Physiol* **35**, 925–930.

Caviness, V. S., Misson, J. P., and Gadisseux, J. F. (1989). Abnormal neuronal migrational patterns and disorders of neocortical development. In Galaburuda, A. M. ed. *From Reading to Neuron.* Cambridge: MIT Press, pp. 405–442.

Charness, M. E., Safaran, R. M., and Perides, G. (1994). Ethanol inhibits neural cell-cell adhesion. *J Biol Chem* **269**, 9304–9309.

Cicchetti, D. and Rogosch, F. A. (1996). Equifinality and multifinality in developmental psychopathology. *Dev Psychopathol* **8**, 597–600.

Clarke, A. S. and Schneider, M. L. (1993). Prenatal stress has long-term effects on behavioral responses to stress in juvenile rhesus monkeys. *Dev Psychobiol* **26**, 293–304.

Clarke, A. S., Wittwer, D. J., Abbott, D. H., and Schneider, M. L. (1994). Long-term effects of prenatal stress on HPA axis activity in juvenile rhesus monkeys. *Dev Psychobiol* **27**, 257–269.

Clarke, A. S., Soto, A., Bergholz, T., and Schneider, M. L. (1996). Maternal gestational stress alters adaptive and social behavior in adolescent rhesus monkey offspring. *Infant Behav Dev* **19**, 451–461.

Cliver, S. P., Goldenberg, R. L., Cutter, G. R. *et al.* (1992). The relationships among psychosocial pro-file, maternal size, and smoking in predicting fetal growth retardation. *Obstet Gynecol* **80**, 262–267.

Coe, C. L. and Lubach, G. R. (2006). Prenatal influences on immunity and the developmental trajec-tory of infant primates. In: Hodgson, D. M. and Coe, C. L. eds. *Perinatal Programming Early Life Determinants of Adult Health and Disease.* London: Taylor and Francis Group, pp. 131–142.

Coe, C. L., Mendoza, S. P., Davidson, J., Smith, E. R., Dallman, M., and Levine, S. (1978). Hormonal response to stress in the squirrel monkey. *Neuroendocrinology* **26**, 367–377.

Coe, C. L., Kramer, M., Czeh, B. *et al.* (2003). Prenatal stress diminishes neurogenesis in the dentate gyrus of juvenile rhesus monkeys. *Biol Psychiatry* **54**, 1025–1034.

Dawson, D. A., Grant, B. F., Chou, S. P., and Pickering, R. P. (1995). Subgroup variation in U.S. drink-ing patterns: Results of the 1992 national longitudinal alcohol epidemiologic study. *J Subst Abuse* **7**, 331–344.

de Kloet, E. R. and Reul, J. M. (1987). Feedback action and tonic influence of corticosteroids on brain function: A concept arising from the heterogeneity of brain. *Psychoneuroendocrinology* **12**, 83–105.

de Kloet, E. R., Vreugdenhil, E., Oitzl, M. S., and Joels, M. (1998). Brain corticosteroid receptor bal-ance in health and disease. *Endocr Rev* **19**, 269–301.

DeJesus, O. T., Flores, L. G., Murali, D. *et al.* (2005). Aromatic L-amino acid decarboxylase turnover *in vivo* in rhesus macaque striatum: A microPET study. *Brain Res* **1054**, 55–60.

Dipietro, J. A., Costigan, K. A., and Gurewitsch, E. D. (2003). Fetal response to induced maternal stress. *Early Hum Dev* **74**, 125–138.

Dipietro, J. A., Caulfield, L. E., Irizarry, R. A., Chen, P., Merialdi, M., and Zavaleta, N. (2006). Prenatal development of intrafetal and maternal-fetal synchrony. *Behav Neurosci* **120**, 687–701.

Dole, N., Savitz, D. A., Hertz-Picciotto, I., Siega-Riz, A. M., McMahon, M. J., and Buekens, P. (2003). Maternal stress and preterm birth. *Am J Epidemiol* **157**, 14–24.

Emde, R., Harmon, R., Metcalf, D., Koenig, K., and Wagonfeld, S. (1971). Stress and neonatal sleep. *Psychosom Med* **33**, 491–497.

Fameli, M., Kitraki, E., and Stylianopoulou, F. (1994). Effects of hyperactivity of the maternal hypo-thalamic-pituitary-adrenal (HPA) axis during pregnancy on the development of the HPA axis and brain monoamines of the offspring. *Int J Dev Neurosci* **12**, 651–659.

Fride, E. and Weinstock, M. (1988). Prenatal stress increases anxiety-related behavior and alters cerebral lateralization of dopamine activity. *Life Sci* **42**, 1059–1065.

Fride, E. and Weinstock, M. (1989). Alterations in behavioral and striatal dopamine asymmetries induced by prenatal stress. *Pharmacol Biochem Behav* **32**, 425–430.

Fride, E., Dan, Y., Feldon, J., Halevy, G., and Weinstock, M. (1986). Effects of prenatal stress on vul-nerability to stress in prepubertal and adult rats. *Physiol Behav* **37**, 681–687.

Fumagalli, F., Bedogni, F., Slotkin, T. A., Racagni, G., and Riva, M. A. (2005). Prenatal stress elicits regionally selective changes in basal FGF-2 gene expression in adulthood and alters the adult response to acute or chronic stress. *Neurobiol Dis* **20**, 731–737.

Galaburuda, A. M., Rosen, G. D., and Sherman, G. F. (1989). The neural origin of developmental dyslexia: Implications for medicine, neurology, and cognition. In: Galaburuda, A. M. ed. *From Reading to Neurons.* Cambridge, MA: MIT Press, pp. 377–404.

Gitau, R., Cameron, A., Fisk, N. M., and Glover, V. (1998). Fetal exposure to maternal cortisol. *Lancet* **352**, 707–708.

Glover, V., O'Connor, T. G., Heron, J., and Golding, J. (2004). Antenatal maternal anxiety is linked with atypical handedness in the child. *Early Hum Dev* **79**, 107–118.

Goodlett, C. R., Leo, J. T., O'Callaghan, J. P., Mahoney, J. C., and West, J. R. (1993). Transient corti-cal astrogliosis induced by alcohol exposure during the neonatal brain growth spurt in rats. *Dev Brain Res* **72**, 85–97.

Gorin, A. A. and Stone, A. A. (2001). Recall biases and cognitive errors in retrospective self-reports: A call for momentary assessments. In: Baum, A., Revenson, T., and Singer, J. eds. *Handbook of Health Psychology.* Mahwah, NJ: Lawrence Erlbaum, pp. 405–413.

Gottlieb, G. and Halpern, C. T. (2002). A relational view of causality in normal and abnormal development. *Dev Psychopathol* **14**, 421–435.

Griffin, W. C., III, Skinner, H. D., and Birkle, D. L. (2005). Prenatal stress influences 8-OH-DPAT modulated startle responding and [3H]-8-OH-DPAT binding in rats. *Pharmacol Biochem Behav* **81**, 601–607.

Gunnar, M. R., Malone, S., Vance, G., and Fisch, R. O. (1985). Coping with aversive stimulation in the neonatal period: Quiet sleep and plasma cortisol levels during recovery from circumcision. *Child Dev* **56**, 824–834.

Gutteling, B. M., de Weerth, C., and Buitelaar, J. K. (2005a). Prenatal stress and children's cortisol reaction to the first day of school. *Psychoneuroendocrinology* **30**, 541–549.

Gutteling, B. M., de Weerth, C., Willemsen-Swinkels, S. H. *et al.* (2005b). The effects of prenatal stress on temperament and problem behavior of 27-month-old toddlers. *Eur Child Adolesc Psychiatry* **14**, 41–51.

Hedegaard, M., Henriksen, T. B., Secher, N. J., Hatch, M. C., and Sabroe, S. (1996). Do stressful life events affect duration of gestation and risk of preterm delivery? *Epidemiology* **7**, 339–345.

Henry, C., Guegant, G., Cador, M. *et al.* (1995). Prenatal stress in rats facilitates amphetamine-induced sensitization and induces long-lasting changes in dopamine receptors in the nucleus accumbens. *Brain Res* **685**, 179–186.

Herrero, M. T., Barcia, C., and Navarro, J. M. (2002). Functional anatomy of thalamus and basal ganglia. *Child's Nervous Syst* **18**, 386–404.

Hudson, H. M. and Larkin, R. S. (1994). Accelerated image reconstruction using ordered subsets of projection data. *IEEE Trans Med Imag* **13**, 601–609.

Huizink, A. C., de Medina, P. G., Mulder, E. J., Visser, G. H., and Buitelaar, J. K. (2002). Psychological measures of prenatal stress as predictors of infant temperament. *J Am Acad Child Adolesc Psychiatry* **41**, 1078–1085.

Huizink, A. C., Robles de Medina, P. G., Mulder, E. J., Visser, G. H., and Buitelaar, J. K. (2003). Stress during pregnancy is associated with developmental outcome in infancy. *J Child Psychol Psychiatry* **44**, 810–818.

Huttunen, M. O. and Niskanen, P. (1978). Prenatal loss of father and psychiatric disorders. *Arch Gen Psychiatry* **35**, 429–431.

Jacobson, L. and Sapolsky, R. (1991). The role of the hippocampus in feedback regulation of the hypothalamic–pituitary–adrenocortical axis. *Endocr Rev* **12**, 118–134.

Kaplan, J. R., Manuck, S. B., and Gatsonis, C. (1990). Heart rate and social status among male cynomolgus monkeys (*Macaca fasicularis*) housed in disrupted social groupings. *Am J Primatol* **21**, 175–187.

Kaufman, I. C. and Rosenblum, L. A. (1967). The reaction to separation in infant monkeys: Anaclitic depression and conservation-withdrawl. *Psychosom Med* **29**, 648–675.

Kotrla, K. J., Sater, A. K., and Weinberger, D. R. (1997). Neuropathology, neurodevelopment and schizophrenia. In: Keshavan, M. S. and Murray, R. M. eds. *Neurodevelopment and Adult Psychopathology.* Cambridge: Cambridge University Press.

Laruelle, M. (1998). Imaging dopamine transmission in schizophrenia: A review and meta-analysis. *Q J Nucl Med* **42**, 211–221.

Lemaire, V., Lamarque, S., Le Moal, M., Piazza, P. V., and Abrous, D. N. (2006). Postnatal stimulation of the pups counteracts prenatal stress-induced deficits in hippocampal neurogenesis. *Biol Psychiatry* **59**, 786–792.

Lobel, M. (1994). Conceptualizations, measurement, and effects of prenatal maternal stress on birth outcomes. *J Behav Med* **17**, 225–272.

Logan, J., Fowler, J. S., Volkow, N. D., Wang, G. J., Ding, Y. S., and Alexoff, D. L. (1996). Distribution volume ratios without blood sampling from graphical analysis of PET data. *J Cerebr Blood Flow Metab* **16**, 834–840.

Lou, H. C., Hansen, D., Nordentoft, M. *et al.* (1994). Prenatal stressors of human life affect fetal brain development. *Dev Med Child Neurol* **36**, 826–832.

Maccari, S., Piazza, P. V., Kabbaj, M., Barbazanges, A., Simon, H., and Le Moal, M. (1995). Adoption reverses the long-term impairment in glucocorticoid feedback induced by prenatal stress. *J Neurosci* **15**, 110–115.

McEwen, B. S., De Kloet, E. R., and Rostene, W. (1986). Adrenal steroid receptors and actions in the nervous system. *Physiol Rev* **66**, 1121–1188.

McIntosh, D. E., Mulkins, R. S., and Dean, R. S. (1995). Utilization of maternal perinatal risk indicators: I. the differential diagnosis of ADHD and UADD children. *Int J Neurosci* **81**, 35–46.

Meijer, A. (1985). Child psychiatric sequelae of maternal war stress. *Acta Psychiatr Scand* **72**, 505–511.

Mendoza, S. P., Coe, C. L., and Levine, S. (1979). Physiological response to group formation in the squirrel monkey. *Psychoneuroendocrinology* **3**, 221–229.

Meyers, R. E. (1975). Maternal psychological stress and fetal asphyxia: A study in the monkey. *Am J Obstetr Gynecol* **122**, 47–59.

Miller, L. J., McIntosh, D. N., McGrath, J. *et al.* (1999). Electrodermal responses to sensory stimuli in individuals with fragile X syndrome: A preliminary report. *Am J Med Genet* **83**, 268–279.

Monk, C., Myers, M. M., Sloan, R. P., Ellman, L. M., and Fifer, W. P. (2003). Effects of women's stress-elicited physiological activity and chronic anxiety on fetal heart rate. *J Dev Behav Pediatr* **24**, 32–38.

Morishima, H. O., Pedersen, H., and Finster, M. (1978). The influence of maternal psychological stress on the fetus. *Am J Obstetr Gynecol* **131**, 286–290.

Mukherjee, J., Yang, Z. Y., Lew, R. *et al.* (1997). Evaluation of d-amphetamine effects on the binding of dopamine D_2 receptor radioligand, ^{18}F-fallypride in nonhuman primates using positron emission tomography *Synapse* **27**, 1–13.

Newell-Morris, L. L., Fahrenbruch, C. E., and Sackett, G. P. (1989). Prenatal psychological stress, dermatoglyphic asymmetry and pregnancy outcome in the pigtailed macaque (*Macaca nemestrina*). *Biol Neonate* **56**, 61–75.

Newell-Morris, L., Carrol, B., Covey, A., Medley, S., and Sackett, G. P. (1991). Postnatal growth and skeletal maturation of experimental preterm macaques (*Macaca nemestrina*). *J Med Primatol* **20**, 17–22.

Novak, M. F. S. X. (2004). Fetal-maternal interactions: Prenatal psychobiological precursors to adaptive infant development. *Curr Top Dev Biol* **59**, 37–60.

Nyirenda, M. J., Dean, S., Lyons, V., Chapman, K. E., and Seckl, J. R. (2006). Prenatal programming of hepatocyte nuclear factor 4alpha in the rat: A key mechanism in the "foetal origins of hyperglycaemia"? *Diabetologia* **49**, 1412–1420.

O'Connor, T. G., Heron, J., and Glover, V. (2002a). Antenatal anxiety predicts child behavioral/emotional problems independently of postnatal depression. *J Am Acad Child Adolesc Psychiatry* **41**, 1470–1477.

O'Connor, T. G., Heron, J., Golding, J., Beveridge, M., and Glover, V. (2002b). Maternal antenatal anxiety and children's behavioural/emotional problems at 4 years. Report from the Avon Longitudinal Study of Parents and Children. *Br J Psychiatry* **180**, 502–508.

O'Connor, T. G., Ben-Shlomo, Y., Heron, J., Golding, J., Adams, D., and Glover, V. (2005). Prenatal anxiety predicts individual differences in cortisol in pre-adolescent children. *Biol Psychiatry* **58**, 211–217.

Oyemade, U. J., Cole, O. J., Johnson, A. A. *et al.* (1994). Prenatal predictors of performance on the Brazelton neonatal behavioral assessment scale. *J Nutr* **124**(suppl 6), 1000S–10005S.

Paarlberg, K. M., Vingerhoets, A. J., Dekker, G. A., and Van Geijn, H. P. (1995). Psychosocial factors and pregnancy outcome: A review with emphasis on methodological issues. *J Psychosom Res* **39**, 563–595.

Patlak, C. S. and Blasberg, R. G. (1985). Graphical evaluation of blood-to-brain transfer constants from multiple-time uptake data: Generalizations. *J Cereb Blood Flow Metab* **5**, 584–590.

Peters, D. A. (1982). Prenatal stress: Effects of brain biogenic amine and plasma corticosterone levels. *Pharmacol Biochem Behav* **17**, 721–725.

Peters, D. A. (1986). Prenatal stress: Effect on development of rat brain serotonergic neurons. *Pharmacol Biochem Behav* **24**, 1377–1382.

Peters, D. A. (1988). Effects of maternal stress during different gestational periods on the serotonergic system in the adult rat offspring. *Pharmacol Biochem Behav* **31**, 839–943.

Peters, D. A. (1990). Maternal stress increases fetal brain and neonatal cerebral cortex 5-hydroxytrypta-mine synthesis in rats: A possible mechanism by which stress influences brain development. *Pharmacol Biochem Behav* **35**, 943–947.

Plotsky, P. M. (1991). Pathways to the secretion of adrenocorticotropin: A view from the portal. *J Neuroendocrinol* **3**, 1–9.

Rakic, P. (1985). Limits of neurogenesis in primates. *Science* **227**, 154–156.

Rakic, P. (1988). Defects of neuronal migration and the pathogenesis of cortical malformations. *Progr Brain Res* **73**, 15–37.

Rakic, P. (1995). Radial versus tangential migration of neuronal clones in the developing cerebral cortex. *Proc Natl Acad Sci USA* **92**, 11323–11327.

Redgrave, P., Prescott, T. J., and Gurney, K. (1999). Is the short-latency dopamine response too short to signal reward error? *Trends Neurosci* **22**, 146–151.

Rimanoczy, A., Slamberova, R., Bar, N., and Vathy, I. (2006). Morphine exposure prevents up-regulation of MR and GR binding sites in the brain of adult male and female rats due to prenatal stress. *Int J Dev Neurosci* **24**, 241–248.

Rini, C. K., Dunkel-Schetter, C., Wadhwa, P. D., and Sandman, C. A. (1999). Psychological adaptation and birth outcomes: The role of personal resources, stress, and sociocultural context in pregnancy. *Health Psychol* **18**, 333–345.

Roberts, A. D., Moore, C. F., DeJesus, O. T. *et al.* (2004). Prenatal stress, moderate fetal alcohol, and dopamine system function in rhesus monkeys. *Neurotoxicol Teratol* **26**, 169–178.

Sanchez, M. M., Ladd, C. O., and Plotsky, P. M. (2001). Early adverse experience as a developmental risk factor for later psychopathology: Evidence from rodent and primate models. *Dev Psychopathol* **13**, 419–449.

Savage, D. D., Montano, C. Y., Otero, M. A., and Paxton, L. L. (1991). Prenatal ethanol exposure decreases hippocampal NMDA-sensitive [3H]-glutamate binding site density in 45-day-old rats. *Alcohol* **8**, 193–201.

Schneider, M. L. (1992a). The effect of mild stress during pregnancy on birth weight and neuromotor maturation in rhesus monkey infants (*Macaca mulatta*). *Infant Behav Dev* **15**, 389–403.

Schneider, M. L. (1992b). Delayed object permanence development in prenatally stressed rhesus monkey infants (*Macaca mulatta*). *Occup Ther J Res* **12**, 96–110.

Schneider, M. L. (1992c). Prenatal stress exposure alters postnatal behavioral expression under conditions of novelty challenge in rhesus monkey infants. *Dev Psychobiol* **25**, 529–540.

Schneider, M. L. and Coe, C. L. (1993). Repeated social stress during pregnancy impairs neuromotor development of the primate infant. *J Dev Behav Pediatr* **14**, 81–87.

Schneider, M. L. and Moore, C. F. (2000). Effect of prenatal stress on development: A nonhuman primate model. In: Nelson, C. A. ed. *The Effects of Early Adversity on Neurobehavioral Development*, Vol 31. Mahwah, NJ: Lawrence Erlbaum Associates, pp. 201–244.

Schneider, M. L. and Suomi, S. J. (1992). Neurobehavioral assessment in rhesus monkey neonates (*Macaca mulatta*): Developmental changes, behavioral stability, and early experience. *Infant Behav Dev* **15**, 155–177.

Schneider, M. L., Moore, C., Suomi, S. J., and Champoux, M. (1991). Laboratory assessment of temperament and environmental enrichment in rhesus monkey infants. (*Macaca mulatta*). *Am J Primatol* **25**, 137–155.

Schneider, M. L., Coe, C. L., and Lubach, G. R. (1992). Endocrine activation mimics the adverse effects of prenatal stress on the neuromotor development of the infant primate. *Dev Psychobiol* **25**, 427–439.

Schneider, M. L., Roughton, E. C., and Lubach, G. R. (1997). Moderate alcohol consumption and psychological stress during pregnancy induces attention and neuromotor impairments in primate infants. *Child Dev* **68**, 747–759.

Schneider, M. L., Clarke, A. S., Kraemer, G. W. *et al.* (1998). Prenatal stress alters brain biogenic amine levels in primates. *Dev Psychopathol* **10**, 427–440.

Schneider, M. L., Roughton, E. C., Koehler, A. J., and Lubach, G. R. (1999). Growth and development following prenatal stress exposure in primates: An examination of ontogenetic vulnerability. *Child Dev* **70**, 263–274.

Selye, H. (1936). A syndrome produced by severe noxious agents. *Nature* **138**, 32–41.

Sjostrom, K., Valentin, L., Thelin, T., and Marsal, K. (1997). Maternal anxiety in late pregnancy and fetal hemodynamics. *Eur J Obstet Gynecol Reprod Biol* **74**, 149–155.

Suomi, S. J. (1997). Early determinants of behaviour: Evidence from primate studies. *Br Med Bull* **53**, 170–184.

Suomi, S. J., Seaman, S. F., Lewis, J. K., DeLizio, R. D., and McKinney, W. T., Jr. (1978). Effects of imipramine treatment of separation-induced social disorders in rhesus monkeys. *Arch Gen Psychiatry* **35**, 321–325.

Sutherland, R. J., McDonald, R. J., and Savage, D. D. (1997). Prenatal exposure to moderate levels of ethanol can have long-lasting effects on hippocampal synaptic plasticity in adult offspring. *Hippocampus* **7**, 232–238.

Swanson, L. W., Sawchenko, P. E., Rivier, J., and Vale, W. (1983). Organization of ovine corticotropin-releasing factor (CRF)- immunoreactive cells and fibers in the rat brain: An immunocytochemical study. *Neuroendocrinology* **36**, 165–186.

Takahashi, L. K., Haglin, C., and Kalin, N. H. (1992). Prenatal stress potentiates stress-induced behavior and reduces the propensitiy to play in juvenile rats. *Physiol Behav* **51**, 319–323.

Takahashi, H., Takada, Y., Nagai, N., Urano, T., and Takada, A. (1998). Effects of nicotine and footshock stress on dopamine release in the striatum and nucleus accumbens. *Brain Res Bull* **45**, 157–162.

Teixeira, J. M., Fisk, N. M., and Glover, V. (1999). Association between maternal anxiety in pregnancy and increased uterine artery resistance index: Cohort based study. *BMJ* **318**, 153–157.

Tsigos, C. and Chrousos, G. P. (2002). Hypothalamic-pituitary-adrenal axis, neuroendocrine factors and stress. *J Psychosom Res* **53**, 865–871.

Uno, H., Lohmiller, L., Thieme, C. *et al.* (1990). Brain damage induced by prenatal exposure to dexamethasone in fetal rhesus macaques 1 Hippocampus. *Brain Res Dev Brain Res* **53**, 157–167.

Van den Bergh, B. R. and Marcoen, A. (2004). High antenatal maternal anxiety is related to ADHD symptoms, externalizing problems, and anxiety in 8- and 9-year-olds. *Child Dev* **75**, 1085–1097.

Van den Bergh, B. R., Mennes, M., Oosterlaan, J. *et al.* (2005). High antenatal maternal anxiety is related to impulsivity during performance on cognitive tasks in 14- and 15-year-olds. *Neurosci Biobehav Rev* **29**, 259–269.

Van den Hove, D. L., Steinbusch, H. W., Scheepens, A. *et al.* (2006). Prenatal stress and neonatal rat brain development. *Neuroscience* **137**, 145–155.

Viltart, O., Mairesse, J., Darnaudery, M. *et al.* (2006). Prenatal stress alters Fos protein expression in hippocampus and locus coeruleus stress-related brain structures. *Psychoneuroendocrinology* **31**, 769–780.

Volkow, N. D., Wang, G. J., Fowler, J. S. *et al.* (2002). Brain DA D$_2$ receptors predict reinforcing effects of stimulants in humans: Replication study. *Synapse* **46**, 79–82.

Wadhwa, P. D. (1998). Prenatal stress and life-span development. In: Friedman, H. S. ed. *Encyclopedia of Mental Health*, Vol 3. San Diego: Academic Press, pp. 265–280.

Wadhwa, P. D. and Federenko, I. S. (2006). Prenatal stress influences human fetal development and birth outcomes: Implications for development origins of health and disease. In: Hodgson, D. M. and Coe, C. L. eds. *Perinatal Programming: Early Life Determinants of Adult Health and Disease*. London: Taylor and Francis Group, pp. 29–46.

Wadhwa, P. D., Sandman, C. A., Proto, M., Dunkel-Schetter, C., and Garite, T. J. (1993). The association between prenatal stress and infant birth weight and gestational age at birth: A prospective investigation. *Am J Obstet Gynecol* **169**, 858–865.

Wasser, S. K., Norton, G. W., Rhine, R. J., Klein, N., and Kleindorfer, S. (1998). Ageing and social rank effects on the reproductive system of free-ranging yellow baboons (*Papio cynocephalus*) at Mikumi National Park, Tanzania. *Hum Reprod Update* **4**, 430–438.

Weinstock, M. (1997). Does prenatal stress impair coping and regulation of hypothalamic-pituitary-adrenal axis? *Neurosci Biobehav Rev* **21**, 1–10.

Weinstock, M. (2006). The role of prenatal stress in the programming of behavior. In: Hodgson, D. M. and Coe, C. L. eds. *Perinatal Programming Early Life Determinants of Adult Health and Disease*. London: Taylor and Francis Group, pp. 241–252.

Wilbarger, J. L. and Wilbarger, P. L. (2002). The Wilbarger approach to treating sensory defensiveness. In: Bundy, A. C., Lane, S. J. and Murray, E. A. eds. *Sensory Integration Theory and Practice*. Philadelphia: F. A. Davis Company, pp. 335–338,

Williams, M. T., Hennessy, M. B., and Davis, H. N. (1995). CRF administered to pregnant rats alters offspring behavior and morphology. *Pharmacol Biochem Behav* **52**, 161–167.

Yang, J., Han, H., Cao, J., Li, L., and Xu, L. (2006). Prenatal stress modifies hippocampal synaptic plasticity and spatial learning in young rat offspring. *Hippocampus* **16**, 431–436.

Zambrana, R. E., Scrimshaw, S. C., Collins, N., and Dunkel-Schetter, C. (1997). Prenatal health behaviors and psychosocial risk factors in pregnant women of Mexican origin: The role of acculturation. *Am J Public Health* **87**, 1022–1026.

CHAPTER 10

Pediatric AIDS: Maternal–Fetal and Maternal–Infant Transmission of Lentiviruses and Effects on Infant Development in Nonhuman Primates

Koen K. A. Van Rompay and Nancy L. Haigwood

INTRODUCTION

Nonhuman primate models for human immunodeficiency virus (HIV) infection and acquired immunodeficiency syndrome (AIDS) have been developed and refined over the last 20 years in an effort to investigate key questions in lentiviral transmission and pathogenesis. With the expansion of the epidemic to a pandemic, there has also developed a greater awareness of affected populations in the developing world. Those most affected include the estimated half million HIV-infected children who are born to infected mothers each year. Vertical transmission of HIV has been studied quite extensively in an effort to understand factors contributing to the timing and route of infection, which can be in utero, intrapartum, or postpartum via breast-milk. The reader is encouraged to consult several outstanding recent reviews on vertical transmission for more comprehensive discussion of the literature (Luzuriaga and Sullivan, 2000; Luzuriaga and Sullivan, 2002; Safrit et al., 2004; Scarlatti, 2004; Wilfert and Fowler, 2007).

It is currently believed that a large portion of vertical transmission occurs around the time of delivery, while earlier in utero transmission accounts for a smaller percentage. The major risk for HIV transmission from mother to child (MTCT) at birth is maternal plasma virus load at the time of birth (Fang et al., 1995), but there is additional risk with breastfeeding (Nduati et al., 2000; Rousseau et al., 2004; reviewed in Nduati, 2000). Thus, infants uninfected at birth who rely on breastmilk for nutrition remain at risk for transmission. Antiretroviral treatment (ART) has shown great benefit for reducing virus load in maternal tissues and blood (Mbori-Ngacha

Primate Models of Children's Health and Developmental Disabilities

et al., 2003) and preventing transmission to infants (Connor *et al.*, 1994; Guay *et al.*, 1999; Musoke *et al.*, 1999; St John *et al.*, 2003). Vertically infected infants are exposed to the virus with a relatively less-developed immune system, and a higher population of CD4-positive cellular targets for virus infection. It is thus not surprising that there is frequently more rapid onset of disease in young patients, with over 80% of infected newborns developing symptoms, AIDS, or dying within the first year, with a median survival of 21 months after AIDS (Bamji *et al.*, 1996). In a more recent study, progression occurred by six months in 15% and by 18 months in 32% of infants (Rich *et al.*, 2000).

The question of which variants are transmitted is highly significant since HIV-1 pathogenesis is in part genetically encoded. In utero versus intrapartum routes of transmission can influence the number of different variants that are acquired by the newborn (Dickover *et al.*, 2001). Transmission occurs in the presence of variable levels of maternal immunity that can be measured *in vitro*, including maternal cytotoxic T cells (CTLs) in blood (Jin *et al.*, 1998) and in milk (Lohman *et al.*, 2003) and passively transferred antibodies, both those with antibody-dependent cellular cytotoxicity (Nag *et al.*, 2004) and neutralizing activity (Dickover *et al.*, 2006; Wu *et al.*, 2006). There is increasing evidence that maternal neutralizing antibodies provide selective pressure and may limit infection (Barin *et al.*, 2006).

The role for each of these immunological components in limiting transmission is an active area of study. ART or HAART (highly active antiretroviral therapy), when present, provides additional selection pressure which can lead to the development of drug-resistant variants if the therapeutic dose is not maintained (Chung *et al.*, 2005; Muro *et al.*, 2005). Several key studies have shown that the genital tract has evidence for compartmentalization, and that these variants include drug-resistant viruses (Kemal *et al.*, 2003; Kemal *et al.*, 2007). This point is even more relevant as we begin to appreciate the level of superinfection and viral recombination that is taking place in patients (Fang *et al.*, 2004; Chohan *et al.*, 2005). Maternal viral variants may reappear in children after several years of infection and could be derived from the reservoirs established during primary infection (Nowak *et al.*, 2002).

In addressing some of these virological and immunological variables in vertical transmission, there were early efforts to develop nonhuman primate models for maternal–fetal and maternal–infant transmission of pathogenic lentiviruses, reviewed recently by Jayaraman and Haigwood (2006) and summarized below. After two decades in development, there are now several models that have been established in Asian macaque species for different stages of MTCT. With these models in hand, research questions can be addressed that would be too difficult or too risky to perform in the clinic. As with all animal models, the nonhuman primate models for AIDS are not perfect replicas of HIV infection in humans, and their expense limits large studies that might derive strongly correlative data such as correlates of immune protection. However, the ability to infect with a defined viral inoculum (Hirsch *et al.*, 1998), coupled with the ability to use well-designed interventions and obtain specimens at necropsy, allows the careful analysis of the fate of the virus and its subsequent

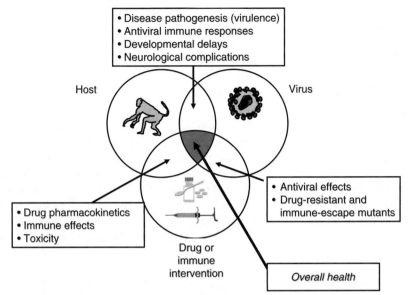

FIGURE 10.1   Overall outcome of antiviral interventions. The ultimate goal of antiviral interventions is to improve the overall health of the host and indefinitely delay disease progression. This outcome is determined by many interactions between the virus, the host, and the intervention strategy, most of which cannot be predicted sufficiently by *in vitro* studies. Potential interventions include antiviral drugs (which target a specific step in the viral cycle), as well as immune-based strategies, such as vaccines and immunomodulators (e.g. cytokines, immune-stimulators and -suppressants). Animal models allow us to control and manipulate many of these variables through experimental approaches that are not feasible in humans, but that allow us to gain further insights into these mechanisms. Examples of such approaches are experimental inoculation of animals with defined virus isolates, *in vivo* depletion of certain immune cells, or administration of monotherapy. (See Plate 4 for the color version of this figure.)

pathology (Figure 10.1). Ironically, the failure of the field to develop vaccines that can deliver "sterilizing immunity" has led to nonhuman primate studies with longer observation times in order to determine whether vaccines or ART have affected acute and steady state virus loads and disease progression (Haigwood, 1999, 2004; Staprans and Feinberg, 2004; Hu, 2005). As a result, the nonhuman primate models have provided an opportunity to investigate developmental and neurological changes, particularly since the lentiviruses were shown to be neurotropic as well as immunosuppressive (Lackner *et al.*, 1991).

Thus, an understanding of the short-term and longer term effects of lentiviral pathogenesis is of major importance. This review analyzes the status of developmental disabilities in humans, the current status of nonhuman primate models for lentivirus infection, and how they have been utilized to study developmental disabilities, and potential treatments and vaccines designed to limit disease and its effects. We conclude with some thoughts about how the models may be used in the future to help inform therapies and vaccines for newborns and children to protect them from the ravages of AIDS.

DEVELOPMENTAL DISABILITIES IN HIV-INFECTED INFANTS AND CHILDREN

Clinical studies have contributed to our understanding of the toll that AIDS takes on health and well-being. The more severe pathogenic effects of HIV-1 on newborns (Rich *et al.*, 2000) compared with juveniles or adults is an important aspect of the disease which has been realized from relatively early in the epidemic, but which has taken on greater significance now that HIV-infected babies and children are living longer with ART. How does this infection impact their neurological development? Are these neurological effects primarily motor, or cognitive? Since our knowledge on the long-term effects of many ARTs is limited, several questions are highly relevant: (1) If ART successfully suppresses viremia, is viral-induced encephalopathy slowed down or completely abrogated? (2) Would years of continuous exposure to antiviral drugs lead to any direct harmful effects on the developing brain?

Early studies documented the significant incidence of encephalopathy in children in the pre-HAART era. HIV encephalopathy in children with perinatally acquired AIDS is a common condition and is associated with severe morbidity evidenced by frequent hospitalizations, severe immunodeficiency, and short survival (Lobato *et al.*, 1995). Both cognitive and motor development effects have been seen in children who acquired HIV via vertical transmission (Blanchette *et al.*, 2001; Blanchette *et al.*, 2002). Using the Bayley Scales of Infant Development, these workers examined 50 infants born to HIV-1-infected mothers, 25 of whom were infected and 25 not. Infected infants were impaired compared with the control group, both on the mental scale and the performance scale used. Using CT scans, they examined 20 HIV-positive infants in this study and observed abnormalities associated with motor development, suggesting the importance of studying myelination and subcortical lesions.

Another group examined the frequency, timing, and factors associated with abnormal cognitive and motor development during the first 30 postnatal months in infants born to HIV-infected mothers. They found that a significant proportion of HIV-infected infants had early and marked cognitive and motor delays or declines (Chase *et al.*, 2000). Importantly, the most current clinical data suggest that children (mean age 11.2 years) with HIV being treated with HAART remain at risk for developing CNS disease (Martin *et al.*, 2006). Although global cognitive functioning among participants was average, children with minimal to moderate CT brain scan abnormalities scored significantly lower than children with normal scans on composite measures of cognitive functioning. This finding was unrelated to viral load, but seemed to track with loss of $CD4^+$ T cells to less than 500 per μL. Thus, conducting neuropsychological assessments in this population remains a key objective to track subtle effects of HIV during slowed but inexorable disease progression.

A key issue in this field is the role of pathogenic effects that are attributed to genetic differences in the unique HIV isolates in each mother and child pair. In part, this has been one of the attractive features of nonhuman primate models, where timing of the infection and genetic identity and pathogenic potential of the infecting virus can be held constant. In the next section, we will briefly review the nonhuman primate models in use today to study pathogenesis.

REVIEW OF LENTIVIRUS MODELS FOR AIDS IN NONHUMAN PRIMATES

The primate lentiviruses include HIV-1, HIV-2, and simian immunodeficiency virus (SIV). The various SIV isolates do not cause clinical disease in their natural reservoir hosts in Africa. SIVcpz, which has been found in chimpanzees, and SIVsm in sooty mangabeys (*Cercocebus atys*) was zoonotically transmitted to humans, resulting in the HIV-1 and HIV-2 epidemic, respectively (Hahn *et al.*, 2000). HIV-1 and HIV-2 both cause an immunodeficiency disease in humans, but the rate of disease progression with HIV-2 is slower than that for HIV-1. It was also discovered that Asian macaque species (*Macaca mulatta*, *Macaca fascicularis*, and *Macaca nemestrina*) develop AIDS after infection with SIV; although the virus first isolated from these macaques was called SIVmac, it was retrospectively found that this transmission occurred accidentally from co-housing asymptomatic SIVsm-infected sooty mangabeys with susceptible *M. mulatta* (rhesus macaques) at primate research facilities in the USA (for a review, see Gardner, 1993). Since then, infection of macaques with any one of a number of SIV isolates (SIVmac, SIVmne, SIVsm) has become an important animal model because it recapitulates many of the events of HIV disease pathogenesis, and the same markers can be used to monitor disease progression.

Some differences exist in timing of pathogenic outcomes and sequelae when comparing SIV infection in rhesus and pig-tailed macaques (*M. nemestrina*) and cynomolgous or long-tailed macaques (*M. fascicularis*), but all can be infected with the various viral isolates in use today. Additional pathogenic virus isolates and derivative molecular clones have been developed by *in vivo* passage of HIV-2-EHO to obtain HIV-2–287 (Watson *et al.*, 1997).

Other *in vivo* passaged viruses include laboratory engineered gene-swapped chimeras of HIV and SIV, termed simian–human immunodeficiency viruses, or SHIV (Hayami *et al.*, 1999). Certain SHIVs designed for vaccine testing bear the HIV *env* gene in a genetic "backbone" of SIV. Other models developed for drug testing include replacing parts of the SIV *pol* gene with that from HIV to obtain reverse transcriptase (RT) SHIVs. The reader is encouraged to consult one or more of several outstanding reviews written about the models, particularly those written more recently to address a number of issues; namely, the severe depletion of immune cells in the gut during the acute stage of infection and its role on disease pathogenesis (Veazey and Lackner, 2005), the role of MHC in susceptibility (Bontrop and Watkins,

2005), the uses of the models for antiviral drug and vaccine research (Haigwood, 2004; Staprans and Feinberg, 2004; Hu, 2005; Van Rompay, 2005), studies on pathogenic effects (Sestak, 2005), the development of low-dose challenge models (Regoes *et al.*, 2005), and MTCT (Ruprecht *et al.*, 1993, 1998, 1999; Jayaraman and Haigwood, 2006).

Routes of infection

While some macaque models studied natural pre- and postnatal transmission from infected mothers to their newborns, other studies used experimental inoculations of the offspring in which the newborn/infant animals are then usually reared in specialized nurseries. Both models have their advantages and disadvantages, and their choice depends largely upon the study question. The natural transmission studies, while ideal to study the pathogenesis and events during transmission, have as disadvantage that, as in humans, transmission occurs only in a portion of the animals. While more "natural," this aspect hampers the ability to reach statistical significance in intervention strategies because animal numbers are limited. In contrast, experimental inoculation of animals with tissue culture-propagated virus can use a virus inoculum selected at achieving 100% infection of untreated animals, facilitating the testing of therapeutic and prophylactic intervention strategies. One caveat of such experimental inoculation studies, however, is that the virus inoculum is generally larger than what is typically observed in human exposures to HIV. This may underestimate the prophylactic efficacy of intervention strategies with moderate potency. In other words, a strategy with moderate efficacy in the animal model may be more effective to reduce transmission in humans. Since the lentiviruses have been shown to be transmitted by several mucosal routes (Trichel *et al.*, 1997), it was reasonable to assume that infection of dams could lead to transmission to their offspring during or after birth via cervical, vaginal, or breastmilk virus and exposure to blood.

Intravenous infection of dams and peripartum transmission

Early work to set up a model for vertical transmission focused on mating SIV-infected females to establish pregnancy in the presence of persistent viremia, with low to moderate rates of live birth due to the late stage of the infection in the dam. Furthermore, rates of transmission to the infants were low and peripartum exposure was eliminated by Cesarean section delivery. These procedures were supplanted by models of intravenous infection of pregnant dams in mid-gestation with SIV (Amedee *et al.*, 1995) and later, with SHIV (reviewed in Jayaraman and Haigwood, 2006; and shown in Jayaraman *et al.*, 2004, 2007) Overall, these models provide significant but variable levels of vertical transmission, in the range of that in humans, if vaginal birth and suckling are allowed. Retention of pregnancy was high (9/10) when infection with pathogenic SHIV was initiated in the second trimester. All three routes of infection (in utero, intrapartum, and postpartum) were recorded with SHIV-SF162P3 infection of dams. Even with the pregnant dam experiencing acute viremia with over 10^7 copies of viral RNA per mL, only 10% in utero transmission was observed, consistent with the early SIV studies (Jayaraman et al., 2007).

Disease progression was more rapid in macaques infected in utero, similar to clinical data for HIV-1 in newborns, and dependent on virus load in all infants. Three infants had infection that was highly controlled to the point of lack of detection in the blood after the acute phase, presumably by their immune responses. These models have been very useful in measuring passive transfer of neutralizing antibodies (Jaspan et al., 2004) and for determining which variants are transmitted, discussed below. This type of model, with a less than 50% transmission rate and relatively slow T cell loss and pathogenesis, could be amenable to analysis of cognitive and developmental outcomes comparing infected with uninfected newborns as they develop.

Catheterization of pregnant dams and intra-amniotic infection

The direct injection of SIV into amniotic fluid during late gestation resulted in six of seven rhesus monkeys infected at birth. All infected neonates were viable and showed signs of disease, including low birth weights, lymphadenopathy, and rashes (Fazely et al., 1993). Ho and colleagues have developed a model where catheters have been implanted in the mother and infant for ease of monitoring the virus in the amniotic fluid and transmission to the infant. Twelve infants were born to dams that had been inoculated and infected with HIV-2–287 in the third trimester of pregnancy (Ho et al., 1996, 2001). Eight of these pregnancies had undergone surgical procedures in the form of maternal amniotic catheters or maternal amniotic and fetal carotid artery and jugular vein catheters. Data indicated that catheterization had little or no impact on behavioral development. Seven infants were vertically infected (Worlein et al., 2005) and five were not infected, as measured by polymerase chain reaction (PCR) and coculture on repeated testing.

Direct oral infection of newborns

To mimic intrapartum HIV transmission, a newborn macaque model has been developed in which the animals are inoculated shortly after birth by the oral route with one or two high doses of SIV aimed at giving 100% infection of untreated animals (Baba et al., 1994). Because HIV transmission through breastfeeding involves repeated exposure of the nursing infant to relatively low amounts of virus in the breastmilk, an infant macaque model has been developed in which the monkeys are hand-held and bottle-fed repeatedly with low amounts of virus (three inoculations per day × 5 days) either at birth and/or at four weeks of age. This model has been used to test the prophylactic efficacy of drugs and neonatal vaccines against SIV (Baba et al., 1994; Van Rompay et al., 2005, 2006). This method of oral inoculation with multiple exposures to establish infection has become more common as investigators have utilized stocks of SIV or SHIV that are transmitted by mucosal routes and which utilize the coreceptor CCR5.

Oral infection with SIV has also been shown to be more readily achieved than mucosal infection by other routes, and these studies demonstrated the differential pathogenesis of SIV strains that are highly attenuated for disease in juveniles, as discussed below (Ruprecht et al., 1998, 1999). SHIV infection by this route also leads to the establishment of high titers of virus and more rapid disease progression (Jayaraman et al., 2007).

Breastmilk transmission models

SIV/DeltaB670 has been used in a model for breastmilk transmission from macaques infected after giving birth and then allowed to suckle their newborns. Transmission occurred at multiple time points throughout the period of lactation. During the chronic stage, SIV infection correlated with a threshold level of virus expression and more persistent shedding in milk (Martin Amedee et al., 1996; Amedee et al., 2004). These data suggest that suckling is a major route of transmission and may be related to maternal virus load, as in humans (Rousseau et al., 2004). The transmitted genotype in the dam typically was found in plasma before milk and was coincident with increased milk viral loads (Rychert et al., 2006). Thus, specific viral genotypes are selectively transmitted to infants through breastfeeding.

Intracerebral infection

Several studies have used intracerebral virus inoculation using macrophage-tropic and neuroadapted SIV isolates, followed by early euthanasia to study the early pathogenesis of SIV encephalopathy (Joag et al., 1994). Brains of animals showed mild to moderate neuropathological changes, characterized by gliosis, microglial nodules, perivascular infiltrates and occasional white matter pallor and low numbers of infected cells. These findings were similar to those observed in animals following intravenous inoculation. These results provided evidence for the low susceptibility of resident microglia to SIV replication during the early stages of infection (Hurtrel et al., 1991, 1993; Smith et al., 2005), so this route of intracerebral inoculation is now rarely used.

Determinants of disease progression in newborn macaques

The pathogenesis of lentiviral disease is dependent upon several factors. Similar to vertically acquired infection of HIV-1, there is a correlation between viral RNA setpoint (i.e. the viral RNA levels in plasma established after the acute viremia stage) and disease progression of infant macaques (Van Rompay et al., 2004b). Accordingly, the factors that do influence time to disease progression consist of viral factors such as its intrinsically encoded pathogenic potential (Marthas *et al.*, 1995) and host factors including age and the genotype of the host (Bontrop and Watkins, 2005). These together determine the host's ability to mount effective antiviral immune responses to control virus replication.

The importance of dose is not fully understood and currently an area of active investigation in these models. SIV and SHIV are both differentially infectious when delivered by different routes, with intravenous infection requiring many log_{10} lower doses to establish infection by this route than by a traumatic mucosal exposure. However, once infection is established, pathogenic outcome is indistinguishable.

Surprisingly, and disturbingly, newborn rhesus macaques were shown to progress rapidly to AIDS upon infection with a highly attenuated vaccine strain of SIVmac that had been nonpathogenic in juvenile and adult rhesus (Baba *et al.*, 1999). Ultimately, adult macaques also succumbed to disease as well but on a longer timeline.

One reason for more rapid disease progression in young nonhuman primates may be the relatively rapid spread to tissues within days of infection (Milush *et al.*, 2004; Abel *et al.*, 2006). As seen with adult HIV (Guadalupe *et al.*, 2003; Betts *et al.*, 2004; Brenchley *et al.*, 2004) and SIV (Heise *et al.*, 1994) infection there is evidence for profound and selective depletion of jejunum lamina propria CD4$^+$ T cells in neonatal macaques within 21 days of infection, preceded by large numbers of SIV-infected cells in this compartment (Veazey *et al.*, 2003). Neonates with less CD4$^+$ T-cell depletion in tissues generally have higher viral loads. These detailed virological and phylogenetic analyses of viral distribution have provided valuable data to better understand tissue distribution of SIV and SHIV in newborns (Miyake *et al.*, 2004).

Certain variants are transmitted from dam to newborn, suggesting a bottleneck for transmission, as seen in humans. The Tulane group has observed evidence for both genotypic and phenotypic selection in transplacental transmission of SIV and suggest a critical role for macrophages in fetal infection in utero (Amedee *et al.*, 1995; Martin Amedee *et al.*, 1996). There is evidence for tissue compartmentaliza-tion in these models that supports the concept of distal site and "protected" site replication that may contribute to the inability of host immunity and ART to fully clear HIV infection. Current work suggests some novel methods to reactivate SIV from latent reservoirs by induction (Shen *et al.*, 2007).

Future studies no doubt will bring additional data to bear on the role of specific variants and the role of host immunity in selection of viral variants and suppression of viremia.

EFFECTS OF INFECTION ON INFANT DEVELOPMENT AND NEUROBIOLOGY

Lentivirus-infected nonhuman primates have been shown to exhibit behavioral and neurological pathology similar to HIV-infected humans, and they offer a means

TABLE 10.1   SIV infection and neurological development: examples of a few representative studies

Host	Virus	Major findings/ concepts	Reference
M. mulatta	SIV/17E-Fr + SIV/DeltaB670	Predictable encephalitis through inoculation of mixture of neurotropic SIV/17E-Fr and immunosuppressive SIV/DeltaB670	Zink et al., 1999; Clements et al., 2002
	SIVmac251	Growth restriction, fetal death; rapid disease, encephalopathy	Tarantal et al., 1993, 1995; Marthas et al., 1995
	DeltavpuSHIV (KU–1bMC33)	Rapid CD4+ depletion and neurological disease	McCormick-Davis et al., 2000
	SIVmac R71/17E	Neuronal degeneration in basal ganglia	Marcario et al., 2004
	SIVmac182	Disturbance of CNS neuronal circuitry (delayed latency of sensory-evoked potentials)	Fox et al., 2000
	SIVmac182, SIVmac230	Impaired neuropsychological test performance	Weed et al., 2003, 2004; Weed and Steward, 2005
	SIVmac239Δ3	Rapid disease in newborns	Baba et al., 1999
	SIVmac1A11	Normal development	Marthas et al., 1995; Tarantal et al., 1995
M. nemestrina	HIV-2-287	Delayed cognitive and motor development	Kinman et al., 2004; Worlein et al., 2005

to examine the effects of lentivirus infection while controlling for confounding factors inherent in human populations. Several key studies in adult macaques have been important to our understanding of the effects of lentivirus infection on the brain. As discussed above, the brain is a key compartment and the obvious major source of virus causing neurological compromise. This factor alone underscores the need for animal models in which it is possible to follow viral dissemination, compartmentalization, local and systemic immunity, fetal and infant development, and effects on behavior. In this section we will summarize the findings in these models, grouped by the timing of the infection. A brief summary of these models is shown in Table 10.1.

Neurological effects in juvenile and adult infection models

Before addressing the effects on infants, we briefly summarize studies that have examined effects on older animals using neurotropic isolates of SIV, summarized in several papers from the Johns Hopkins group, which was the first to establish these isolates (Clements et al., 1994; Zink and Clements, 2002; Zink et al., 2006). One of these studies (Clements *et al.*, 2002) demonstrated that neurotropic isolates of SIV show viral RNA in brain during the acute phase, but viral DNA persistence continues and may be the source, based on phylogenetic data of recrudescing virus throughout the body later in infection. Other recent studies in the SIV model have utilized a combination of low-dose wild-type SIV (DeltaB670 or mac) and high-dose SIV/17E-Fr, a dual infection that leads to rapid development of AIDS and a high frequency of CNS lesions (Amedee *et al.*, 1995).

An examination of encephalitic and nonencephalitic brains of macaques infected with a neurovirulent, neuroendotheliotropic strain of SIV demonstrated the presence of DNA damage indicative of apoptosis in neurons, endothelial cells, and glial cells of the CNS (Adamson *et al.*, 1996). This model has allowed more detailed analysis of the roles of specific genes as pathogenic determinants. For example, truncated Vpu in one SHIV isolate (McCormick-Davis *et al.*) led to rapid CD4$^+$ T-cell loss and neurological disease (McCormick-Davis *et al.*, 2000). Other studies have focused on mechanisms of pathogenesis, implicating the glucose transporter protein (Mankowski *et al.*, 1999).

Dopamine has been implicated in neuro-AIDS, since HIV-infected patients and SIV-infected macaques show decreases in dopamine and dopamine transporter (Marcario *et al.*, 2004). Additional data suggest that cognitive impairments due to dopamine dysfunction are involved in the cognitive impairments observed (Gray *et al.*, 2006). Consistent with HIV-infected patients, SIV-infected monkeys tend to be impaired in tasks dependent upon intact frontal corical and/or subcortical functioning (Weed *et al.*, 2003, 2004; Weed and Steward, 2005). The role of the virus in causing neurophysiological and movement abnormalities has been investigated by infecting rhesus macaques with a microglia-grown SIV stock. This resulted in delayed latency of sensory-evoked potentials, a measure of CNS neuronal circuitry (Fox *et al.*, 2000).

Fetal infection

Ultrasound-guided intraperitoneal inoculation of fetal rhesus macaques has been performed as a model to investigate the effects of viral infection on fetal development (Tarantal *et al.*, 1993, 1995). Variables in these studies included the timing of inoculation and the virulence of the virus inoculum. Inoculation with virulent uncloned SIVmac251 at each of the three trimesters of gestation led to intrauterine growth retardation and/or fetal death, with the most severe adverse events for those fetuses inoculated during the first and second trimester of the pregnancy. The surviving fetuses developed disease within nine months after birth (Tarantal *et al.*, 1993, 1995). In contrast, fetal macaques that were inoculated with the clone SIVmac1A11, which was previously found to induce transient low-level viremia and no disease in juvenile and adult macaques (Marthas *et al.*, 1989), had normal growth and no disease (Tarantal *et al.*, 1995).

Peripartum or in utero infection

A group at the University of Washington (Worlein *et al.*, 2005) demonstrated that cognitive and motor deficits in HIV-2-infected infant macaques closely resemble those observed in human infants and children infected with HIV. They examined cognitive and motor development in infant macaques vertically infected with HIV-2–287 after maternal–infant catheterization. Subjects were 20 infant pigtail macaques (*Macaca nemestrina*); 8 controls born to uninfected dams and 12 born to infected dams. Infected infants attained cognitive and motor milestones at significantly later ages than controls. Uninfected infants born to infected dams attained developmental milestones at later ages than controls on all tasks, but this reached statistical significance only for the fine motor task. Attainment of milestones was not correlated with viral dose, maternal $CD4^+$ levels at parturition or infant viral RNA levels at birth. Attainment of milestones was negatively correlated with infants' proportions of $CD4^+$ lymphocytes at birth and significantly correlated with proportions of $CD4^+$ lymphocytes two weeks after birth, indicating poorer performance in those infants with a more rapid $CD4^+$ depletion. Defects were observed after necropsy in cortex degeneration.

These results are similar to those seen in adult macaques, where neuron death and morphological alterations in the basal ganglia of rapid progressors may contribute to the motor impairments similar to those seen in human neuro-AIDS (Marcario *et al.*, 2004).

Infant infection

The potential of three genetically distinct SIV isolates to induce simian AIDS was investigated in newborn macaques that were inoculated within 3 days after birth (Marthas *et al.*, 1995). The purpose was to determine how viral variants may affect disease progression in human pediatric AIDS. The three virus isolates were previously shown to range from pathogenic (SIVmac251 and SIVmac239) to nonpathogenic (SIVmac1A11) when inoculated intravenously into juvenile and adult rhesus macaques. Newborn macaques infected with virulent SIVmac251 had persistently high virus levels in peripheral blood, had poor antibody responses to SIV and to test antigens due to rapid immunosuppression, and exhibited poor weight gain that was already evident during the first 10 weeks of life. Most SIVmac251-infected infant macaques animals developed clinical disease (AIDS) within 3–4 months of infection, which is much faster than the disease course that is typically seen in adult macaques infected with SIVmac251 (Marthas *et al.*, 1995; Otsyula *et al.*, 1996).

Infection with SIVmac239 also resulted in persistently high viremia, but animals developed antibody responses to SIV and test antigens, had initially normal weight gain, but eventually developed disease. In contrast, animals inoculated with SIVmac1A11 had transient low-level viremia, seroconverted, had normal weight gain and no clinical disease (Marthas *et al.*, 1995; Otsyula *et al.*, 1996). Thus, this study demonstrated that when different SIV isolates are used, neonatal macaques exhibit patterns of infection, virus levels, growth and clinical disease progression that are very similar to those observed in HIV-infected children, ranging from rapid progressors to slow or long-term nonprogressors. This provides support for utilizing this model to study the mechanisms underlying the differences in disease progression in HIV-infected human infants and to test intervention strategies.

Intrathecal transmission

To compare pathogenic outcomes of direct blood and CNS inoculation, three newborns (*M. nemestrina*) were infected with HIV-2–287 by each route (Kinman *et al.*, 2004). There was detectable viral RNA in CSF and productive infection in blood, concomitant with a severe and rapid decline in $CD4^+$ T cells by 10 weeks post infection. There were delays in reaching cognitive and motor milestones, which paralleled neuropathological changes. Deficits in neurobehavioral development were particularly evident in infants infected by the intravenous route. This small study suggests that additional work with this virus may be important for evaluating drugs to limit developmental defects.

APPLICATIONS OF THE MODELS FOR ANTIVIRAL INTERVENTION STRATEGIES TO LIMIT VIRAL SPREAD AND MAINTAIN CD4 CELLS

For most of the last 20 years, research emphasis has been placed on the development of antiviral treatments and prophylactic vaccines for adults. Thus the vast majority of experiments in nonhuman primates has followed this paradigm, and only recently has there been a more concerted effort to study vaccines and drug therapies in newborns. An exception to this is chemoprophylaxis, as drug studies aimed at preventing infection were already initiated and demonstrated to be effective in human and macaque infants since the early 1990s. The goal of ART is to prevent loss of T cells in the gut and in the periphery, and studies performed in adult macaques indicate that this is achievable and that timing is important (George *et al.*, 2005).

Antiviral drug prophylaxis and therapy

Over the past decade, the application of ART, particularly the nucleoside RT inhibitor zidovudine (AZT) and the non-nucleoside reverse transcriptase inhibitor nevirapine, has achieved significant reductions in vertical HIV-1 transmission in developed and resource-poor areas (for review, see Newell, 2000). This is an interesting case in point, as zidovudine and nevirapine were shown first to have prophylactic antiviral effects *in vivo* in the nonhuman primate (Van Rompay *et al.*, 1992; Grob *et al.*, 1997).

The infant macaque model has been used to study the therapeutic effects of antiviral therapy on established infection. While untreated infant macaques that were infected at birth with virulent SIVmac251 demonstrated growth retardation and rapid disease course (within 3–6 months), several studies demonstrated that early antiviral drug therapy with compounds such as zidovudine (AZT), and tenofovir (PMPA) reduced viremia, and improved growth and clinical outcome (Van Rompay *et al.*, 1995, 1996). Tenofovir was more effective than zidovudine, as some of the SIV-infected infant macaques that received prolonged tenofovir monotherapy have achievedlow/undetectable viremia and remained healthy for more than 7–12 years (Van Rompay *et al.*, 2004a; unpublished data). In another study, zidovudine treatment of SIVsmm/B670-infected infant macaques led to improved survival, a delay in the occurrence of motor impairment, and lower virus levels and quinolinic acid levels in cerebrospinal fluid (Rausch *et al.*, 1994, 1995).

Primate models have also used drugs to examine questions related to viral reservoirs during ART (Shen *et al.*, 2003), and the emergence and clinical implications of drug-resistant mutants (reviewed in Van Rompay, 2005). The effects of drug treatment on neurophysiological and movement abnormalities was investigated by infecting macaques with the microglia-grown stock described above and then treating with PMPA. During two months' duration of drug treatment, plasma and CSF virus loads were reduced and there was improvement in sensory-evoked potentials, but there was no effect upon the SIV-induced decline in movement; PMPA in uninfected controls had no effect on gross motor activity (Fox *et al.*, 2000).

While antiviral drugs are expected to improve clinical markers by reducing virus replication, antiviral drugs may also have toxic effects that directly impact fetal and postnatal development. Very few studies, however, have investigated the biological effects of long-term administration of anti-HIV drugs in primate models. When pregnant cynomolgus macaques were treated early in gestation with efavirenz at a regimen that gives plasma levels similar to the human regimen, approximately a quarter of the offspring had severe birth defects. These findings contributed to the clinical recommendation that pregnant women should avoid taking efavirenz (Chersich *et al.*, 2006).

Prolonged treatment of infant macaques with a high dose of the antiviral drug tenofovir led to a Fanconi-like syndrome (proximal renal tubular disorder) with glucosuria, hypophosphatemia, growth restriction, and bone pathology (osteomalacia), that was largely reversible upon dose reduction or withdrawal. Growth restriction was also reported in some newborn macaques born to adult female macaques that were treated during pregnancy with a high dose of tenofovir (30 mg/kg subcutaneously once daily). At first, this may be surprising since drug levels in the fetus were 10-fold lower than maternal drug levels (Tarantal *et al.*, 1999, 2002). However, as explained previously (Van Rompay *et al.*, 2004a), this growth restriction most likely occurred because this high-dose tenofovir regimen induced a proximal renal tubular disorder with severe phosphate depletion in the mothers. The reduced transplacental transfer of phosphate led to fetal deprivation, rather than a direct transplacental effect of tenofovir on the growing fetus.

In other studies, prolonged treatment of infant macaques starting at birth with a lower dose of tenofovir, still higher than the currently used human regimen, proved to be safe. The study included follow-up of animals for more than 10 years, with continued treatment during pregnancy and follow-up of their offspring for up to 4 years (Van Rompay et al., 2004a; Van Rompay, unpublished data).

One recent study utilized minocycline, an antibiotic with potent anti-inflammatory and neuroprotective properties, to test its effectiveness in preventing encephalitis and neurodegeneration caused by a neurotropic SIV infection (Zink et al., 2005). Although a small pilot study, there was evidence that the minocycline treatment inhibited SIV replication in the brain, reduced the severity of encephalitis, and decreased CNS inflammatory markers. This is an example of the benefits of testing of novel therapies in the nonhuman primate model to support new concepts prior to clinical work.

Immuno-prophylactic and -therapeutic interventions

Due to a relatively short half-life (hours to days), drug-based approaches are costly and require frequent administration of the drug regimen. Another approach to attempt to prevent or treat infection is by immune-based approaches, which may offer the benefit of prolonged antiviral activity (weeks to months). A number of studies have investigated passive or active immunization strategies aimed at preventing infection or, if infection is not prevented, lowering viremia and delaying disease progression. Such strategies may be useful to reduce perinatal and postnatal HIV transmission.

Several research groups have demonstrated that passive immunization with monoclonal antibodies or SIV hyperimmune serum was able to protect infant macaques against infection following oral inoculation with virulent SIV or SHIV isolates (Van Rompay et al., 1998; Ferrantelli et al., 2003, 2004). Purified polyclonal immunoglobulin (IgG) with a high titer of neutralizing antibody against SIV, termed SIVIG, given to juvenile macaques as a therapeutic one day and two weeks post infection led to significant delays in time to onset of AIDS and evidence for accelerated neutralizing antibody responses that may have contributed to viral control (Haigwood et al., 2004).

These studies were followed by observation of low-level, possibly occult, virus infection in newborns born to SHIV-infected dams and allowed to suckle (Jayaraman et al., 2007). Transmission occurred in the presence of passively transferred maternal neutralizing antibodies, which may again have had a role in limiting viral replication and/or spread in vivo. There was evidence for selection of maternal neutralization escape variants, as seen in humans (Wu et al., 2006).

Active immunization studies have been performed in which newborn macaques were immunized on a rapid immunization schedule consisting of a primary immunization at birth, and a booster immunization at two and/or three weeks later (Van Rompay *et al.*, 2003, 2005). The animals were challenged orally with virulent SIV at four weeks of age. Animals that remained uninfected were re-inoculated with virus again as juveniles. Attenuated poxvirus-based vaccines (MVA, ALVAC) were shown to be safe and immunogenic and they provided partial protection against infection following repeated low-dose oral exposures to SIV. Those animals that became infected fared better than unimmunized control animals (Van Rompay *et al.*, 2005). Based on these results the HPTN-027 trial is currently testing an ALVAC-vector based HIV-1 vaccine in breastfeeding infants of HIV-1-infected women in Uganda (http://www.hptn.org).

Combined antiviral drug and immune-based interventions

Although HAART has led to significant advances in the treatment of HIV infection, it is currently not able to eradicate infection. The prolonged use of these drugs is often associated with problems of costs, compliance, toxicity, and resistance. Withdrawing drug treatment usually leads to rapid viral rebound and eventual disease progression (Chun *et al.*, 1999). Since antiviral immune responses contribute to controlling virus replication, a number of approaches have also been tested that combine both drug therapy and immune-based interventions. The ultimate goal is boosting antiviral immune responses that can achieve immunologic control on virus replication so that drugs can be withdrawn for prolonged periods. Such immunization strategies include: (1) structured treatment interruptions, aimed at inducing progressively smaller viral rebounds that boost immune responses against autologous virus, and (2) a number of active immunization strategies including adoptive transfer (Hel *et al.*, 2000; Lori *et al.*, 2000; Lisziewicz *et al.*, 2005). While these studies demonstrated a benefit of the immunotherapy, it has also become clear that these strategies are most effective in inducing immunologic control of virus replication when initiated during the early stages of infection – prior to the severe depletion of antiviral immune cells (Veazey *et al.*, 1998) and with virus isolates that are of moderate virulence. When initiated during chronic infection or with the use of the most virulent SIV isolates, sustained immunological control was generally not observed in the absence of drug therapy (Van Rompay *et al.*, 2006).

These findings are consistent with those obtained in macaques that are infected with viral mutants with reduced *in vitro* susceptibility to tenofovir. Both continued tenofovir administration and antiviral immune responses were required to achieve prolonged suppression of viremia to undetectable levels, as either tenofovir withdrawal or $CD8^+$ immune cell depletion resulted in a viral rebound (reviewed in Van Rompay, 2005).

SUMMARY AND FUTURE DIRECTIONS TO
REDUCE DEVELOPMENT DISABILITIES

Prevention of neurological and developmental disabilities in children exposed to HIV-1 can best be limited by reducing the risk of infection, and in cases of infection limiting virus replication and disease development. In the preceding sections we have presented evidence from nonhuman primate models showing that developmental disabilities stem directly from viral pathogenesis, and thus efforts effective in limiting pathogenesis are of critical importance to benefit children. The nonhuman primate models can continue to play a critically important role in this endeavor, particularly as access to ART becomes more widespread. Ultimately, the overall health of the nonhuman primate is influenced by the host, the virus, and the treatment – drug or immune intervention – which is ideally beneficial but may be limited in its efficacy due to toxicities or pharmacokinetics (Figure 10.1). Although host and virus would not be controllable in human populations, if the effects of the virus can be minimized and the interventions maximized the area of health can be envisioned as increasing and developmental disabilities concomitantly decreasing.

There are several key questions that remain to be addressed. These are issues that can be challenging to study in human newborns either due to sample access or due to risk of perturbing health by frequent sampling. Prevention of peripartum transmission remains a key objective worldwide, and the availability of less-expensive, fast-acting ART has been an important tool to limit the rate of HIV-1 infection where applied. However, additional strategies are needed, especially in resource poor areas with limited healthcare facilities. Most families in these areas have more than one child. Thus, the use of nevirapine to reduce intrapartum transmission will raise the risk of drug-resistant variant selection both for these mothers, which can affect their future treatment options, and their subsequent infants (Eshleman *et al.*, 2005; Lockman *et al.*, 2007).

Prevention strategies to limit breastmilk transmission are another priority area (Chersich and Gray, 2005). Mothers and infants in the developing world have severely limited alternatives to breastfeeding, which besides offering good nutrition has the value of providing protective immunity to endemic pathogens. Accordingly, affordable and simple drug- or immune-based intervention strategies are needed to reduce HIV transmission through breastmilk (Gaillard *et al.*, 2004). Once effective vaccines are developed they will also be important to apply to the breastfeeding population.

Finally, there have been reports over the years of very low-level or "transient" infection in newborns (Bryson *et al.*, 1995), a finding that has been difficult to substantiate in some cases but may be akin to the very low level infections seen in "exposed seronegative" patients with evidence for CTL responses (Zhu *et al.*, 2003). An understanding of "exposed uninfected" newborns – and whether they are infected and at risk for developmental disabilities – is an area for future diagnostic research.

In conclusion, progress in the last two decades in the development of lentiviral nonhuman primate models for vertical transmission, combined with progress in noninvasive imaging and cognitive testing for these valuable animals should lead to further important insights in our understanding of the risks to HIV-infected newborns and children and ultimately to vaccines and therapies that can provide the promise of a healthy childhood worldwide.

Dedication

The authors wish to dedicate this chapter to the many dedicated animal caretakers, researchers, and their nonhuman primate subjects, which have together provided this level of understanding of lentiviral disease and its neurological sequelae.

REFERENCES

Abel, K., Pahar, B., Van Rompay, K. K. *et al.* (2006). Rapid virus dissemination in infant macaques after oral simian immunodeficiency virus exposure in the presence of local innate immune responses. *J Virol* **80**, 6357–6367.

Adamson, D. C., Dawson, T. M., Zink, M. C., Clements, J. E., and Dawson, V. L. (1996). Neurovirulent simian immunodeficiency virus infection induces neuronal, endothelial, and glial apoptosis. *Mol Med* **2**, 417–428.

Amedee, A. M., Lacour, N., Gierman, J. L. *et al.* (1995). Genotypic selection of simian immunodeficiency virus in macaque infants infected transplacentally. *J Virol* **69**, 7982–7990.

Amedee, A. M., Rychert, J., Lacour, N., Fresh, L., and Ratterree, M. (2004). Viral and immunological factors associated with breast milk transmission of SIV in rhesus macaques. *Retrovirology* **1**, 17.

Baba, T. W., Koch, J., Mittler, E. S. *et al.* (1994). Mucosal infection of neonatal rhesus monkeys with cell-free SIV. *AIDS Res Hum Retroviruses* **10**, 351–357.

Baba, T. W., Liska, V., Khimani, A. H. *et al.* (1999). Live attenuated, multiply deleted simian immunodeficiency virus causes AIDS in infant and adult macaques. *Nat Med* **5**, 194–203.

Bamji, M., Thea, D. M., Weedon, J. *et al.* (1996). Prospective study of human immunodeficiency virus 1-related disease among 512 infants born to infected women in New York City. The New York City Perinatal HIV Transmission Collaborative Study Group. *Pediatr Infect Dis J* **15**, 891–898.

Barin, F., Jourdain, G., Brunet, S. *et al.* (2006). Revisiting the role of neutralizing antibodies in mother-to-child transmission of HIV-1. *J Infect Dis* **193**, 1504–1511.

Betts, M. R., Price, D. A., Brenchley, J. M. *et al.* (2004). The functional profile of primary human antiviral CD8+ T cell effector activity is dictated by cognate peptide concentration. *J Immunol* **172**, 6407–6417.

Blanchette, N., Smith, M. L., Fernandes-Penney, A., King, S., and Read, S. (2001). Cognitive and motor development in children with vertically transmitted HIV infection. *Brain Cogn* **46**, 50–53.

Blanchette, N., Smith, M. L., King, S., Fernandes-Penney, A., and Read, S. (2002). Cognitive development in school-age children with vertically transmitted HIV infection. *Dev Neuropsychol* **21**, 223–241.

Bontrop, R. E. and Watkins, D. I. (2005). MHC polymorphism: AIDS susceptibility in non-human primates. *Trends Immunol* **26**, 227–233.

Brenchley, J. M., Schacker, T. W., Ruff, L. E. *et al.* (2004). CD4+ T cell depletion during all stages of HIV disease occurs predominantly in the gastrointestinal tract. *J Exp Med* **200**, 749–759.

Bryson, Y. J., Pang, S., Wei, L. S., Dickover, R., Diagne, A., and Chen, I. S. (1995). Clearance of HIV infection in a perinatally infected infant. *N Engl J Med* **332**, 833–838.

Chase, C., Ware, J., Hittelman, J. et al. (2000). Early cognitive and motor development among infants born to women infected with human immunodeficiency virus. Women and Infants Transmission Study Group. *Pediatrics* **106**, E25.

Chersich, M. F. and Gray, G. E. (2005). Progress and emerging challenges in preventing mother-to-child transmission. *Curr Infect Dis Rep* **7**, 393–400.

Chersich, M. F., Urban, M. F., Venter, F. W. et al. (2006). Efavirenz use during pregnancy and for women of child-bearing potential. *AIDS Res Ther* **3**, 11.

Chohan, B., Lavreys, L., Rainwater, S. M., and Overbaugh, J. (2005). Evidence for frequent reinfection with human immunodeficiency virus type 1 of a different subtype. *J Virol* **79**, 10701–10708.

Chun, T. W., Davey, R. T., Jr., Engel, D., Lane, H. C., and Fauci, A. S. (1999). Re-emergence of HIV after stopping therapy. *Nature* **401**, 874–875.

Chung, M. H., Kiarie, J. N., Richardson, B. A., Lehman, D. A., Overbaugh, J., and John-Stewart, G. C. (2005). Breast milk HIV-1 suppression and decreased transmission: a randomized trial comparing HIVNET 012 nevirapine versus short-course zidovudine. *AIDS* **19**, 1415–1422.

Clements, J. E., Anderson, M. G., Zink, M. C., Joag, S. V., and Narayan, O. (1994). The SIV model of AIDS encephalopathy. Role of neurotropic viruses in diseases. *Res Publ Assoc Res Nerv Ment Dis* **72**, 147–157.

Clements, J. E., Babas, T., Mankowski, J. L. et al. (2002). The central nervous system as a reservoir for simian immunodeficiency virus (SIV): steady-state levels of SIV DNA in brain from acute through asymptomatic infection. *J Infect Dis* **186**, 905–913.

Connor, E. M., Sperling, R. S., Gelber, R. et al. (1994). Reduction of maternal-infant transmission of human immunodeficiency virus type 1 with zidovudine treatment. Pediatric AIDS Clinical Trials Group Protocol 076 Study Group. *N Engl J Med* **331**, 1173–1180.

Dickover, R. E., Garratty, E. M., Plaeger, S., and Bryson, Y. J. (2001). Perinatal transmission of major, minor, and multiple maternal human immunodeficiency virus type 1 variants in utero and intra-partum. *J Virol* **75**, 2194–2203.

Dickover, R., Garratty, E., Yusim, K., Miller, C., Korber, B., and Bryson, Y. (2006). Role of maternal autologous neutralizing antibody in selective perinatal transmission of human immunodeficiency virus type 1 escape variants. *J Virol* **80**, 6525–6533.

Eshleman, S. H., Hoover, D. R., Chen, S. et al. (2005). Resistance after single-dose nevirapine prophylaxis emerges in a high proportion of Malawian newborns. *AIDS* **19**, 2167–2169.

Fang, G., Burger, H., Grimson, R. et al. (1995). Maternal plasma human immunodeficiency virus type 1 RNA level: a determinant and projected threshold for mother-to-child transmission. *Proc Natl Acad Sci USA* **92**, 12100–12104.

Fang, G., Weiser, B., Kuiken, C. et al. (2004). Recombination following superinfection by HIV-1. *AIDS* **18**, 153–159.

Fazely, F., Sharma, P. L., Fratazzi, C. et al. (1993). Simian immunodeficiency virus infection via amniotic fluid: a model to study fetal immunopathogenesis and prophylaxis. *J Acquir Immune Defic Syndr* **6**, 107–114.

Ferrantelli, F., Hofmann-Lehmann, R., Rasmussen, R. A. et al. (2003). Post-exposure prophylaxis with human monoclonal antibodies prevented SHIV89.6P infection or disease in neonatal macaques. *AIDS* **17**, 301–309.

Ferrantelli, F., Rasmussen, R. A., Buckley, K. A. et al. (2004). Complete protection of neonatal rhesus macaques against oral exposure to pathogenic simian-human immunodeficiency virus by human anti-HIV monoclonal antibodies. *J Infect Dis* **189**, 2167–2173.

Fox, H. S., Weed, M. R., Huitron-Resendiz, S. et al. (2000). Antiviral treatment normalizes neurophysiological but not movement abnormalities in simian immunodeficiency virus-infected monkeys. *J Clin Invest* **106**, 37–45.

Gaillard, P., Fowler, M. G., Dabis, F. et al. (2004). Use of antiretroviral drugs to prevent HIV-1 transmission through breast-feeding: from animal studies to randomized clinical trials. *J Acquir Immune Defic Syndr* **35**, 178–187.

Gardner, M. B. (1993). The importance of nonhuman primate research in the battle against AIDS: a historical perspective. *J Med Primatol* **22**, 86–91.

George, M. D., Reay, E., Sankaran, S., and Dandekar, S. (2005). Early antiretroviral therapy for simian immunodeficiency virus infection leads to mucosal CD4+ T-cell restoration and enhanced gene expression regulating mucosal repair and regeneration. *J Virol* **79**, 2709–2719.

Gray, R. A., Wilcox, K. M., Zink, M. C., and Weed, M. R. (2006). Impaired performance on the object retrieval-detour test of executive function in the SIV/macaque model of AIDS. *AIDS Res Hum Retroviruses* **22**, 1031–1035.

Grob, P. M., Cao, Y., Muchmore, E. *et al.* (1997). Prophylaxis against HIV-1 infection in chimpanzees by nevirapine, a nonnucleoside inhibitor of reverse transcriptase. *Nat Med* **3**, 665–670.

Guadalupe, M., Reay, E., Sankaran, S. *et al.* (2003). Severe CD4+ T-cell depletion in gut lymphoid tissue during primary human immunodeficiency virus type 1 infection and substantial delay in restoration following highly active antiretroviral therapy. *J Virol* **77**, 11708–11717.

Guay, L. A., Musoke, P., Fleming, T. *et al.* (1999). Intrapartum and neonatal single-dose nevirapine compared with zidovudine for prevention of mother-to-child transmission of HIV-1 in Kampala, Uganda: HIVNET 012 randomised trial. *Lancet* **354**, 795–802.

Hahn, B. H., Shaw, G. M., De Cock, K. M., and Sharp, P. M. (2000). AIDS as a zoonosis: scientific and public health implications. *Science* **287**, 607–614.

Haigwood, N. L. (1999). Progress and challenges in therapies for AIDS in nonhuman primate models. *J Med Primatol* **28**, 154–163.

Haigwood, N. L. (2004). Predictive value of primate models for AIDS. *AIDS Rev* **6**, 187–198.

Haigwood, N. L., Montefiori, D. C., Sutton, W. F. *et al.* (2004). Passive immunotherapy in simian immunodeficiency virus-infected macaques accelerates the development of neutralizing antibodies. *J Virol* **78**, 5983–5995.

Hayami, M., Igarashi, T., Kuwata, T. *et al.* (1999). Gene-mutated HIV-1/SIV chimeric viruses as AIDS live attenuated vaccines for potential human use. *Leukemia* **13**(suppl 1), S42–47.

Heise, C., Miller, C. J., Lackner, A., and Dandekar, S. (1994). Primary acute simian immunodeficiency virus infection of intestinal lymphoid tissue is associated with gastrointestinal dysfunction. *J Infect Dis* **169**, 1116–1120.

Hel, Z., Venzon, D., Poudyal, M. *et al.* (2000). Viremia control following antiretroviral treatment and therapeutic immunization during primary SIV251 infection of macaques. *Nat Med* **6**, 1140–1146.

Hirsch, V. M., Dapolito, G., Hahn, A. *et al.* (1998). Viral genetic evolution in macaques infected with molecularly cloned simian immunodeficiency virus correlates with the extent of persistent viremia. *J Virol* **72**, 6482–6489.

Ho, R. J., Agy, M. B., Morton, W. R. *et al.* (1996). Development of a chronically catheterized maternal-fetal macaque model to study in utero mother-to-fetus HIV transmission: a preliminary report. *J Med Primatol* **25**, 218–224.

Ho, R. J., Larsen, K., Kinman, L. *et al.* (2001). Characterization of a maternal-fetal HIV transmission model using pregnant macaques infected with HIV-2(287). *J Med Primatol* **30**, 131–140.

Hu, S. L. (2005). Non-human primate models for AIDS vaccine research. *Curr Drug Targets Infect Disord* **5**, 193–201.

Hurtrel, B., Chakrabarti, L., Hurtrel, M., Maire, M. A., Dormont, D., and Montagnier, L. (1991). Early SIV encephalopathy. *J Med Primatol* **20**, 159–166.

Hurtrel, B., Chakrabarti, L., Hurtrel, M., and Montagnier, L. (1993). Target cells during early SIV encephalopathy. *Res Virol* **144**, 41–46.

Jaspan, H. B., Robinson, J. E., Amedee, A. M., Van Dyke, R. B., and Garry, R. F. (2004). Amniotic fluid has higher relative levels of lentivirus-specific antibodies than plasma and can contain neutralizing antibodies. *J Clin Virol* **31**, 190–197.

Jayaraman, P., Mohan, D., Polacino, P. *et al.* (2004). Perinatal transmission of SHIV-SF162P3 in *Macaca nemestrina*. *J Med Primatol* **33**, 243–250.

Jayaraman, P. and Haigwood, N. L. (2006). Animal models for perinatal transmission of HIV-1. *Front Biosci* **11**, 2828–2844.

Jayaraman, P., Zhu, T., Misher, L. *et al.* (2007). Evidence for persistent, occult infection in neonatal macaques following perinatal transmission of simian-human immunodeficiency virus SF162P3. *J Virol* **81**, 822–834.

Jin, X., Roberts, C. G., Nixon, D. F. *et al.* (1998). Longitudinal and cross-sectional analysis of cytotoxic T lymphocyte responses and their relationship to vertical human immunodeficiency virus transmission. ARIEL Project Investigators. *J Infect Dis* **178**, 1317–1326.

Joag, S. V., Adams, R. J., Pinson, D. M., Adany, I., and Narayan, O. (1994). Intracerebral infusion of TNF-alpha and IL-6 failed to activate latent SIV infection in the brains of macaques inoculated with macrophage-tropic neuroadapted SIVmac. *J Leukoc Biol* **56**, 353–357.

Kemal, K. S., Foley, B., Burger, H. *et al.* (2003). HIV-1 in genital tract and plasma of women: compartmentalization of viral sequences, coreceptor usage, and glycosylation. *Proc Natl Acad Sci USA* **100**, 12972–12977.

Kemal, K. S., Burger, H., Mayers, D. *et al.* (2007). HIV-1 drug resistance in variants from the female genital tract and plasma. *J Infect Dis* **195**, 535–545.

Kinman, L. M., Worlein, J. M., Leigh, J. *et al.* (2004). HIV in central nervous system and behavioral development: an HIV-2287 macaque model of AIDS. *AIDS* **18**, 1363–1370.

Lackner, A. A., Dandekar, S., and Gardner, M. B. (1991). Neurobiology of simian and feline immunodeficiency virus infections. *Brain Pathol* **1**, 201–212.

Lisziewicz, J., Trocio, J., Xu, J. *et al.* (2005). Control of viral rebound through therapeutic immunization with DermaVir. *AIDS* **19**, 35–43.

Lobato, M. N., Caldwell, M. B., Ng, P., and Oxtoby, M. J. (1995). Encephalopathy in children with perinatally acquired human immunodeficiency virus infection. Pediatric Spectrum of Disease Clinical Consortium. *J Pediatr* **126**, 710–715.

Lockman, S., Shapiro, R. L., Smeaton, L. M. *et al.* (2007). Response to antiretroviral therapy after a single, peripartum dose of nevirapine. *N Engl J Med* **356**, 135–147.

Lohman, B. L., Slyker, J., Mbori-Ngacha, D. *et al.* (2003). Prevalence and magnitude of human immunodeficiency virus (HIV) type 1-specific lymphocyte responses in breast milk from HIV-1-seropositive women. *J Infect Dis* **188**, 1666–1674.

Lori, F., Lewis, M. G., Xu, J. *et al.* (2000). Control of SIV rebound through structured treatment interruptions during early infection. *Science* **290**, 1591–1593.

Luzuriaga, K. and Sullivan, J. L. (2000). Viral and immunopathogenesis of vertical HIV-1 infection. *Pediatr Clin North Am* **47**, 65–78.

Luzuriaga, K. and Sullivan, J. L. (2002). Pediatric HIV-1 infection: advances and remaining challenges. *AIDS Rev* **4**, 21–26.

Mankowski, J. L., Queen, S. E., Kirstein, L. M. *et al.* (1999). Alterations in blood-brain barrier glucose transport in SIV-infected macaques. *J Neurovirol* **5**, 695–702.

Marcario, J. K., Manaye, K. F., SantaCruz, K. S., Mouton, P. R., Berman, N. E., and Cheney, P. D. (2004). Severe subcortical degeneration in macaques infected with neurovirulent simian immunodeficiency virus. *J Neurovirol* **10**, 387–399.

Marthas, M. L., Banapour, B., Sutjipto, S. *et al.* (1989). Rhesus macaques inoculated with molecularly cloned simian immunodeficiency virus. *J Med Primatol* **18**, 311–319.

Marthas, M. L., van Rompay, K. K., Otsyula, M. *et al.* (1995). Viral factors determine progression to AIDS in simian immunodeficiency virus-infected newborn rhesus macaques. *J Virol* **69**, 4198–4205.

Martin Amedee, A., Lacour, N., Martin, L. N. *et al.* (1996). Genotypic analysis of infant macaques infected transplacentally and orally. *J Med Primatol* **25**, 225–235.

Martin, S. C., Wolters, P. L., Toledo-Tamula, M. A., Zeichner, S. L., Hazra, R., and Civitello, L. (2006). Cognitive functioning in school-aged children with vertically acquired HIV infection being treated with highly active antiretroviral therapy (HAART). *Dev Neuropsychol* **30**, 633–657.

Mbori-Ngacha, D., Richardson, B. A., Overbaugh, J. *et al.* (2003). Short-term effect of zidovudine on plasma and genital human immunodeficiency virus type 1 and viral turnover in these compartments. *J Virol* **77**, 7702–7705.

McCormick-Davis, C., Dalton, S. B., Hout, D. R. *et al.* (2000). A molecular clone of simian-human immunodeficiency virus (DeltavpuSHIV(KU-1bMC33)) with a truncated, non-membrane-bound vpu results in rapid CD4(+) T cell loss and neuro-AIDS in pig-tailed macaques. *Virology* **272**, 112–126.

Milush, J. M., Kosub, D., Marthas, M. *et al.* (2004). Rapid dissemination of SIV following oral inoculation. *AIDS* **18**, 2371–2380.

Miyake, A., Enose, Y., Ohkura, S. *et al.* (2004). The quantity and diversity of infectious viruses in various tissues of SHIV-infected monkeys at the early and AIDS stages. *Arch Virol* **149**, 943–955.

Muro, E., Droste, J. A., Hofstede, H. T., Bosch, M., Dolmans, W., and Burger, D. M. (2005). Nevirapine plasma concentrations are still detectable after more than 2 weeks in the majority of women receiving single-dose nevirapine: implications for intervention studies. *J Acquir Immune Defic Syndr* **39**, 419–421.

Musoke, P., Guay, L. A., Bagenda, D. *et al.* (1999). A phase I/II study of the safety and pharmacokinetics of nevirapine in HIV-1-infected pregnant Ugandan women and their neonates (HIVNET 006). *AIDS* **13**, 479–486.

Nag, P., Kim, J., Sapiega, V. *et al.* (2004). Women with cervicovaginal antibody-dependent cell-mediated cytotoxicity have lower genital HIV-1 RNA loads. *J Infect Dis* **190**, 1970–1978.

Nduati, R. (2000). Breastfeeding and HIV-1 infection. A review of current literature. *Adv Exp Med Biol* **478**, 201–210.

Nduati, R., John, G., Mbori-Ngacha, D. *et al.* (2000). Effect of breastfeeding and formula feeding on transmission of HIV-1: a randomized clinical trial. *JAMA* **283**, 1167–1174.

Newell, M. L. (2000). Vertical transmission of HIV-1 infection. *Trans R Soc Trop Med Hyg* **94**, 1–2.

Nowak, P., Karlsson, A. C., Naver, L., Bohlin, A. B., Piasek, A., and Sonnerborg, A. (2002). The selection and evolution of viral quasispecies in HIV-1 infected children. *HIV Med* **3**, 1–11.

Otsyula, M. G., Miller, C. J., Tarantal, A. F. *et al.* (1996). Fetal or neonatal infection with attenuated simian immunodeficiency virus results in protective immunity against oral challenge with pathogenic SIVmac251. *Virology* **222**, 275–278.

Rausch, D. M., Heyes, M., and Eiden, L. E. (1994). Effects of chronic zidovudine administration on CNS function and virus burden after perinatal SIV infection in rhesus monkeys. *Adv Neuroimmunol* **4**, 233–237.

Rausch, D. M., Heyes, M. P., Murray, E. A., and Eiden, L. E. (1995). Zidovudine treatment prolongs survival and decreases virus load in the central nervous system of rhesus macaques infected perinatally with simian immunodeficiency virus. *J Infect Dis* **172**, 59–69.

Regoes, R. R., Longini, I. M., Feinberg, M. B., and Staprans, S. I. (2005). Preclinical assessment of HIV vaccines and microbicides by repeated low-dose virus challenges. *PLoS Med* **2**, e249.

Rich, K. C., Fowler, M. G., Mofenson, L. M. *et al.* (2000). Maternal and infant factors predicting disease progression in human immunodeficiency virus type 1-infected infants. Women and Infants Transmission Study Group. *Pediatrics* **105**, e8.

Rousseau, C. M., Nduati, R. W., Richardson, B. A. *et al.* (2004). Association of levels of HIV-1-infected breast milk cells and risk of mother-to-child transmission. *J Infect Dis* **190**, 1880–1888.

Ruprecht, R. M., Fratazzi, C., Sharma, P. L., Greene, M. F., Penninck, D., and Wyand, M. (1993). Animal models for perinatal transmission of pathogenic viruses. *Ann N Y Acad Sci* **693**, 213–228.

Ruprecht, R. M., Baba, T. W., Liska, V. *et al.* (1998). Oral SIV, SHIV, and HIV type 1 infection. *AIDS Res Hum Retroviruses* **14**(suppl 1), S97–103.

Ruprecht, R. M., Baba, T. W., Liska, V. *et al.* (1999). Oral transmission of primate lentiviruses. *J Infect Dis* **179**(suppl 3), S408–412.

Rychert, J., Lacour, N., and Amedee, A. M. (2006). Genetic analysis of simian immunodeficiency virus expressed in milk and selectively transmitted through breastfeeding. *J Virol* **80**, 3721–3731.

Safrit, J. T., Ruprecht, R., Ferrantelli, F. *et al.* (2004). Immunoprophylaxis to prevent mother-to-child transmission of HIV-1. *J Acquir Immune Defic Syndr* **35**, 169–177.

Scarlatti, G. (2004). Mother-to-child transmission of HIV-1: advances and controversies of the twentieth centuries. *AIDS Rev* **6**, 67–78.

Sestak, K. (2005). Chronic diarrhea and AIDS: insights into studies with non-human primates. *Curr HIV Res* **3**, 199–205.

Shen, A., Zink, M. C., Mankowski, J. L. *et al.* (2003). Resting CD4+ T lymphocytes but not thymocytes provide a latent viral reservoir in a simian immunodeficiency virus-*Macaca nemestrina* model of human immunodeficiency virus type 1-infected patients on highly active antiretroviral therapy. *J Virol* **77**, 4938–4949.

Shen, A., Yang, H. C., Zhou, Y. *et al.* (2007). Novel pathway for induction of latent virus from resting CD4(+) T cells in the simian immunodeficiency virus/macaque model of human immunodeficiency virus type 1 latency. *J Virol* **81**, 1660–1670.

Smith, M. S., Niu, Y., Buch, S. *et al.* (2005). Active simian immunodeficiency virus (strain smmPGm) infection in macaque central nervous system correlates with neurologic disease. *J Acquir Immune Defic Syndr* **38**, 518–530.

St John, A. M., Kumar, A., and Cave, C. (2003). Reduction in perinatal transmission and mortality from human immunodeficiency virus after intervention with zidovudine in Barbados. *Pediatr Infect Dis J* **22**, 422–426.

Staprans, S. I. and Feinberg, M. B. (2004). The roles of nonhuman primates in the preclinical evaluation of candidate AIDS vaccines. *Expert Rev Vaccines* **3**(suppl), S5–32.

Tarantal, A. F., Marthas, M. L., McChesney, M. D. *et al.* (1993). Effects of SIV infection on fetal development and prenancy outcome in the rhesus macaque (*Macaca mulatta*). *Pediatr AIDS HIV Infect Fetus Adolesc* **4**, 373–380.

Tarantal, A. F., Marthas, M. L., Gargosky, S. E. *et al.* (1995). Effects of viral virulence on intrauterine growth in SIV-infected fetal rhesus macaques (*Macaca mulatta*). *J Acquir Immune Defic Syndr Hum Retrovirol* **10**, 129–138.

Tarantal, A. F., Castillo, A., Ekert, J. E., Bischofberger, N., and Martin, R. B. (2002). Fetal and maternal outcome after administration of tenofovir to gravid rhesus monkeys (*Macaca mulatta*). *J Acquir Immune Defic Syndr* **29**, 207–220.

Tarantal, A. F., Marthas, M. L., Shaw, J. P., Cundy, K., and Bischofberger, N. (1999). Administration of 9-[2-(R)-(phosphonomethoxy)propyl]adenine (PMPA) to gravid and infant rhesus macaques (*Macaca mulatta*): safety and efficacy studies. *J Acquir Immune Defic Syndr Hum Retrovirol* **20**, 323–333.

Trichel, A. M., Roberts, E. D., Wilson, L. A., Martin, L. N., Ruprecht, R. M., and Murphey-Corb, M. (1997). SIV/DeltaB670 transmission across oral, colonic, and vaginal mucosae in the macaque. *J Med Primatol* **26**, 3–10.

Van Rompay, K. K. (2005). Antiretroviral drug studies in nonhuman primates: a valid animal model for innovative drug efficacy and pathogenesis experiments. *AIDS Rev* **7**, 67–83.

Van Rompay, K. K., Marthas, M. L., Ramos, R. A. *et al.* (1992). Simian immunodeficiency virus (SIV) infection of infant rhesus macaques as a model to test antiretroviral drug prophylaxis and therapy: oral 3′ azido-3′ -deoxythymidine prevents SIV infection. *Antimicrob Agents Chemother* **36**, 2381–2386.

Van Rompay, K. K. A., Otsyula, M. G., Marthas, M. L. *et al.* (1995). Immediate zidovudine treatment protects simian immunodeficiency virus-infected newborn macaques against rapid onset of AIDS. *Antimicrob Agents Chemother* **39**, 125–131.

Van Rompay, K. K. A., Cherrington, J. M., Marthas, M. L. *et al.* (1996). 9-[2-(Phosphonomethoxy)propyl]adenine therapy of established simian immunodeficiency virus infection in infant rhesus macaques. *Antimicrob Agents Chemother* **40**, 2586–2591.

Van Rompay, K. K. A., Berardi, C. J., Dillard-Telm, S. *et al.* (1998). Passive immunization of newborn rhesus macaques prevents oral simian immunodeficiency virus infection. *J Infect Dis* **177**, 1247–1259.

Van Rompay, K. K., Greenier, J. L., Cole, K. S. *et al.* (2003). Immunization of newborn rhesus macaques with simian immunodeficiency virus (SIV) vaccines prolongs survival after oral challenge with virulent SIVmac251. *J Virol* **77**, 179–190.

Van Rompay, K. K., Brignolo, L. L., Meyer, D. J. *et al.* (2004a). Biological effects of short-term or prolonged administration of 9-[2-(phosphonomethoxy)propyl]adenine (tenofovir) to newborn and infant rhesus macaques. *Antimicrob Agents Chemother* **48**, 1469–1487.

Van Rompay, K. K., Singh, R. P., Brignolo, L. L. *et al.* (2004b). The clinical benefits of tenofovir for simian immunodeficiency virus-infected macaques are larger than predicted by its effects on standard viral and immunologic parameters. *J Acquir Immune Defic Syndr* **36**, 900–914.

Van Rompay, K. K., Abel, K., Lawson, J. R. *et al.* (2005). Attenuated poxvirus-based simian immunodeficiency virus (SIV) vaccines given in infancy partially protect infant and juvenile macaques against repeated oral challenge with virulent SIV. *J Acquir Immune Defic Syndr* **38**, 124–134.

Van Rompay, K. K., Singh, R. P., Heneine, W. *et al.* (2006a). Structured treatment interruptions with tenofovir monotherapy for simian immunodeficiency virus-infected newborn macaques. *J Virol* **80**, 6399–6410.

Van Rompay, K. K. A., Kearney, B. P., Sexton, J. J. *et al.* (2006b). Evaluation of oral tenofovir disoproxil fumarate and topical tenofovir GS-7340 to protect infant macaques against repeated oral challenges with virulent simian immunodeficiency virus. *J Acquir Immune Defic Syndr* **43**, 6–14.

Veazey, R. S. and Lackner, A. A. (2005). HIV swiftly guts the immune system. *Nat Med* **11**, 469–470.

Veazey, R. S., DeMaria, M., Chalifoux, L. V. *et al.* (1998). Gastrointestinal tract as a major site of CD4+ T-cell depletion and viral replication in SIV infection. *Science* **280**, 427–431.

Veazey, R. S., Lifson, J. D., Pandrea, I., Purcell, J., Piatak, M., Jr., and Lackner, A. A. (2003). Simian immunodeficiency virus infection in neonatal macaques. *J Virol* **77**, 8783–8792.

Watson, A., McClure, J., Ranchalis, J. *et al.* (1997). Early postinfection antiviral treatment reduces viral load and prevents CD4+ cell decline in HIV type 2-infected macaques. *AIDS Res Hum Retroviruses* **13**, 1375–1381.

Weed, M. R. and Steward, D. J. (2005). Neuropsychopathology in the SIV/macaque model of AIDS. *Front Biosci* **10**, 710–727.

Weed, M. R., Hienz, R. D., Brady, J. V. *et al.* (2003). Central nervous system correlates of behavioral deficits following simian immunodeficiency virus infection. *J Neurovirol* **9**, 452–464.

Weed, M. R., Gold, L. H., Polis, I., Koob, G. F., Fox, H. S., and Taffe, M. A. (2004). Impaired performance on a rhesus monkey neuropsychological testing battery following simian immunodeficiency virus infection. *AIDS Res Hum Retroviruses* **20**, 77–89.

Wilfert, C. M. and Fowler, M. G. (2007). Balancing maternal and infant benefits and the consequences of breast-feeding in the developing world during the era of HIV infection. *J Infect Dis* **195**, 165–167.

Worlein, J. M., Leigh, J., Larsen, K. *et al.* (2005). Cognitive and motor deficits associated with HIV-2(287) infection in infant pigtailed macaques: a nonhuman primate model of pediatric neuro-AIDS. *J Neurovirol* **11**, 34–45.

Wu, X., Parast, A. B., Richardson, B. A. *et al.* (2006). Neutralization escape variants of human immunodeficiency virus type 1 are transmitted from mother to infant. *J Virol* **80**, 835–844.

Zhu, T., Corey, L., Hwangbo, Y. *et al.* (2003). Persistence of extraordinarily low levels of genetically homogeneous human immunodeficiency virus type 1 in exposed seronegative individuals. *J Virol* **77**, 6108–6116.

Zink, M. C. and Clements, J. E. (2002). A novel simian immunodeficiency virus model that provides insight into mechanisms of human immunodeficiency virus central nervous system disease. *J Neurovirol* **8**(suppl 2), 42–48.

Zink, M. C., Suryanarayana, K., Mankowski, J. L. *et al.* (1999). High viral load in the cerebrospinal fluid and brain correlates with severity of simian immunodeficiency virus encephalitis. *J Virol* **73**, 10480–10488.

Zink, M. C., Uhrlaub, J., DeWitt, J. *et al.* (2005). Neuroprotective and anti-human immunodeficiency virus activity of minocycline. *JAMA* **293**, 2003–2011.

Zink, M. C., Laast, V. A., Helke, K. L. *et al.* (2006). From mice to macaques – animal models of HIV nervous system disease. *Curr HIV Res* **4**, 293–305.

CHAPTER 11

Endocrine Disruption during Brain Development of Nonhuman Primates

Mari S. Golub

INTRODUCTION

The endocrine system regulates many biological processes including gender determination, physical growth, sexual maturation, and reproduction. There are three primary components to the endocrine system: (1) glands located throughout the body (e.g. thyroid, ovaries, testes, pituitary, adrenal), (2) hormones that act as chemical messengers, and (3) specialized receptors that bind with hormones and initiate programmed biological actions. In recent years, scientists have noted that some chemicals are capable of mimicking the biological action of endogenous hormones. Endocrine disrupting chemicals act by changing the structure of endocrine glands and/or interfering with the production or function of endogenous hormones. These agents, collectively known as endocrine disruptors (EDs), have been associated with a continuum of health effects in human and wildlife populations.

The far reaching effects of endocrine-disrupting chemicals were brought into focus as a research area by a 1991 consensus statement from a Wingspread conference held in Racine, Wisconsin, USA (Colborn and Clement, 1992) and the popular book *Our Stolen Future: Are We Threatening our Fertility, Intelligence and Survival – A Scientific Detective Story* (Colborn *et al.*, 1997). Initially observed in wildlife, effects included thyroid dysfunction, reduced fertility, physical malformations, demasculinization and feminization in males, defeminization and masculinization of females, and impaired immune function. Both of these publications address the potential danger that EDs pose to human and animal health, emphasizing the enhanced vulnerability of the fetus to adverse effects of exposure. At present, the United States, the European Union and Japan have federally mandated programs to identify agents that are endocrine disruptors (Office of Pesticides Pollutants and Toxic Substances, 1998; Vos *et al.*, 2000; Longnecker *et al.*, 2003; Gelbke *et al.*, 2004; Matthiessen and Johnson, 2006), and research programs to determine their potential impact on human health and wildlife populations (Taylor *et al.*, 1999; Longnecker *et al.*, 2003; Harding *et al.*, 2006).

Primate Models of Children's Health and Developmental Disabilities

The United States Environmental Agency has defined an endocrine disruptor as "an exogenous agent that interferes with the synthesis, secretion, transport, binding, action, or elimination of natural hormones in the body which are responsible for maintenance or homeostasis, reproduction, development and or behavior" (Kavlock *et al.*, 1996). Despite this broad definition, research and concern have focused primarily on agents that are estrogenic or estrogen mimics, on anti-androgens, and on agents that lead to hypothyroid conditions. Examples of chemicals currently under intense research interest for their ED effects are phthalates, PCBs, polyphenols, soy phytoestrogens, and antiandrogenic pesticides (vinclozolin). Lists of endocrine disruptors can be found at http://www.ourstolenfuture.org/Basics/chemlist.htm.

The effects of EDs on reproduction and development are potentially dramatic. Endocrine disruption has been posited as a factor in the worldwide decline in frog populations, in reproductive tract malformations of mollusks, fish, alligators, and polar bears, and in human health problems such as obesity, early pubertal development, and reproductive tract cancer. In addition, from the earliest consideration of this issue, there has been an emphasis on brain development and the possible role of EDs on behavioral competence, including cognitive abilities, after exposure of fetuses, infants, and children (Schantz and Widholm, 2001; Weiss, 2002; Colborn, 2004, 2006). It is in investigating ED effects on brain development that nonhuman primate models can provide a particularly valuable research model.

It is commonly understood that prior to the onset of reproductive maturity, one important function of endogenous steroidal hormones is to elicit sexual differentiation in the brain. This topic has been extensively studied in nonhuman primates. Abnormalities in the sexual differentiation of the brain, such as those associated with endocrine dysfunction, can have far-reaching effects on normal physical and behavioral development in exposed offspring.

SEXUAL DIFFERENTIATION OF THE BRAIN AND NEURODEVELOPMENTAL DISORDERS

Abnormal sexual differentiation of the brain has been implicated in the etiology of childhood behavior disorders in the Extreme Male Brain theory of autism (Baron-Cohen *et al.*, 2005). According to the conceptual framework of this theory, social behavior is sex differentiated to provide differences in empathizing versus systematizing in women versus men. According to this theory, 6.1% of normal males, but 47% of males with Asperger's syndrome or autism, show the most extreme version of the systematizing phenotype, which is attributed to abnormal exposure to testosterone during fetal life. This theory is currently being tested in human studies that relate testosterone concentrations in amniotic fluid to incidence of autism-related traits in children (Knickmeyer *et al.*, 2005a, 2005b, 2006).

An association between disruption of sexual differentiation of the brain and childhood behavior disorders could also be mediated by altered age at puberty.

Mann and colleagues (Mann, 2005; Mann *et al.*, 1998) have suggested a link between later age at puberty with suppression of developmental testosterone and earlier puberty with exogenous testosterone in male monkeys. In humans, early and late onset of puberty are associated with behavioral problems of adolescence such as substance abuse, anorexia nervosa, depression, and conduct disorder (Kaltiala-Heino *et al.*, 2001, 2003a, 2003b). Sexual behavior prior to age 16 was found to be more prevalent in young people who were diagnosed with depression, eating disorders, substance abuse, antisocial disorders, and schizophrenia spectrum disorders (Ramrakha *et al.*, 2000). These associations may be mediated by psychosocial factors, such as age-inappropriate appearance and peer interactions, but they could also have a biological origin in altered sexual differentiation of the brain.

Inadequate or disrupted sexual differentiation of the brain could contribute to a variety of personality disorders and crimes (sex offenses) that involve inappropriate or abnormal sexual behavior. Although the psychosocial origins of these disorders are most often studied, biology is also known to be important. Little attention has been directed at chemical agent exposure during development as part of the etiology of these disorders; no research in this area was located for this review.

ARE NONHUMAN PRIMATE MODELS NEEDED TO UNDERSTAND THE IMPACT OF ENDOCRINE DISRUPTION ON SEXUAL DIFFERENTIATION OF THE BRAIN IN HUMANS?

There are several reasons why nonhuman primates are a more appropriate model than commonly used laboratory rodents for studying endocrine disruption during brain development.

Much of the brain development that takes place prenatally in primates occurs postnatally in rodents. Understanding the impact of exposure to environmental chemicals during pregnancy on human fetal brain development is thus difficult from rodent studies. If the agent is administered postnatally to simulate at an equivalent stage of brain development, the mediation of the maternal system will be much different. While EDs are not unique in this regard, the fairly clear-cut developmental time periods for sexual differentiation of the brain make this an important consideration.

Primates also differ from rodents in the role of protein binding and aromatization in mediating hormone influences on brain differentiation. As discussed below, protein binding of estrogen to alpha-fetoprotein (AFP) in circulation plays a critical role in preventing masculinization of the brain in female rodents (rats and mice) by preventing ovarian estrogen from reaching cell targets in the hypothalamus. The relative AFP binding of endocrine-disrupting agents would largely determine their potential to affect sexual differentiation of the brain in rodents but would not be relevant to humans. On the other hand, sex differentiation of the fetal gonadotropin activation is the factor protecting female brain from masculinization in monkeys, and the same may be true in human primates.

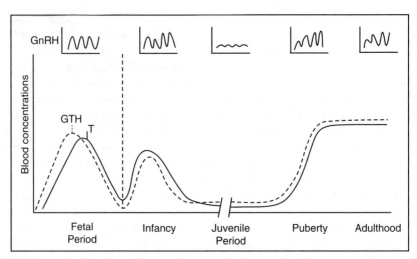

FIGURE 11.1   Activation of the hypothalamic–pituitary–gonadal axis prior to puberty in male rhesus macaques. From Mann (2005). GnRH, gonadotropin-releasing hormone; GTH, gonadotropic hormone; T, testosterone.

Goy and colleagues (Goy and Deputte, 1996) have pointed out several discrepancies between primate and rodent studies of endocrine disruption and sexual differentiation, including the finding that dihydrotestosterone, an androgen that cannot be aromatized to estrogen, was effective in producing brain masculinization in female rhesus fetuses (Pomerantz et al., 1985), although it is ineffective in rodents.

In most mammals there are discrete periods of hypothalamic-pituitary-gonadal (HPG) activity during fetal and neonatal life when pulsatile gonadotropin-releasing hormone (GnRH) occurs and gonads produce steroidal hormones, although ovulation, sperm production and reproduction do not occur (Figure 11.1). These periods are sensitive to disruption of hormone-dependent brain differentiation.

The initiation of HPG activity prior to puberty differs in laboratory rodents and primates. In humans, and in nonhuman primates commonly studied in the laboratory setting, puberty is marked by the onset of pulsatile secretion of GnRH, after a period of HPG quiescence extending from infancy through the prolonged juvenile phase (Perera and Plant, 1992; Terasawa, 1995; Mann, 2005). In contrast, a gradual change in HPG activity occurs during the brief juvenile stage of standard laboratory rodents (Kavlock et al., 1996). Thus the consequences of exposure to EDs during the juvenile period are likely to differ between laboratory rodents and human/nonhuman primates.

OVERVIEW OF RELEVANT NONHUMAN PRIMATE STUDIES

A number of studies in monkeys have explored the consequences of endocrine disruption during brain development (see Table 11.1). These studies use pharmacological

TABLE 11.1   Studies of endocrine disruption and sexually differentiated behavior in monkeys. All studies were performed in rhesus monkeys

Agent	Time period	Sex	Behavior reports
Testosterone	gd 40–64, or gd 115–139	F F	Goy et al., 1988
Testosterone, or Dihydrotestosterone, or Castration	gd 42–97, 122 gd 42–102 Birth	F F M	Pomerantz et al., 1985
DES	gd 40–birth gd 115–140	F, M F	Goy and Deputte, 1996
GnRH agonist	2 weeks–4 months of age	M	Mann et al., 1993
Antide (GnRH antagonist), or Antide + testosterone	Birth–4 months of age	M M	Wallen et al., 1995
Testosterone Flutamide	gd 35, 40–70 or gd 110, 115–145	M F	Herman et al., 2003
Testosterone	gd 39–79, or pnd 1–46, or pnd 75–120, or pnd 540–586	F F F F	Clark and Goldman- Rakic, 1989
Ovariectomy + testosterone, or Ovariectomy + dihydrotestosterone, or Orchiectomy	Birth	F F M	Hagger and Bachevalier, 1991

gd, gestation day; pnd, postnatal day.

agents developed as hormone agonists or antagonists, rather than environmental chemicals, to disrupt the pathway of HPG activation (Figure 11.2). However to the extent that environmental agents mimic or block the actions of endogenous gonadal hormones, the findings provide a framework for anticipating the consequences of endocrine disruption by exogenous chemicals during brain development. The major focus of most these studies is maturation of the reproductive tract, including abnormalities of the external genitalia. However, studies of social and cognitive behavior were also sometimes included.

Interestingly, the monkey studies were stimulated by, and patterned after, reports of syndromes in humans associated with genetic abnormalities (such as congenital adrenal hyperplasia) or pharmacological disruptions (therapeutic use of diethylstilbestrol in pregnancy) that were shown to interfere with sexual differentiation of the genitals at birth and in sexually differentiated behaviors in children (Ehrhardt and Meyer-Bahlburg, 1981; Meyer-Bahlburg and Ehrhardt, 1986; Meyer-Bahlburg et al., 2004). By using hormonal manipulations under direct experimental control in otherwise normal animals, the nonhuman primate studies have already contributed

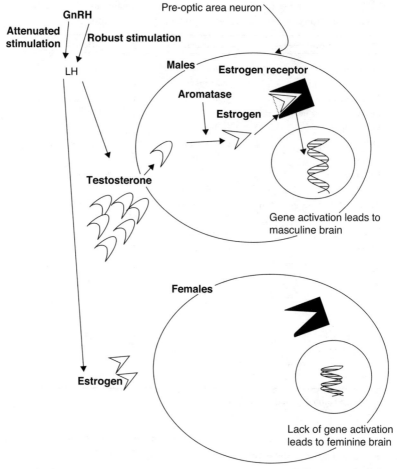

FIGURE 11.2   Schematic of sexual differentiation of the brain showing agents used in monkey experiments to interfere with this process. GnRH, gonadotropin-releasing hormone; GTH, gonadotropic hormone; LH, luteinizing hormone.

to understanding of these human syndromes, and now have the possibility of adding an important dimension to contemporary research on environmental estrogens and antiandrogens.

Figure 11.2 outlines the currently understood concept of sexual maturation of the brain, demonstrating steps in the process that can be disrupted by endocrine active agents. Pulsatile GnRH production stimulates luteinizing hormone (LH) release from the pituitary, which in turn stimulates the ovary to produce estrogen or the testes to produce testosterone. Testosterone enter neurons in the preoptic area of the hypothalamus. Here the testosterone is converted to estrogen via the enzyme aromatase. Estrogen binds to cytoplasmic estrogen receptors which translocate to the nucleus and initiate patterns of gene expression that lead to different morphological and functional properties of this area that are characteristic of males. In the absence of the LH stimulation, testosterone production, and/or aromatization, the brain develops the morphological and functional characteristics of the female. Considerable research indicates that the process is more complex and species-dependent, but the general outline of the process has been effective in explaining a large body of experimental and clinical research.

It follows that exogenous testosterone, or exogenous estrogen in sufficient amounts, can masculinize the brain. Dihydrotestosterone, an androgen agent that does not aromatize to estrogen, would not have this effect. GnRH antagonists would also be anticipated to block masculinization. Notably, GnRH agonists, as well as antagonists, suppress the HPG axis. HPG suppression is thought to result from GnRH agonist actions because, after an initial burst of gonadal hormone production, negative feedback shuts down GnRH production. However, direct effects of the agonist at brain GnRH receptors, or indirect effects related to the initial though transient burst of gonadal stimulation cannot be disregarded in experiments using GnRH agonists. Antiandrogens that act at the androgen receptor would not be expected to have direct effects on this process, but could act indirectly by upregulating testosterone production.

SOCIAL INTERACTIONS – PRENATAL INTERVENTIONS

A study that supported the role of estrogen in masculinization of the primate brain was reported by Goy and colleagues (Goy and Deputte, 1996). In this study, diethylstilbestrol (DES), a synthetic nonsteroidal estrogen, was found to masculinize the play and immature sexual behavior of juvenile (3–12 months old) female monkeys when administered to their mothers from the first trimester (gestation day (gd) 40) until term. A later, more abbreviated treatment (gd 115–140) was not effective. DES led to more play initiation, and specifically more play initiations with male partners, and to more rough play bouts in the DES-treated females than control females. The play behavior of the DES-treated females was very similar to that of control males. In contrast, although DES-treated females displayed more mounting than control females, this behavior had a significantly lower incidence than in control males. Mounting in immature monkeys is considered as part of the sex-differentiated play repertoire. A further qualitative difference was in the proportion of footclasp mounts (complete mounts). DES-treated females were similar to control females in having a larger proportion of mounts as incomplete mounts. There was also a small group of three DES-treated males in this experiment; they did not appear to differ from the control males. Effects of the DES on the reproductive tract were not discussed.

The hypothesis, developed from rodent studies (Tarttelin and Gorski, 1988), was that the high levels of estrogen substituted for the testosterone aromatized to estrogen which accomplishes brain masculinization in males. In rodents, DES has been shown to accomplish brain masculinization in females presumably because it is not bound to alpha-fetoprotein (AFP). AFP is a serum-binding protein produced during fetal life that binds estrogen in rodents and prevents endogenous estrogen from entering the neurons of the sexually differentiated nucleus of the preoptic area. As demonstrated recently in the AFP knockout mouse, even endogenous estrogen masculinizes the mouse brain in the absence of the serum-binding protein (Bakker *et al.*, 2006). However, human AFP does not have the estrogen-binding site, although it can have antiestrogenic properties (Allen *et al.*, 1993). AFP has been identified in maternal and fetal serum and amniotic fluid of humans and maternal serum of monkeys (Mattison and King, 1983), but very little is known about the role of this protein in primate species (Mizejewski, 2004). Sex hormone-binding globulin (SHBG) is the major estrogen-binding plasma protein in monkeys as in humans (Anderson *et al.*, 1976; Hotchkiss, 1985). The failure of endogenous estrogen to masculinize the brain in female primates is presumably due to the sex differentiation of LH release at the time of fetal HPG activation; it has been demonstrated that the LH pulse in fetal primate males is about twice as great as that in females (Herman *et al.*, 2000) (see Figure 11.2).

In addition to directly demonstrating brain masculinization by exogenous estrogen treatment during sensitive fetal periods, Goy and colleagues (1988) also demonstrated that disrupted sexual differentiation of genitalia and behavior can occur independently. Testosterone was administered to rhesus monkey dams with female fetuses on either gd 40–46, during organogenesis, or gd 115–140, during the early fetal period. The former treatment led to complete genital masculinization, while the latter did not. However, indications of brain masculinization were seen with the later treatment. The monkeys were observed throughout the juvenile period, from 3 to 27 months of age, and were compared with untreated male and female juveniles living in the same social groups. An outline of the behavioral findings is provided in Table 11.2.

TABLE 11.2   Results of study by Goy *et al.* (1988) with prenatal testosterone administration in rhesus monkeys

Behavior category	Group comparisons
Rough play	M > BA > GA = F
Play initiation partner of control males	M = BA > GA = F
Grooming (by mother)	M = GA < BA = F
Mounting	M > GA = BA > F

M, normal males; F, normal females; GA, genital androgenization, females treated in the early fetal period; BA, brain androgenization, females treated in the late fetal period.

Thus the incidence of rough play and the choice of gender in play partners was not altered by testosterone treatment which produced genital masculinization in female monkeys. However, a later testosterone treatment which did not influence the genitals did lead to a more masculine pattern of play behavior. Both the earlier and later treatments led to an increase in complete (footclasp) mounts above the level of female controls, but it was statistically lower than in male controls.

A similar study design, using early and late pregnancy manipulation of testosterone, focused in detail on sex-differentiated interactions with infants (<10 months of age) in juvenile rhesus monkeys (Herman *et al.*, 2003). In addition to groups treated with exogenous testosterone at these two periods of gestation, flutamide, an androgen receptor antagonist, was also administered to separate groups at the same periods. There were 4–7 juveniles of each gender in each of the four treatment groups and also in the vehicle-treated control group. Neither androgen treatment nor androgen blockade in utero affected the sex-differentiated behavior of the male juveniles. Genitalia of male, but not female, infants were altered by the treatments. Notably, both androgen and androgen blockade induced behavioral masculinization in the female juveniles, with markedly greater masculinization in the late-treated flutamide group. This group differed from control females in showing lower incidences of infant-directed observational categories of "contact," "embrace," and "groom," and also of "harass" and "kidnap." A composite of infant-directed behaviors, an Index of Infant Interest, clearly demonstrated masculinization of behavior in the late-treated flutamide group as a significantly lower infant interest relative to control females. However, the late flutamide-treated females also differed significantly from control males.

The authors provide several possible explanations of the counterintuitive masculinizing effects of androgen receptor blockade by flutamide. One is that the blockade led to compensatory increase in testosterone production which acted to masculinize the females immediately after the blockade was removed by cessation of flutamide treatment. Another possible explanation is differential access of flutamide and testosterone to brain areas involved in sex differentiation. If more feedback-stimulated testosterone than receptor-blocking flutamide reached these areas the net result could be masculinization. A third explanation is an as yet unknown action of flutamide on the brain that is independent of its androgen receptor-blocking properties.

SOCIAL INTERACTIONS – POSTNATAL INTERVENTIONS

More recent studies demonstrate that although major sex-differentiated behavior patterns in juvenile monkeys are established prenatally, some aspects of these behaviors can be influenced by postnatal endocrine disruption. In studies using early postnatal treatment with the GnRH antagonist antide, male monkeys were observed in stable social groups between 12 and 15 months of age (Wallen *et al.* 1995). Half of the antide-treated males received testosterone replacement resulting in three levels of early testosterone, low (antide), intermediate (no antide or testosterone) and high (antide with supplementary testosterone). The behavioral categories were affiliative behaviors, agonistic behavior, play, immature sexual behavior, and infant (<five months old) directed behavior. To determine changes in sex-differentiated patterns of these behaviors, the treated and control males were compared with females of the same age.

As anticipated, untreated male and female juvenile monkeys differed most clearly in play behavior and immature sexual behavior. Males initiated and received more brief contact, chase, and rough and tumble play, but less frequently engaged in quiet solitary play, than females. Minimal effects of treatment were found on play behaviors; neonatally treated male juveniles, as well as control males, differed from the control females, but the treated males did not differ from control males. The only detectable effect was on reception of brief contact play. Males treated with antide and androgen, unlike the other males, did not differ from females in the frequency of brief contact play directed at them. As regards to immature sexual behavior, males in treated groups, as well as control males, showed a higher frequency of hip touches and footclasp mounts than females and did not differ from control males on these measures. Thus sex-differentiated play and immature sexual behavior, shown previously to be influenced by estrogen and androgen treatments during the late fetal period, were not affected by HPG suppression, and resulting lowering of neonatal testosterone, in the early postnatal period. Presumably this reflects a difference in the sensitive period for exogenous hormone effects on sexual differentiation of brain areas regulating these behaviors; however, as treatments were not identical, this conclusion must be qualified.

In contrast to play behavior, affiliative social behaviors (following, proximity, contact, grooming) did show a more feminine pattern in the GnRH-suppressed males. Affiliative behaviors, particularly proximity, following and infant-directed behavior, were generally higher in incidence in control females than control males. The HPG-suppressed males had similar frequencies of initiated proximity to other juveniles as did the females (although they did not differ significantly from control males). In examining proximity categories in more detail, the authors noted that proximity to the mother, the major proximity partner, was particularly sensitive to treatment. They reported a testosterone dose-related pattern of means for the duration of time spent in proximity to the mother (as a percentage of total proximity for an individual). The group with the highest testosterone as neonates (antide/androgen) spent the least time with their mothers, followed by the control males, the HPG-suppressed males, and the control females. Further analysis indicated that this was due to infant, rather than mother-controlled proximity interactions. The authors suggested that this abnormal degree of proximity to their mothers may have represented a delay in independence from mother, which is normally greater in males than females at this age, or that it may have represented a more subtle but permanent adjustment of male social interaction with females.

PRE/POSTNATAL INTERVENTIONS AND COGNITION

The experiments reported above were all based on observation of infants raised in social groups. In connection with their studies of differential effects of developmental brain lesions in nursery-reared male and female rhesus infants, investigators at NIH undertook some experiments with gonadal hormones and cognitive abilities tested beginning at about three months of age (Table 11.3) (Hagger and Bachevalier, 1991).

Clark and Goldman-Rakic (1989) noted that male infant rhesus performed better in a discrimination reversal task than females when tested beginning at 75 days of age. They found that performance of females could be improved to the level of males by administration of testosterone propionate during prenatal or early postnatal life (see Table 11.1 for treatment times). As anticipated, prenatally treated females had fully virilized genitalia, but postnatally treated females had only slight changes in genitalia. Nonetheless, the test performance of prenatal and postnatally treated females did not differ, and the two groups were combined for statistical comparison to controls. Graphs indicate that control females took longer to develop reversal skills than the control males, and testosterone-treated females, although all groups

TABLE 11.3   Comparison of two research programs that included testosterone treatment during development and cognitive behaviors

	Investigators	
	Hagger and Bachevalier (1991)	Clark and Goldman-Rakic (1989)
Task	Concurrent object discrimination	Discrimination reversal
Sex differentiation in normal infants	Females better than males (sessions to criterion)	Males better than females (errors to criterion)
Effect of brain lesion	Inferior temporal cortex: Females: Lesioned better than control Males: no effect	Orbitoprefrontal cortex: Females: no effect Males: lesioned more errors than controls
Effect of testosterone	Females: more errors	Females: fewer errors than nontreated females Males: no effect
Effect of orchiectomy	Males: fewer errors	n/a
Effect of ovariectomy + testosterone	Females: no effects	n/a
Effect of ovariectomy + dihydrotestosterone	Females: more errors	n/a

had similar low error rates by the sixth reversal. The authors suggest that the effects were due to sexual differentiation of the timing of brain maturation, and in particular of the cerebral cortex. This was supported by the finding that early orbitofrontal lesions had an adverse effect on male infant, but not female infant discrimination reversal performance. Presumably, males had an earlier dependence on frontal cortex in performing the discrimination reversal task.

The pooling of the various times of testosterone treatment for the statistical analysis may seem contrary to the concept of sensitive periods for sexual differentiation of the brain. However, in these experiments the hypothesis did not concern sexual differentiation of brain functions, but rather "sex differences in the emergence of a specific cognitive function" (which sex matured first). Further, the sexual differentiation did not involve the ability of the males and females to perform discrimination reversals but rather their early improvement during learning of this task. Thus this information is relevant to endocrine disruption but not necessarily to mechanism pathways that involve sensitive periods for sexual differentiation of the brain.

In a similar study, Hagger and Bachevalier (1991) noted that female infant rhesus monkeys performed the concurrent object discrimination (COD) task better than males. To explore the effects of early gonadal hormones, they ovariectomized or orchiectomized (castrated) infants within 48 hours of birth and then administered either testosterone or dihydrotestosterone daily to the ovariectomized females from immediately after the surgery to 3.5 months of age. Despite the small group sizes ($n = 3 - 8$) the authors identified significant effects of group for both errors and sessions to criterion during a COD test conducted from 1.5 to 3.5 months of age, as well as significant post-hoc comparisons of control males to orchiectomized males and control females to testosterone-treated females. This experiment indicated that removal of testosterone from genetic males in the early postnatal period "feminized" cognitive behavior, while administration of dihydrotestosterone to genetic, ovariectomized females "masculinized" test behavior. Recall that these treatments had minimal effects on sexually differentiated play behavior in the studies by Wallen et al. (1995). The authors thus suggest that binding to the androgen receptor, rather than aromatization of testosterone to estrogen, was the critical factor. Further, they reported that testosterone in normal males was significantly correlated with COD performance. Once again it is important to note that this study had to do with the concurrent effects of circulating testosterone on performance of cognitive tasks by infants, not with effects on sexual differentiation of the brain. Like the previous study it is relevant to endocrine disruption but not necessarily to mechanisms that involve action of steroid hormones during critical periods for sexual differentiation.

In addition to these two research programs, a number of experiments have measured cognitive function in infant and juvenile monkeys. However, there is limited information on sex differentiation in these tests. Commonly, male and female monkeys are both tested and treatment group sizes are usually not large enough to detect statistically significant sex differences. For example in reviewing studies of novelty preference, or visual recognition memory, the most commonly used cognitive test in monkeys under three months of age, most of the studies did not describe the sex distribution of the comparison groups, and often when the sex distribution was stated sex was not used as a variable in the analysis.

In contrast, extensive and elegant experiments in rats have shown that, in addition to influencing reproductive behavior and social interaction, manipulation of hormone levels during sensitive periods of brain development alters sex-differentiated performance of learning and memory tasks, particularly those that involve spatial memory. Thus spatial tasks have become a standard approach to detecting effects of endocrine disruption on sexual differentiation of the brain in humans and rodents. Mental rotation and targeting tasks are commonly used in humans (Kimura, 2002), and maze tasks with spatial cues in rats and mice (Williams et al., 1990). Although information on sexually differentiation of spatial cognition in nonhuman primates would be valuable, we identified only one paper directly addressing this issue.

In this experiment (LaCreuse et al., 1999), 112 rhesus monkeys of both sexes and in three age groups (young, middle-aged, old) were trained in a spatial memory task, the Delayed Recognition Span Test. In this test, an array of identical objects, increasing in number over trials, is presented to the monkeys. On each trial a new object is added at a new spatial location and needs to be selected by the animal in order to receive the reward. In a sample of 90 monkeys, an effect of sex was found at $P < 0.01$, with males demonstrating better performance. Working memory, but not reference memory, was sex differentiated, which is similar to findings in rats (Williams et al., 1990). The sex differences were mainly seen in the younger monkeys (4–14 years of age, $n = 8$ females and 27 males). Further work with this task may provide a sensitive assay for sex differences in spatial cognitive behavior similar to the mental rotation test in humans or the radial maze test in rats. Use of computer-generated "virtual" mazes in both humans (Astur et al., 2004) and nonhuman primates (Washburn and Astur, 2003) may also help bring rodent and human research in closer contact.

INTERVENTIONS IN THE JUVENILE PERIOD

Very little information is available on the consequences of endocrine disruption in juvenile monkeys. The juvenile period extends from the end of infancy (weaning) to puberty, typically considered in macaque species to be 8/12 months to 36 months for females and to 48 months for males. Recently, Mann et al. (2006) used the antithyroid agent methimazole to determine the effect of hypothyroid condition in juvenile male rhesus on puberty. The juvenile monkeys were orchiectomized to assess the effects on the hypothalamus without the complication of peripheral hormones. The endpoint in the study was the pubertal rise in plasma LH. With this approach, the authors were able to conclude that the hypothyroid condition delays the onset of puberty at the hypothalamic level. Implications for neurobehavioral development were not explored. In a study in female rhesus, the nonsteroidal estrogen DES and the estrogenic pesticide methoxychlor (MXC) were administered prior to and during puberty (Golub *et al.*, 2003, 2004). Both DES and MXC led to premature emergence of secondary sex characteristics. Nipple development and menarche were delayed by DES. Thus the estrogenic agents could not be said to either accelerate or delay puberty. The juvenile monkeys were tested for cognitive function throughout the one year dosing period. Some aspects of performance, such as rate of acquisition, were influenced by MXC, but not by the more potent estrogen DES. This study addresses the potential concurrent effects of estrogenic agents on brain function, rather than the effects on sexual differentiation, since only females were tested and sex-differentiated behaviors were not assessed.

IMPORTANT DATA GAPS

So what are the important data gaps in our understanding of endocrine disruptor effects on sex-differentiated aspects of neurobehavioral development in nonhuman primates? Play and immature sexual behavior in juvenile monkeys, and cognitive tasks in infants and juveniles, are the only endpoints explored thus far in connection with endocrine disruption during brain development in nonhuman primates.

- There are no studies of sexually differentiated nonreproductive behavior in *adult* nonhuman primates after endocrine disruption during brain development. Such studies would demonstrate the permanent effect of "organizational" exposures.
- There are no studies of sexually differentiated cognitive behavior in *juvenile* nonhuman primates. The changes in infant cognitive behavior have been interpreted as developmental delay, but longer term consequences, or later delays in maturation of cognitive ability, have not been studied.
- There are no studies of cognitive behavior in nonhuman primates using *tasks that are comparable to sexually differentiated cognition in humans.* In particular, studies of spatial cognition would be valuable in this regard.
- The potential role of androgenic adrenal steroids (DHEA/DHEAS) in fetal brain differentiation have not been explored. Dehydroepiandrosterone sulfate (DHEAS) is a steroidal hormone unique to primate species and is involved in the congenital adrenal hyperplasia syndrome.

In conclusion, a solid groundwork has been established for studies of endocrine disruption and its contribution to neurodevelopmental disorders in children. Such studies in a nonhuman primate will be critical in integrating findings from ongoing studies in human populations exposed to endocrine disrupting agents like polychlorinated biphenyls (PCBs), polybrominated diphenyl ethers (PBDEs), phthalates and polyphenols and basic research in laboratory rodents.

Acknowledgments

This chapter is based on a presentation made at the May 2006 Children's Environmental Health Symposium, sponsored by the Office of Environmental Health Hazard Assessment, California Environmental Protection Agency.

Disclaimer

Opinions expressed are those of the authors and do not represent those of the California Environmental Protection Agency.

REFERENCES

Allen, S. H., Bennett, J. A., Mizejewski, G. J., Andersen, T. T., Ferraris, S., and Jacobson, H. I. (1993). Purification of alpha-fetoprotein from human cord serum with demonstration of its antiestrogenic activity. *Biochim Biophys Acta* **1202**, 135–142.

Anderson, D. C., Lasley, B. L., Risher, R. A., Shepherd, J. H., Newman, L., and Hendrickx, A. G. (1976). Transplacental gradients of sex-hormone-binding globulin in human and simian pregnancy. *Clin Endocrinol (Oxf)* **5**, 657–669.

Astur, R. S., Tropp, J., Sava, S., Constable, R. T., and Markus, E. J. (2004). Sex differences and correlations in a virtual Morris water task, a virtual radial arm maze, and mental rotation. *Behav Brain Res* **151**, 103–115.

Bakker, J., De Mees, C., Douhard, Q. *et al.* (2006). Alpha-fetoprotein protects the developing female mouse brain from masculinization and defeminization by estrogens. *Nat Neurosci* **9**, 220–226.

Baron-Cohen, S., Knickmeyer, R. C., and Belmonte, M. K. (2005). Sex differences in the brain: implications for explaining autism. *Science* **310**, 819–823.

Clark, A. S. and Goldman-Rakic, P. S. (1989). Gonadal hormones influence the emergence of cortical function in nonhuman primates. *Behav Neurosci* **103**, 1287–1295.

Colborn, T. (2004). Neurodevelopment and endocrine disruption. *Environ Health Perspect* **112**, 944–949.

Colborn, T. (2006). A case for revisiting the safety of pesticides: a closer look at neurodevelopment. *Environ Health Perspect* **114**, 10–17.

Colborn, T. and Clement, C. (1992). *Chemically-induced Alterations in Sexual and Functional Development: The Wildlife/Human Connection.* Princeton, NJ: Princeton Scientific Publishing Co.

Colborn, T., Dumanoski, D., and Meyer, J. (1997). *Our Stolen Future: How we are Threatening our Fertiity, Intelligence and Survival. A Scientific Detective Story.* New York: Penguin Books.

Ehrhardt, A. A. and Meyer-Bahlburg, H. F. (1981). Effects of prenatal sex hormones on gender-related behavior. *Science* **211**, 1312–1318.

Gelbke, H. P., Kayser, M., and Poole, A. (2004). OECD test strategies and methods for endocrine disruptors. *Toxicology* 205, 17–25.

Golub, M. S., Hogrefe, C. E., Germann, S. L., Lasley, B. L., Natarajan, K., and Tarantal, A. F. (2003). Effects of exogenous estrogenic agents on pubertal growth and reproductive system maturation in female rhesus monkeys. *Toxicol Sci* **74**, 103–113.

Golub, M. S., Germann, S. L., and Hogrefe, C. E. (2004). Endocrine disruption and cognitive function in adolescent female rhesus monkeys. *Neurotoxicol Teratol* **26**, 799–809.

Goy, R. W. and Deputte, B. L. (1996). The effects of diethylstilbestrol (DES) before birth on the development of masculine behavior in juvenile female rhesus monkeys. *Horm Behav* **30**, 379–386.

Goy, R. W., Bercovitch, F. B., and McBrair, M. C. (1988). Behavioral masculinization is independent of genital masculinization in prenatally androgenized female rhesus macaques. *Horm Behav* **22**, 552–571.

Hagger, C. and Bachevalier, J. (1991). Visual habit formation in 3-month-old monkeys (*Macaca mulatta*): reversal of sex difference following neonatal manipulations of androgens. *Behav Brain Res* **45**, 57–63.

Harding, A. K., Daston, G. P., Boyd, G. R. *et al.* (2006). Endocrine disrupting chemicals research program of the U.S. Environmental Protection Agency: summary of a peer-review report. *Environ Health Perspect* **114**, 1276–1282.

Herman, R. A., Jones, B., Mann, D. R., and Wallen, K. (2000). Timing of prenatal androgen exposure: anatomical and endocrine effects on juvenile male and female rhesus monkeys. *Horm Behav* **38**, 52–66.

Herman, R. A., Measday, M. A., and Wallen, K. (2003). Sex differences in interest in infants in juvenile rhesus monkeys: relationship to prenatal androgen. *Horm Behav* **43**, 573–583.

Hotchkiss, J. (1985). Changes in sex hormone-binding globulin binding capacity and percent free estradiol during development in the female rhesus monkey (*Macaca mulatta*): relation to the metabolic clearance rate of estradiol. *J Clin Endocrinol Metab* **60**, 786–792.

Kaltiala-Heino, R., Rimpela, M., Rissanen, A., and Rantanen, P. (2001). Early puberty and early sexual activity are associated with bulimic-type eating pathology in middle adolescence. *J Adolesc Health* **28**, 346–352.

Kaltiala-Heino, R., Kosunen, E., and Rimpela, M. (2003a). Pubertal timing, sexual behaviour and self-reported depression in middle adolescence. *J Adolesc* **26**, 531–545.

Kaltiala-Heino, R., Marttunen, M., Rantanen, P., and Rimpela, M. (2003b). Early puberty is associated with mental health problems in middle adolescence. *Soc Sci Med* **57**, 1055–1064.

Kavlock, R. J., Daston, G. P., DeRosa, C. *et al.* (1996). Research needs for the risk assessment of health and environmental effects of endocrine disruptors: a report of the U.S. EPA-sponsored workshop. *Environ Health Perspect* **104**(suppl 4), 715–740.

Kimura, D. (2002). REVIEW. Sex Hormones Influence Human Cognitive Pattern. *Neuro Endocrinol Lett* **23**(suppl 4), 67–77.

Knickmeyer, R., Baron-Cohen, S., Raggatt, P., and Taylor, K. (2005a). Foetal testosterone, social relationships, and restricted interests in children. *J Child Psychol Psychiatry* **46**, 198–210.

Knickmeyer, R. C., Wheelwright, S., Taylor, K., Raggatt, P., Hackett, G., and Baron-Cohen, S. (2005b). Gender-typed play and amniotic testosterone. *Dev Psychol* **41**, 517–528.

Knickmeyer, R., Baron-Cohen, S., Raggatt, P., Taylor, K., and Hackett, G. (2006). Fetal testosterone and empathy. *Horm Behav* **49**, 282–292.

Lacreuse, A., Hendon, J. G., Killiany, R. J., Rosens, D. L., and Moss, M. B. (1999). Spatial cognition in rhesus monkeys: Male superiority declines with age. *Horm Behav* **36**, 70–76.

Longnecker, M. P., Bellinger, D. C., Crews, D. *et al.* (2003). An approach to assessment of endocrine disruption in the National Children's Study. *Environ Health Perspect* **111**, 1691–1697.

Mann, D. R. (2005). Neonatal endocrine activation and development of the primate reproductive and immune system. In: Weinbauer, G. F. B. E., Muller, W., and Vogel, F. eds. *New Developments and Challenges in Primate Toxicology.* Munster: Waxmann Munster, pp. 33–62.

Mann, D. R., Akinbami, M. A., Gould, K. G., Tanner, J. M., and Wallen, K. (1993). Neonatal treatment of male monkeys with a gonadotropin-releasing hormone agonist alters differentiation of central nervous system centers that regulate sexual and skeletal development. *J Clin Endocrinol Metab* **76**, 1319–1324.

Mann, D. R., Akinbami, M. A., Gould, K. G., Paul, K., and Wallen, K. (1998). Sexual maturation in male rhesus monkeys, importance of neonatal testosterone exposure and social rank. *J Endocrinol* **156**, 493–501.

Mann, D. R., Bhat, G. K., Stah, C. D., Pohl, C.R., and Plant, T. M. (2006). Induction of a hypothyroid state during juvenile development delays pubertal reactivation of the neuroendocrine system governing luteinising hormone secretion in the male rhesus monkey (*Macaca mulatta*). *J Neuroendocrinol* **18**, 662–671.

Matthiessen, P. and Johnson, I. (2006). Implications of research on endocrine disruption for the environmental risk assessment, regulation and monitoring of chemicals in the European Union. *Environ Pollut* **146**, 9–18.

Mattison, D. R. and King, J. C. (1983). Development of a nonhuman primate model for fetoscopy. *J Med Primatol* **12**, 319–330.

Meyer-Bahlburg, H. F. and Ehrhardt, A. A. (1986). Prenatal diethylstilbestrol exposure: behavioral consequences in humans. *Monogr Neural Sci* **12**, 90–95.

Meyer-Bahlburg, H. F., Dolezal, C., Baker, S. W., Carlson, A. D., Obeid, J. S., and New, M. I. (2004). Cognitive and motor development of children with and without congenital adrenal hyperplasia after early-prenatal dexamethasone. *J Clin Endocrinol Metab* **89**, 610–614.

Mizejewski, G. J. (2004). Biological roles of alpha-fetoprotein during pregnancy and perinatal development. *Exp Biol Med (Maywood)* **229**, 439–463.

Office of Pesticides Pollutants and Toxic Substances USEPA. (1998). Endocrine Disruptor Screening and Testing Advisory Committee (EDSTAC): Final Report.

Perera, A. D. and Plant, T. M. (1992). The neurobiology of primate puberty. *CIBA Found Symp* **168**, 252–262.

Pomerantz, S. M., Roy, M. M., Thornton, J. E., and Goy, R. W. (1985). Expression of adult female patterns of sexual behavior by male, female, and pseudohermaphroditic female rhesus monkeys. *Biol Reprod* **33**, 878–889.

Ramrakha, S., Caspi, A., Dickson, N., Moffitt, T. E., and Paul, C. (2000). Psychiatric disorders and risky sexual behaviour in young adulthood: cross sectional study in birth cohort. *BMJ* **321**, 263–266.

Schantz, S. L. and Widholm, J. J. (2001). Cognitive effects of endocrine-disrupting chemicals in animals. *Environ Health Perspect* **109**, 1197–1206.

Tarttelin, M. F. and Gorski, R. A. (1988). Postnatal influence of diethylstilbestrol on the differentiation of the sexually dimorphic nucleus in the rat is as effective as perinatal treatment. *Brain Res* **456**, 271–274.

Taylor, M. R., Holmes, P., Duarte-Davidson, R., Humfrey, C. D., and Harrison, P. T. (1999). A research strategy for investigating the ecological significance of endocrine disruption: report of a UK workshop. *Sci Total Environ* **233**, 181–191.

Terasawa, E. (1995). Control of luteinizing hormone-releasing hormone pulse generation in nonhuman primates. *Cell Mol Neurobiol* **15**, 141–164.

Vos, J. G., Dybing, E., Greim, H. A. *et al.* (2000). Health effects of endocrine-disrupting chemicals on wildlife, with special reference to the European situation. *Crit Rev Toxicol* **30**, 71–133.

Wallen, K., Maestripieri, D., and Mann, D. R. (1995). Effects of neonatal testicular suppression with a GnRH antagonist on social behavior in group-living juvenile rhesus monkeys. *Horm Behav* **29**, 322–337.

Washburn, D. A. and Astur, R. S. (2003). Exploration of virtual mazes by rhesus monkeys (*Macaca mulatta*). *Anim Cogn* **6**, 161–168.

Weiss, B. (2002). Sexually dimorphic nonreproductive behaviors as indicators of endocrine disruption. *Environ Health Perspect* **110**(suppl 3), 387–391.

Williams, C. L., Barnett, A. M., and Meck, W. H. (1990). Organizational effects of early gonadal secretions on sexual differentiation in spatial memory. *Behav Neurosci* **104**, 84–97.

CHAPTER 12

Exposure to Drugs of Abuse: Alterations in Nonhuman Primate Development as Models of Adverse Consequences

Merle G. Paule

Examples of the use of nonhuman primates as models for determining the effects of developmental exposure to drugs of abuse are, unfortunately, all too rare. Given the apparent utility and relevance of these unique models, it seems that the research community is failing to take advantage of these invaluable resources and, thus, the public for whom we toil is not provided timely access to valuable information waiting to be discovered. Use of these models has repeatedly demonstrated or confirmed the effects of abused drugs on the developing nervous system. Gestational exposure to cocaine can lead to a decrease in the ability of offspring to adjust to important changes in their environment and to a decrease in sensitivity to the behavioral effects of cocaine as adults. Chronic marijuana use during pubescence decreases aspects of motivation, but complete recovery can occur within a few months of drug withdrawal. Opiates routinely used as analgesics during the peripartum period can cause changes in behavior that are detectable for at least a year after exposure. Exposure to ketamine during critical periods of brain growth can significantly alter the natural pattern of programmed apoptotic cell death in addition to causing necrotic cell death. The true value of the nonhuman primate in such studies has yet to be realized.

INTRODUCTION

This chapter will provide an overview of our work and that of others in which the consequences of exposures to drugs of abuse have been studied in immature nonhuman primates. In reviewing the literature on this topic, it is very surprising that so little work has been done in what is arguably the most appropriate animal model available for studying the consequences of exposure to drugs of abuse during development. Given the magnitude of human exposures to abused drugs that can occur during important formative periods, it only seems prudent that substantial efforts to understand the consequences of such exposure in nonhuman primates should be a scientific and societal priority. Unfortunately, that has not been the case. The current acknowledgment that an apparently increasing proportion of our offspring are diagnosed with a variety of behavioral/functional problems such as autism and related disorders, attention deficit/hyperactivity disorder, and restless leg syndrome, suggests that environmental factors are likely contributing factors. The extent to which abused substances and related compounds might contribute to these clinical entities is not yet understood and much more research needs to be conducted in order to address these issues. Here, examples of both acute (short-term) and chronic (long-term) drug exposures will be provided, with the focus in all cases being on subsequent residual or "down-stream" functional consequences and not on physical abnormalities or acute effects. In all cases, exposures utilized are considered to be very relevant (similar) to those experienced by humans. Likewise, many of the behavioral instruments utilized to assess brain function in these animal models have been shown in human subjects to correlate with important clinical measures of intellect such as IQ scores (Paule et al., 1990, 1999b; Paule, 2001). The developmental effects of ethanol will not be discussed here, since the literature on that topic alone (particularly with respect to the anatomical abnormalities caused by alcohol exposure during pregnancy) is considerable and has been addressed elsewhere (i.e. Clarren et al., 1990, 1992; Astley et al., 1999; Shively et al., 2002; Roberts et al., 2004; Schneider et al., 2004, 2005). Burbacher and Grant (2006) have also recently reviewed the topic of the neurodevelopmental effects of both ethanol and methanol, covering both the human and monkey literature. Important findings on the effects of the interaction of ethanol with prenatal stress are detailed in a chapter in this publication (Schneider et al., 2007) and a recent review on the interactions between genes, early experience and alcohol intake in adolescent macaques has also been published (Barr et al., 2004)

A noted presumption here is that the need for – and relevance of – animal models in biomedical research is absolute. Preclinical data from animal models are required for drug discovery and approval and to determine the safety or toxicity of environmental chemicals. Disease processes and interventions are most efficiently studied when appropriate animal models exist. The slow progress made toward finding effective treatments for Alzheimer's disease and other brain disorders is primarily due to the lack of appropriate animal models that could greatly expedite such research. The absolute requirement for animal studies results from the great difficulty in conducting definitive studies in humans. In the case of studying the effects of in utero drug exposure on human offspring, for example, difficulties in the techniques of exposure measurement preclude accurate determination of the type, dose, and pattern of drug use (Day and Robles, 1989; Bandstra and Burkett, 1991; Lindenberg *et al.*, 1991; Nair and Watson, 1991; Slutsker 1992). Likewise, difficulties in controlling for a host of confounding variables such as race, socioeconomic status, other drug use, quality and frequency of prenatal care (Bandstra and Burkett, 1991; Lindenberg *et al.*, 1991; Slutsker 1992) often make interpretation of findings problematic at best. While more recent studies are attempting to take these confounds into consideration (e.g. Chiriboga 1998; Richardson 1998; Scher *et al.*, 2000), limitations like these seriously undermine assessments of chronic drug exposures on growth and development in human studies.

The phylogenetic proximity of nonhuman primates to humans generally qualifies them as the animals most closely approximating the human condition and their ethical use in research has been addressed previously (Evans 1990). In this chapter, the laboratory rhesus monkey (*Macaca mulatta*) will be the primary species discussed, since most of the work relevant to drugs of abuse has been conducted in this animal. This chapter will focus on several aspects of complex brain function observed during and/or after drug exposures that occur during development because they provide important metrics of functional derangements that can accompany such exposures.

METHODS FOR ASSESSING COMPLEX BRAIN FUNCTION IN NONHUMAN PRIMATES

Since the focus of this chapter will revolve around a discussion of the functional consequences of drug exposure(s) during development, it will be important to provide some description of the methods utilized in assessing important cognitive domains in these animals. Descriptions of a variety of behavioral tasks thought to depend upon specific brain functions will be provided and, inasmuch as specific functions are subserved by specific brain areas, those areas will be mentioned, when known.

While the broader topic of behavioral methods utilized in toxicological and teratological studies in nonhuman primates has been recently discussed in some detail (Burbacher and Grant, 2000), most of the studies to be described here have employed a specific battery of operant behavioral tasks (see Paule *et al.*, 1988, 1992; Schulze *et al.*, 1988, 1989; Paule 2001, 2005). This instrument is known as the National Center for Toxicological Research (NCTR) operant test battery or OTB, where the term operant simply means that subjects have to operate something in their environment (e.g. levers or press-plates) in order to obtain reinforcers (in our studies, banana-flavored food pellets). Operant tasks typically require extensive training and therefore differ from spontaneous or ethological behaviors that can also serve as metrics of brain function. The utility of operant behaviors derives from the fact that they can be made extremely specific, allowing for the isolation of brain functions of special importance or interest (i.e. learning, time perception, counting) and they can be generated at the will of the experimenter after appropriate training (see Paule, 2005). Operant tasks are also easily automated, a feature which eliminates subjective interpretation of responses and easily provides for repeated testing under identical conditions. And, perhaps most importantly, operant tasks are easily utilized with human subjects and OTB performance is, in many instances, significantly correlated with IQ in children (Paule *et al.*, 1999b). This observation alone demonstrates direct relevance to the human condition and eliminates assumptions about this issue in risk-assessment procedures.

Utilizing identical endpoints across species minimizes the need to employ large safety factors when extrapolating data from laboratory animals to humans and presumably provides more precise estimates of risk associated with human exposure to chemicals. Additionally, the effects of several drugs on OTB performance by monkeys have been shown to be predictive of drug effects in humans (Paule, 2001). For example, when rhesus monkeys are exposed acutely to pure delta-9-tetrahydro-cannabinol (THC, the primary psychoactive ingredient in marijuana smoke) they overestimate the passage of time, responding as though 8 or 9 seconds is perceived as 10 seconds or more. When exposed to marijuana smoke, short-term memory is disrupted along with time perception. Both of these observations are important because the same effects of THC and marijuana smoke are seen in human subjects and at similar exposure levels. Where data are available, similar findings hold for other drugs (Paule, 2001). Brief descriptions of the OTB tasks, as well as other tests that have been used to study the functional consequences of exposure to drugs of abuse in monkeys, will be provided here.

Motivation

It is very important to have some measure of a subject's motivation to perform tasks that are being used to assess the integrity of the brain. If the reinforcer being used to elicit the behavior of interest is ineffective, then the data obtained from such a task will be difficult to interpret. Progressive ratio tasks (initially described by Hodos, 1961; Hodos and Kalman, 1963), are often employed to determine how much effort subjects are willing to put in to earn reinforcers. For all of the operant studies to be discussed here, the reinforcers used are food pellets. In the progressive ratio task as used in the NCTR OTB, responses are made on a single response lever and the number of lever presses required to obtain a reinforcer (the response/reinforcer ratio) progresses throughout each test session. Initially, some small number of lever presses (e.g. two) is required to obtain the first reinforcer while the next reinforcer "costs" four lever presses, the next six and so on. In this manner, the work required for each subsequent reinforcer is quickly ramped up, and task performance provides metrics (response rates, number of reinforcers earned, etc.) of motivation. Given that many, if not all, of the tasks utilized in studies of the functional assessment of drug effects during development employ some type of reinforcement, it is critical to know what effect drug treatment might have on a subjects' motivation for the reinforcer employed. Typically, performance on these tasks over time is very consistent within a given subject, but can vary considerably between subjects.

Importantly, for food reinforcers, body weight – and not recent feeding episodes – is the more important variable in controlling progressive ratio performance (Ferguson and Paule, 1995, 1997). Brain areas likely to be involved in the performance of this type of task include the "reward" centers (e.g. the nucleus accumbens) and the hypothalamic feeding centers.

Visual discrimination

To determine how well subjects discriminate colors, we have employed a conditioned position responding task. In this task, a red, yellow, blue, or green color is presented to the subject. The subject indicates that it has seen the color by pressing the colored stimulus. If the initial color had been red or yellow, then a left choice response is reinforced; if it had been blue or green, then a right choice response is reinforced. In well-trained subjects, task performance is characterized by rapid responding and average choice accuracies of greater than 90%. Processes underlying these types of abilities are thought to reside in frontal-cortical brain areas (Goldman et al., 1970; Kojima et al., 1982).

Learning

The learning task used as part of the NCTR OTB is an incremental repeated acquisition task that is a modification of more traditional repeated acquisition procedures (Cohn and Paule, 1995) and is very similar to the children's game "Simon." Here, subjects repeatedly acquire knowledge in an incremental fashion each test session. Four response levers, arranged horizontally, are used in this task and each session starts with the presentation of a one-lever response "sequence": a response to the correct one of the four levers results in reinforcer delivery. After this sequence has been mastered, the task difficulty (required response sequence length) is incremented to a two-lever sequence in which the subject must learn which of the four levers is the "new" lever for the "incremented" sequence and remember to follow a response to the new lever with a response to the lever that was correct in the previously learned one-lever "sequence." Once this two-lever sequence has been learned, the response requirement is again incremented to a three-lever sequence and so on up to a maximum six-lever sequence. In each test session, then, several learning curves can be captured, one for each lever sequence length mastered. Response accuracy, speed, errors, and length of sequence mastered are metrics of learning. While there is a considerable training period during which animals come to learn the rules of reinforcement (task contingencies), asymptotic performance, at least for short response sequences, can be obtained after only a few weeks of training. After this time, the process of new learning can be observed each test session.

In other forms of learning tasks, subjects are assessed using nonautomated procedures (see again, Burbacher and Grant, 2000) in which subjects come to learn conditional discriminations. Generally in these procedures – usually performed using the Wisconsin General Test Apparatus (WGTA) – two different stimuli are used to cover baited wells in which food reinforcers have been placed. One stimulus (a black square block for example) is designated as the correct or reinforced stimulus, whereas another stimulus (a red square block) is designated as the incorrect stimulus. Here, the number of trials needed for subjects to learn the correct discrimination becomes the primary metric of learning. Once the discrimination has been learned, a new set of stimuli must be used, or the problem can be reversed. In such reversal learning paradigms, the previously incorrect stimulus becomes the correct stimulus and vice versa and the number of trials to learn the new discrimination becomes the metric of learning. Performance of learning tasks is thought to be heavily dependent upon the integrity of the hippocampus and reversal learning involves orbitofrontal cortical function (see Jentsch *et al.*, 2002).

Short-term memory

A variety of tasks are used with nonhuman primates for assessing short-term memory. These include delayed matching-to-sample (DMTS) procedures (see Paule *et al.*, 1998a for an overview) and other delayed recall procedures (see Burbacher and Grant, 2000 for additional examples). Typically, each trial in these tasks begins with the presentation of a "sample" stimulus that is "acknowledged" by the subject (they touch it or otherwise indicate that they have seen it). After this acknowledgment, random recall delays occur after which two or more "choice" stimuli are presented, only one of which matches the initial sample stimulus. A response to the "matching" stimulus results in reinforcer delivery. Accuracy of matching after no or very short delays (i.e. with no or little opportunity to forget) is thought to represent a measure of an organism's ability to attend to the task and to encode the information to be remembered and also represents the ability of the subject to learn the conceptual basis of the matching-to-sample principle. Typically, response accuracies at very short delays are quite high. As recall delays increase, response accuracy decreases, with the slope of the decrease in accuracy serving as a metric of memory decay or a "forgetting" function.

Other delayed response tasks that employ the WGTA can also be used to assess short-term memory. In delayed alternation tasks, for example, the correct or reinforced location alternates from left to right and subjects are required to remember the location of the last reinforced location from trial to trial. Imposing delays between trials invokes the need to utilize short-term memory. The performance of short-term memory tasks is thought to depend upon the hippocampus, subiculum, and prefrontal cortical areas. (Deadwyler and Hampson, 2004).

Time perception

Timing behavior, or temporal discrimination, can be quantified using several different tasks (see Paule *et al.*, 1999a for a review of issues concerning experimental aspects of timing ability). In the examples to be discussed here, a temporal response differentiation (TRD) task has been utilized which requires subjects to press and hold a response lever down for at least 10 but not more than 14 seconds. Thus, subjects must hit a 4-second window of opportunity to obtain a reinforcer. The data obtained from this task include a variety of measures associated with the distribution of lever-hold durations (time production) which are typically characterized by Gaussian distributions. It is thought that the distribution means of "timed" responses represent timing accuracy and that the spread or standard deviation of the response distributions represents timing precision. Alterations in the characteristics of the response duration distribution are thought to provide insights into the mechanisms of timing such as the speed of an "internal clock" (Meck, 1996). Shifts to shorter means in the response duration distribution have been interpreted as increases in the speed of the internal clock (8 seconds is interpreted as 10 seconds) and shifts toward longer means suggests a slowing of the internal clock (12 seconds seems like 10 seconds). It has recently been demonstrated that timing mechanisms appear at around 6 years of age in children (Chelonis *et al.*, 2004). While the specific brain structures associated with time perception have not been studied extensively, recent data suggest that the basal ganglia, right parietal cortex and frontal-striatal systems are involved (Rao *et al.*, 2001).

Relevance to the human experience

Data obtained from children performing NCTR OTB tasks – for coins instead of food – have provided important comparative information: OTB performance of children is generally indistinguishable from that of well-trained monkeys (Figure 12.1) (Paule *et al.*, 1990). And, as mentioned earlier, performance of most OTB tasks correlates significantly with measures of intelligence in kids (Paule *et al.*, 1999b). Some data have also been published concerning OTB performance in children as a function of age (e.g. Chelonis *et al.*, 2000, 2004).

ALTERED BRAIN FUNCTION AFTER EXPOSURE TO DRUGS OF ABUSE DURING DEVELOPMENT

Cocaine

Gestational exposure

In studies designed to model human pregnancies, young adult female rhesus monkeys were exposed to cocaine once pregnancy was established (ca. gestation day 30–40) and exposure continued until birth (see Morris *et al.*, 1996a, 1996b, 1997 for exposure

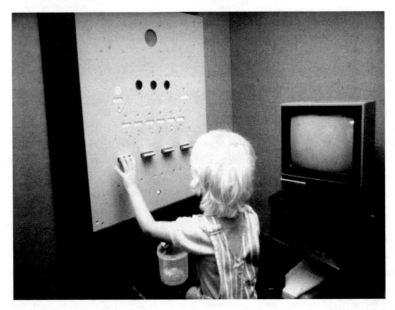

FIGURE 12.1   A four-year-old boy ready to perform operant test battery tasks (for nickel reinforcers). Video-taped instructions are provided via the adjacent monitor prior to each task. The manipulanda include retractable levers and press-plates and reinforcers (nickels) are delivered into the plastic
bucket below the panel.

details). Initial groups ($n = 3$) were exposed to doses equivalent to human
exposures of about one-tenth to a quarter of a gram of cocaine hydrochloride per day
and a Monday through Friday dosing regimen that modeled the binge-use typical of
human cocaine users was used. Cocaine binges are often characterized by several days
of drug-taking followed by 1–2 days of recovery in between binges. For these studies,
the intramuscular route of administration was used since the pharmacokinetics of
cocaine via this route of exposure nicely modeled those seen after intranasal administration (snorting) in humans (Morris *et al.*, 1996a). Once it was demonstrated that
these dosing regimens were well tolerated and pregnancy outcomes remained good,
an additional treatment group was given progressively increasing doses throughout
pregnancy: the dose was increased every two weeks to allow tolerance to the appetite-
suppressing effects of cocaine to develop and ensure adequate nutrition. By term,
some subjects were receiving doses equivalent to about 1.5–1.75 g of cocaine HCl (the
form typically snorted) per day. Once it was clear that this escalating dosing regimen
was also well tolerated, dosing was begun weeks to months prior to mating to obtain
a larger group ($n = 10$) of pregnancies that would experience exposure throughout
gestation (Paule *et al.*, 1996; Morris *et al.*, 1997). Since the focus of these efforts was
to determine the effects of in utero cocaine exposure on the integrity of offspring
brain function, no exposures occurred after birth.

While no significant effects of cocaine exposure were found in the smaller groups of animals in which exposure began after the detection of pregnancy, the offspring exposed to cocaine throughout the entire pregnancy weighed significantly less, were shorter (crown–rump lengths were less) and had smaller head circumferences than controls (Morris *et al.*, 1997). These findings were important because they replicated those reported for children exposed to cocaine during gestation. The monkey infants remained with their natural mothers for six months, after which they were weaned, singly housed, and began OTB training. Acquisition of OTB responding was monitored for over a year and no exposure-related effects on task learning curves were observed (Morris *et al.*, 1996b).

These findings are of interest given that others have reported neurobehavioral deficits in rhesus monkey offspring exposed similarly to cocaine during gestation (He *et al.*, 2004). These authors utilized a nonhuman primate adaptation of the Neonatal Behavioral Assessment Scale (NBAS; described in Schneider *et al.*, 1991 and Schneider and Suomi, 1992) to assess offspring weekly for the first month of life. The NBAS provides a fairly comprehensive assessment of alertness, general physical tone, responses to a variety of stimuli and major reflexes. Exposure to cocaine in utero was associated with increased tremulousness during weeks 1 and 2, and alterations in orientation, state control, and motor maturity during weeks 2–4. Testing beyond this age in these animals has not been reported.

Drug challenges

For 6 years after a year of OTB training, a number of psychoactive drugs were given to the monkey offspring in the Morris *et al.* studies (1996 a and b; 1997) in efforts to determine whether specific neurotransmitter systems might have been altered by gestational cocaine exposure (see Chelonis *et al.*, 2003 for exposure details). In particular, the focus has been on the dopamine system since cocaine is known to cause its typical behavioral effects via its interaction with it. In these acute dose–response studies, no differences in drug sensitivities were noted among the smaller treatment groups, but, while most of those data have yet to be analyzed for the larger treatment group, preliminary results suggest that animals exposed to cocaine in utero are less sensitive as adults (ca. 6 years of age) to the behavioral effects of cocaine to disrupt behavior in the OTB timing task (Paule *et al.*, 2005a, 2005b). This finding indicates that gestational cocaine exposure alters the function of the dopamine system and that these effects may represent permanent alterations in neurochemistry.

Other investigators have shown that similar gestational cocaine exposures in rhesus monkeys cause a reduction in the number of cortical neurons, alter the normal migration pattern of cortical cells, and change glial morphology (Lidow 1995, 1998; Lidow and Song, 2001a, 2001b). These changes, however, occur only if the exposure occurs during the period of neocortical neuronogenesis (Lidow *et al.*, 2001). In addition, cocaine exposure late in the first trimester of pregnancy induces an increase in cell death (presumably via apoptotic mechanisms) in the cerebral wall of fetal monkeys

(He *et al.*, 1999; Lidow and Song, 2001a, 2001b). In yet other studies, dopaminergic and opioidergic systems were examined in similarly exposed rhesus monkey fetuses. Here it was demonstrated that in utero cocaine exposure reduced the levels of mu-opiate receptor mRNA in the diencephalon (Chai *et al.*, 1999). Cocaine exposure also reduced the levels of tyrosine hydroxylase mRNA in the substantia nigra and the ventral tegmental area (Ronnekleiv and Naylor, 1995; Ronnekleiv *et al.*, 1998), increased dopamine D1, D2, and D5 receptor subtype mRNAs in the frontal cortex/striatal area (Choi and Ronnekleiv, 1996; Ronnekleiv *et al.*, 1998), and increased dopamine transporter mRNA expression within midbrain dopamine neurons (Fang and Ronnekleiv, 1999). In addition, endogenous opioid systems (presumably in dopamine target neurons) were altered in these same animals: dynorphin and enkephalin mRNA expression was increased in the striatum and enkephalin mRNA also increased in the frontal cortex. These observations suggest an upregulation of certain aspects of dopaminergic systems, presumably because of prolonged hypoactivity caused by prolonged cocaine exposure (Fang and Ronnekleiv, 1999). Thus, the OTB behavioral observations of hyposensitivity to cocaine seen in gestationally exposed adults may represent the functional consequences of such cellular effects.

Age-related sensitivity to dopaminergic compounds

One interesting observation noted during the acute drug challenge experiments was the discovery that, irrespective of treatment group, monkeys become increasingly sensitive to the behavioral effects of cocaine to disrupt progressive ratio responding as they mature (Paule *et al.*, 1995, 1998b; Morris *et al.*, 1996c). Animals about $1\frac{1}{2}$ years of age are 10–30 times less sensitive to an intravenous injection of cocaine than are 10- to 11-year-old adults: juveniles at about 3 years of age are intermediate in sensitivity. Thus, irrespective of gestational cocaine exposure, rhesus monkeys become more sensitive to the behavioral effects of cocaine simply as a function of age. These observations of drug effects on motivation task performance demonstrate that the young primate brain is quite different from the mature brain in its response to the acute effects of cocaine. Subsequent studies have shown similar age-dependent sensitivities to methylphenidate and amphetamine, suggesting that this phenomenon likely relates to the maturation of the dopaminergic system (Morris *et al.*, 1996c).

This developmental time-course of the sensitivity of the dopamine system and related physiology likely has important implications for the abuse of these drugs since abuse of these substances generally occurs after puberty. It is also possible that altered functions of dopamine systems that occur as a function of in utero cocaine exposure may not become apparent until those systems transition to their adult forms.

Behavioral plasticity

The lack of effects of gestational cocaine exposure on the ability of the young monkeys in our study to learn to perform the OTB tasks seems remarkable in light of the effects of similar exposures to alter development of the frontal cortex (Lidow, 1998; Lidow and Song, 2001a, 2001b), dopamine neurons (Ronnekleiv and Naylor, 1995; Choi and Ronnekleiv, 1996; Ronnekleiv et al., 1998), and the levels of dynorphin and enkephalin mRNA (Chai et al., 1997). It is possible that the operant behavioral assessments occurred too early or too late in life to show effects or that the highly practiced, food-reinforced tasks were simply insensitive to the effects of in utero cocaine exposure.

Since reversal learning tasks are thought to provide greater behavioral challenges than initial learning procedures because the new behaviors to be learned require the extinction of previously acquired responses (Schmajuk and Blair, 1995; Means and Holsten, 1992; Hilson and Strupp, 1997; Li and Shao, 1998), we instituted a task reversal in the OTB color and position discrimination task as a behavioral challenge. Instead of a left choice being correct after presentation of a red or yellow color and a right choice being correct after presentation of a blue or green color, the correct positions were reversed (Chelonis et al., 2003). This reversal occurred when the animals were 7 years of age, after they had over 6 years of experience with the original task. As expected, all animals showed impaired reversal perform-ance initially and all were relatively slow in adapting their behavior to match the new task rules. All cocaine-exposed groups took more sessions to attain – or never attained – prereversal-like responding than did the control animals. After $2\frac{1}{2}$ years, animals from our escalating dose group improved only up to the point where they were obtaining reinforcers by chance (50% choice accuracy), suggest-ing that the escalating dosing regimen produced long-lasting – likely permanent – deficits in behavioral plasticity.

Reversal data from the other treatment groups showed that in utero cocaine expo-sure caused dose-related deficits in behavioral adaptation (Chelonis et al., 2003). Motoric abilities were not affected (rates of responding did not show a systematic effect of exposure), thus, the reversal effects primarily unmasked the inability of sub-jects to extinguish a heavily over-practiced behavior and/or to adapt to environmen-tal requirements. Although there were very few subjects in this study, the results were striking. These findings are not unlike those seen in rats exposed prenatally to cocaine where subjects have difficulty in performing serial reversal and extradimensional set shifting tasks (Garavan et al., 2000).

More recently, we have employed reversal-type procedures when our delayed matching-to-sample task was changed to a delayed nonmatching-to-sample task. In this case, the rather striking deficits that were observed in these same animals for the conditioned position responding reversal were not observed: there was no signifi-cant difference in postreversal acquisition between treatment groups (Dimova et al., 2007). The lack of a significant treatment effect in these studies may be due to the unique procedural aspects of this DMTS/DNMTS reversal wherein the "different" stimuli become the correct stimuli, and attests to the fairly specific cognitive deficits that seem to be caused by gestational cocaine exposure and to the need to survey multiple cognitive domains when assessing the long-lasting effects of developmental drug effects. Future plans for these animals include assessing whether gestational cocaine exposure has made them more prone to drug-taking behaviors.

Marijuana

The teenage model

In earlier studies designed to model marijuana smoke exposure in the human teenage population, 2–3 year old rhesus monkeys served in studies to examine the effects of marijuana smoke exposure on complex brain function and structure (Paule et al., 1992). All subjects were trained to perform the NCTR OTB tasks for one year prior to the beginning of marijuana smoke exposure. To minimize the acute behavioral effects of marijuana smoke, daily exposures were withheld until after behavioral assessments were complete such that subjects were behaviorally assessed 22–23 hours after their last exposure. Studies on the acute effects of marijuana smoke on OTB performance (Schulze et al., 1988) demonstrated that time perception (TRD) and short-term memory (DMTS) tasks were more sensitive (affected at lower doses) than the learning (IRA) and color and position discrimination (CPR) tasks. The motivation (PR) task was the least sensitive. For the chronic studies, the exposure groups included daily marijuana smoke exposure, weekend-only marijuana smoke exposure, daily placebo marijuana smoke exposure, and daily sham exposures. Half of the subjects were behaviorally assessed using the OTB throughout an entire year of exposure and for seven months following the cessation of exposure and half of the subjects were not behaviorally assessed during the year of exposure and for two months following the last exposure.

Motivational effects

There were no differences in OTB performance between any of the treatment groups prior to the start of treatment. Over the entire year of exposure, subjects in both of the control groups (the sham and extracted marijuana smoke groups) exhibited steady increases in responding in the motivation task (response rates increased, the number of food pellets earned increased, etc.). By the end of the exposure year, the control animals were emitting about three times as much effort in the motivation task as they were prior to the start of exposure. In contrast, performance by subjects in the weekend or daily marijuana smoke groups remained static over this same period. At about one month after cessation of exposure, all measures of performance in the motivation task began to increase for both marijuana groups and stabilized about 2–3 months after the last exposure at levels that were no different from those for the control groups. It was clear that during periods of active marijuana exposure in "teenage" monkeys (whether exposures occurred daily or just on weekends), an "amotivational" syndrome was evident. In addition, several months of abstinence were required for this effect to completely abate. In the animals that were not behaviorally assessed during the year of exposure (or for two months afterward), there was no evidence of a lingering amotivational effect.

The finding that exposure to marijuana smoke only on weekends was sufficient to elicit such an effect on motivation was particularly interesting in that it demonstrated that such an effect can occur with relatively infrequent exposures when they occur over a protracted period. That the effect was as large as that seen in daily "smokers" was also noteworthy and would seem to suggest that there is a slow accumulation of some compound (or metabolites) in marijuana smoke that affects performance for an extended period of time. This latter suggestion is consistent with reports of a long half-life for THC in blood (Johansson et al., 1988a, 1988b).

Individual sensitivity

While there were no clear effects of chronic marijuana smoke exposure on response rates or accuracies in the other OTB tasks, the percentage of a given task completed was generally lower for the daily marijuana smoke group. Examination of data from individual subjects in this group revealed that, at about three months after exposure began, one of the animals exhibited a large decrease in percentage task completed in the color and position discrimination task. The adverse performance of this subject manifest as decreases in response rate in the absence of any effects on accuracy. After the cessation of marijuana smoke exposure, the performance of this animal recovered substantially but it never returned to pre-exposure levels. It thus appears that individual subjects may exhibit very different sensitivities to the effects of marijuana smoke.

Concordance with human data

In reviewing the human literature, one can find little experimental evidence of an amotivational syndrome that is associated with marijuana use in adults (Brill et al., 1971; Brill and Christie 1974; Carter and Doughty, 1976; Comitas, 1976). The data supporting such an effect in humans comes from studies in teenagers and young adults (Lantner, 1982; Smith, 1968). Thus, the use of the "teenage" monkey model seems to have validated the observations reported for teenage and young adult humans. Notable increases in the motivation behavior of control monkeys began at about 3–4 years of age, and appeared to be developmental in nature. It may be that this increase in motivation occurred in concert with the subjects' natural maturation into or through puberty, which would be expected to occur at about this same age. The effect of marijuana smoke exposure to suppress this slowly increasing expression of motivation would be difficult to monitor and document in humans.

Opiates

Opiates are compounds – both natural and synthetic – that share morphine-like analgesic properties. Heroin and methadone are among the most common examples of such drugs that are used/abused for prolonged periods during pregnancy in humans. The most widely reported finding of maternal opiate use during pregnancy in humans is a neonatal withdrawal syndrome that results in a drug addiction/physical dependence in the fetus that is evident by withdrawal symptoms in the neonate. Generally, long-lasting functional consequences (i.e. changes in Bayley Scales of Mental Development, IQ) of gestational opiate exposure in humans have not been observed (Hutchings *et al.*, 1993; Kaltenbach and Finnegan, 1987, 1989). Some have suggested, however, that obstetric opiate analgesia may cause the imprinting of later addictive behavior (Jacobson *et al.*, 1990) and concerns over the consequences of perinatal analgesia, in general remain (Nencini and Nencini, 2005). Morphine, meperidine, and alfentanil are routinely used for analgesia during labor and data concerning the effects of such exposures are extremely pertinent to the issue of developmental opiate effects since all of these agents interact with the same family of subcellular receptors.

Of direct relevance to this issue is the demonstration of significant behavioral effects in rhesus monkeys caused by the perinatal (intrapartum) administration of the opiate analgesics meperidine or alfentanil (Golub *et al.*, 1988a, 1988b; Golub and Donald, 1995). The striking feature of these studies is the finding that functional changes (behavioral effects) were noted not only during the neonatal period but, in the case of meperidine, out to 12 months of age. The pattern of development of spontaneous behaviors (e.g. motor activity) and the performance of several learning, memory, and attention tasks (discrimination/reversals, delayed spatial alternation, and continuous performance) were altered by acute exposure to meperidine during labor.

These findings clearly suggest a potential for opiates to alter normal patterns of brain development when administered during critical periods. It is very important to note that these observations of lingering or residual behavioral effects occurred after acute treatments during labor, not after long-term exposures during which adaptive processes may intercede to attenuate such effects. Given the frequency of opiate use during the peripartum period in humans, it is truly surprising that these observations have not been followed up.

Ketamine and related compounds

Abused drugs and anesthetic agents

Ketamine (vitamin K, special K) – a phencyclidine (PCP, angel dust) derivative – and phencyclidine share the pharmacological property of being antagonists at n-methyl-D-aspartate (NMDA) excitatory amino acid receptors and both are abused substances.

The NMDA receptor participates in the neural phenomenon of long-term potentiation or LTP, which is a stimulus-induced increase in synaptic efficiency (Collingridge et al., 1983) that manifests as an increase in synaptic efficiency (Collingridge and Lester, 1989; Tomita et al., 1990) and which is thought to play an integral role in learning and memory processes (Huang and Stevens, 1998). Excitatory amino acids also play critical roles during development by regulating the structure and survival of neurons and participating in synaptogenesis and plasticity (McDonald and Johnston, 1993). Studies in humans have indicated significant differences in excitatory amino acid receptor sites between newborns and adults out to the 10th decade of life (D'Souza et al., 1992; Court et al., 1993; Johnson et al., 1993; Slater et al., 1993) and have led to the speculation that young brains may be more responsive to agents that affect NMDA receptors than are older brains (D'Souza et al., 1992). Compounds that are capable of interacting with the NMDA receptor could potentially affect a variety of important neural processes that likely would vary as a function of age.

Ketamine, in addition to being a drug of abuse, is also used routinely as a pediatric anesthetic, often being used in neonatal intensive care and burn units. Both ketamine and PCP produce dose-related analgesia and unconsciousness commonly referred to as dissociative anesthesia (Kohrs and Durieux, 1998). Recent studies have shown that clinically relevant doses of ketamine trigger massive and widespread apoptotic neurodegeneration during the brain growth-spurt period in the postnatal rat (Ikonomidou et al., 1999; Scallet et al., 2004). Such changes can result in apparently permanent alterations in brain function as evidenced by altered behavioral performance in animals when tested as adults (Jevtovic-Todorovic et al., 2003).

In order to better assess the clinical relevance of these observations, a nonhuman primate model that more closely mimics the pediatric population (Haberny et al., 2002; Wang et al., 2006) has recently been used in similar studies (Zou et al., 2006; Slikker et al., 2007). Whether ketamine-induced neurodegeneration occurs in primates has important and widespread implications for the pediatric use of such compounds and for ketamine-abusing pregnant women and nursing mothers. Recent efforts have focused on determining whether ketamine anesthesia produces elevated neurodegeneration in the developing rhesus monkey and determining the most sensitive stages of development during which ketamine might increase neuronal cell death (Slikker et al., 2007). In addition, the durations of ketamine exposure that might be needed to cause significant neurodegeneration are being defined.

Anesthetic durations of 24 hours have been employed in preliminary studies to determine whether ketamine causes neurodegeneration similar to that observed in rodents. While anesthetic procedures lasting as long as 24 hours do not occur as frequently as shorter duration anesthetic procedures in humans, they are not rare events, particularly in neonatal intensive care and burn units. In addition, it is feasible that ketamine self-administration may extend for relatively long periods in drug abusers.

The results of these early studies have demonstrated that in 5-day-old animals, keta-mine can cause increases in neuronal cell death in nonhuman primates. The suscep-tibility of the monkey to such effects appears to occur during a sensitive period of development that has yet to be fully defined (Slikker *et al.*, 2007). Ongoing studies are underway to not only define this sensitive period but also to determine a thresh-old duration of ketamine exposure needed to cause significant nerve cell death.

It is important to note that the topography of ketamine-induced neurodegener-ation observed in the monkey is quite different from that seen in rats. In the rat, ketamine induces an increase in apoptosis in several brain areas, particularly in the thalamus and amygdala. In the monkey, it seems the primary lesions occur in the cortex. In addition, the mechanism of neuronal cell death in the rat appears to be primarily apoptotic, while that in the monkey appears to be both apoptotic and necrotic (Slikker *et al.*, 2007). Thus, there are clear differences in primate and rodent responses to the neurotoxic effects of ketamine exposure during the brain growth spurt. It remains to be determined whether the ketamine-induced neu-ronal cell death that occurs in the developing primate results in permanent and/or long-lasting alterations in brain function as has been reported for the rat model. While studies to examine this possibility are currently underway, it will yet be sev-eral years before the answers to such questions are known.

Related compounds

Compounds sharing pharmacological properties with ketamine will likely have the potential to cause effects similar to those seen for ketamine. Certainly, phencyclidine would fall into this category but primate data are currently lacking for this compound. Another related compound, remacemide, is used therapeutically as an adjunct to antiepileptic drugs for reducing the frequency of seizures in adult humans (Crawford *et al.*, 1992). The mechanisms thought to underlie the neuroactive properties of remacemide involve non-competitive antagonism of NMDA receptors and the block-ade of fast sodium channels. Given its interaction with the NMDA receptor, concern about administering remacemide chronically to epileptic children was heightened and prompted studies in the rhesus monkey model (see Popke *et al.*, 2001a, 2001b, 2002). The study design modeled anticipated human pediatric consumption and sought to determine if such treatment might pose risks to normal cognitive development. The emphasis in these studies was on the ability of young (~9-month-old) subjects to learn to perform OTB tasks while undergoing daily drug treatment. Chronic treat-ment continued for 18 months, followed by a six-month washout period. Dizocilpine (MK-801) was used in this study as a relatively "pure" NMDA receptor antagonist. A striking finding of these studies was that daily treatment with the high dose of remacemide (plasma levels were clinically relevant) completely prevented the ability of these young animals to learn to perform the OTB learning task: no increase in task accuracy was apparent after 18 months of training during treatment and no improve-ment was noted during the six-month washout period.

There was also a significant effect of remacemide to delay the acquisition of color and position discrimination task performance. However, by the end of treatment CPR performance by these animals was no different from any other group (Popke *et al.*, 2001b). There was also no adverse effect of remacemide on the acquisition of either the motivation or short-term memory tasks, and, very importantly, there were no effects of any drug treatment on systems and endpoints that typically serve as the focus of routine toxicity testing (general comportment, spontaneous activity, hematological and clinical chemistry measures, ophthalmology, pharmacokinetics, etc., Popke *et al.*, 2002). Thus, the effect of remacemide on learning was quite specific and has been considered an example of a chemically induced mental retardation (Paule, 2005). Had only routine toxicity testing occurred, remacemide would have shown no adverse effects. Quite unexpectedly, MK-801 was without any significant adverse effects on any of the measures taken.

A role for sodium channel blockade in the effects of remacemide is likely. However, it is also likely that its effects resulted in part from its desglycinated metabolite that has a greater affinity for the NMDA receptor than does remacemide. Thus, although the half-lives for MK-801 and remacemide are similar, the presence of an active remacemide metabolite may have resulted in longer blockade of NMDA receptors than that caused by MK-801. This difference in functional NMDA receptor blockade may have accounted for differences in the effects of these two agents.

COMMENTS

While several examples of studies on exposures to drugs of abuse (or related compounds) in developing nonhuman primates have been presented here, the lack of additional, similar studies is remarkable. This is particularly true given the apparent ability of the monkey model to predict both acute and chronic drug effects in humans and because of the availability of behavioral instruments that can be used in both humans and monkeys to assess a variety of important and relevant cognitive domains. These behavioral instruments are useful – in fact necessary – for the kinds of longitudinal studies needed to determine the long-term consequences of drug exposure in that they can be used repeatedly in the same subject(s), can often be automated, and can be tailored to minimize or eliminate the influence of the tester on the testee.

Acknowledgments

The author wishes to dedicate this chapter to the memory of Andrew C. Scallet, Ph.D. Andy was a constant source of enthusiasm and hope and a wonderful colleague, collaborator, and friend. His ever-positive outlook on life, science and the world in which we found ourselves together was, and remains, a constant source of inspiration. I would also like to acknowledge the financial and other support of a number of entities that include: the National Institute on Drug Abuse, The National Institute of Child Health and Human Development, The Food and Drug Administration''s National Center for Toxicological Research, The University of Arkansas for Medical Sciences and Arkansas Children''s Hospital, AstraZeneca, and a host of dedicated collaborators and colleagues who gave freely of their time, resources and encouragement. The views presented herein are solely those of the author and are not meant to reflect those of the Food and Drug Administration.

REFERENCES

Astley, S. J., Magnuson, S. I., Omnell, L. M., and Clarren, S. K. (1999). Fetal alcohol syndrome: changes in craniofacial form with age, cognition, and timing of ethanol exposure in the macaque. *Teratology* **59**, 163–172.

Bandstra, E. S. and Burkett, G. (1991). Maternal-fetal and neonatal effects of in-utero cocaine exposure. *Semin Perinat* **15**, 288–301.

Barr, C. S., Schwandt, M. L., Newman, T. K., and Higley, J. D. (2004). The use of adolescent nonhuman primates to model human alcohol intake: neurobiological, genetic, and psychological variables. *Ann N Y Acad Sci* **1021**, 221–233.

Brill, N. Q. and Christie, R. L. (1974). Marijuana use and psychosocial adaptation: follow-up study of a collegiate population. *Arch Gen Psychiatry* **31**, 713–719.

Brill, N. Q., Crumpton, E., and Grayson, H. M. (1971). Personality factors in marijuana use: a preliminary report. *Arch Gen Psychiatry* **24**, 163–165.

Burbacher, T. M. and Grant, K. S. (2006). Neurodevelopmental effects of alcohol. *Int Rev Res Ment Retard* **30**, 1–45.

Burbacher, T. M. and Grant, K. S. (2000). Methods for studying nonhuman primates in neurobehavioral toxicology and teratology. *Neurotoxicol Teratol* **22**(4), 475–486.

Carter, W. E. and Doughty, P. L. (1976). Social and cultural aspects of cannabis use in Costa Rica. *Ann N Y Acad Sci* **282**, 2–16.

Chai, L., Choi, W. S., and Ronnekleiv, O. K. (1997). Maternal cocaine treatment alters dynorphin and enkephalin mRNA expression in brains of fetal rhesus macaques. *J Neurosci* **17**, 1112–1121.

Chai, L., Bosch, M. A., Moore, J. M., and Ronnekleiv, O. K. (1999). Chronic prenatal cocaine treatment down-regulates mu-opioid receptor mRNA expression in the brain of fetal Rhesus Macaque. *Neurosci Lett* **261**, 45–48.

Chelonis, J. J., Daniels-Shaw, J. L., Blake, D. J., and Paule, M. G. (2000). Developmental aspects of delayed matching-to-sample task performance in children. *Neurotoxicol Teratol* **22**, 683–694.

Chelonis, J. J., Gillam, M. P., and Paule, M. G. (2003). The effects of prenatal cocaine exposure on reversal learning using a simple visual discrimination task in rhesus monkeys. *Neurotoxicol Teratol* **25**, 437–446.

Chelonis, J. J., Flake, R. A., Baldwin, R. L., Blake, D. J., and Paule, M. G. (2004). Developmental aspects of timing behavior in children. *Neurotoxicol Teratol* **26**, 461–476.

Chiriboga, C. A. (1998). Neurological Correlates of Fetal Cocaine Exposure. *Ann N Y Acad Sci* **846**, 109–125.

Choi, W. S. and Ronnekleiv, O. K. (1996). Effects of *in utero* cocaine exposure on the expression of mRNAs encoding the dopamine transporter and the D1, D2 and D5 dopamine receptor subtypes in fetal rhesus monkey. *Dev Brain Res* **96**, 249–260.

Clarren, S. K., Astley, S. J., Bowden, D. M. *et al.* (1990). Neuroanatomic and neurochemical abnormalities in nonhuman primate infants exposed to weekly doses of ethanol during gestation. *Alcohol Clin Exp Res* **14**, 674–683.

Clarren, S. K., Astley, S. J., Gunderson, V. M., and Spellman, D. (1992). Cognitive and behavioral deficits in nonhuman primates associated with very early embryonic binge exposures to ethanol. *J Pediatr* **121**, 789–796.

Cohn, J. and Paule, M. G. (1995). Repeated acquisition: the analysis of behavior in transition. *Neurosci Biobehav Rev* **19**, 397–406.

Collingridge, G. L. and Lester, R. A. J. (1989). Excitatory amino acid receptors in the vertebrate central nervous system. *Pharm Rev* **40**, 143–210,

Collingridge, G. L.,Kehl, S. J., and McLennan, H. (1983). Excitatory amino acids in synaptic transmission in the Schaffer collateral-commissural pathway of the rat hippocampus. *J Physiol* **334**, 33–46.

Comitas, L. (1976). Cannabis and work in Jamaica: A refutation of the amotivational syndrome. *Ann N Y Acad Sci* **282**, 24–32.

Court, J. A., Perry, E. K., Johnson, M. *et al.* (1993). Regional patterns of cholinergic and glutamate activity in the developing and aging human brain. *Dev Brain Res* **71**, 73–82.

Crawford, P. , Richens, A., Mawer, G., Cooper, P., and Hutchinson, J. B. (1992). A double-blind placebo-controlled crossover study of remacemide hydrochloride on adjunct therapy in patients with refractory epilepsy. *Epilepsy* **1**, 7–17.

Day, N. L. and Robles, N. (1989). Methodological issues in the measurement of substance abuse. *Ann N Y Acad Sci* **562**, 8–13.

Deadwyler, S. A. and Hampson, R. E. (2004). Differential but complementary mnemonic functions of the hippocampus and subiculum. *Neuron* **42**, 465–476.

Dimova, J. G., Chelonis, J. J., and Paule, M. G. (2007). Effects of prenatal cocaine exposure on DMTS task reversal performance in monkeys. *Neurotoxicology* (submitted).

D'Souza, S. W., McConnell, S. E., Slater, P., and Barson, A. J. (1992). N-methyl-D-aspartate binding sites in neonatal and adult brain. *Lancet* **339**, 1240.

Evans, H. L. (1990). Nonhuman primates in behavioral toxicology: issues of validity, ethics and public health. *Neurotoxicol Teratol* **12**, 531–536.

Fang, Y. and Ronnekleiv, O. K. (1999). Cocaine upregulates the dopamine receptor in fetal rhesus monkey brain. *J. Neurosci.* **19**, 8966–8978.

Ferguson, S. A. and Paule, M. G. (1995). Lack of effect of prefeeding on food-reinforced temporal response differentiation and progressive ratio responding. *Behav Process* **34**, 153–160.

Ferguson, S. A. and Paule, M. G. (1997). Progressive ratio performance varies with body weight in rats. *Behav Process* **40**, 177–182.

Garavan, H., Morgan, R. E., Mactutus, C. F., Levitsky, D. A., Booze, R. M., and Strupp, B. J. (2000). Prenatal cocaine exposure impairs selective attention: evidence from serial reversal and extradimensional shift tasks. *Behav Neurosci* **114**, 725–738.

Goldman, P. S., Rosvold, H. E., and Mishkin M. (1970). Selective sparing of function following prefrontal lobectomy in infant monkeys. *Exp Neurol* **29**, 221–226.

Golub, M. S. and Donald, J. M. (1995). Effect of intrapartum meperidine on behavior of 3- to 12-month-old infant rhesus monkeys. *Biol Neonate* **67**, 140–148.

Golub, M. S., Eisele, J. H., and Donald, J. M. (1988a). Obstetric analgesia and infant outcome in monkeys: neonatal measures after intrapartum exposure to meperidine or alfentanil. *Am J Obstet Gynecol* **158**, 1219–1225.

Golub, M. S., Eisele, J. H., and Donald, J. M. (1988b). Obstetric analgesia and infant outcome in monkeys: infant development after intrapartum exposure to meperidine or alfentanil. *Am J Obstet Gynecol* **159**, 1280–1286.

Haberny, K. A., Paule, M. G., Scallet, A. C., Sistare, F. D., Lester, D. S., Hanig, J. P., and William Slikker, Jr. (2002). Ontogeny of the N-methyl-D-aspartate (NMDA) receptor system and susceptibility to neurotoxicity. *Tox Sci* **68**, 9–17.

He, N., Song, Z. M., and Lidow, M. S. (1999). Cocaine induces cell death within the primate fetal cerebral wall. *Neuropathol Appl Neurobiol* **25**, 504–512.

He, N., Bai, J., Champoux, M., Suomi, S.J., and Lidow, M. S. (2004). Neurobehavioral deficits in neonatal rhesus monkeys exposed to cocaine in utero. *Neurotoxicol Teratol* **26**, 13–21.

Hilson, J. A. and Strupp, B. J. (1997). Analyses of response patterns clarify lead effects in olfactory reversal and extradimensional shift tasks: assessment of inhibitory control, associative ability, and memory. *Behav Neurosci* **111**, 532–542.

Hodos, W. (1961). Progressive ratio as a measure of reward strength. *Science* **134**, 943–944.

Hodos, W. and Kalman, G. (1963). Effects of increment size and reinforcer volume on progressive ratio performance. *J Exp Anal Behav* **6**, 387–392.

Huang, E. P. and Stevens, C. E. (1998). The matter of mind: molecular control of memory. *Essays Biochem* **33**, 165–178.

Hutchings, D. E., Zmitrovich, A. C., Brake, S. C., Church, S. H., and Malowany, D. (1993). Prenatal administration of methadone in the rat increases offspring acoustic startle amplitude at age 3 weeks. *Neurotoxicol Teratol* **15**(3), 157–164.

Ikonomidou, C., Bosch, F., Miksa, M. *et al.* (1999). Blockade of NMDA receptors and apoptotic neurodegeneration in the developing brain. *Science* **283**, 70–74.

Jacobson, B., Nyberg, K. Gronbladh, L., Eklund G., Bygdeman, M., and Rydberg, U. (1990). Opiate addiction in adult offspring through possible imprinting after obstetric treatment. *BMJ* **301**, 1067–1070.

Jentsch, J. D., Olausson, P., De La Garza, R., and Taylor, J. R. (2002). Impairments of reversal learning and response perseveration after repeated, intermittent cocaine administrations to monkeys. *Neuropsychopharmacology* **26**, 183–190.

Jevtovic-Todorovic, V., Hartman, R. E., Izumi, Y. *et al.* (2003). Early exposure to common anesthetic agents causes widespread neurodegeneration in the developing rat brain and persistent learning deficits. *J Neurosci* **23**, 876–882.

Johansson, E., Agurell, S., Hollister, L. E., and Halldin, M. M. (1988a). Prolonged apparent half-life of delta-1-tetrahydrocannabinol in plasma of chronic marijuana users. *J Pharm Pharmacol* 40, 374–375.

Johansson, E., Sjovall, J., Noren, K., Agurell, S., Hollister, L. E., and Halldin, M. M. (1988b). Analysis of delta-1-tetrahydrocannabinol (delta-1-THC). in human plasma and fat after smoking. In: Chester, G., Consroe, P. Musty eds. *Marijuana: An International Research Report.* Canberra: Australian Government Publication Service, pp. 291–296.

Johnson, M., Perry, E. K., Ince, P. G., Shaw, P. J., and Perry, R. H. (1993). Autoradiographic comparison of the distribution of [3H] MK801 and [3H] CNQX in the human cerebellum during development and aging. *Brain Res* **615**, 259–266.

Kaltenbach, K. and Finnegan, L. P. (1987). Perinatal and developmental outcome of infants exposed to methadone in utero. *Neurotoxicol Teratol* **9**, 311–313.

Kaltenbach, K. and Finnegan, L. P. (1989). Children exposed to methadone in utero. *Ann N Y Acad Sci* **562**, 360–362.

Kohrs, R. and Durieux, M. E. (1998). Ketamine: teaching an old drug new tricks. *Anesth Analg* **87**, 1186–1193.

Kojima, S., Kojima, M., and Goldman-Rakic, P. S. (1982). Operant behavioral analysis of memory loss in monkeys with prefrontal lesions. *Brain Res* **248**, 51–59.

Lantner, I. L. (1982). Marijuana use by children and teenagers: A pediatrician's view. In: *Marijuana and Youth: Clinical Observations on Motivation and Learning.* DHHS Publication No. ADM 82–1186. US Government Printing Office, Washington, D.C., pp. 84–92.

Li, L. and Shao, J. (1998). Restricted lesions to ventral prefrontal subareas bock reversal learning but not visual discrimination learning in rats. *Physiol Behav* **65**, 371–379.

Lidow, M. S. (1995). Prenatal cocaine exposure adversely affects development of the primate cerebral cortex. *Synapse* **21**, 332–341.

Lidow, M. S. (1998). Nonhuman primate model of the effect of prenatal cocaine exposure on cerebral cortical development. *Ann N Y Acad Sci* **846**, 182–193.

Lidow, M. S. and Song, Z. M. (2001a). Primates exposed to cocaine in utero display reduced density and number of cerebral cortical neurons. *J Comp Neurol* **453**, 263–275.

Lidow, M. S. and Song, Z. M. (2001b). Effect of cocaine on cell proliferation in the cerebral wall of monkey fetuses. *Cereb Cortex* **11**, 545–551.

Lidow, M. S., Bozian, D., and Song, Z. M. (2001). Cocaine affects cerebral neocortical cytoarchitecture in primates only if administered during neocortical neuronogenesis. *Brain Res Dev Brain Res* **128**, 45–52.

Lindenberg, C. S., Alexander, E. M., Gendrop, S. C., Nencioli, M., and Williams, D. G. (1991). A review of the literature on cocaine abuse in pregnancy. *Nurs Res* **40**, 69–75.

McDonald, J. W. and Johnston, M. V. (1993). Excitatory amino acid neurotoxicity in the developing brain. *NIDA Res Monogr* **133**, 185–205.

Means, L. W. and Holsten, R. D. (1992). Individual aged rats are impaired on repeated reversal due to loss of different behavioral patterns. *Physiol Behav* **52**, 959–963.

Meck, W. H. (1996). Neuropharmacology of timing and time perception. *Cogn Brain Res* **3**, 227–242.

Morris, P., Binienda, Z., Gillam, M. P. *et al.* (1996a). The effect of chronic cocaine exposure during pregnancy on maternal and infant outcomes in the rhesus monkey. *Neurotoxicol Teratol* **18**, 147–154.

Morris, P., Gillam, M. P., Allen, R. R., and Paule, M. G. (1996b). The effects of chronic cocaine exposure during pregnancy on the acquisition of operant behaviors by rhesus monkey offspring. *Neurotox Teratol* **18**, 155–166.

Morris, P., Gillam, M., Lensing, S., Allen, R. R., Schulze, G. E., and Paule, M. G. (1996c). Age-dependent effects of amphetamine on several complex behaviors in rhesus monkeys, *Soc Neurosci Abstr* **22**, 705.

Morris, P., Binienda, Z., Gillam, M. P. *et al.* (1997). The effect of chronic cocaine exposure throughout pregnancy on maternal and infant outcomes in the rhesus monkey. *Neurotoxicol Teratol* **19**, 47–57.

Nair, B. S. and Watson, R. R. (1991). Cocaine and the pregnant woman. *J Reprod Med* **36**, 862–867.

Nencini, C. and Nencini, P. (2005). Toxicological aspects of perinatal analgesia. *Min Anesthesiol* **72**, 527–532.

Paule, M. G. (2001). Validation of a behavioral test battery for monkeys. In: Buccafusco, J. J. ed. *Methods of Behavioral Analysis in Neuroscience*. Boca Raton, FL: CRC Press, pp. 281–294.

Paule, M. G. (2005). Chronic drug exposures during development in nonhuman primates: models of brain dysfunction in humans. In: Taffe, M. and Weed, M. R. eds. *Frontiers in Bioscience Special Issue: Nonhuman Primate Models of Neuropsychopathology, Frontiers in Bioscience*, Vol 10, pp. 2240–2249.

Paule, M. G., Schulze, G. E., and Slikker, W. Jr. (1988). Complex brain function in monkeys as a baseline for studying the effects of exogenous compounds. *Neurotoxicology* **9**, 463–470.

Paule, M. G., Forrester, T. M., Maher, M. A., Cranmer, J. M., and Allen, R. R. (1990). Monkey versus human performance in the NCTR operant test battery. *Neurotoxicol Teratol* **12**, 503–507.

Paule, M. G., Allen, R. R., Bailey, J. R. *et al.* (1992). Chronic marijuana smoke exposure in the rhesus monkey II: Effects on progressive ratio and conditioned position responding. *J Pharmacol Exp Ther* **260**, 210–222.

Paule, M. G., Gillam, M. P., Allen, R. R., and Morris, P. (1995). Age-dependent effects of cocaine on several complex behaviors in rhesus monkeys. *Soc Neurosci Abstr* **21**, 707.

Paule, M. G., Gillam, M. P., Binienda, Z., and Morris, P. (1996). Chronic cocaine exposure throughout gestation in the rhesus monkey: pregnancy outcomes and offspring behavior. *Ann N Y Acad Sci* **801**, 301–309.

Paule, M. G., Bushnell, P. J., Maurissen, J. P. J. *et al.* (1998a). Symposium overview: the use of delayed matching-to-sample procedures in studies of short-term memory in animals and humans. *Neurotoxicol Teratol* **20**, 493–502.

Paule, M. G., Gillam, M. P., and Morris, P. (1998b). The effects of cocaine on nonhuman primate brain function are age-dependent. *Ann N Y Acad Sci* **844**, 178–182.

Paule, M. G., Meck, W. H., McMillan, D. E. *et al.* (1999a). Symposium overview: the use of timing behaviors in animals and humans to detect drug and/or toxicant effects. *Neurotoxicol Teratol* **21**, 491–502.

Paule, M. G., Chelonis, J. J., Buffalo, E. A., Blake, D. J., and Casey, P. H. (1999b). Operant test battery performance in children: correlation with IQ. *Neurotoxicol Teratol* **21**, 223–230.

Paule, M. G., Gillam, M. P., Graham, S. A., and Chelonis, J. J. (2005a). Exposure of rhesus monkeys to cocaine throughout gestation results in decreased sensitivity to cocaine in adulthood: effects of cocaine on timing behavior. *The Toxicologist.*

Paule, M. G., Chelonis, J. J., Gillam, M. P., and Graham, S. A. (2005b). Cocaine exposure throughout gestation results in decreased sensitivity to cocaine in adulthood: effects on timing behavior in rhesus monkeys, *Neurotoxicol Teratol.*

Popke, E. J., Allen, R. R., Pearson, E. C., Hammond, T. G., and Paule, M. G. (2001a). Differential effects of two NMDA receptor antagonists on cognitive-behavioral development in non-human primates II. *Neurotoxicol Teratol* **23**, 333–347.

Popke, E. J., Allen, R. R., Pearson, E. C., Hammond, T. G., and Paule, M. G. (2001b). Differential effects of two NMDA receptor antagonists on cognitive-behavioral development in non-human primates I. *Neurotoxicol Teratol* **23**, 319–332.

Popke, E. J., Patton, R., Newport, G. D. *et al.* (2002). Assessing the potential toxicity of mk-801 and remacemide: chronic exposure in juvenile rhesus monkeys. *Neurotoxicol Teratol* 24, 193–207.

Rao, S. M., Mayer, A. R., and Harrington, D. L. (2001). The evolution of brain activation during temporal processing. *Nat Neurosci* **4**, 317–323.

Richardson, G. A. (1998). Prenatal cocaine exposure: a longitudinal study of development. In: Harvey, J. A. and Kosofsky, B. E. eds. *Cocaine: Effects on the Developing Brain. Ann N Y Acad Sci* **846**, 144–152.

Roberts, A. D., Moore, C. F., DeJesus, O. T. *et al.* (2004). Prenatal stress, moderate fetal alcohol, and dopamine system function in rhesus monkeys. *Neurotoxicol Teratol* **26**, 169–178.

Ronnekleiv, O. K. and Naylor, B. R. (1995). Chronic cocaine exposure in the fetal rhesus monkey: consequences for early development of dopamine neurons. *J Neurosci* **15**, 7330–7343.

Ronnekleiv, O. K., Fang, Y., Choi, W. S., and Chai, L. (1998). Changes in the midbrain-rostral forebrain dopamine circuitry in the cocaine-exposed primate fetal brain. *Ann N Y Acad Sci* **846**, 165–181.

Scallet, A. C., Schmued, L. C., Slikker, W., Jr. *et al.* (2004). Developmental neurotoxicity of ketamine: morphometric confirmation, exposure parameters, and multiple fluorescent labeling of apoptotic neurons. *Toxicol Sci* **81**, 364–370.

Scher, M. S., Richardson, G. A., and Day, N. L. (2000). Effects of prenatal cocaine/crack and other drug exposure on electroencephalographic sleep studies at birth and one year. *Pediatrics* **105**, 39–48.

Schmajuk, N. A. and Blair, H. T. (1995). Time, space, and the hippocampus. In: Spear, N. E., Spear, L. P., and Woodruff, M. L. eds. *Neurobehavioral Plasticity.* Hillsdale, NJ: Lawrence Erlbaum Associates, pp. 33–56.

Schneider, M. L., Moore, C. F., Suomi, S. J., and Champoux, M. (1991). Laboratory assessment of temperament and environmental enrichment in rhesus monkey infants (*Macaca mulatta*). *Am J Primatol* **25**(3), 137–155.

Schneider, M. L., and Suomi, S. J. (1992). Neurobehavioral assessment in rhesus monkey neonates (*Macaca mulatta*): developmental changes, behavioral stability, and early experience. *Infant Behav & Dev* **15**(2) 155–177.

Schneider, M. J., Moore, C. F., and Kraemer, G. W. (2004). Moderate level alcohol during pregnancy, prenatal stress, or both and limbic-hypothalamic-pituitary-adrenocortical axis response to stress in rhesus monkeys. *Child Dev* **75**, 96–109.

Schneider, M. J., Moore, C. F., Barnhart, T. E. *et al.* (2005). Moderate level prenatal alcohol exposure alters striatal dopamine system function in rhesus monkeys. *Alcohol Clin Exp Res* **29**, 1685–1697.

Schneider, M. L., Moore, C. F., DeJesus, O. T., and Converse, A. K. (2007). Prenatal stress: Influences on neurobehavior, stress reactivity, and dopaminergic function in rhesus monkeys.

Schulze, G. E., McMillan, D. E., Bailey, J. R. *et al.* (1988). Acute effects of delta-9-tetrahydrocannabinol in rhesus monkeys as measured by performance in a battery of complex operant tests. *J Pharmacol Exp Ther* **245**, 178–186.

Schulze, G. E., McMillan, D. E., Bailey, J. R. *et al.* (1989). Effects of marijuana smoke on complex operant behavior in rhesus monkeys. *Life Sci* **45**, 465–475.

Shively, C. A., Grant, K. A., and Register, T. C. (2002). Effects of long-term moderate alcohol consumption on agonistic and affiliative behavior of socially housed female cynomolgus monkeys (*Macaca fascicularis*). *Psychopharmacology* **165**, 1–8.

Slater, P., McConnell, S. E., D'Souza, S. W., and Barson, A. J. (1993). Postnatal changes in N-methyl-D-aspartate receptor binding and stimulation by glutamate and glycine of [3H]-MK-801 binding in human temporal cortex. *Br J Pharmacol* **108**, 1143–1149.

Slikker, W. Jr., Zou, X., Hotchkiss, C. E. *et al.* (2007). Anesthetic-induced neurodegeneration in the perinatal rhesus monkey. *Toxicol Sci*

Slutsker, L. (1992). Risks associated with cocaine use during pregnancy. *Obstet Gynecol* **79**, 778–789.

Smith, D. E. (1968). Acute and chronic toxicity of marijuana. *J Psychedelic Drugs* **2**, 37–47.

Tomita, J., Shibata, Y., Sakurai, T., and Okada, Y. (1990). Involvement of a protein kinase C-dependent process in long-term potentiation formation in guinea pig superior colliculus slices. *Brain Res* **536**, 146–152.

Wang, C., Sadovova, N., Zou, X. *et al.* (2006). Ketamine produces oxidative DNA damage and loss of monkey frontal cortical neurons in culture, *Neurotoxicology* **27**, abstracts page 44.

Zou, X., Divine, B., Sadovova, N. *et al.* (2006). Ketamine-induced neurotoxicity in developing monkeys: a histochemical study. *Soc Neurosci Abstr*.

CHAPTER 13

The Use of Nonhuman Primates in Evaluating the Safety of Therapeutic Medications Used During Pregnancy

Nina Isoherranen and Thomas M. Burbacher

INTRODUCTION

In the United States, approximately 3–5% of babies are born with a congenital anomaly and birth defects remain the leading cause of infant mortality (Detrait et al., 2005). The conditions with the highest prevalence include orofacial clefts, which affect approximately 6800 infants annually, and Down syndrome, which affects approximately 5500 infants annually (CDC, 2006). In addition, 10–30% of pregnancies are lost due to miscarriages (Wilcox et al., 1988; Gindler et al., 2001). The primary mechanisms that lead to reproductive loss and birth defects are still largely unknown although significant advances have been made.

During the past five decades, scientific research has increasingly focused on the possible link between maternal use of medicinal agents and birth outcomes in exposed children. The greatest progress in defining fetal risk from maternal drug exposure has come from (1) studies of the teratogenic effects of xenobiotics in animal models and (2) the scientific review of retrospective fetal outcome data in human populations. Recently, several groups have conducted prospective studies of the safety of certain classes of therapeutic agents following in utero exposures at different stages of gestation. It has also become standard medical practise for new therapeutic entities used by women of childbearing age to be tracked for reproductive and developmental effects. All such efforts have greatly increased our understanding of the relative safety of drug exposures during pregnancy and demonstrated that not all chemical entities are harmful when consumed during pregnancy. However, experiences with a variety of agents have illustrated the complexities of assessing developmental effects and demonstrated the great variability in the phenotype and relative severity of effects.

Primate Models of Children's Health and Developmental Disabilities

This chapter will focus on the safety of drugs used to treat major diseases in pregnant women and will review data on the reproductive and developmental consequences of therapeutic drug exposures in human and nonhuman primates. To this end, classical teratogens and their effects on development are reviewed. Dose–response effects in the developing embryo and fetus are presented to provide the reader with an overview of the severity of effects caused by xenobiotic exposure in both humans and animals. Finally, an opinion on the usefulness of primate models to evaluate drug safety during pregnancy in the future is provided.

THERAPEUTIC USES OF DRUGS DURING HUMAN PREGNANCY

Clinical need for drug treatment

The use of prescription and nonprescription drugs during pregnancy is surprisingly high. On average, a pregnant woman will ingest three different drugs for various therapeutic implications on a daily basis. Drugs are consumed during pregnancy to manage pre-existing chronic illnesses, to treat pregnancy-related diseases and to cure acute bacterial and fungal infections or other conditions that occur during gestation. The major pregnancy-related medical problems that affect large numbers of women include pregnancy induced hypertension and preeclampsia, gestational diabetes, and depression. Approximately 6–8% of US pregnancies are complicated by preeclampsia and a similar percentage is affected by gestational diabetes (Creasy and Resnik, 2004). About 10% of pregnant women suffer from major depression. Because pregnancy may change the natural course of a pre-existing chronic disease, disorders such as epilepsy, autoimmune diseases, thyroid problems, and human immunodeficiency virus/acquired immune deficiency syndrome (HIV/AIDS) commonly require close monitoring and treatment during pregnancy. All of these conditions, if left untreated, can have detrimental effects on the developing fetus and on the mother and are therefore, generally treated with drugs throughout pregnancy.

Despite the widespread use of drugs during pregnancy, about 66% of the drugs administered to pregnant women have never been studied in pregnant women (Sannerstedt et al., 1996). This is of great concern as inevitably, administration of drugs to the pregnant woman leads to administration of these drugs to the fetus as well. Pregnant women are often treated off-label and physicians frequently lack adequate knowledge of safe and efficacious dosages at different stages of gestation. The fact that the effects of drugs on fetal development are poorly understood constitutes a major concern relating to off-label use of drugs in pregnant women.

Dose–exposure relationships during pregnancy

It is well established that pregnancy alters the responsiveness to certain drugs. To maintain therapeutic efficacy and safety; dosages must be adjusted during pregnancy

(Little, 1999). Dosage adjustments may be necessary because drug metabolism and excretion is altered by pregnancy and the pharmacological target functions differently during pregnancy. Published studies of pharmacokinetics in pregnancy are limited, often contradictory and almost always fail to provide clinically relevant guidelines (Mirochnick and Capparelli, 2004). Despite the fact that the disposition of nearly all drugs studied in pregnant women changes when compared to nonpregnant controls, systematic studies of the quantitative changes leading to recommendations of dosage adjustments or mechanistic studies allowing extrapolations from drug-to-drug have been limited (Little, 1999). Of the few drugs studied, it is known that if dosages are not adjusted during gestation, some drugs, such as lamotrigine, metoprolol, phenytoin, and atenolol have greatly decreased plasma concentrations during pregnancy, whereas others (caffeine, theophylline) achieve plasma levels higher than those in nonpregnant women. Recently, pharmacokinetic studies in pregnant women have been extended to probe drugs, which has allowed identification of potential clearance pathways that are selectively affected. For example, renal clearance is increased due to the increased blood flow to the kidneys during pregnancy. Of liver enzymes, the activity of uridinyl-glucuronosyltransferases (UGTs) and some cytochrome P450 enzymes (CYP2D6, CYP3A4) is increased during pregnancy while the activity of others (CYP1A2) is decreased.

From a toxicological perspective, the poor characterization of drug disposition during pregnancy is of great concern because studies of the dose–exposure relationship in males and nonpregnant females cannot be extrapolated to pregnant females. There is also great species variability in the effects of pregnancy on the pharmacokinetics of a specific drug and the dose–exposure relationships in animal studies may not reflect those seen in humans. Altered metabolism during pregnancy may lead to higher or lower exposures to potentially harmful metabolites when compared to the nonpregnant state in a species-specific manner. To adequately address the difficulties associated with dose–exposure parameters during pregnancy and cross-species extrapolation, a better understanding of the mechanisms that contribute to the special changes that occur during pregnancy is needed. This is especially important in the field of predictive toxicology where one wants to eliminate human exposures to potentially harmful agents.

Given the current understanding of changes in drug clearance during human pregnancy, it is clear that any studies that address developmental outcomes must measure exposure to the therapeutic compound and its metabolites. However, maternal exposure may not be a sufficient marker of fetal exposure. The maternal liver and kidneys regulate the overall elimination of xenobiotics but the extent of placental barrier determines what fraction of maternal concentrations the fetus is exposed to. Despite the early literature that evaluated elimination and metabolism of drugs within the feto-placental unit, it is now well accepted that the expression of drug-metabolizing enzymes is too small in the fetal liver to contribute significantly to the overall drug clearance. In the placenta, the major factor limiting fetal exposures to xenobiotics is the expression of various drug transporters that may either contribute to active uptake of compounds by the fetus or may efflux compounds from the fetal side to the maternal circulation. The expression and function of transport proteins in the placenta has been thoroughly reviewed elsewhere (Ganapathy et al., 2000; Syme et al., 2004; Unadkat et al., 2004). Placental development in different model species and in humans is reviewed in this chapter.

If a drug molecule is highly permeable and readily crosses biological membranes, it will usually cross the placenta easily. It is generally believed that only the drug molecules that are free (unbound to proteins such as albumin) in plasma cross the placenta. Consequently, many authors have argued that a high degree of plasma protein binding will prevent drug access to the fetus. This is, however, only correct if the duration of exposure is so short that distribution equilibrium is not achieved. In steady state conditions (distribution equilibrium reached), the free drug concentration on both sides of the placental barrier will be equal regardless of the protein binding in the fetal and maternal compartment unless active transport in the placenta contributes to drug disposition. An active uptake transporter will cause a greater free concentration of the drug molecule in the fetus whereas an efflux transporter will reduce fetal exposure. Because fetal circulation is separate from maternal circulation, the binding proteins in plasma may be present at different concentrations on the fetal and maternal sides and result in different total concentrations while free concentrations are equal. Given the belief that only the unbound drug is pharmacologically and toxicologically active, measurement of free concentrations from both the maternal and fetal compartments is important to understanding the pharmacological effects of the drug on the mother and fetus.

FETAL SAFETY AND IMPACT OF DRUGS ON FETAL DEVELOPMENT

Basic principles

Birth defects are the leading cause of death in babies under one year of age and approximately 3–5% of babies born in the US suffer from congenital birth defects (Detrait et al., 2005). Congenital heart defects and neural tube defects are the most common defects affecting approximately 8/1000 and 1/1000 live births in the US, respectively (Detrait et al., 2005; McBride et al., 2005). In addition, 10–30% of all pregnancies are lost due to spontaneous abortions (Wilcox et al., 1988; Gindler et al., 2001). The exact etiology for the majority of these adverse outcomes is unknown, but both environmental and genetic factors are likely to be involved in the pathogenesis (Cabrera et al., 2004; McBride et al., 2005; Piacentini et al., 2005). It has been estimated that 65–70% of birth defects are of unknown etiology, 20% are genetic, 3–5% chromosomal defects, 2–3% caused by maternal infection or viruses and 2–3% are caused by teratogen exposure (Finnell, 1999). Observed species differences in animal models and difficulty in controlling for environmental factors in human populations has hindered the progress in understanding the mechanisms that cause human birth defects. Both maternal and fetal factors as well as the placenta, may contribute to susceptibility of congenital malformations.

From a clinical and toxicological point of view, the risks of drug-induced malformations may be related to exaggerated pharmacology, secondary pharmacology, hypersensitivity, and direct toxicity usually related to generation of reactive metabolites. The effect of a therapeutic agent on the developing fetus should be evaluated in light of the six basic principles of teratology (Wilson, 1977; Finnell 1999), which are as follows:

1. Susceptibility to teratogenesis depends on the genotype of the conceptus and the manner in which this interacts with environmental factors.
2. Susceptibility to a teratogenic agent varies with the developmental stage at time of exposure.
3. Teratogenic agents act in specific ways (mechanisms) on developing cells and tissues to initiate abnormal embryogenesis (pathogenesis).
4. The final manifestations of abnormal development are death, malformation, growth retardation, and functional disorder.
5. Access of an adverse environmental agent to developing tissues depends on the nature of the agent.
6. The manifestations of deviant development increase in degree as dosage increases from no effect to the lethal level.

When one considers the effects of therapeutic drugs on the developing fetus, the primary factors that can be controlled are the dose of the agent (principle 6) and the time at which the fetus is exposed (principle 2). Principle 1 is clearly illustrated in the context of drug exposures by the fact that not all infants exposed to thalidomide, alcohol, or antiepileptic drugs suffer from birth defects and that in affected infants, the phenotype varies although the overall exposure of the developing embryo has been the same. Despite the evidence that the genotype of the embryo affects its susceptibility to teratogenic insults, the therapeutic applications of genotyping individuals for teratogenic effects of xenobiotics are yet to be established. This principle is commonly applied to research by use of genetically modified animals in teratology studies. Studying the genetic basis of teratogenic insults offers unique insight into the mechanisms by which certain compounds cause developmental defects.

As stated by principle 2, the teratogenic insult depends on the specific time that exposure occurs in relation to the specific developmental stage. Insults that occur during the preimplantation period will either be sufficient to cause death of the conceptus or kill only a fraction of the cells that allow further healthy development and normal organogenesis. The greatest risk for teratogenic insult is the period of organogenesis, which lasts from implantation until approximately 60 days after conception in humans. Once the major organ systems have developed, later exposures cannot alter their formation. Details of sensitive periods in terms of organogenesis in human, macaque and baboon development are summarized below. For certain therapeutic agents, such as antihypertensives and antidiabetic drugs, human exposures most commonly occur during the second and third trimester of pregnancy due to the general etiology of these pregnancy-induced conditions. Little information is available on the safety of these drugs when used during the period of embryogenesis. In contrast, antiepileptics, antiretrovirals, and antidepressants represent drugs that are used to treat chronic conditions and exposures to these agents occur as commonly during the first trimester as during later gestation. It should be noted that embryogenesis occurs in humans during a period of time when most women are not yet aware they are pregnant. Therefore alterations of drug therapy based on safety during pregnancy may be necessary in women of childbearing age who are not using reliable birth control methods.

Drug exposures during the fetal period (from approximately postconception day 60 to term in humans and monkeys) are most likely to impact the growth and functional maturation of the fetus and the effects may persist after birth. In terms of therapeutic agents, such exposures are common in the clinic but understudied from a scientific perspective. The effect of specific drugs on child health and development are difficult to identify in humans because of the impact of other mediating variables such as nutrition, socio-economic status, and familial mental and physical health. Also, as is discussed below, adverse effects on functional outcome are likely to occur at much lower doses than outright structural malformations. Functional effects, reflecting injury to the nervous system, may occur at dosage levels that are commonly used in therapeutic settings and do not cause side-effects in the mother.

Figure 13.1 shows the dose–response relationships for the final manifestations of abnormal development (principle 4) and illustrates how the degree of deviant development increases with increasing dosages (principle 6). Initial studies with

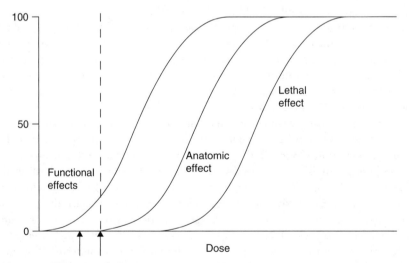

FIGURE 13.1   Dose–response relationship for agents teratogenic to the central nervous system (from Butcher *et al.*, 1975).

hydroxyurea and acetazolamide (Butcher *et al.*, 1975) showed that learning impairments and deficits in locomotion could be observed at dose levels that did not cause skeletal or muscular malformations. Later studies of numerous other compounds have reported similar findings for both drug (see Chapter 12) and environmental exposures (see Chapter 14). It is notable that outcomes documented in standard studies of the teratogenic potential of drug entities include fetal viability and growth retardation as well as soft tissue, skeletal and central nervous system malformations. Typically, these effects are observed at doses that exceed recommended maximum human doses.

SELECTION OF APPROPRIATE ANIMAL MODEL

Sensitivity of the species

One of the most important methodological aspects of studies designed to investigate developmental drug exposure is the identification of the appropriate animal model. For studies investigating the relationship between drug exposure and structural malformations, the selection is frequently based on the species most likely to exhibit the adverse effects that parallel those observed in humans. A report by Brown and Fabro (1983) reviewing 38 drugs that were known human teratogens indicated that the guinea-pig was the most sensitive species to identify teratogenic effects, followed by the mouse and the rat with the rabbit and primate being approximately equal but less sensitive than the rat (mouse > rat > rabbit ~ primate). The mouse model accurately identified about 85% of the human teratogens while the nonhuman primate model identified approximately 30%. One important reason for the observed lower concordance for the nonhuman primate may be the diminished statistical power that is a result of small sample sizes (single fetus per mother) available for such experiments. Although monkeys were not the most sensitive species for modeling drug-induced anatomical changes in this review, positive concordance has been documented for important human teratogens such as alcohol, androgens, anticonvulsants, chemotherapeutic agents, retinoids, and thalidomide (Schardein, 1988). In the same report, Brown and Fabro (1983) reviewed 165 drugs that were known to be nonteratogenic in humans. For this analysis, the rank order of the most sensitive species was (primate ~ rabbit > rat > mouse) and monkeys correctly identified over 80% of drugs that were not associated with birth defects in humans (Brown and Fabro, 1983).

The strength of the monkey model may rest largely in studies less focused on structural malformations but on the neurodevelopmental effects of xenobiotic exposure. Therapeutic levels of exposure that are not associated with frank malformations can result in subtle injuries to the central nervous system that are manifested as functional alterations in behavioral development (see discussion above). Neurobehavioral parallels between monkeys and humans include highly developed intelligence and binding social relationships. The complex behavioral repertoire of these animals makes them useful models for research on the developmental consequences of fetal xenobiotic exposure.

Fetal development and sensitivity periods in humans and nonhuman primates

Fetal development in rodents and rabbits is relatively fast and the entire gestation in rodents and rabbits is short when compared to humans (16–68 days versus 270 days). Most importantly, the period of organogenesis is about two-thirds of the entire gestation in rodents and rabbits whereas in humans, this period is only one quarter of the total length of gestation. This difference may have important consequences in developmental toxicity studies since consequences associated with third trimester exposures would have to be mimicked during the postnatal period. In contrast, the developmental periods observed in humans are somewhat better mimicked in nonhuman primates although the overall gestation is still shorter than that observed in the human.

Table 13.1 summarizes the gestational days of major developmental milestones in humans, macaques, and baboons during organogenesis. These values are presented for reference of time periods when certain organ systems are developing and thus can be damaged by xenobiotic exposure. Generally, after organogenesis is

TABLE 13.1   Developmental time-scale (in days after fertilization) for human, rhesus monkey and baboon[a]

Event	Human	Rhesus	Baboon
Implantation	6–7.5	9	9
Amniotic cavity	8	10	
Neural folds	18–21	20–21	
Vascularization of yolk sac	19–20	16–18	
Start of somite phase	19–21	20–21	
Fusing heart tubes	21	22	
Fusion of neural folds	22–24	21–23	24–26
Anterior neuropore closes	26	25–30	
Anterior limb bud appears	26	25–28	28
Both neuropores closed	25–28	28–31	28–30
Hind limb bud appears	28–32	28–30	28–30
Histologic differentiation of testes	46–48	38–39	
Completion of organogenesis	60	50	47
Birth	280	170	

[a]Data abstracted from Butler and Juurlink (1987), Hood (2005), and Hendrickx (1971a).

complete, a human fetus is approximately 5–15 days older than a rhesus fetus of equivalent crown–rump length. This difference is maintained until approximately gestational day 170 when a macaque is born, whereas the human fetus continues to grow in the uterus for an additional 100 days. Figure 13.2 depicts the comparative growth curves of the macaque and human until post-conception age of 270 days. As can be seen, the human fetus grows much larger by the time of birth than the macaque. This, however, does not reflect the relative maturity of the fetus at a given period of time. For example, the macaque is much more mature at birth than the human infant: it has more advanced dental development, skeletal ossification and brain growth.

In the context of this chapter the most notable difference between the human and macaque development is the great difference in brain "maturity" at birth. The macaque attains 76% of its adult brain weight by birth whereas humans reach only 27% of adult brain weight prenatally. The question whether larger portion of macaque behavioral and cognitive development has already occurred during prenatal development than in humans remains to be answered.

Drug disposition during pregnancy:

As stated above, significant changes occur in drug disposition during pregnancy causing altered dose–exposure relationships that also change in a gestational age-specific manner. The nonhuman primate may be the most appropriate model for determining fetal exposure levels of xenobiotics and the changes in disposition of

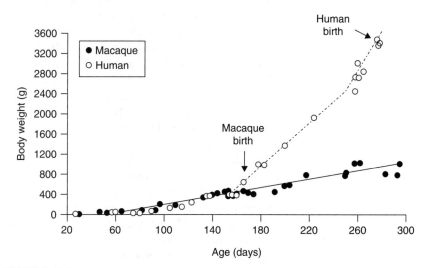

FIGURE 13.2   Comparitive growth curves (body weight) of the macaque and human from conception to 270 days post-conception.

xenobiotics during pregnancy, because the physiological changes that occur during human pregnancy are poorly reflected in the rodent. For example, the liver of mice and rats increases significantly in size during pregnancy, a phenomenon not observed in humans or in rabbits and nonhuman primates. Unpublished data from the author's lab have shown that the concentrations of various "pregnancy-related hormones," such as estrogens and progesterone, do not follow similar concentration profiles during pregnancy in rodents and in humans, potentially changing the regulation of enzyme expression. Finally, the regulation of drug-metabolizing enzyme expression in rodents has different functional determinants than that in humans and other primates.

Placental development

The placenta is the interface between the embryo and the maternal environment and serves the function of delivering nutrients to the fetus and disposing of fetal metabolic waste products. As such, it is responsible also for the transfer of foreign compounds from the mother to the fetus. Because the placenta delivers nutrients and waste products between the two circulatory systems, it is only truly established once a competent embryonic circulatory system is operative. Basically, the placenta consists of fetal membranes and parts of the uterus and the exact shape, morphology, and composition depends on the species in question. The gross appearance, mode of implantation, type of modification of the chorionic surface and the way the embryo is embedded into maternal tissues varies between species. Because of the critical role the placenta plays in providing a barrier between maternal and fetal circulation, it is important to understand the stages of placental development and the differences between species.

The early placenta in rodents is the inverted yolk sac placenta. The rodent placenta maintains characteristics of this type of placenta throughout gestation together with the chorioallantoic placenta that develops later in gestation. The important characteristic of the inverted yolk sac placenta in terms of xenobiotics passing through from maternal to fetal circulation is that it delivers nutrients to the developing embryo by pinocytosis followed by digestion of macromolecules within lysosomal vacuoles and diffusion of resulting products to the embryo. In humans and monkeys the placenta is chorioallantoic throughout gestation and the embryonic tissue projects into maternal circulation as villi.

One may conclude that due to the differences in early placental development, rodents may not be a good model to evaluate the extent of fetal exposures to xenobiotics, especially at early gestation. However, the history of experiments of teratogenic exposures has demonstrated that rodents do effectively transfer xenobiotics from maternal circulation to the fetus, although quantitatively the extent of transfer may differ from humans. Nevertheless, due to the differences in placental anatomy and mechanisms of transfer of nutrients, studies of placental physiology in rodents may poorly represent human placental function. Thus, for such studies, nonhuman primates have clear advantages due to the similar anatomical development and time-course of placental differentiation in relation to fetal development. In addition, the fetal plasma concentrations of xenobiotics can be measured in the primate during gestation. For example, morphine and morphine glucuronides have been successfully measured in the fetal compartment of baboons and the metabolic clearance and drug passage to both directions through the placenta was modeled using *in vivo* measurements (Garland *et al.*, 2005). Such studies provide invaluable insight into the processes that mediate transfer and exposure of the fetus to xenobiotics present in the mother. It should be noted that conducting such studies in rodent models is almost impossible due to the size of the fetus. Typically, rodent studies yield only total concentrations of xenobiotics, which may not reflect the true pharmacologically active concentrations when one assumes that only free drug contributes to pharmacological activity and toxicity.

EFFECTS OF DRUG EXPOSURES VIA BREASTMILK

Most drugs are present in breastmilk at some levels. However, because drug concentrations in breastmilk are typically around the plasma concentrations of the therapeutic agents, the total dose that the infant is exposed to by drinking breastmilk is minimal. It is possible to calculate the maximum exposure by measuring the concentration of the drug in breastmilk and multiplying that with the approximate maximum daily consumption of breastmilk (30 ounces or 900 mL). For example, for a drug that has milk concentration of 1 mg/L, a total daily dose of less than 1 mg would be obtained by the infant over a 24-hour period, of which not all would necessarily be absorbed. Such doses are very unlikely to yield measurable concentrations of the parent drug in infant circulation. For example, fluoxetine is present in breastmilk but even in fully breastfed infants, the amount absorbed by the infant is not sufficient to maintain infant plasma levels. However, there have been reports that antibiotics in the mother's milk can cause gastrointestinal effects in the infant due to the impact on the gut microflora. Given the positive effects of breastfeeding on overall infant health and development, breastfeeding is frequently recommended in mothers taking therapeutic drugs.

TERATOGENS OF SPECIAL INTEREST

Discoveries with some classical teratogens have contributed the most to our understanding of how xenobiotics impair normal development. Of these, the two classical examples are the retinoic acid isomers (the naturally occurring all-trans-retinoic acid and the drug Accutane (i.e. 13-*cis*-retinoic acid)) and thalidomide. In adddition, diethylstibestrol (DES) provides a classic example of latent teratogenic (and carcinogenic) effects.

Retinoids

Vitamin A and its biologically active form all-trans-retinoic acid are essential for normal reproduction including spermatogenesis, oogenesis, conception and placental development (Maden, 2000; Tzimas and Nau, 2001). All-*trans*-Retinoic acid is a critical regulator of gene expression during embryonic development, affecting nervous system development, patterning of the body axis and digitation. It also appears to have critical roles in cognitive and behavioral development (Tzimas and Nau, 2001). In the developing mammalian embryo, exposure to either too much or too little all-*trans*-retinoic acid has been shown to give similar patterns of birth defects including neural tube defects, cleft palate, heart defects, malformations of the ear (microtia, anotia), and limb malformations (Lammer *et al.*, 1985; Rosa *et al.*, 1986; Clagett-Dame and Deluca, 2002; Tzimas and Nau, 2001). Numerous studies have shown that embryos of every animal species tested are susceptible to the effects of excess vitamin A at doses that do not cause maternal toxicity (Tzimas and Nau, 2001).

Adverse effects observed after *consumption* of 13-*cis*-retinoic acid (Accutane) during pregnancy have also demonstrated the significance of retinoic acid in development. Exposure has been related to an increase in the incidence of spontaneous abortions was increased and developmental effects in the exposed fetuses including hydrocephaly, microcephaly, mental retardation (Nau *et al.*, 1994), and cardiac malformations (Lammer *et al.*, 1985; Rosa *et al.*, 1986). Exposure to accutane during pregnancy results in a 40% spontaneous abortion rate, a 25% risk for a major malformation and an additional 52% risk for impairment in cognition or development in the offspring (Finnell, 1999).

The teratogenic effects associated with excess vitamin A intake as well as effects associated with the use of the drug Accutane (13-*cis*-retinoic acid) have been demonstrated in several studies using nonhuman primates. Tables 13.2 and 13.3 show a summary of the results of studies in nonhuman primates investigating all-*trans*-retinoic acid and 13-*cis*-retinoic acid. Studies investigating all-*trans*-retinoic acid have reported craniofacial malformations similar to those described in humans (Lammer *et al.*, 1985), involving craniofacial malformations such as micrognathia, cleft palate, external ear defects such as microtia and anotia, and cardiac malformations (Wilson, 1974; Fantel *et al.*, 1977; Hendrickx *et al.*, 1980, 2000; Hendrickx and Hummler, 1992; Tzimas *et al.*, 1996). Studies have examined all-*trans*-retinoic acid exposures beginning around day 20 of gestation and typically focus on the first trimester of pregnancy. Dosages used in studies of all-*trans*-retinoic acid teratogenicity range from 2 mg/kg per day to over 50 mg/kg per day. The lowest dose that has been associated with the effects described above in nonhuman primates is approximately 5 mg/kg per day.

Studies investigating 13-*cis*-retinoic acid have also reported teratogenic effects consistent with those observed in humans (Lammer *et al.*, 1985; Rosa *et al.*, 1986), involving craniofacial malformations, ear defects, and cardiac, cerebellar, and thymic

TABLE 13.2 Primate developmental toxicity studies with all-*trans*-retinoic acid

	Wilson (1974)	Fantel et al. (1977)*	Hendrickx et al. (1980)	Hendrickx and Hummler (1992)	Tzimas et al. (1996)	Hendrickx et al. (2000)
Dose (mg/kg per day)	10–80	7.5–10	20–40	5–20	5–10	2.25–24
Treatment days	20–46 (variable)	18–44	17–45 (4–8 days)	10–24	16–31	18–60 (variable)
Maternal toxicity						
Weight loss	–	–	–	X	–	X
Gastrointestinal	–	–	–	X	–	X
Facial	–	–	–	X	–	X
Embryo/fetal lethality	X	X	X	X	(All normal)	X
Malformations						
Craniofacial						
Ears	X	X	X	X		X
Mandible		X	X	X		X
Palate	X	X	X	X		X
Skeletal		X	X	X		X
Thymus	X		X			X
Heart	X[a]	X[a]				X
Brain	X[a]					X

X, present; –, not reported.

[a] n = 1.

*Also described in Newell-Morris et al., 1980; Yip et al., 1980.

TABLE 13.3 Developmental toxicity of 13-*cis*-retinoic acid in the cynomologus monkey

	Dose (mg/kg per day)	Treatment days	Maternal toxicity			Embryo/fetal lethality	Malformations						
							Craniofacial						
			Weight loss	Gastrointestinal	Facial		External ears	Temporal bone	Mandible	Palate	Thymus	Heart	Brain
Hummler et al. (1990)*	2, 10, 25	18–28	X	X	X	X							
	2.5	21–24											
	2.5 (2 × daily)	25–27				X							
	2.5 plus	10–25				X	X	X			X	X	
	2.5 (2 × daily)	26–27											
Korte et al. (1993)*	2.5 plus	16–25					X	X					X
	2.5	26–27											
	(2 × daily) 2.5 plus 10–20						X	X	X			X	
	2.5 (2 × daily)	21–24											
Hendrickx et al. (1998)*	2.5	12–27				X	X	X	X			X	X
	2.5	20–27				X		X					X
	2.5	28–30											
	2.5 (2 × daily)	26–27	(All normal)										
Hendrickx et al. (2000)	0.5	16–27	(All normal)										
	5.0	16–27				X	X		X		X	X	X

* Also described in Wei et al., 1999.

defects (Hummler *et al.*, 1990; Korte *et al.*, 1993; Hendrickx *et al.*, 1998, 2000). Studies of 13-*cis*-retinoic acid have examined exposures beginning around day 12 of gestation and have also focused on the first trimester of pregnancy. Dosages used in studies of 13-*cis*-retinoic acid teratogenicity range from 0.5 mg/kg per day to over 50 mg/kg per day. The lowest dose that has been associated with the effects described above in nonhuman primates is approximately 2 mg/kg per day (close to the therapeutic dose for humans, 0.5–1.5 mg/kg per day). The malformation syndromes associated with all-*trans*- and 13-*cis*-retinoic acid are similar in the nonhuman primate model, although there are some differences (visceral and cerebellar defects). There is close concordance between the effects observed in the nonhuman primate model and human cases of retinoid teratogenicity.

Thalidomide

The thalidomide disaster of the early 1960s demonstrates the importance of epidemiological studies focused on drug use during pregnancy. There is a clear-cut relationship between the sales of thalidomide and the incidence of limb malformations (Figure 13.3). It has been estimated that 12 000 infants were born with defects caused by thalidomide (Randall, 1990). In addition to the classical signs of teratogenicity (phocomelia, absence of limbs, and abnormal small and short limbs), abnormalities of other organs such as absence of external and internal ears, hemangioma on the forehead, heart defects, and anomalies of the urinary and alimentary systems have also been reported with thalidomide use.

The thalidomide syndrome has been demonstrated in numerous nonhuman primate species. Over 30 years ago, Wilson (1973a) summarized the results of thalidomide studies in seven different species (see update in Table 13.4). The results of these

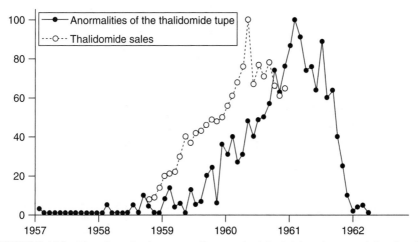

FIGURE 13.3   The relationship between malformation's of the thalidomide type and the sales of thalidomide in Germany (excluding Hamburg).

TABLE 13.4 Experimental demonstration of the thalidomide syndrome in simian primates

Common name	Scientific name	Treatment Dose (mg/kg per day)	Gestational age (days)	No. and condition of offspring	Reference
Baboon	Papio sp.	5	18–36 (var.)[a]	2 typical syndrome/2 aborted or resorbed	Hendrickx et al., 1966
Cynomologus	Macaca irus	10	30–40 22–32	1 normal 4 typical syndrome/2 aborted	Delahunt and Lessen, 1964
Cynomologus	Macaca irus	5 10 10 30	25–27 24–29 (one day) 51 25 or 28	1 typical syndrome 6 typical syndrome/5 normal 1 normal 1 typical syndrome	Hendrickx, 1973
Rhesus	Macaca mulatta	8–50 (var.) 17–100 (var.)	50–60 22–30 (var.) 32	1 normal 6 typical syndrome/5 normal 3 normal	Wilson and Gavan, 1967
Rhesus	Macaca mulatta	~20	24, 25, 27 27–29 30	1 typical syndrome 1 typical lower limbs 1 normal	Barrow et al., 1969
Bonnet	Macaca radiate	10	24–29 26 or 28	7 typical upper limb 2 normal	Hendrickx, 1971b

Bonnet	*Macaca radiate*	5	25–27	1 typical syndrome	Hendrickx and Newman, 1973★
		10	24–28 (one day)	12 normal/7 typical syndrome	
Japanese	*Macaca fuscata*	20	24–26	2 typical syndrome	Tanimura, 1972
Stumptail	*Macaca arctoides*	5	24–30 (var.)	3 typical syndrome	Vondruska *et al.*, 1971
		10	25–27	2 typical syndrome/1 aborted	
			23–30	3 aborted	
Marmoset	*Callithrix jacchus*	7.5	25–35 (alt.)[b]	10 typical syndrome/1 aborted	Poswillo *et al.*, 1972
			35–45	10 normal	
Green (vervets)	*Cercopithecus aethiops*	10	25	1 normal/1 minor malformation	Hendrickx and Sawyer, 1978
		30	28–30	1 abortion/2 typical syndrome	
			31–33	1 abortion/2 typical syndrome	
			41–48	1 abortion	
			25–40 (one day)	3 abortions/2 typical syndrome, visceral malformation/2 normal	

Adapted from Wilson (1973b).

[a] var., dosage or the time of treatment varied within the range indicated.

[b] alt., treatment given on alternate days.

★ Also described in Newman and Hendrickx, 1981, 1985.

studies, and studies conducted thereafter, reveal a pattern of appendage reduction defects and other malformations similar to that described in human cases (phocomelia, polydactyly, syndactyly, ear malformations). Dosages used in studies of thalidomide teratogenicity range from 5 mg/kg per day to over 50 mg/kg per day. The lowest dose that has been associated with the effects described above in nonhuman primates is approximately 5 mg/kg per day. The timing of the exposure to produce these effects is also similar in the nonhuman primate and human cases, with a critical period from 20 to 30–35 days gestation (Nishimura *et al.*, 1968).

Diethylstibestrol (DES)

The use of DES for the prevention of abortion in high-risk pregnancies resulted in another disaster in obstetrics (Herbst *et al.*, 1971). For women exposed in utero to DES, an increase in the occurrence of cervical hooding, vaginal ridging, and vaginal adenosis have been reported at puberty (Herbst *et al.*, 1972; Hart *et al.*, 1976; Bibbo *et al.*, 1977). Adenocarcinoma has also been reported in a number of cases following in utero exposure to DES (Herbst *et al.*, 1972, 1975; Lanier *et al.*, 1973; Hart *et al.*, 1976). According to Hendrickx *et al.* (1979), the occurrence for these effects has been estimated to range from 10 to 45% for cervical hooding and vaginal ridging, 33–90% for vaginal adenosis, and 0.4% for adenocarcinoma; with 65–80% of adeno-carcinoma cases reporting prior history of in utero exposure to DES. For male off-spring exposed in utero to DES, increased risk of epididymal cysts, urethral obstructions, and cryptorchidism, testicular hypoplasia, and poor-quality semen have been reported (Gill *et al.*, 1976, 1977, 1979; Henderson *et al.*, 1976; Hoefnagel, 1976; Bibbo *et al.*, 1977; Cosgrove *et al.*, 1977).

Studies in nonhuman primates have examined the teratogenic and offspring carcinogenic effects of DES. Studies have also described the disposition, biotransformation, metabolism, and biliary excretion of DES in adult nonhuman primate models (Mroszczak and Riegelman, 1975; Metzler *et al.*, 1977; Helton *et al.*, 1978, Mroszczak and Riegelman, 1978). Hendrickx *et al.* (1979) administered 1 mg/day DES to adult female rhesus monkeys beginning on gestation day 21 (period of gonadal development and differentiation), gestation day 100 (period of vaginal plate breakdown), or gestation day 130 (latter period of vaginal development and vaginal differentiation) and continuing until delivery (gestation day 155–175). Teratogenic effects similar to those reported in women exposed in utero to DES were observed in seven of eight DES-exposed female offspring at 5 years of age (vaginal ridging and/or cervical hooding) and three of the offspring exhibited vaginal adenosis. DES, however, was not carcinogenic as no evidence of adenocarcinoma was observed at this time. Teratogenic effects were not related to any one exposure period; effects were observed regardless of the time exposure began. A follow-up study of these females at 12 years of age (Hendrickx *et al.*, 1987) reported similar findings (teratogenic effects but no carcinogenic effects) and also reported a lower pregnancy rate in DES exposed females. Teratogenic effects for male offspring were also similar to those reported in humans exposed in utero to DES. Testicular hypoplasia, undescended testes, and abnormal semen quality were observed. Similar to effects reported in humans (Bibbo et al., 1977), these effects were independent of treatment period.

While no carcinogenic effects have been reported in nonhuman primate models following in utero exposure to DES, carcinogenic effects have been reported in adult DES-exposed nonhuman primates (McClure and Graham, 1973). Female squirrel monkeys implated with four 60 mg pellets of DES developed malignant lesions only five months after exposure, with extensive lesions observed after 11–14 months. Early lesions were restricted to "hyperplasia and hypertrophy of the serosal cells and superficial invasion of the subserosal area." More advanced lesions included "extensive myometrial invasion that extended into the endometrium." The tumors originated from the uterine serosa and were classified as mesotheliomas.

The monkey model has also been used to study the disposition of DES in the maternal–fetal unit or in the mother and fetus (Hill et al., 1980). Single doses of radiolabeled DES were injected into pregnant rhesus monkeys (gestation day 119–134) and maternal and fetal blood was collected over a 2-hour sampling period. DES readily crossed the placenta and the estimates of the half-life in the fetus were 2–10 times longer than the average half-life for the mother (174 minutes). The data indicated that, in the mother, DES was quickly converted to conjugated metabolites and eliminated in the urine. DES that crosses the placenta is also biotransformed to conjugated metabolites, but these metabolites are "trapped in the fetal circulation by selective permeability of the placenta." According to the authors, this prolongs the exposure of the fetus to DES and may be related to the fetotoxic effects.

SAFETY OF DRUGS USED DURING PREGNANCY

The drugs commonly used by pregnant women and the major findings of studies of their safety in humans, rodents, and nonhuman primate models are summarized in Table 13.5. Studies in humans and nonhuman primates will be discussed. Data from studies using rodents are provided for comparison purposes. Anti-HIV drugs are not included in this review as they are the topic of Chapter 10.

Antiepileptics

One in every 250 newborns is exposed to antiepileptic drugs in utero (Lindhout and Omtzigt, 1994). The absolute risk of major malformations in these infants is 7–10%, 3–5% higher than in the general population. Several lines of evidence suggest that the specific pattern of malformations observed in these exposed infants is due to the exposure to antiepileptic drugs rather than maternal epilepsy: First, malformations related to antiepileptic drugs can be reproduced in nonepileptic animals, second, inbred mice with uncontrolled seizures produce healthy offspring whereas mice

TABLE 13.5   Comparison of the major findings of developmental safety of common drugs used in pregnant women between humans, rodents and nonhuman primates

Drug	Human data	Rodent and rabbit data	Primate data
Antiepileptics:			
Carbamazepine	↑ Major and minor malformations ↔ Global IQ, verbal comprehension at 18–36 months	Rats and mice: ↑ Major and minor malformations	↔ Hyperexcitability
Phenytoin	↑ Major and minor malformations, fetal hydantoin syndrome ↑ Growth retardation ↑ Reduced global IQ, verbal comprehension at 18–36 months	Rats and mice: ↑ Major and minor malformations	(Maternal plasma 5–15 µg/mL) ↑ Hyperexcitability ↑ Abnormal/weak reflexes ↑ Retarded motor development (Maternal plasma >30 µg/mL) ↑ Maternal toxicity ↑ Embryolethality
Phenobarbital	↑ Major and minor malformations ↑ Reduced verbal and nonverbal IQ	Mice: ↑ Major and minor malformations	↑ Glucuronyl transferase ↓ Hyperbilirubinemia
Valproic acid	↑ Major and minor malformations, especially neural tube defects, fetal valproate syndrome ↑ Hyperexcitability at age 6 years	Mice: ↑ Major and minor malformations	↑ Birth defects (1 × human dose) ↑ Birth defects (5 × human dose) ↑ Embryo deaths, birth defects (10×) ↑ Embryo deaths, maternal tox (30×) (Birth defects = craniofacial, limb defects)
Topiramate	Insufficient data, used in combination with other teratogenic antiepileptics	Mice: ↑ Major malformations, fetal growth retardation Rats: ↑ Major malformations, delayed physical development, fetal growth retardation	No data reported

Medication	Human data	Animal data	Primate/other
Lamotrigine	Insufficient data	Rabbits: ↑ Major malformations v fetal deaths	↔ Reduction in signs of anxiety or depression in young treated monkeys
Oxcarbazepine	Insufficient data, used in combination with other teratogenic antiepileptics	Mice, rats and rabbits: ↔ Major malformations ↑ Delayed ossification, reduced fetal weight, fetal deaths	No data reported
Antidepressants:			
Fluoxetine	Prospective studies: ↔ Risk for major birth defects and major malformations ↔ Spontaneous abortions (relative risk 0.92–3.92) ↑ Three or more minor anomalies ↑ Perinatal complications, persistent pulmonary hypertension, serotonin toxicity/fluoxetine toxicity	Rats: ↑ Major malformations, delayed physical development, fetal growth retardation Rabbits: ↔ Major malformations ↑ Embryo and fetal death Rats: ↑ Stillbirths, growth restriction, decrease in pup survival (MRHD) Rats and rabbits: ↔ Teratogenicity (1.5–3.6 × MRHD) (product information)	↑ Permeability blood–brain and blood–CSF barrier ↑ Baseline immunoreactivity ↑ Baseline cortisol ↓ Antibody response in young treated monkeys 2–5 years after treatment
Sertraline	Major or minor malformations ↑ Prematurity, neonatal transition difficulty and admission to special care nursery	Rats and rabbits: ↔ Teratogenicity (4 × MRHD), delayed ossification ↑ Stillbirths ↓ Pup survival and pup weight (1 × MRHD)	No data reported

(Continued)

TABLE 13.5   (Continued)

Drug	Human data	Rodent and rabbit data	Primate data
Citalopram	↔ Major malformations ↑ Neurobehavioral disruptions	Rats: ↑ Growth retardation, reduced survival and cardiovascular and skeletal defects (18× MRHD), no effect dose 9 × MRHD Rabbits: No developmental effects (5 × MRHD)	↔ Reduction in signs of anxiety or depression in young treated monkeys
Paroxetine	↔ Major malformations ↑ Need for intensive care and prolonged hospitalization after birth ↑ Respiratory distress, "withdrawal symptoms," tremulousness ↓ Delayed psychomotor development, behavior motor quality	Rats: ↔ Major malformations (9.7 × MRHD ↑ Pup deaths Rabbits: ↔ Major malformations (2.2 × MRHD) (product information) Mice: ↔ Major malformations ↔ Pregnancy duration, litter size ↓ Body weight ↑ Anxiety in pups	No data reported
Imipramine	↑ Suggested cardiovascular defects Withdrawal effect	Rats, mice and rabbits: ↔ Major malformations	
Amitriptyline	↑ Limb reduction anomalies (inconsistent) *Inconclusive major malformations*	Rats: ↓ Skeletal malformations Rats mice, rabbits: ↑ Malformations (> 13 × MRHD)	↑ Permeability blood–brain and blood–CSF barrier ↑ Baseline immunoreactivity ↑ Baseline cortisol ↓ Antibody response in young treated monkeys 2–5 years after treatment
Antihypertensives: Methyldopa	↔ Major malformations ↔ Mental development	Rats, mice and rabbits: ↔ Major malformations	No data reported

(*Continued*)

Drug			
Atenolol	↑ Possible association with developmental defects ↑ Fetal growth retardation	Rats and rabbits: ↔ Major malformations ↑ Growth retardation, fetal resorptions (25 × MRHD)	No data reported
Labetalol	↑ Possible association with developmental defects ↑ Bradycardia and infant hypotension ↑ Fetal growth retardation	Rats and rabbits: ↔ Major malformations ↑ Growth retardation, fetal resorptions (4–6 × MRHD)	No data available
Metoprolol	↔ Major malformations ↑ ? Fetal growth retardation	Rats and mice: ↔ Major malformations ↑ Fetal resorptions and neonatal loss (55 × MRHD)	↓ Bioavailability during pregnancy ↔ Half-life ↑ Oral clearance rate
Hydralazine	↔ Major malformations	—	No data available
Furosemide	↔ ? Major malformations	Rats, mice and rabbits: ↑ Malformations	No data available
Antidiabetic:			
Insulin	Insufficient data	No data reported	
Glipizide	↔ Major malformations	Rats and rabbits: ↔ Major malformations Rats: ↑ Fetal resorptions	No data available No data available
Metformin	↔ Major malformations	Rats and rabbits: ↔ Major malformations (2 × MRHD) Rats and mice: ↑ Neural tube defects, embryotoxicity	No data available
Glyburide (glibenclamide)	↔ Major malformations	Rats, mice and rabbits: ↔ Major malformations, fetal resorptions	No data available

TABLE 13.5   (Continued)

Drug	Human data	Rodent and rabbit data	Primate data
Antibiotics:			
Ciprofloxacin	↔ ? Major and minor malformations[b]	Mice, rats and rabbits: ↔ Major malformations Rats and dogs: ↑ Lesions and erosion of cartilage	↔ Abortions
Norfloxacin	↔ ? Major and minor malformations[b]	Rats: ↔ Major malformations Rabbits: ↑ Embryolethality	↑ Maternal toxicity, embryo lethality ↔ Birth defects
Penicillin	↔ Major and minor malformations	No data	No data available
Ampicillin	↔ Major and minor malformations	Mice and rats: ↔ Major malformations or fetal harm	No data available
Amoxicillin	↔ Major and minor malformations	No data	No data available
Cephalexin	Insufficient data[b]	↔ Major malformations	No data available
Cefazolin	Insufficient data[b]	Mice, rats, and rabbits: ↔ Major malformations	No data available
Cefdinir	No data[b]	Rats and rabbits: ↔ Major malformations ↑ Decreased fetal weight	No data available
Cefixime	No data[b]	Mice and rats: ↔ Major malformations	No data available
Sulfamethoxazole–trimethoprim	↑ Jaundice, hyperbilirubinemia, hemolytic anemia	Rats: ↑ Major malformations, cleft palate	No data available
Tetracyclin	↑ Minor malformations		No data available
Streptomycin	↑ Minor malformations		No data available

Drug	Human	Animal	Other
Gentamicin,	↔ Major malformations[b]	Rats: ↑ Nephrotoxicity	No data available
Tobramycin	↔ Major malformations[b]	Rats: ↑ Nephrotoxicity	No data available
Erythromycin	↔ Major malformations	Rats: ↔ Major malformations	No data available
Spiramycin	↔ ?: Major and minor malformations	No data available	↑ Maternal plasma levels ↑ Placental levels ↓ Fetal plasma levels
Others:			
Warfarin	↑ Malformations ↑ Mental retardation ↓ Fetal growth ↑ Spontaneous abortions, stillbirths, neonatal deaths		No data available
Lithium	↑ Major malformations[b]	Rats: ↑ Major malformations Mice and rabbits: ↔ Major malformations	↔ Weight, blood measurements ↔ Mortality, birth defects
Methadone	↔ Major malformations ↑ Withdrawal symptoms in infants ↑ Growth retardation, mortality, SIDS, jaundice, thrombocytosis (confounded by other substance abuse)	↔ Major malformations	↑ Low birth weight ↓ Maternal metabolism during pregnancy
Bendectin	↑ Malformations (early reports) ↔ Malformations (later reports)		↑ Ventricular septal defects in preterm fetuses (delay closure of ventricular-septum)

[a]Data for human and animal studies adapted from Briggs *et al.* (2005).
[b]See text for details.
↔ No change in risk; ↑ increased risk; ↓ decreased risk.
MRHD, maximum recommended human daily dose on a body surface area basis.

treated with antiepileptic drugs to reduce seizure frequency exhibit an increase in the incidence of malformations (Finnell and Chernoff, 1982), and third, each antiepileptic drug causes a characteristic pattern of malformations independent of the types of seizures it is used to treat. Due to the large number of exposed pregnancies every year around the world, antiepileptic drugs represent the best-characterized group of human teratogens and they are also well studied in various animal models.

The four "old" or "first-line" antiepileptic drugs include carbamazepine, phenytoin, phenobarbital, and valproic acid. Exposure to each one of these drugs during sensitive periods of development leads to a different pattern of malformations (Lindhout and Omtzigt, 1994; Samren and Lindhout, 1997). The best known are the fetal hydantoin syndrome cased by phenytoin exposures and the neural tube defects that follow valproate exposures. Common effects of in utero phenytoin exposure include cleft lip and palate and heart defects (Lindhout and Omtzigt, 1994; Samren and Lindhout, 1997). Valproate monotherapy is associated with increased risk for spina bifida, skeletal, cardiovascular, and genitourinary defects (Lindhout and Omtzigt 1994, Samren and Lindhout 1997; Artama et al., 2005; Kini et al., 2006). Phenobarbital is associated with heart defects, facial clefts, and craniofacial and limb abnormalities. Carbamazepine exposure results in soft tissue malformations and abnormal growth together with neural tube defects (Samren and Lindhout, 1997).

It seems clear that exposure to antiepileptic drugs in utero is associated with major malformations. However, it is still not clear whether antiepileptic drug exposures cause significant effects on long-term behavioral and psychomotor development of the offspring. Several authors have argued that maternal seizures do affect the long-term cognitive development of the offspring (Granstrom and Gaily, 1992) but the data on the effects of maternal use of antiepileptic drugs and uncontrolled epilepsy on long-term development in the offspring are controversial. One may argue that uncontrolled seizures in the mother have an effect on the parenting skills of the mother and thus indirectly effect the development of the infant/child. Hirano et al. (2004) found that when assessed at age 1.5 years, maternal seizures, high dose of antiepileptic drugs in utero and small head circumference at birth affected development quotient scores of motor and linguistic abilities. The effects were less when the same children were retested at the age of 3 years (Hirano et al., 2004). In a study by Koch et al. (1996) neonates exposed to valproate, phenobarbitone, and phenytoin were tested for apathy and hyperexitability for 28 days after birth and again at age 6 years. Valproic acid-exposed children were the highest compromised, except for apathy, which was most common in phenobarbitone-exposed neonates. Valproate exposure was associated with hyperexcitability in the children when tested at infancy and with neurological dysfunction when children were re-examined at the age of 6 years.

Interestingly, Koch et al. (1999) also studied the long-term neurological development (school age and adolescents) in children exposed to antiepileptic drugs. They found in a cohort of 67 children that minor neurologic dysfunction and compromised intelligence score increased with increasing exposure to antiepileptic drugs.

The authors concluded that maternal epilepsy and antiepileptic drug use appear to have long-term effects on the development of the offspring well into adolescence (Koch *et al.*, 1999).

Several studies have focused on changes in the pharmacokinetics of certain antiepileptic drugs during pregnancy. These changes may be important for maintaining the therapeutic dose of the drug during pregnancy. Changes in the pharmacokinetics of phenytoin during pregnancy have been reported (Swift *et al.*, 1989; Dickinson *et al.*, 1989; Lander and Eadie, 1991; Tomson *et al.*, 1994a; Jarvis *et al.*, 1999). An increased clearance and decreased half-life of phenytoin were reported during pregnancy by Dickinson *et al.* (1989) and Tomson *et al.* (1994b) and consequently phenytoin dosage had to be increased in 85% of pregnancies to maintain therapeutic efficacy (Lander and Eadie, 1991). The mechanisms underlying the changes in phenytoin pharmacokinetics are currently not understood. Phenytoin is extensively bound to plasma proteins (90%) and it is possible that a decrease in protein binding during pregnancy results in increased plasma clearance (Johannessen, 1990). However, attempts to determine the role of plasma protein binding in altered phenytoin disposition during pregnancy have been equivocal. Yerby *et al.* (1990) reported 56% decrease in total plasma concentrations of phenytoin whereas the unbound concentration was decreased only 31%. In another study, total phenytoin concentrations decreased steadily as pregnancy progressed, being only 39% of the baseline level in the third trimester (Tomson *et al.*, 1994a). Unbound phenytoin levels decreased less and the change was significant only during the third trimester. The changes in the unbound as well as in total phenytoin steady-state concentrations suggest that metabolism of phenytoin is increased during pregnancy. These changes are most likely due to increased activity of CYP2C9.

Over the last decade, several new antiepileptic drugs have been introduced to the market including lamotrigine, topiramate, and oxcarbazepine. Of these, lamotrigine was considered safe when administered during pregnancy but recent reports have questioned its relative safety (FDA-Medwatch, 2006). It is possible that early absence of developmental toxicity in humans was due to the fact that the clearance of lamotrigine (mainly cleared via glucuronidation) increases significantly during human pregnancy and thus without dose adjustment exposures are almost nonexistant. With increasing awareness of this pharmacokinetic change during pregnancy dose adjustments of lamotrigine during pregnancy have become common practise, assuring sufficient plasma concentrations of lamotrigine to control maternal epilepsy but also increasing exposure to the fetus.

There has been considerable effort to test whether it is possible to develop an antiepileptic compound that is not teratogenic. This has been successful in mice, when animals genetically sensitive to the malformations caused by valproic acid and other antiepileptics were used. Amide derivatives and analogs of valproic acid that were very effective anticonvulsants did not induce developmental effects even at doses that were toxic to the mother (Isoherranen *et al.*, 2002, 2003). Whether these compounds would be teratogenic in humans is not known.

A gestational monkey model was developed by Phillips and Lockard in the early 1980s to "ascertain the potential effects of gestational antiepileptic drug concentrations and/or maternal seizures on the neonate" (Phillips and Lockard, 1985a). Studies using phenytion, stiripentol, and carbamazepine were described in a series of articles and abstracts (see below). Initial studies utilized an experimental epilepsy monkey model previously developed by Lockard and Barensten (1967) using unilateral aluminum hydroxide injections into the left pre- and postcentral gyrus sensorimotor hand and face areas. Following treatment, animals exhibit EEG spikes and contralateral focal-motor seizures within two months after the injection and secondary generalized tonic-clonic seizures by four months post injection. The model was developed to mimic patients with partial motor epilepsy and previous studies using this model demonstrated that efficacious plasma drug levels overlap with those observed in these patients (Lockard et al., 1975). The results of studies with these animals indicated that epileptic females who were not treated with drugs during their pregnancy experienced multiple seizures but there were no indications of morphologic, growth, or behavioral problems in their offspring (Lockard, 1980a).

Later studies of epileptic and nonepileptic (normal) female macaques treated with phenytoin during pregnancy did indicate drug treatment-related effects on offspring (Phillips and Lockard, 1985a, 1985b). Therapeutic plasma levels of phenytoin have been reported to be in the range of 10–12 µg/mL. Three epileptic females received approximately 20 mg/kg of phenytoin twice daily. Plasma phenytoin levels in two of the females were 8–9 µg/mL during the first trimester. The third female did not receive phenytoin until the second trimester. The plasma phenytoin levels decreased during the second and third trimester for all three females (range = 1.8–8.3 µg/mL).

In addition to the above, two normal ($N = 4$ pregnancies) and two epileptic ($N = 2$ pregnancies) females received phenytoin twice daily at doses aimed at maintaining a steady-state plasma phenytoin level of 8–15 µg/mL during pregnancy. Infants were evaluated at birth and were observed with their mothers over a 12-week period. One of the epileptic females required a cesarean section to deliver a full-term fetus that had died in utero (stillbirth). An abnormally high maternal plasma phenytoin level (over 20 µg/mL) was observed in this female ~3 days prior to the death of the fetus. Another infant was born with an upper lip anomaly (from a nonepileptic female). The plasma phenytoin levels for this female during pregnancy were between 5 and 14 µg/mL. All of the neonates displayed weak or abnormal reflexes (weak grasping, sucking or rooting, no clasping, tremors). Weight gain for all of the infants appeared normal and was not associated with maternal phenytoin levels or seizure exposure. Observations of mother/infant interactions over the first 12 weeks of life indicated significant inverse correlations between third trimester phenytoin levels and motor development. Infants exposed to higher phenytoin levels late in pregnancy broke contact with their mothers less often, and walked, hopped, and jumped less often. First trimester plasma phenytoin levels and seizure frequency were not related to these behavioral outcomes. The effects were observed in offspring of both epileptic and normal females exposed to phenytoin during pregnancy and the results were not associated with seizures in epileptic females. The pattern of results indicates a direct effect of prenatal phenytoin exposure on infant development.

Additional studies using normal female macaques treated during pregnancy with phenytoin, stiripentol, carbamazepine or a polydrug treatment of phenytoin and stiripentol, or carbamazepine and stiripentol were conducted by Phillips and Lockard (1993, 1996). The focus of these studies was on evaluating "hyperexcitability" in infants following in utero drug exposure. In the first study, adult female monkeys were administered phenytoin, stiripentol or the two drugs in combination (poly-therapy) to maintain plasma levels during pregnancy between 4 and 12 μg/mL (phenytoin) or 4 and 10 μg/mL (stiripentol). Infants were separated from their mothers at birth and nursery reared. A 10-point hyperexcitability rating scale was devel-oped to evaluate the behavior of infants while they were being tested on a series of cognitive assessments between two weeks and three months of age. Animals with a rating of 1 were asleep, a rating of 2–7 indicated cooperative behavior during the assessment, and a rating of 8–10 indicated that the animal was difficult to test and was hyperexcitable. The results of the study indicated a significantly higher rate of hyperexcitable ratings for the phenytoin (60%) and the phenytoin + stiripentol (57%)-exposed infants when compared with the infants that were exposed to stiripentol alone (2%). The results indicate that infants exposed in utero to phenytoin have a more difficult time attending to a cognitive task and that coadministration of stiripentol does not reduce this behavior. In utero exposure to stiripentol alone did not result in increased hyperexcitable ratings; nearly all of the stiripentol-exposed animals were "remarkably cooperative" during testing.

A follow-up study of the same epileptic drugs as well as carbamazepine alone or in combination with stiripentol again indicated increased hyperexcitabilty in infants prenatally exposed to phenytoin. Carbamazepine exposure did not result in increased ratings of hyperexcitability when given alone or in combination with stiripentol. Consistent with the results of the previous study, infants exposed to stiripentol alone also did not exhibit increased rates of hyperexcitability.

Studies focused on the developmental toxicity and pharmacokinetics of pheny-toin in rhesus monkeys were conducted by Hendrie et al. (1990). Pregnant females were given one of five doses of phenytoin orally (60–600 mg/kg), once daily from gestation day 21 to gestation day 50. Pharmacokinetic studies were conducted fol-lowing the initial dose on day 21 and after the last dose on day 50. Fetal ultrasounds were conducted every 10 days from gestation day 21 until gestation day 100. Viable fetuses were removed by hysterotomy on gestation day 100 and were weighed and evaluated for the presence of gross abnormalities. There was a significant decrease in the half-life and an increase in the clearance of phenytoin during pregnancy. The half-life at gestation day 21 ranged from 69 to 31 hours, depending on the dose, while the half-life at gestation day 50 ranged from 8 to 19 hours. Maternal toxic-ity was observed at all doses. Central nervous system effects increased with increas-ing dose and were related to plasma levels in excess of 30 μg/mL. Gastrointestinal toxicity (emesis, anorexia, constipation) was observed in nearly all of the animals regardless of dose. The incidence of embryonic loss was high and related to the first two weeks of treatment when maternal plasma phenytoin levels were high. Fetal body weights and organ weights of viable fetuses were normal and there was no increase in fetal malformations. The authors concluded that plasma phenytion levels approximating the human therapeutic range (10–20 μg/mL) were not teratogenic in surviving fetuses and that the risk of birth defects in human populations may be related to an interaction between factors such as genetics, socioeconomics, and drug therapy.

Using a similar study design, Hendrickx and colleagues (Mast *et al.*, 1986; Hendrickx *et al.*, 1988) examined the developmental toxicity and pharmacokinetics of valproic acid in rhesus monkeys. In the first study (Mast *et al.*, 1986), rhesus monkeys were given valproic acid by gavage daily at the human therapeutic dose (20 mg/kg per day) or at doses 10 and 30 times the human therapeutic dose (200 and 600 mg/kg per day). Monkeys were treated during organogenesis, on gestation days 21–50. Pharmacokinetic studies were conducted after the first and last exposure using females from the 10× dose group. For all groups, viable fetuses were removed by hysterotomy on gestation day 100 and were weighed and evaluated for the presence of gross abnormalities. The highest dosage group (30×) was embryolethal in all three pregnancies studied. Maternal toxicity was also apparent (anorexia, general malaise) in all three females. The middle dosage group (10×) was also embryolethal in three of five pregnancies and birth defects were observed in all embryos and fetuses recovered. Craniofacial defects included exophthalmia and mandibular hypoplasia was observed as well as lower limb defects and shortened digits on the hands and feet. For the lowest dosage group (1×), there was no embryo or fetal deaths but one of the three fetuses exhibited craniofacial defects similar to that described above. The results of the pharmacokinetic studies indicated that the blood half-life of valproic acid doubled during the 30-day treatment (average, 1.6 hours to 3.2 hours) and the clearance rate was decreased by nearly half (average, 172 mL/h per kg to 93 mL/h per kg). The blood half-life reported in this study is shorter than that observed in human subjects (8–16 hours). The decline in blood levels for the monkey appeared to be biphasic, indicating the presence of a longer half-life. This was also observed in rodents and humans (Gugler and von Unruh, 1980).

A more extensive study of valproic acid was reported by Hendrickx *et al.* (1988), using a similar design and dosage range to the study described above. Prenatal loss increased with increasing dose (0% for 20 and 75 mg/kg per day, 14% for 100 mg/kg per day to 83% for 600 mg/kg per day). Craniofacial defects similar to those described above were observed at all dosages but increased in frequency with increasing doses. Limb defects were observed at dosage levels of 100 mg/kg per day (5×) and above and also increased with increasing doses. The average blood half-life of valproic acid observed in this study was similar to that reported above (2–4 hours), but a change in blood half-life with repeated exposures was not observed.

Gartner *et al.* (1977) used rhesus monkeys to study the effects of late gestation phenobarbital treatment on newborn bilirubin transport and metabolism. Phenobarbital treatment late in pregnancy (six weeks prior to delivery) prevented the occurrence of hyperbilirubinemia in newborns. A threefold increase in glucuronyl transferase activity enhanced bilirubin conjugation and accounted for the prevention of hyperbilirubinemia. Similar effects of antenatal pheonobarbital treatment have been reported in human newborns (Ramboer *et al.*, 1969; Valaes *et al.*, 1980; Rayburn *et al.*, 1988; Trevett *et al.*, 2005).

Lamotrigine, as well as several other antiepileptic drugs, have been used to treat pediatric cases of epilepsy. A recent report by Trevathan *et al.* (2006) on a randomized, blinded, placebo-controlled study of the efficacy and tolerability of lamotrigine indicated that the drug was effective in treating of generalized absence seizures as well as partial seizures in childhood. While side-effects including an increased risk of serious rash have been reported with lamotrigine (Messenheimer, 1998; Guberman *et al.*, 1999) when rapid dose-escalation schedules are used, no such side-effects were reported in this study using dose-escalation schedules recommended by the manufacturer.

Data from nonhuman primate models for the newer antiepileptic drugs such as lamotrigine, topiramate, and oxcarbazepine is quite limited. Lamotrigine has been tested in conjuction with the evaluation of psychotropic medication in young (<1 year) vervet monkeys to examine changes in behavior following maternal separation (Marais *et al.*, 2006). Maternal separation models in young monkeys typically produce behaviors indicative of separation anxiety (increased activity, stereotypical behaviors) and depression (decreased huddling and exploration). Lamotrigine was administered daily (1.4 mg/kg) for four weeks prior to maternal separation and for three weeks afterwards. Animals were observed pre-weaning as they interacted with their mothers. Post-weaning observations took place when animals were in social groups of three or four animals. A scoring system that rated behaviors such as huddling, exploration, general activity, and stereotypy was used to measure anxiety and depression. Nontreated animals displayed behaviors indicative of separation anxiety and depression (see above). Lamotrigine treatment had no effect on these behaviors. Lamotrigine-treated monkeys displayed anxiety and depressive behaviors similar to nontreated controls.

Another drug, oxcarbazepine has been used in conjunction with the adult experimental epilepsy monkey model described above (Schmutz *et al.*, 1994). Treatment with 50 mg/kg p.o. or 20 mg/kg i.m. protected against recurring partial seizures. The authors hypothesized that the effect was most likely due to a direct effect of oxcarbazepine on sodium channels. Studies of drug use during pregnancy in nonhuman primate models have not been reported for these newer antiepilepics.

Antidepressants

Major depression during pregnancy can be life-threatening and impair normal life. It is usually treated with antidepressant drugs such as selective serotonin reuptake inhibitors (SSRIs). Antidepressant drugs are taken chronically throughout pregnancy and there is accumulating evidence that their use, especially during the third trimester, delays the growth of the baby and causes adverse reactions in the newborn such as poor neonatal adaptation. However, based on evaluation of available clinical data, it is not evident whether these effects are specific to individual SSRIs and whether there is a definite relationship between drug exposure and infant outcome. Human data are additionally complicated because uncontrolled depression in the mother is associated with pregnancy complications and low birth weight and preterm delivery (Steer *et al.*, 1992; Kurki *et al.*, 2000). Despite the widespread use of SSRIs during pregnancy, it is not known how the efficacy and adverse effects relate to the exposure (i.e. plasma concentrations during pregnancy).

The effects of antidepressant drugs on the developing fetus can be summarized as potential congenital malformations, retardation of growth and neurological development and postnatal withdrawal symptoms (poor neonatal adaptation). Until recently, SSRIs and tricyclic antidepressants as a group have been considered to be devoid of teratogenic potential. Multiple studies have failed to show a connection between increased rates of major or minor congenital malformations and exposure to SSRIs during first trimester of pregnancy (Einarson and Einarson, 2005; Gentile, 2005). However, in a recent study evaluating 3581 women exposed to SSRI antidepressants during the first trimester, increased rates of overall major congenital malformations were associated with use of the SSRI paroxetine when compared with other antidepressants (odds ratio (OR) 2.2) (Williams and Wooltorton, 2005). In the same study, the SSRI antidepressants fluoxetine and sertraline showed no increased risk of birth defects, whereas citalopram showed a modest increase in risk (OR 1.39). Based on these results, one may conclude that each antidepressant drug should be evaluated separately for its teratogenic potential since the mechanisms of teratogenicity are probably not related to the common mechanism of action for this class of drugs.

Many clinical studies in humans have shown that the use of SSRIs during the third trimester is associated with lower birth weights and preterm labor, but the evidence of fetal adverse effects following SSRI use during late pregnancy (after 20 weeks) is controversial. The most likely explanation for the variability of outcomes reported is the lack of control of maternal depression and drug exposure, the heterogeneous group of SSRIs used and small sample size. A meta-analysis of the various studies evaluating neonatal outcomes in infants exposed to SSRIs during late pregnancy showed that these infants had significantly lower birth weights (OR 3.6, $P = 0.04$), a significantly higher rate of admissions to neonatal intensive care units or specialized nurseries (OR 3.3, $P = 0.02$) and significantly poorer neonatal adaptation scores (OR 4.1, $P = 0.07$) (Lattimore *et al.*, 2005). The rate of prematurity was not significantly increased in SSRI-exposed pregnancies in the meta-analysis. In addition, according to a recent case–control study, maternal use of SSRIs after 20 weeks of gestation significantly increases the risk for persistent pulmonary hypertension in the newborn (OR = 6.1) but there was no analysis of which SSRIs may pose a greater risk than others (Chambers *et al.*, 2006). The poor neonatal adaptation, also referred to as SSRI withdrawal syndrome, is characterized by jitterness, tachypnea, hypoglycemia, hypothermia, poor tone, respiratory distress, weak or absent cry, and desaturation during feeding (Moses-Kolko *et al.*, 2005). Severe cases of withdrawal may also include seizures. Paroxetine is most commonly associated with the infant withdrawal syndrome after exposure during the last trimester of pregnancy, but reports of infant withdrawal syndrome exist for all SSRIs (Moses-Kolko et al., 2005; Sanz et al., 2005). Whether these effects have long-term consequences on the neurological development of the infant is currently unknown (Gentile, 2005).

It is extremely difficult to determine the reproductive and developmental effects associated with specific SSRIs. The major shortcomings of the human data are the fact that studies evaluate SSRIs as a group and individual SSRIs are not systematically evaluated, maternal or newborn drug plasma concentrations are not documented or dosages controlled, and maternal depression status during late pregnancy is not known. Controlled clinical studies are exceptionally difficult to conduct and usually require clinical experience for numerous years after drug approval.

Teratogenic studies using nonhuman primates have been reported for the tricyclic antidepressant imipramine (Hendrickx, 1975). Imipramine was administered to bonnet and rhesus monkeys twice daily by stomach intubation for 1–3 days or 14–22 days starting early in pregnancy (days 23–31). Maternal doses were 5, 40, and 120 times greater than the prescribed human dosage on a milligram per kilogram basis. The acute treatment (1–3 days) was designed to test the effects of imipramine during critical periods of limb development, while the chronic treatment (14–22 days) was chosen to examine the periods of organogenesis including the period of palate closure. Maternal toxicity was observed in animals given the highest dose after just one exposure. Ataxia and grand mal-like seizures were observed immediately after the first treatment. These effects disappeared after 24 hours. Seventy to 100-day fetuses were examined and no evidence of teratogenic effects were found. The authors concluded that the teratogenic potential of imipramine was low and there was no evidence to support an association between imipramine treatment and reduction deformities of the limbs.

SSRI antidepressant drugs are used to treat depression in children and adolescents (Wong et al., 2004; Hjalmarsson et al., 2005). The SSRI drug fluoxetine has been studied in young nonhuman primates. Investigators examined the long-term effects of fluoxetine treatment (2 mg/kg) administered by nasogastric tube 7 days/week for 12 weeks beginning at eight months of age. Therapeutic doses of fluoxetine for humans are in the range of 10–60 mg. Coe et al. (1996) reported an increase in the leukocyte count and albumin in the CSF for fluoxetine-treated monkeys more than 2 years after treatment had stopped. The data indicated, according to the authors, a long-term (possibly permanent) change in the permeability of the blood–brain or blood–CFS barrier due to the early fluoxetine treatment. Laudenslager and Clarke (2000) examined immune and endocrine responses in the same group of monkeys. At 6 years, baseline levels of immunoreactive plasma IgM, IgG, C3, and C4 were obtained as well as total and % free cortisol. Animals were then immunized with tetanus toxoid (2.5 IU intramuscularly) and the above parameters were measured again. Fluoxetine-treated monkeys showed higher baseline immunoreactive IgM, IgG, C3, and C4 levels as well as elevated levels of plasma cortisol. Treated monkeys showed a reduced antibody response following immunization. The authors concluded that the drug treatment prior to 1 year of age disrupted the organization and long-term regulation of markers of the immune response. While the significance of these disruptions was unclear, the authors pointed out that changes that were observed in these animals could contribute to autoimmune disease pathogenesis.

Studies of the short-term effects of fluoxetine treatment (2 mg/kg, 7 days/week for 16 weeks) have also reported increases in cortisol levels and levels of ACTH after just two weeks of treatment (Clarke *et al.*, 1998).

Citalopram has also been tested in young nonhuman primates using the maternal separation model described above (see lamotrigine). Citalopram was administered to young vervet monkeys daily (1 mg/kg) for four weeks prior to maternal separation and for three weeks afterwards. Therapeutic doses of citalopram for humans is in the range of 20–40 mg/day. Citalopram treatment had no effect on behaviors indicative of separation anxiety and depression. Citalopram-treated monkeys displayed anxiety and depressive behaviors similar to nontreated controls.

Studies examining the antidepressant drugs sertraline, paroxetine, and amitriptyline have been conducted in adult nonhuman primates. Sertraline (like many of the other antidepressant drugs) has been found to be effective in altering nicotine or cocaine self-administration behaviors (Sannerud *et al.*, 1994; Kleven and Woolverton, 1993). A study by Petersen *et al.* (1978) examined the relationship between paroxetine dose, paroxetine levels in whole blood and depletion of plasma 5-hyproxy-tryptamine (5-HT) in adult rhesus monkeys. Paroxetine depleted plasma 5-HT levels in a dose-dependent fashion. Whole blood paroxetine levels below 2 ng/mL (dose of 1 mg/kg/day for 13 weeks) were associated with a 30% depletion of 5-HT; blood levels at approximately 5 ng/mL (2.5 mg/kg/day dose) with a 85% depletion, and paroxetine blood levels ranging from 100 to 450 ng/mL (7.5 mg/kg per day dose) were associated with a 93% depletion of 5-HT. Studies of amitriptyline have focused on the reinforcement properties of the drug in adult monkeys using operant conditioning procedures (Hoffmeister, 1977; McKearney, 1982). Studies of the effects of drug use during pregnancy in nonhuman primates have not been reported for these antidepressant drugs.

Antihypertensives

Despite the widespread use of antihypertensive medications in pregnant women, their reproductive safety has been inadequately evaluated in humans. All of the antihypertensive medications cross the placenta and fetal concentrations are equal to maternal concentrations. The major effects of antihypertensive drugs, such as atenolol, labetalol, and metoprolol, when taken during pregnancy appear to be retardation of growth and decreased birth weight. The common mechanism for these effects is decreased placental and fetal circulation due to vasoconstriction. Growth retardation and decreased birth weight have been observed after third trimester exposures to these beta-blockers. However, the degree of growth retardation can probably be controlled by appropriate dosing and close monitoring of the patients. Interestingly, the severity of growth retardation correlates with the duration of exposure not the dose: early exposures during the second trimester and thereafter result in the greatest growth retardation. Despite the concerns of effects on fetal growth, beta-blockers are generally considered safe for use during gestation. These drugs are not typically used during the first trimester and thus their association with major malformations is unclear.

While no studies have been reported in nonhuman primates concerning the effects of antihypertensive drugs on offspring growth, maternal pharmacokinetic studies have been reported for some of the drugs. Studies have been conducted to examine whether pregnancy changes the pharmacokinetics of the antihypertensive drug metoprolol (Rane et al., 1984; Hogstedt et al., 1990). Rhesus monkeys were given an oral dose of metoprolol (9 mg/kg) via nasogastric catheter during the last 2–6 weeks of pregnancy and again 1–4 months post partum. The oral bioavailability of metoprolol decreased during pregnancy (from a range of 9–49% for nonpregnant state to a range of 6–22% during pregnancy). Metoprolol half-life did not change significantly (range between 1 and 2.5 hours) during pregnancy but oral clearance rates increased with pregnancy (43–80 mL/min per kg for nonpregnant state to a range of 95–107 mL/min per kg during pregnancy). Similar effects have been observed during pregnancy in humans. Reports indicated that the oral clearance of metoprolol increases sixfold and the bioavailability decreases by half when values at 26–30 weeks gestation are compared with those post partum (Hogstedt et al., 1985). Since no changes in plasma protein binding were observed, the increased oral clearance relates to a sixfold increase in the intrinsic clearance of metoprolol and based on enzyme kinetic principles a sixfold increase in CYP2D6 expression.

Studies of furosemide pharmacokinetics have also been reported in nonhuman primates, although no data are available for pregnant animals. Yakatan et al. (1976) reported that 24% of a single oral dose of 5 mg/kg furosemide was excreted in the urine of rhesus monkeys in 24 hours. Repeated oral dosing at 5 mg/kg per day did not change this excretion rate. Daily average plasma levels at 2 and 24 hours post dosing were 0.250 and 0.044 respectively and the half-life of furosemide was 11 days (Yakatan et al., 1979). A study by Doyle et al. (1982) compared the pharmacokinetics of furosemide across three nonhuman primate species: the rhesus monkey, the cynomolgus monkey, and the baboon. A single intravenous dose of 3 mg/kg of furosemide resulted in an average half-life of 26, 28, and 14 days respectively for the rhesus, cynomolgus, and baboon. Clearance rates were 18, 10, and 23 mL/min. The authors concluded that the pharmacokinetics of furosemide for humans were more closely reflected in the cynomolgus monkey than in the rhesus, baboon, or "other common laboratory animal species."

Finally, studies using adult nonhuman primates have examined the cardiovascular effects of hypertensive drugs such as methyldopa (Walson et al., 1975; Spence, 1977; Spence et al., 1977), atenolol (Banka et al., 1984), and hydralazine (Spence et al., 1977), although none have been tested in pregnant or young animals.

Antidiabetic drugs

Evaluation of the safety of antidiabetic compounds in humans is complicated because gestational diabetes itself can cause teratogenicity and a multitude of malformations (risk 3–5 times that of controls). Congenital malformations are now the most common cause of perinatal death in infants of diabetic mothers (Dignan, 1981, Schwartz and Teramo, 2000; Temple *et al.*, 2002). The frequency of both major malformations and multiple malformations (affecting more than one organ system) is increased as a result of hyperglycemia. Organ systems affected include cardiovascular, renal, and gastrointestinal, and neural tube defects are observed (Casson *et al.*, 1997; Temple *et al.*, 2002). In rodents, episodes of hypoglycemia during organogenesis are also associated with skeletal and cardiovascular malformations and reduced growth (Tanigawa *et al.*, 1991; Kawaguchi *et al.*, 1994). Consequently, any treatment that offers good control of maternal blood sugar levels is likely to reduce the overall malformation rates.

The gold standard of diabetes treatment during pregnancy is still insulin. Surprisingly, essentially no studies have assessed the safety of insulin in humans, perhaps because for a long time it was believed that insulin does not cross the placental barrier due to its size. It has, however, been demonstrated that insulin of animal origin does cross from maternal to fetal circulation as an antibody complex (Menon *et al.*, 1990). Despite the presence of the maternal antibodies, the insulin that passes to the fetus appears to have biological activity. Cord blood insulin concentrations have been associated with fetal macrosomia (Menon *et al.*, 1990), although this finding is somewhat controversial.

The two sulfonylurea drugs glipizide and glyburide are increasingly used to control gestational diabetes but inadequate data exist to evaluate their safety during pregnancy. In general they are believed to be safe for use during the first trimester. Recent studies have suggested that glyburide (and glipizide) is a substrate of efflux transporters in the placenta and thus its passage to the fetus may be limited, making it a potentially safe compound for use during pregnancy. However, more data are needed to confirm that the sulfonylureas truly are safe to use during pregnancy.

Models of diabetes mellitus have been developed in pregnant nonhuman primates. Mintz *et al.* (1972) developed a streptozotocin-induced diabetes model in the pregnant rhesus monkey. Offspring and placentas of diabetic monkeys were significantly heavier than average for their gestational age (macro-somia) and cases of polyhydramnios and third trimester stillbirths were increased for the diabetic pregnancies. Streptozotocin-induced diabetic females exhibited lower intravenous glucose tolerance and decreased glucose mediated insulin release. Hyperinsulinemia was found in both late-term fetuses and neonates of diabetic mothers.

Schwartz and his colleagues have published a series of reports using a rhesus monkey chronic fetal hyperinsulinemia model (McCormick *et al.*, 1979; Susa *et al.*, 1979; Schwartz and Susa, 1980; Widness *et al.*, 1981; Rooney *et al.*, 1983; Susa *et al.*, 1984a, 1984b, 1984c, 1992a, 1992b). According to the authors the model "provides an opportunity to study the metabolic effects of hyperinsulinemia separate from those of hyperglycemia on the primate fetus," making it a useful model for the study of fetal pathologic conditions in diabetic pregnancies. To date, no studies using these or other nonhuman primate models have been conducted to examine the antidiabetic drugs listed in Table 13.2.

Antibiotics

Antibiotics are perhaps the most commonly used drugs during pregnancy, although official statistics of their use are not available. Ciprofloxacin and its primary metabolite norfloxacin are two of the fluoroquinolone class of antibiotics. A number of birth defects have occurred in offspring of women who had taken fluoroquinolones during pregnancy, but there was no pattern of malformations observed (Briggs *et al.*, 2005). There have been some suggestions of fluoroquinolone-induced fetal cartilage damage and that fluoroquinolones may be mutagenic (Briggs *et al.*, 2005) but no consensus has been reached in the matter. Penicillin, ampicillin, amoxicillin, and other cephalosporin antibiotics are generally considered to be safe to consume during pregnancy, although they do cross the placenta (Briggs *et al.*, 2005). There are essentially no studies that address the safety of individual cephalosporin antibiotics in humans and as such the relative safety of these antibiotics is extrapolated from the class that they belong to. The major risk for use of penicillins during gestation is the potential for allergic reaction in the mother that may lead to anaphylactic shock in the mother and metabolic acidosis in the infant (Briggs *et al.*, 2005).

The aminoglycoside antibiotics (streptomycin, gentamycin, and tobramycin) are associated with nephrotoxicity and ototoxicity in adults and it has been assumed that as a class they may impair kidney and ear development. However, deafness or ototoxicity has not been observed in infants exposed in utero (Briggs *et al.*, 2005). It is well documented that fetal exposure to aminoglycosides is associated with toxicity to the eighth cranial nerve.

Of the antibiotics available for treatment of pregnant women, sulfamethoxazole and tetracycline are the two that have clearly been associated with adverse outcomes in the infant. The major concern with sulfonamides is that when administered close to term they can cause severe jaundice in the baby that may lead to kenicterus (Briggs *et al.*, 2005). Sulfonamides compete with bilirubin for binding to plasma albumin and thus presence of sulfonamides increases free bilirubin concentrations. In terms of major malformations, although teratogenic in the rat (Briggs *et al.*, 2005), sulfonamides are not believed to cause malformations in humans. In contrast, tetracyclines are contraindicated during pregnancy due to their teratogenic effects. They have adverse effects on fetal teeth and bones and cause congenital defects including neural tube defects, cardiovascular defects and cleft palate (Briggs *et al.*, 2005).

Cynomolgus monkeys have been used to study the developmental toxicity and maternal pharmacokinetics of norfloxacin (Cukierski *et al.*, 1989, 1992). Pregnant monkeys were given norfloxacin by nasogastric gavage at daily doses of 50–300 mg/kg per day during organogenesis (gestation days 21–50). For all groups, viable fetuses were removed by hysterotomy on gestation day 100 and were weighed and evaluated for the presence of gross abnormalities. Significant maternal toxicity and embryolethality was observed in the highest dosage group, 200/300 mg/kg per day. Embryonic loss was also apparent at a dosage of 150 mg/kg per day. Dosages of 50 and 100 mg/kg per day did not result in an increase in maternal toxicity or embryolethality. No indications of teratogenicity were observed at any dose. Studies of later gestation norfloxacin exposures (gd 35–45, gd 71–80, and gd 111–120) were also conducted. Oral administration of norflaxacin at 200 mg/kg per day during these gestation periods did not produce signs of maternal toxicity, or embro or fetal toxicity. The authors indicated that the effects observed during early pregnancy are likely due to changes in placental-derived progesterone production. Maternal kinetic studies indicated that the average maximum plasma concentrations were 20–40% lower during pregnancy. The authors indicated that the cynomolgus monkey appeared to be a good model for norfloxacin metabolism, although less drug is absorbed by the model (<25% compared with ~40% in humans) and that 150 mg/kg per day is the threshold of effects. The authors indicated that the plasma levels of norfloxacin in the monkey model are approximately threefold higher than the levels observed in humans taking the maximum recommended therapeutic dose (approximately 6 mg/kg twice daily). The authors concluded that this would provide a threefold margin of safety for women taking therapeutic doses of norfloxacin.

A brief report of a study to examine the potential for ciprofloxacin to act as an abortifacient in monkeys was published by Schluter (1989). Oral doses of 0–200 mg/kg per day ciprofloxacin were given to cynomolgus monkeys from days 20 to 50 of pregnancy. Pregnant animals tolerated the drug at all doses; there were no increases in abortions and there ciprofloxacin did not "influence the physiological development of the embryo or fetus."

Maternal–fetal pharmacokinetic studies of spiramycin using nonhuman primates have been reported (Schoondermark-Van de Ven et al., 1994a, 1994b). Transplacental passage and tissue distribution in the mother and fetus were examined. At a single intravenous dose of 50 mg, the serum half-life of spiramycin was approximately 2 hours and renal clearance was 15 mL/min. Fetal serum levels of spiramycin were only 5–7% of maternal levels after approximately 3 hours after administration. This level increased to over 50% when females were exposed for at least three weeks. Placental levels of spiramycin were 10–20 times higher then fetal serum levels, which may account for the low fetal–maternal serum ratios. Spiramycin concentrated mostly in the liver and spleen in the mother and fetus and no spiramycin was found in the brain. Fetal tissue levels were 5–28 times higher than serum levels but were still 11–16 times lower than the tissue levels found in the mother.

Pharmacokinetic studies or studies of serum or tissue levels of antibiotics following administration to adult nonhuman primates have been reported for ciprofloxacin

(Siefert *et al.*, 1986; Kelly *et al.*, 1992; Hummler *et al.*, 1993) norfloxacin (Hummler *et al.*, 1993), penicillin (Kelly *et al.*, 1992), cefazolin (Fare *et al.*, 1974), or sulfamethoxazole trimethoprim (Craig and Kunin, 1973).

OTHER DRUGS OF INTEREST

Warfarin

The most commonly used anticoagulant warfarin is a human teratogen. All anticoagulants (coumarin derivatives) except heparin cross the placental barrier and can subsequently cause hemorrhage in the embryo (Creasy and Resnik, 2004; Briggs *et al.*, 2005). Exposure to warfarin in 6–9 weeks of gestation results in a fetal warfarin syndrome characterized by hypoplasia of nasal cartilage and stippled epiphyses and incidence up to 25% in the exposed fetuses. Effects before or after this period may cause various CNS defects. Exposure to warfarin during second and third trimester may result in mental retardation, optic athrophy, and microcephaly. In addition, fetal growth retardation, spontaneous abortions, stillbirths, and neonatal deaths are associated with exposure to warfarin in utero. (Creasy and Resnik, 2004; Briggs *et al.*, 2005).

Studies of the reproductive and/or offspring developmental effects of warfarin in monkeys were not found.

Lithium

Lithium, used to treat manic episodes of manic-depressive disease, is considered teratogenic in humans. Lithium readily crosses the placenta and can be detected in the amniotic fluid and in cord blood. The fetal effects of lithium have been documented by the Lithium Baby Register started in Denmark, and by several other prospective, retrospective, and surveillance studies (Briggs *et al.*, 2005). The major congenital malformations after lithium administration occur mainly in the heart and great vessels. The incidence of rare Ebstein's anomaly has been reported to be increased in babies exposed to lithium during first trimester (Briggs *et al.*, 2005), but some authors have argued that no clear association is shown. At therapeutic concentrations in humans, lithium can cause major cardiac malformations and may be associated with neonatal toxicity (Weinstein and Goldfield, 1975; Weinstein, 1976; Kallen and Tandberg, 1983).

A developmental toxicology study of lithium carbonate was conducted in rhesus monkeys by Gralla and McIlhenny (1972). Six females were dosed with 0.67 meq/kg per day during organogenesis (days 14–35). Plasma levels of lithium were within the therapeutic range for humans (0.2–1.4 meq/L). Offspring were examined at birth and again at 7 and 30 days of age. Weights, body measures (cranial and limb), and blood measures (hematocrit, hemoglobin, etc.) were obtained. All offspring parameters were normal throughout the first 12–15 months of age. The results of the study do not indicate that the use of lithium during pregnancy results in developmental toxicity in exposed offspring.

Other studies of lithium exposure in nonhuman primates have focused on the effects of this drug on various behavioral parameters in adults (Slikker *et al.*, 1976; Bergman and Glowa, 1986; Welsh and Moore-Ede, 1990).

Methadone

Methadone is used in pregnant women to treat heroin addiction. As such, the developmental outcome data are complicated due to potential multisubstance abuse (alcohol, smoking, etc.). Infants of drug-addicted mothers are often small for gestational age so it is perhaps not surprising that newborns of methadone-treated women have higher birth weights than offspring of heroin addicts but are still low for gestational age (Briggs *et al.*, 2005). The major adverse outcome of methadone use during pregnancy is that the infants typically suffer from withdrawal symptoms that start within 48 hours of delivery and may last for 7–14 days. There are also reports of increased incidence of sudden infant death syndrome (SIDS), neonatal death, and stillbirths (Briggs *et al.*, 2005). Long-term effects on psychomotor and behavioral development are not known.

Methadone clearance has been found to increase during human pregnancy (Jarvis *et al.*, 1999; Wolff *et al.*, 2005) Trough mean plasma methadone concentrations reduced as the pregnancies progressed from 0.12 mg/L (first trimester) to 0.07 mg/L (third trimester). The weight-adjusted clearance rates gradually increased from a mean of 0.17–0.21 L/h per kg during pregnancy (Wolff *et al.*, 2005). With or without normalization for dose and body weight, trough plasma concentrations of methadone were significantly lower and total or unbound methadone clearances greater during pregnancy than after delivery (Pond *et al.*, 1985).

Nonhuman primate models have been used to study the association between maternal methadone use during pregnancy and low birth weight offspring (Hein *et al.*, 1988). Methadone was administered to cynomolgus monkeys in their food (40 mg/day) on a daily basis throughout pregnancy. The range of therapeutic doses for women during pregnancy is typically 50–150 mg/day (Drozdick *et al.*, 2002). Ten methadone pregnancies and six controls were studied and offspring size at birth was determined. There were no differences in the food intake between the methadone and control females. The duration of pregnancy was shorter for the methadone group (157 days versus 162 days) but the difference was not statistically significant. The average birth weight of the offspring from methadone females was significantly lower (320 grams) when compared to the controls (408 grams). The results of the study indicated that gestation exposure to methadone results in intra-uterine growth retardation (IUGR) and low birth weight in exposed offspring. Further studies of these pregnancies did not indicate that the effects were due to changes in maternal hormone level during pregnancy but via a direct effect of methadone on growth (Hein *et al.*, 1991).

Nonhuman primate models have also been used to study the placental transfer and maternal–fetal distribution of methadone. Pregnant rhesus monkeys were examined to determine the placental transfer of unchanged methadone or methadone metabolites during early and late pregnancy (Davis and Fenimore, 1978). Four pregnant females were injected i.m. with methadone, two early in pregnancy (first trimester or second trimester) and two late in pregnancy (late third trimester). Animals were then sacrificed either 1 or 6 hours after the injection ($N = 1$ per time point). Methadone and metabolite levels were significantly higher at both time points (1 and 6 hours) when injections occurred late in pregnancy. Mothers who received methadone late in pregnancy had 40% (6 hour sacrifice) to 50% (1 hour sacrifice) higher levels of unchanged methadone in their tissue and fluids. Similar results were seen for the fetal tissue. Fetal tissue levels following early gestation exposure were mostly near the detection limit while levels following late gestation exposure were much higher and near to those found in the mother (e.g. maternal brain 172 ng/g, fetal brain 123 ng/g). The data suggest a slowing of methadone metabolism in late pregnancy.

Bendectin

Bendectin use was widespread during the 1960s and 1970s to control nausea and vomiting during pregnancy (Kutcher *et al.*, 2003). Studies relating the use of Bendectin during pregnancy to congenital malformations appeared in the literature in the early 1980s (Eskenazi and Bracken, 1982; Golding *et al.*, 1983; Rothman *et al.*, 1995). These studies reported a positive association between Bendictin use during pregnancy and congenital heart disease, pyloric stenosis, and cleft lip and palate. Additional studies prompted by these reports failed to find an association between Bendectin and congenital defects in children (see McKeigue *et al.*, 1994 for review). In 1983, the manufacturer of Bendectin discontinued production of the drug worldwide, citing increased costs associated with litigation. At the time of writing, discussions are underway focused on the return of Bendectin as an effective therapy for nausea and vomiting (Brent, 2003).

During the height of the controversy over Bendectin, Hendrickx *et al.* (1985a, 1985b) examined the embryotoxicity of the drug in three nonhuman primate species. In the first study, Bendectin was administered via nasogastric intubation to rhesus monkeys, cynomolgus monkeys, or baboons. The dosages of Bendectin were 10–40 times the therapeutic dose for humans and exposure occurred during organogenesis either from 22 to 50 days gestation or for 4-day periods beginning on day gestation days 22–38. Preterm fetuses were examined at 100 days gestation and some animals were examined near delivery (~150–160 days). For the preterm fetuses exposed to Bendectin throughout organogenesis, the incidence of ventricular septal defects was increased in all species, 40% for the cynomolgus, 23% for the baboons, and 18% for the rhesus. Defects were observed at all doses and no other cardiac or other defects were observed. Preterm fetuses exposed to Bendectin for 4-day periods during organogenesis did not exhibit ventricular septal defects or other defects. Ventricular septal defects were not observed in animals examined near term regardless of their exposure history. The authors indicated that the results were consistent with a delay in the closure of the ventricular septum due to Bendectin. The results would indicate that this delay would not result in an increase in ventricular septal defects at birth.

In a follow-up study, Hendrickx *et al.* (1985b) administered Bendectin to cynomolgus monkeys at dosages 2, 5, or 20 times the human therapeutic dose during organogenesis (20–50 days gestation). Monkeys were delivered by cesarean section near term and examined for malformations. Consistent with the results from above, no ventricular septal defects or other defects were observed. The authors indicated that the results support the notion that Bendectin has "no, or very little, teratogenic potential."

CONCLUSIONS AND FUTURE DIRECTIONS

Of the many drugs commonly used during human pregnancy, only a few have been tested for their effects on long-term behavioral development. For those studies that have been conducted, many are confounded by the potential effects of the maternal disease on the infant. As such, there would be a great value for an animal model, such as the nonhuman primate, that would allow controlled testing of infant development following in utero exposures.

For new drug therapies, clinicians are typically reluctant to use potentially more effective drugs to control maternal disease during pregnancy as insufficient data about their fetal safety and developmental effects are available. Validation of an animal model that mimics well the effects seen in humans would improve the clinical treatment of pregnant women. It is clear that more studies are needed in the nonhuman primate model to fully evaluate the potential of this model for preclinical testing of developmental effects of drugs. However, based on the data available on antiepileptic drugs and other developmental neurotoxicants (see Chapter 14), it is likely that effects on infant development can be detected in this model. As such, one may suggest that widely used drugs such as the antidepressants, antihypertensive drugs, and antidiabetes treatments would be evaluated in the nonhuman primate because of the broad use of the drugs in pregnant women and the indications of potential developmental effects in humans.

REFERENCES

Artama, M., Auvinen, A., Raudaskoski, T., Isojarvi, I., and Isojarvi, J. (2005). Antiepileptic drug use of women with epilepsy and congenital malformations in offspring. *Neurology* **64**, 1874–1878.

Banka, N., Anand, I. S., Chakravarti, R. N., and Sharma, P. L. (1984). Effect of atenolol, nifedipine & oxyfedrine on experimental myocardial infarct size in rhesus monkeys. *Indian J Med Res* **79**, 426–431.

Barrow, M. V., Steffek, A. J., and King, C. T. (1969). Thalidomide syndrome in rhesus monkeys (*Macaca mulatta*). *Folia Primatol (Basel)* **10**, 195–203.

Bergman, J. and Glowa, J. R. (1986). Suppression of behavior by food pellet-lithium chloride pairings in squirrel monkeys. *Pharmacol Biochem Behav* **25**, 973–978.

Bibbo, M., Gill, W. B., Azizi, F. *et al.* (1977). Follow-up study of male and female offspring of DES-exposed mothers. *Obstet Gynecol* **49**, 1–8.

Brent, R. (2003). Bendectin and birth defects: hopefully, the final chapter. *Birth Defects Res A Clin Mol Teratol* **67**, 79–87.

Briggs GG., Freeman RK, and Yaffe SJ. (2005) *Drugs in Pregnancy and Lactation, A Reference Guide to Fetal and Neonatal Risk*, 7th edn. Philadelphia: Lippincott Williams & Wilkins.

Brown, N. A. and Fabro, S. (1983). The value of animal teratogenicity testing for predicting human risk. *Clin Obstet Gynecol* **26**, 467–477.

Butcher, R. E., Hawver, K., Burbacher, T., and Scott, W. (1975). Behavioral effects from antenatal exposure to teratogens. In: Ellis, N. R. ed. *Aberrant Development in Infancy, Human and Animal Studies*. Chichester: John Wiley and Sons, pp. 161–167.

Butler, H. and Juurlink, B. H. J. (1987). *An Atlas for Staging Mammalian and Chick Embryos*. Boca Raton, FL: CRC Press.

Cabrera, R. M., Hill, D. S., Etheredge, A. J., and Finnell, R. H. (2004). Investigations into the etiology of neural tube defects. *Birth Defects Res C* **72**, 330–344.

Casson, I. F., Clarke, C. A., Howard, C. V. *et al.* (1997). Outcomes of pregnancy in insulin dependent diabetic women: results of a five year population cohort study. *BMJ* **315**, 275–278.

CDC. Improved national prevalence estimates for 18 selected major birth defects – United States, 1999–2001. *MMWR* 2006. **54**, 1301–1305.

Chambers, C. D., Hernandez-Diaz, S., Van Marter, L. J. *et al.* (2006). Selective serotonin-reuptake inhibitors and risk of persistent pulmonary hypertension of the newborn. *N Engl J Med* **354**, 579–587.

Clagett-Dame, M. and DeLuca, H. F. (2002). The role of vitamin A in mammalian reproduction and embryonic development. *Annu Rev Nutr* **22**, 347–381.

Clarke, A. S., Kraemer, G. W., and Kupfer, D. J. (1998). Effects of rearing condition on HPA axis response to fluoxetine and desipramine treatment over repeated social separations in young rhesus monkeys. *Psychiatry Res* **79**, 91–104.

Coe, C. L., Hou, F. Y., and Clarke, A. S. (1996). Fluoxetine treatment alters leukocyte trafficking in the intrathecal compartment of the young primate. *Biol Psychiatry* **40**, 361–367.

Cosgrove, M. D., Benton, B., and Henderson, B. E. (1977). Male genitourinary abnormalities and maternal diethylstilbestrol. *J Urol* **117**.

Craig, W. A. and Kunin, C. M. (1973). Distribution of trimethoprim-sulfamethoxazole in tissues of rhesus monkeys. *J Infect Dis* **128**(suppl), 575–579.

Creasy, R. K. and Resnik, R. (2004). *Maternal-Fetal Medicine, Principles and Practice*, 5th edn. Philadelphia: Saunders.

Cukierski, M. A., Prahalada, S., Zacchei, A. G. *et al.* (1989). Embryotoxicity studies of norfloxacin in cynomolgus monkeys: I. Teratology studies and norfloxacin plasma concentration in pregnant and nonpregnant monkeys. *Teratology* **39**, 39–52.

Cukierski, M. A., Hendrickx, A. G., Prahalada, S. *et al.* (1992). Embryotoxicity studies of norfloxacin in cynomolgus monkeys. II. Role of progesterone. *Teratology* **46**, 429–438.

Davis, C. M. and Fenimore, D. C. (1978). The placental transfer and materno-fetal disposition of methadone in monkeys. *J Pharmacol Exp Ther* **205**, 577–586.

368   Primate Models of Children's Health and Developmental Disabilities

Delahunt, C. S. and Lassen, L. J. (1964). Thalidomide syndrome in monkeys. *Science* **146**, 1300–1305.

Detrait, E. R., George, T. M., Etchevers, H. C., Gilbert, J. R., Vekemans, M., and Speer, M. C. (2005). Human neural tube defects: developmental biology, epidemiology, and genetics. *Neurotoxicol Teratol* **27**, 515–524.

Dickinson, R. G., Hooper, W. D., Wood, B., Lander, C. M., and Eadie, M. J. (1989). The effects of pregnancy in humans on the pharmacokinetics of stable isotope labelled phenytoin. *Br J Clin Pharmacol* **28**, 17–27.

Dignan, P. S. (1981). Teratogenic risk and counseling in diabetes *Clin Obstet Gynecol* **24**, 149–159.

Doyle, E., Chasseaud, L. F., and Miller, J. N. (1982). Comparative pharmacokinetics of frusemide in female rhesus monkeys, cynomolgus monkeys and baboons. *Comp Biochem Physiol C* **71C**, 89–93.

Drozdick, J. III, Berghella, V., Hill, M., and Kaltenbach, K. (2002). Methadone trough levels in pregnancy. *Am J Obstet Gynecol* **187**, 1184–1188.

Einarson, T. R. and Einarson, A. (2005). Newer antidepressants in pregnancy and rates of major malformations: a meta-analysis of prospective conparative studies. *Pharmacoepidemiol Drug Saf* **14**, 823–827.

Eskenazi, B. and Bracken, M. B. (1982). Bendectin (Debendox) as a risk factor for pyloric stenosis. *Am J Obstet Gynecol* **144**, 919–924.

Fantel, A. G., Shepard, T. H., Newell-Morris, L. L., and Moffett, B. C. (1977). Teratogenic effects of retinoic acid in pigtail monkeys (*Macaca nemestrina*). I. General features. *Teratology* **15**, 65–71.

Fare, L. R., Actor, P., Sachs, C., Phillips, L., Joloza, M., Pauls, J. F., and Weisbach, J. A. (1974). Comparative serum levels and protective activity of parenterally administered cephalosporins in experimental animals. *Antimicrob Agents Chemother* **6**, 150–155.

FDA-Medwatch (2006). http://www.fda.gov/medwatch/safety/2006/safety06.htm#Lamictal

Finnell, R. H. (1999). Teratology: General considerations and principles. *J Allergy Immunol* S337–S342

Finnell, R. H. and Chernoff, G. F. (1982) Mouse fetal hydantoin syndrome: effects of maternal seizures. *Epilepsia* **23**, 423–429.

Ganapathy, V., Prasad, P. D., Ganapathy, M. E., and Leibach, F. H. (2000). Placental transporters relevant to drug distribution across the maternal-fetal interface. *J Pharmacol Exp Ther* **294**, 413–420.

Garland, M., Abildskov, K. M., Kiu, T. W., Daniel, S. S., and Stark, R. I. (2005). The contribution of fetal metabolism to the disposition of morphine. *Drug Metab Dispos* **33**, 68–76.

Gartner, L. M., Lee, K. S., Vaisman, S., Lane, D., and Zarafu, I. (1977). Development of bilirubin transport and metabolism in the newborn rhesus monkey. *J Pediatr* **90**, 513–531.

Gentile, S. (2005). The safety of newer antidepressants in pregnancy and breastfeeding. *Drug Saf* **28**, 137–152.

Gill, W. B., Schumacher, G. F., and Bibbo, M. (1976). Structural and functional abnormalities in the sex organs of male offspring of mothers treated with diethylstilbestrol (DES). *J Reprod Med* **16**, 147–153.

Gill, W. B., Schumacher, G. F., and Bibbo, M. (1977). Pathological semen and anatomical abnormalities of the genital tract in human male subjects exposed to diethylstilbestrol in utero. *J Urol* **117**, 477–480.

Gill, W. B., Schumacher, G. F., Bibbo, M., Straus, F. H., II, and Schoenberg, H. W. (1979). Association of diethylstilbestrol exposure in utero with cryptorchidism, testicular hypoplasia and semen abnormalities. *J Urol* **122**, 36–39.

Gindler, J., Li, Z., Berry, R. J. *et al.* (2001). Folic acid supplements during pregnancy and risk of miscarriage. *Lancet* **358**, 796–800.

Golding, J., Vivian, S., and Baldwin, J. A. (1983). Maternal anti-nauseants and clefts of lip and palate. *Hum Toxicol* **2**, 63–73.

Gralla, E. J. and McIlhenny, H. M. (1972). Studies in pregnant rats, rabbits and monkeys with lithium carbonate. *Toxicol Appl Pharmacol* **21**, 428–433.

Granstrom, M. -L. and Gaily, E. (1992) Psychomotor development in children with epilepsy. *Neurology* **42**, 144–148.

Guberman, A. H., Besag, F. M., Brodie, M. J. *et al.* (1999). Lamotrigine-associated rash: risk/benefit considerations in adults and children. *Epilepsia* **40**, 985–991.

Gugler, R. and von Unruh, G. E. (1980). Clinical pharmacokinetics of valproic acid. *Clin Pharmacokinet* **5**, 67–83.

Hart, W. R., Townsend, D. E., Aldrich, J. O., Henderson, B. E., Roy, M., and Benton, B. (1976). Histopathologic spectrum of vaginal adenosis and related changes in stilbestrol-exposed females. *Cancer* **37**, 763–775.

Hein, P. R., Schatorje, J. S., and Frencken, H. J. (1988). The effect of chronic methadone treatment on intra-uterine growth of the cynomolgus monkey (*Macaca fascicularis*). *Eur J Obstet Gynecol Reprod Biol* **27**, 81–85.

Hein, P. R., Schatorje, J. S., Frencken, H. J., Segers, M. F., and Thomas, C. M. (1991). The effect of chronic oral methadone treatment on monkey chorionic gonadotropin, estradiol, dehydroepiandrosterone sulfate, progesterone, prolactin and cortisol levels during pregnancy in the cynomolgus monkey (*Macaca fascicularis*). *Eur J Obstet Gynecol Reprod Biol* **38**, 145–150.

Helton, E. D., Hill, D. E., Lipe, G. W., Sziszak, T. J., and King, J. W., Jr. (1978). The metabolism of diethylstilbestrol in the rhesus monkey and chimpanzee. *J Environ Pathol Toxicol* **2**, 521–537.

Henderson, B. E., Benton, B., Cosgrove, M. *et al.* (1976). Urogenital tract abnormalities in sons of women treated with diethylstilbestrol. *Pediatrics* **58**, 505–507.

Hendrickx, A. G. (1971a). *Embryology of the Baboon*, Chicago: The University of Chicago Press.

Hendrickx, A. G, (1971b) Teratogenic effects of thalidomide in bonnet monkey (*Macaca radiate*) and cynomologus monkey (*Macaca irus*). *Teratology* **4**.

Hendrickx, A. G. (1973). The sensitive period and malformation syndrome produced by thalidomide in crab-eating monkey (*Macaca fascicularis*). *J Med Primatol* **2**, 267–276.

Hendrickx, A. G. (1975). Teratologic evaluation of imipramine hydrochloride in bonnet (*Macaca radiata*) and rhesus monkeys (*Macaca mulatta*). *Teratology* **11**, 219–221.

Hendrickx, A. G. and Hummler, H. (1992). Teratogenicity of all-trans retinoic acid during early embryonic development in the cynomolgus monkey (*Macaca fascicularis*). *Teratology* **45**, 65–74.

Hendrickx, A. G. and Newman, L. (1973). Appendicular skeletal and visceral malformations induced by thalidomide in bonnet monkeys. *Teratology* **7**, 151–159.

Hendrickx, A. G. and Sawyer, R. H. (1978). Developmental staging and thalidomide teratogenicity in the green monkey (*Cercopithecus aethiops*). *Teratology* **18**, 393–404.

Hendrickx, A. G., Axelrod, L. R., and Clayborn, L. D. (1966). 'Thalidomide' syndrome in baboons. *Nature* **210**, 958–959.

Hendrickx, A. G., Benirschke, K., Thompson, R. S., Ahern, J. K., Lucas, W. E., and Oi, R. H. (1979). The effects of prenatal diethylstilbestrol (DES) exposure on the genitalia of pubertal *Macaca mulatta*. I. Female offspring. *J Reprod Med* **22**, 233–240.

Hendrickx, A. G., Silverman, S., Pellegrini, M., and Steffek, A. J. (1980). Teratological and radiocephalometric analysis of craniofacial malformations induced with retinoic acid in rhesus monkeys (*Macaca mulatta*). *Teratology* **22**, 13–22.

Hendrickx, A. G., Cukierski, M., Prahalada, S., Janos, G., and Rowland, J. (1985a). Evaluation of bendectin embryotoxicity in nonhuman primates: I. Ventricular septal defects in prenatal macaques and baboon. *Teratology* **32**, 179–189.

Hendrickx, A. G., Cukierski, M., Prahalada, S., Janos, G., Booher, S., and Nyland, T. (1985b). Evaluation of bendectin embryotoxicity in nonhuman primates: II. Double-blind study in term cynomolgus monkeys. *Teratology* **32**, 191–194.

Hendrickx, A. G., Prahalada, S., and Binkerd, P. E. (1987). Long-term evaluation of the diethylstilbestrol (DES) syndrome in adult female rhesus monkeys (*Macaca mulatta*). *Reprod Toxicol* **1**, 253–261.

Hendrickx, A. G., Nau, H., Binkerd, P. *et al.* (1988). Valproic acid developmental toxicity and pharmacokinetics in the rhesus monkey: an interspecies comparison. *Teratology* **38**, 329–345.

Hendrickx, A. G., Tzimas, G., Korte, R., and Hummler, H. (1998). Retinoid teratogenicity in the macaque: verification of dosing regimen. *J Med Primatol* **27**, 310–318.

Hendrickx, A. G., Peterson, P., Hartmann, D., and Hummler, H. (2000). Vitamin A teratogenicity and risk assessment in the macaque retinoid model. *Reprod Toxicol* **14**, 311–323.

Hendrie, T. A., Rowland, J. R., Binkerd, P. E., and Hendrickx, A. G. (1990). Developmental toxicity and pharmacokinetics of phenytoin in the rhesus macaque: an interspecies comparison. *Reprod Toxicol* **4**, 257–266.

Herbst, A. L., Ulfelder, H., and Poskanzer, D. (1971). Adenocarcinoma of the vagina. *N Engl J Med* **284**, 878–881.

Herbst, A. L., Kurman, R. J., and Scully, R. E. (1972). Vaginal and cervical abnormalities after exposure to stilbestrol in utero. *Obstet Gynecol* **40**, 287–298.

Herbst, A. L., Poskanzer, D. C., Robboy, S. J., Friedlander, L., and Scully, R. E. (1975). Prenatal exposure to stilbestrol. A prospective comparison of exposed female offspring with unexposed controls. *N Engl J Med* **292**, 334–339.

Hill, D. E., Slikker, W., Jr., Helton, E. D. *et al.* (1980). Transplacental pharmacokinetics and metabolism of diethylstilbestrol and 17 beta-estradiol in the pregnant rhesus monkey. *J Clin Endocrinol Metab* **50**, 811–818.

Hirano, T., Fujioka, K., Okada, M., Iwasa, H., and Kaneko, S. (2004). Physical and psychomotor development in the offspring born to mothers with epilepsy. *Epilepsia* **45**, 53–57.

Hjalmarsson, L., Corcos, M., and Jeammet, P. (2005). [Selective serotonin reuptake inhibitors in major depressive disorder in children and adolescents (ratio of benefits/risks)]. *Encephale* **31**, 309–316.

Hoefnagel, D. (1976). Letter: Prenatal diethylstilboestrol exposure and male hypogonadism. *Lancet* **1**, 152–153.

Hoffmeister, F. (1977). Reinforcing properties of perphenazine, haloperidol and amitryptiline in rhesus monkeys. *J Pharmacol Exp Ther* **200**, 516–522.

Hogstedt, S., Londberg, B., Peng, D. R., Regardh, C. -G., and Rane, A. (1985). Pregnancy-induced increase in metoprolol metabolism. *Clin Pharmacol Ther* **37**, 688–692.

Hogstedt, S., Lindberg, B. S., Regardh, C. G., Mostrom, U., and Rane, A. (1990). The rhesus monkey as a model for studies of pregnancy induced changes in metoprolol metabolism. *Pharmacol Toxicol* **66**, 32–36.

Hood, R. D. (2005). *Developmental and Reproductive Toxicology. A Practical Approach.* London: Taylor and Francis.

Hummler, H., Korte, R., and Hendrickx, A. G. (1990). Induction of malformations in the cynomolgus monkey with 13-cis retinoic acid. *Teratology* **42**, 263–272.

Hummler, H., Richter, W. F., and Hendrickx, A. G. (1993). Developmental toxicity of fleroxacin and comparative pharmacokinetics of four fluoroquinolones in the cynomolgus macaque (*Macaca fascicularis*). *Toxicol Appl Pharmacol* **122**, 34–45.

Isoherranen, N., White, H. S., Finnell, R. H. *et al.* (2002). Anticonvulsant profile and teratogenicity of N-methyl-tetramethylcyclopropyl carboxamide: a new antiepileptic drug. *Epilepsia* **43**, 115–126.

Isoherranen, N., Yagen B., and Bialer M. (2003). New antiepileptic and CNS drugs that are second generation valproic acid. Can they lead to the development of a magic bullet? *Curr Opin Neurol* **16**, 203–211.

Jarvis, M. A., Wu-Pong, S., Kniseley, J. S., and Schnoll, S. H. (1999) Alterations in methadone metabolism during late pregnancy. *J Addict Dis* **18**, 51–61.

Johannessen, S. I. (1997). Pharmacokinetics of antiepileptic drugs in pregnant women. In: Tomson, T., Gram, L., Sillanpaa, M., and Johannessen, S. I. eds. *Epilepsy and Pregnancy*. Petersfield: Wrightson Biomedical, pp. 71–80.

Kallen, B. and Tandberg, A. (1983). Lithium and pregnancy. A cohort study on manic-depressive women. *Acta Psychiatr Scand* **68**, 134–139.

Kawaguchi, M., Tanigawa, K., Tanaka, O., and Kato, Y. (1994). Embryonic growth impaired by maternal hypoglycemia during early organogenesis in normal and diabetic rats. *Acta Diabetol* **31**, 141–146.

Kelly, D. J., Chulay, J. D., Mikesell, P., and Friedlander, A. M. (1992). Serum concentrations of penicillin, doxycycline, and ciprofloxacin during prolonged therapy in rhesus monkeys. *J Infect Dis* **166**, 1184–1187.

Kini, U., Adab, N., Vinten, J., Fryer, A., and Clayton-Smith, J. (2006). Dysmorphic features: an important clue to the diagnosis and severity of fetal anticonvulsant syndromes. *Arch Dis Child Fetal Neonatal Ed* **91**, F90–95.

Kleven, M. S. and Woolverton, W. L. (1993). Effects of three monoamine uptake inhibitors on behavior maintained by cocaine or food presentation in rhesus monkeys. *Drug Alcohol Depend* **31**, 149–158.

Koch, S., Jager-Roman, E., Losche, G., Nau, H., Rating, D., and Helge, H. (1996). Antiepileptic drug treatment in pregnancy: drug side effects in the neonate and neurological outcome. *Acta Pediatr.* **8**, 739–746.

Koch, S., Titze, K., Zimmermann, R. B., Schroder, M., Lehmkuhl, U., and Rauh, H. (1999). Long-term neuropsychological consequences on maternal epilepsy and anticonvulsant treatment during pregnancy for school-age children and adolescents. *Epilepsia* **40**, 1237–1243.

Korte, R., Hummler, H., and Hendrickx, A. G. (1993). Importance of early exposure to 13-cis retinoic acid to induce teratogenicity in the cynomolgus monkey. *Teratology* **47**, 37–45.

Kurki, T., Hiilesmaa, V., Raitasalo, R., Mattila, H., and Ylikorkala, O. (2000). Depression and anxiety in early pregnancy and risk for preeclampsia. *Obstet Gynecol* **95**, 487–490.

Kutcher, J. S., Engle, A., Firth, J., and Lamm, S. H. (2003). Bendectin and birth defects. II: Ecological analyses. *Birth Defects Res A Clin Mol Teratol* **67**, 88–97.

Lammer, E. J., Chen, D. T., Hoar, R. M. et al. (1985). Retinoic acid embryopathy. *N Engl J Med* **313**, 837–841.

Lander, C. M. and Eadie, M. J. (1991). Plasma antiepileptic drug concentrations during pregnancy. *Epilepsia* **32**, 257–266.

Lanier, A. P., Noller, K. L., Decker, D. G., Elveback, L. R., and Kurland, L. T. (1973). Cancer and stilbestrol. A follow-up of 1,719 persons exposed to estrogens in utero and born 1943–1959. *Mayo Clin Proc* **48**, 793–799.

Lattimore, K. A., Donn, S. M., Kaciroti, N., Kemper, A. R., Neal, C. R. Jr, and Vazquez, D. M. (2005). Selective serotonin reuptake inhibitor (SSRI) use during pregnancy and effects on the fetus and newborn: a meta-analysis. *J Perinatol* **25**, 595–604.

Laudenslager, M. L. and Clarke, A. S. (2000). Antidepressant treatment during social challenge prior to 1 year of age affects immune and endocrine responses in adult macaques. *Psychiatry Res* **95**, 25–34.

Lindhout, D. and Omtzigt, J. G. C. (1994) Teratogenic effects of antiepileptic drugs: Implications for the management of epilepsy in women of childbearing age. *Epilepsia* **35**, 19–28.

Little, B. B. (1999). Pharmacokinetics during pregnancy: Evidence-based maternal dose formulation. *Obstet Gynecol* **93**, 858–868.

Lockard, J. S. and Barensten, R. I. (1967). Behavioral experimental epilepsy in monkeys. I. Clinical seizure recording apparatus and initial data. *Electroencephalogr Clin Neurophysiol* **22**, 482–486.

Lockard, J. S., Uhlir, V., DuCharme, L. L., Farquhar, J. A., and Huntsman, B. J. (1975). Efficacy of standard anticonvulsants in monkey model with spontaneous motor seizures. *Epilepsia* **16**, 301–317.

Lockard, J. S. and Arthur A. Ward, J., eds. (1980). *Epilepsy: A Window to Brain Mechanisms*. New York: Raven Press.

Maden, M. (2000). The role of retinoic acid in embryonic and post-embryonic development. *Proc Nutr Soc* **59**, 65–73.

Marais, L., Daniels, W., Brand, L., Viljoen, F., Hugo, C., and Stein, D. J. (2006). Psychopharmacology of maternal separation anxiety in vervet monkeys. *Metab Brain Dis* **21**, 201–210.

Mast, T. J., Cukierski, M. A., Nau, H., and Hendrickx, A. G. (1986). Predicting the human teratogenic potential of the anticonvulsant, valproic acid, from a non-human primate model. *Toxicology* **39**, 111–119.

McBride, K. L., Pignatelli, R., Lewin, M. et al. (2005). Inheritance analysis of congenital left ventricular outflow tract obstruction malformations: Segregation, multiplex relative risk, and heritability. *Am J Med Genet* **134A**, 180–186.

McClure, H. M. and Graham, C. E. (1973). Malignant uterine mesotheliomas in squirrel monkeys following diethylstilbestrol administration. *Lab Anim Sci* **23**, 493–498.

McCormick, K. L., Susa, J. B., Widness, J. A., Singer, D. B., Adamsons, K., and Schwartz, R. (1979). Chronic hyperinsulinemia in the fetal rhesus monkey: effects on hepatic enzymes active in lipogenesis and carbohydrate metabolism. *Diabetes* **28**, 1064–1068.

McKearney, J. W. (1982). Effects of tricyclic antidepressant and anticholinergic drugs on fixed-interval responding in the squirrel monkey. *J Pharmacol Exp Ther* **222**, 215–219.

McKeigue, P. M., Lamm, S. H., Linn, S., and Kutcher, J. S. (1994). Bendectin and birth defects: I. A meta-analysis of the epidemiologic studies. *Teratology* **50**, 27–37.

Menon, R. K., Cohen, R. M., Sperling, M. A., Cutfield, W. S., Mimouni, F., and Khoury, J. C. (1990). Transplacental passage of insulin in pregnant women with insulin-dependent diabetes mellitus. Its role in fetal macrosomia. *N Engl J Med* **323**, 309–315.

Messenheimer, J. A. (1998). Rash in adult and pediatric patients treated with lamotrigine. *Can J Neurol Sci* **25**, S14–S18.

Metzler, M., Muller, W., and Hobson, W. C. (1977). Biotransformation of diethylstilbestrol in the rhesus monkey and the chimpanzee. *J Toxicol Environ Health* **3**, 439–450.

Mintz, D. H., Chez, R. A., and Hutchinson, D. L. (1972). Subhuman primate pregnancy complicated by streptozotocin-induced diabetes mellitus. *J Clin Invest* **51**, 837–847.

Mirochnick, M. and Capparelli, E. (2004). Pharmacokinetic of antiretrovirals in pregnant women. *Clin Pharmacokinet* **43**, 1071–1087.

Moses-Kolko, E. L., Bogen, D., Perel, J. *et al.* (2005). Neonatal signs after late in utero exposure to serotonin reuptake inhibitors. Literature review and implications for clinical applications. *JAMA* **293**, 2372–2383.

Mroszczak, E. J. and Riegelman, S. (1975). Disposition of diethylstilbestrol in the rhesus monkey. *J Pharmacokinet Biopharm* **3**, 303–327.

Mroszczak, E. J. and Riegelman, S. (1978). Biliary excretion of diethylstilbestrol in the rhesus monkey. *J Pharmacokinet Biopharm* **6**, 339–354.

Nau, H., Chahoud, I., Dencker, L., Lammer, E. J., and Scott, W. J. (1994). Teratogenicity of vitamin A and retinoids. In: Blomhoff, R., ed. *Vitamin A in Health and Disease*. New York: Marcel Dekker, pp. 615–663.

Newell-Morris, L., Sirianni, J. E., Shepard, T. H., Fantel, A. G., and Moffett, B. C. (1980). Teratogenic effects of retinoic acid in pigtail monkeys (*Macaca nemestrina*). II. Craniofacial features. *Teratology* **22**, 87–101.

Newman, L. M. and Hendrickx, A. G. (1981). Fetal ear malformations induced by maternal ingestion of thalidomide in the bonnet monkey (*Macaca radiata*). *Teratology* **23**, 351–364.

Newman, L. M. and Hendrickx, A. G. (1985). Temporomandibular malformations in the bonnet monkey (*Macaca radiata*) fetus following maternal ingestion of thalidomide. *J Craniofac Genet Dev Biol* **5**, 147–157.

Nishimura, H., Takana, K., Tanimura, T., and Yasuda, M. (1968). Normal and abnormal development of human embryos: First report of the analysis of 1,213 intact embryos. *Teratology* 281–290.

Petersen, E. N., Bechgaard, E., Sortwell, R. J., and Wetterberg, L. (1978). Potent depletion of 5HT from monkey whole blood by a new 5HT uptake inhibitor, paroxetine (FG 7051). *Eur J Pharmacol* **52**, 115–119.

Phillips, N. K. and Lockard, J. S. (1985a). A gestational monkey model: effects of phenytoin versus seizures on neonatal outcome. *Epilepsia* **26**, 697–703.

Phillips, N. K. and Lockard, J. S. (1985b). Social and locomotor behavior after phenytoin exposure in neonatal monkeys. *Epilepsia* **26**, 546.

Phillips, N. K. and Lockard, J. S. (1993). Phenytoin and/or stiripentol in pregnancy: infant monkey hyperexcitability. *Epilepsia* **34**, 1117–1122.

Phillips, N. K. and Lockard, J. S. (1996). Infant monkey hyperexcitability after prenatal exposure to antiepileptic compounds. *Epilepsia* **37**, 991–999.

Piacentini, G., Digilio, M. C., Capolino, R. *et al.* (2005). Familial recurrence of heart defects in subjects with congenitally corrected transposition of the great arteries. *Am J Med Genet* **137A**, 176–180.

Pond, S. M., Kreek, M. J., Tong, T. G., Raghunath, J., and Benowitz, N. L. (1985). Altered methadone pharmacokinetics in methadone-maintained pregnant women. *J Pharmacol Exp Ther* **233**, 1–6.

Poswillo, D. E., Hamilton, W. J., and Sopher, D. (1972). The marmoset as an animal model for teratological research. *Nature* **239**, 460–462.

Ramboer, C., Thompson, R. P., and Williams, R. (1969). Controlled trials of phenobarbitone therapy of neonatal jaundice. *Lancet* **1**, 966–968.

Randall, T. (1990). Thalidomide's back in the news, but in more favorable circumstances. *JAMA* **263**, 1467–1468.

Rane, A., Hogstedt, S., Lindberg, B., Regardh, C. G., and Jorulf, H. (1984). Comparison of different clearance estimates for metoprolol in the rhesus monkey. *J Pharmacol Exp Ther* **228**, 774–778.

Rayburn, W., Donn, S., Piehl, E., and Compton, A. (1988). Antenatal phenobarbital and bilirubin metabolism in the very low birth weight infant. *Am J Obstet Gynecol* **159**, 1491–1493.

Rooney, S. A., Chu, A. J., Gross, I. *et al.* (1983). Lung surfactant in the hyperinsulinemic fetal monkey. *Lung* **161**, 313–317.

Rosa, F. W., Wilk, A. L., and Kelsey, F. O. (1986). Teratogen update: vitamin A congeners. *Teratology* **33**, 355–364.

Rothman, K. J., Moore, L. L., Singer, M. R., Nguyen, U. S., Manninno, S., and Milunsky, A. (1995). Teratogenicity of high vitamin A intake. *N Engl J Med* **333**, 1369–1373.

Samren, E. B. and Lindhout, D. (1997). Major malformations associated with maternal use of antiepileptic drugs. In: Tomson, T., Gram, L., Sillanpaa, M., and Johannessen, S. I. eds. *Epilepsy and Pregnancy*. Petersfield: Wrightson Biomedical.

Sannerstedt, R., Lundborg, P., Danielsson, B. R. *et al.* (1996). Drugs during pregnancy: an issue of risk classification and information to prescribers. *Drug Saf* **14**, 69–77.

Sannerud, C. A., Prada, J., Goldberg, D. M., and Goldberg, S. R. (1994). The effects of sertraline on nicotine self-administration and food-maintained responding in squirrel monkeys. *Eur J Pharmacol* **271**, 461–469.

Sanz, E. J., De-las-Cuevas, C., Kiuru, A., Bate, A., and Edwards, R. (2005). Selective serotonin reuptake inhibitors in pregnant women and neonatal withdrawal syndrome: a database analysis. *Lancet* **365**, 482–487.

Schardein, J. L. (1988). Teratologic testing: status and issues after two decades of evolution. *Rev. Environ. Contam. Toxicol.* **102**, 1–78.

Schluter, G. (1989). Ciprofloxacin: toxicologic evaluation of additional safety data. *Am J Med* **87**, 37S–39S.

Schmutz, M., Brugger, F., Gentsch, C., McLean, M. J., and Olpe, H. R. (1994). Oxcarbazepine: preclinical anticonvulsant profile and putative mechanisms of action. *Epilepsia* **35**(suppl 5), S47–50.

Schoondermark-Van de Ven, E., Galama, J., Camps, W. *et al.* (1994a). Pharmacokinetics of spiramycin in the rhesus monkey: transplacental passage and distribution in tissue in the fetus. *Antimicrob Agents Chemother* **38**, 1922–1929.

Schoondermark-Van de Ven, E., Melchers, W., Camps, W., Eskes, T., Meuwissen, J., and Galama, J. (1994b). Effectiveness of spiramycin for treatment of congenital *Toxoplasma gondii* infection in rhesus monkeys. *Antimicrob Agents Chemother* **38**, 1930–1936.

Schwartz, R. and Susa, J. (1980). Fetal macrosomia–animal models. *Diabetes Care* **3**, 430–432.

Schwartz, R. and Teramo, K. A. (2000). Effects of diabetic pregnancy on the fetus and newborn. *Semin Perinatol* **24**, 120–135.

Shapiro, S., Hartz, S. C., Siskind, V. *et al.* (1976), Anticonvulsants and parental epilepsy in the development of birth defects. *Lancet* **1**, 272–275.

Siefert, H. M., Maruhn, D., Maul, W., Forster, D., and Ritter, W. (1986). Pharmacokinetics of ciprofloxacin. 1st communication: absorption, concentrations in plasma, metabolism and excretion after a single administration of [14C]ciprofloxacin in albino rats and rhesus monkeys. *Arzneimittelforschung* **36**, 1496–1502.

Slikker, W., Jr., Brocco, M. J., and Killam, K. F., Jr. (1976). Comparison of the effects of lithium chloride and chlorpromazine on normal and isolate monkeys. *Proc West Pharmacol Soc* **19**, 424–427.

Spence, J. D. (1977). Effects of antihypertensive drugs on blood velocity: implications for prevention of cerebral vascular disease. *Can J Neurol Sci* **4**, 93–97.

Spence, J. D., Pesout, A. B., and Melmon, K. L. (1977). Effects of antihypertensive drugs on blood velocity in rhesus monkeys. *Stroke* **8**, 589–594.

Steer, R. A., Scholl, T. O., Hediger, M. L., and Fischer, R. L. (1992). Self-reported depression and negative pregnancy outcomes. *J Clin Epidemiol* **45**, 1093–1099.

Susa, J. B., McCormick, K. L., Widness, J. A. *et al.* (1979). Chronic hyperinsulinemia in the fetal rhesus monkey: effects on fetal growth and composition. *Diabetes* **28**, 1058–1063.

Susa, J. B., Gruppuso, P. A., Widness, J. A. *et al.* (1984a). Chronic hyperinsulinemia in the fetal rhesus monkey: effects of physiologic hyperinsulinemia on fetal substrates, hormones, and hepatic enzymes. *Am J Obstet Gynecol* **150**, 415–420.

Susa, J. B., Neave, C., Sehgal, P., Singer, D. B., Zeller, W. P., and Schwartz, R. (1984b). Chronic hyperinsulinemia in the fetal rhesus monkey. Effects of physiologic hyperinsulinemia on fetal growth and composition. *Diabetes* **33**, 656–660.

Susa, J. B., Widness, J. A., Hintz, R., Liu, F., Sehgal, P., and Schwartz, R. (1984c). Somatomedins and insulin in diabetic pregnancies: effects on fetal macrosomia in the human and rhesus monkey. *J Clin Endocrinol Metab* **58**, 1099–1105.

Susa, J. B., Boylan, J. M., Sehgal, P., and Schwartz, R. (1992a). Impaired insulin secretion after intravenous glucose in neonatal rhesus monkeys that had been chronically hyperinsulinemic in utero. *Proc Soc Exp Biol Med* **199**, 327–331.

Susa, J. B., Boylan, J. M., Sehgal, P., and Schwartz, R. (1992b). Persistence of impaired insulin secretion in infant rhesus monkeys that had been hyperinsulinemic in utero. *J Clin Endocrinol Metab* **75**, 265–269.

Swift, R. M., Dudley, M., DePetrillo, P., Camara, P., and Griffiths, W. (1989). Altered methadone pharmacokinetics in pregnancy: implications for dosing. *J Subst Abuse* **1**, 453–460.

Syme, M. R., Paxton, J. W., and Keelan, J. A. (2004). Drug transfer and metabolism by the human placenta. *Clin Pharmacokinet* **43**, 487–514.

Tanigawa, K., Kawaguchi, M., Tanaka, O., and Kato, Y. (1991). Skeletal malformations in rat offspring. Long-term effect of maternal insulin-induced hypoglycemia during organogenesis. *Diabetes* **40**, 1115–1121.

Tanimura, T. (1972). Effects on macaque embryos of drugs reported or suspected to be teratogenic in humans. In: Diczfalusy, E. and Standley, C. C. eds. *The Use of Nonhuman Primates in Research on Human Reproduction*. Stockholm: WHO Research and Training Center on Human Reproduction, pp. 293–308

Temple, R., Aldridge, V., Greenwood, R., Heyburn, P., Sampson, M., and Stanley, K. (2002). Association between outcome of pregnancy and glycaemic control in early pregnancy in type 1 diabetes: population based study. *BMJ* **325**, 1275–1276.

Tomson, T., Lindbom, U., Ekqvist, B., and Sundqvist, A. (1994a). Disposition of carbamazepine and phenytoin in pregnancy. *Epilepsia* **35**, 131–135.

Tomson, T., Lindbom, U., Ekqvist, B., and Sundqvist, A. (1994b). Epilepsy and pregnancy: a prospective study of seizure control in relation to free and total plasma concentrations of carbamazepine and phenytoin. *Epilepsia* **35**, 122–130.

Trevathan, E., Kerls, S. P., Hammer, A. E., Vuong, A., and Messenheimer, J. A. (2006). Lamotrigine adjunctive therapy among children and adolescents with primary generalized tonic-clonic seizures. *Pediatrics* **118**, e371–378.

Trevett, T. N., Jr., Dorman, K., Lamvu, G., and Moise, K. J., Jr. (2005). Antenatal maternal administration of phenobarbital for the prevention of exchange transfusion in neonates with hemolytic disease of the fetus and newborn. *Am J Obstet Gynecol* **192**, 478–482.

Tzimas, G. and Nau, H. (2001). The role of metabolism and toxicokinetics in retinoid teratogenesis. *Curr Pharmaceut Res* **7**, 803–831.

Tzimas, G., Nau, H., Hendrickx, A. G., Peterson, P. E., and Hummler, H. (1996). Retinoid metabolism and transplacental pharmacokinetics in the cynomolgus monkey following a nonteratogenic dosing regimen with all-trans–retinoic acid. *Teratology* **54**, 255–265.

Unadkat, J. D., Dahlin, A., and Vijay, S. (2004). Placental drug transporters. *Curr Drug Metab* **5**, 125–131.

Valaes, T., Kipouros, K., Petmezaki, S., Solman, M., and Doxiadis, S. A. (1980). Effectiveness and safety of prenatal phenobarbital for the prevention of neonatal jaundice. *Pediatr Res* **14**, 947–952.

Vondruska, J. F., Fancher, O. E., and Calandra, J. C. (1971). An investigation into the teratogenic potential of captan, folpet, and Difolatan in nonhuman primates. *Toxicol Appl Pharmacol* **18**, 619–624.

Walson, P. D., Marshall, K. S., Forsyth, R. P., Rapoport, R., Melmon, K. L., and Castagnoli, N., Jr. (1975). Metabolic disposition and cardiovascular effects of methyldopa in unanesthetized rhesus monkeys. *J Pharmacol Exp Ther* **195**, 151–158.

Wei, X., Makori, N., Peterson, P. E., Hummler, H., and Hendrickx, A. G. (1999). Pathogenesis of retinoic acid-induced ear malformations in primate model. *Teratology* **60**, 83–92.

Weinstein, M. R. (1976). The international register of lithium babies. *Drug Inf J* **10**, 94–100.

Weinstein, M. R. and Goldfield, M. (1975). Cardiovascular malformations with lithium use during pregnancy. *Am J Psychiatry* **132**, 529–531.

Welsh, D. K. and Moore-Ede, M. C. (1990). Lithium lengthens circadian period in a diurnal primate, Saimiri sciureus. *Biol Psychiatry* **28**, 117–126.

Widness, J. A., Susa, J. B., Garcia, J. F. *et al.* (1981). Increased erythropoiesis and elevated erythropoietin in infants born to diabetic mothers and in hyperinsulinemic rhesus fetuses. *J Clin Invest* **67**, 637–642.

Wilcox, A. J., Weinberg, C. R., O'Connor, J. F. *et al.* (1988). Incidence of early loss of pregnancy. *N Engl J Med* **319**, 189–194.

Williams, M. and Wooltorton, E. (2005). Paroxetine (Paxil) and congenital malformations. *CMAJ* **173**, 1320–1321.

Wilson, J. G. (1973a). Present status of drugs as teratogens in man. *Teratology* **7**, 3–15.

Wilson, J. G. (1973b). An animal model of human disease: Thalidomide embryopathy in primates. *Comp Pathol Bull* **5**, 3–4.

Wilson, J. G. (1974). Teratologic causation in man and its evaluation in non-human primates. In: Motulsky, A. G. ed. *Birth Defects*. New York: American Elsevier Publishing, pp. 191–203.

Wilson, J. G. (1977). Current status of teratology. General principles and mechanisms derived from animal studies. In: *Handbook of Teratology*. New York: Plenum Press, pp. 1–47.

Wilson, J. G. and Gavan, J. A. (1967). Congenital malformations in nonhuman primates: spontaneous and experimentally induced. *Anat Rec* **158**, 99–109.

Wolff, K., Boys, A., Rostami-Hodjegan, A., Hay, A., and Raistrick, D. (2005). Changes to methadone clearance during pregnancy. *Eur J Clin Pharmacol* **61**, 763–768.

Wong, I. C., Besag, F. M., Santosh, P. J., and Murray, M. L. (2004). Use of selective serotonin reuptake inhibitors in children and adolescents. *Drug Saf* **27**, 991–1000.

Yakatan, G. J., Maness, D. D., Scholler, J., Novick, W. J., Jr, and Doluisio, J. T. (1976). Absorption, distribution, metabolism, and excretion of furosemide in dogs and monkeys I: analytical methodology, metabolism, and urinary excretion. *J Pharm Sci* **65**, 1456–1460.

Yakatan, G. J., Maness, D. D., Scholler, J., Johnston, J. T., Novick, W. J., Jr, and Doluisio, J. T. (1979). Plasma and tissue levels of furosemide in dogs and monkeys following single and multiple oral doses. *Res Commun Chem Pathol Pharmacol* **24**, 465–482.

Yerby, M. S., Friel, P. N., McCormick, K. *et al.* (1990) Pharmacokinetics of anticonvulsants in pregnancy: alterations in plasma protein binding. *Epilepsy Res.* **5**, 223–228.

Yip, J. E., Kokich, V. G., and Shepard, T. H. (1980). The effect of high doses of retinoic acid on prenatal craniofacial development in *Macaca nemestrina*. *Teratology* **21**, 29–38.

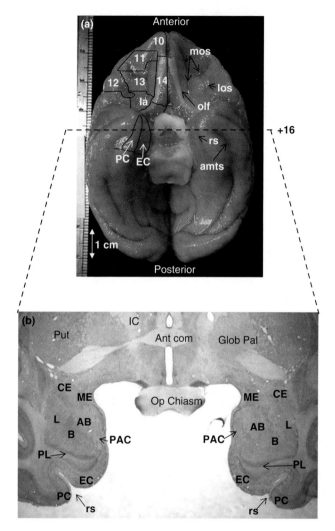

PLATE 1 Anatomical localization of the orbital frontal cortex and amygdala in the rhesus macaque (*Macaca mulatta*) brain. Photograph of a ventral view of a macaque brain (a) identifying the borders (black lines) of the orbital frontal cortex cytoarchitectonic fields (e.g. Broadman areas 10, 11, 12, 13, and 14 from Carmichael and Price, 1994; Barbas, 1995; Öngür and Price, 2000; Petrides and Pandya, 2002) on the right hemisphere (left on the photograph). The borders of the entorhinal (EC) and perirhinal (PC) cortices in the temporal lobe are also shown on the right hemisphere. The sulci on the orbital and temporal surfaces of the brain are indicated by arrows on the left hemisphere (right on the photograph). (b) Photomicrograph of a Nissl-stained coronal section through the medial temporal lobe (at +16 mm from the interaural plane) of a macaque brain, showing the amygdala nuclei and the entorhinal and perirhinal cortices. Amts, anterior medial temporal sulcus; Ant com, anterior commissure; AB, accessory basal nucleus; B, basal nucleus; CE, central nucleus; Glob Pal, globus pallidus; Ia, Insular agranular cortex; IC, internal capsule; L, lateral nucleus; los, lateral orbital sulcus; ME, medial nucleus; mos, medial orbital sulcus; olf, olfactory sulcus; Op Chiasm, optic chiasm; PAC, periamygdaloid nucleus; PL, paralaminar nucleus; Put, putamen; rs, rhinal sulcus.

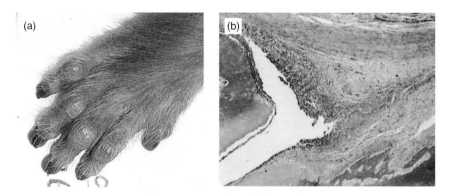

PLATE 2 Clinical manifestation and histopathology of arthritic joints. (a) Outward clinical signs of collagen-induced arthritis can be severe. (b) Histology of an affected proximal interphalangeal joint shows a hyperplastic synovium resulting in pannus formation producing factors as cytokines and matrix metalloproteinases (MMPs) mediating the destruction of the cartilage.

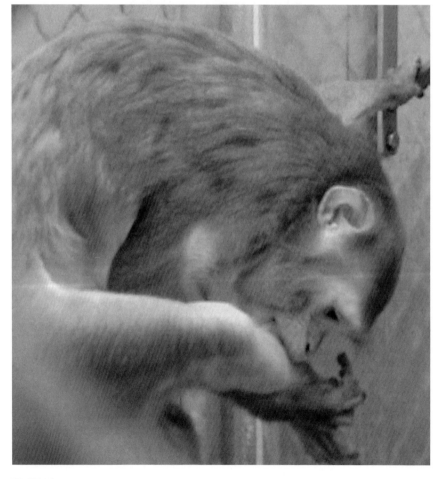

PLATE 3 An adult female rhesus macaque exhibiting self-biting behavior. Photo courtesy of Ernie Davis.

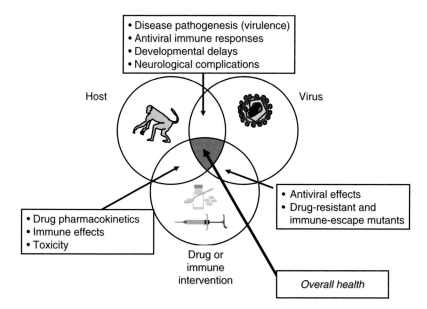

PLATE 4 Overall outcome of antiviral interventions. The ultimate goal of antiviral interventions is to improve the overall health of the host and indefinitely delay disease progression. This outcome is determined by many interactions between the virus, the host, and the intervention strategy, most of which cannot be predicted sufficiently by *in vitro* studies. Potential interventions include antiviral drugs (which target a specific step in the viral cycle), as well as immune-based strategies, such as vaccines and immunomodulators (e.g. cytokines, immune-stimulators and -suppressants). Animal models allow us to control and manipulate many of these variables through experimental approaches that are not feasible in humans, but that allow us to gain further insights into these mechanisms. Examples of such approaches are experimental inoculation of animals with defined virus isolates, *in vivo* depletion of certain immune cells, or administration of monotherapy.

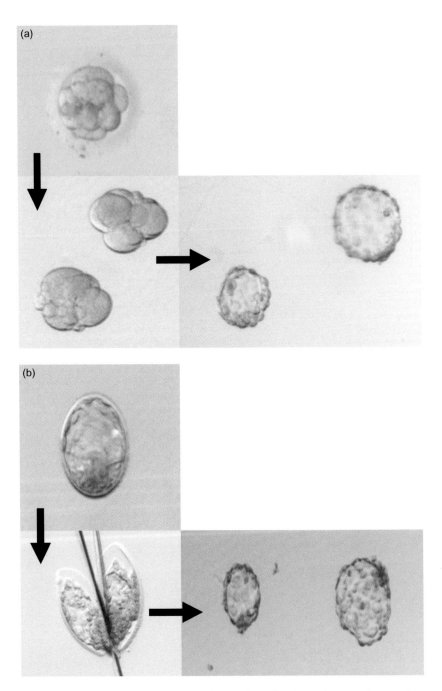

PLATE 5 Two common methods for producing identical twin nonhuman primate embryos. (a) Embryo disaggregation and re-aggregation involves the separation of a single embryo into individual blastomeres, re-aggregation of individual blastomeres into twin pairs and culture to the blastocyst stage prior to transfer. (b) Embryo splitting involves bisection of a single blastocyst stage embryo through the middle of the inner cell mass to produce twin pairs that are allowed to re-expand in culture prior to transfer.

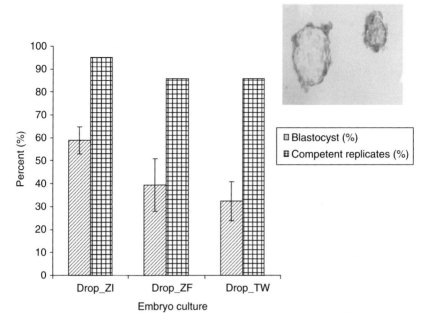

PLATE 6   The effects of micro-drop culture (drop) of twin embryos on blastocyst development rates (% of cleaved embryos; diagonal stripe) of zona-intact (ZI), zona-free (ZF), and twin (TW) embryos produced by *in vitro* fertilization. Data are expressed as mean ± SEM for 57–399 embryos from 7–21 replicates. The proportion of blastocyst competent replicates is expressed as a percentage (cross-hatch). Inset shows the discordant development of identical twin embryo pairs using these techniques.

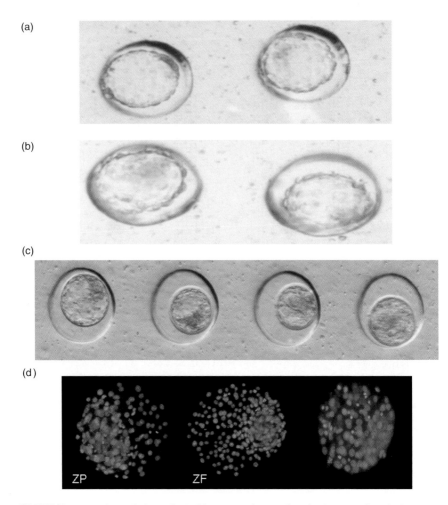

(a)

(b)

(c)

(d)

ZP   ZF

PLATE 7 Size and morphology of twin blastocyst embryos cultured using a novel synthetic micro-well device in the absence (a) or presence (b) of mitogen, and (c) zona-intact control embryos cultured in the absence of mitogen. Although the image sizes are different the micro-well dimensions are the same in each image (200 μm). Cellular development of zona-intact (ZP), zona-free (ZF), and twin (TW) embryos produced using the novel embryo production platform is indicated in (d). Arrows indicate inner cell mass cells as determined by differential staining with Hoescht and propidium iodide.

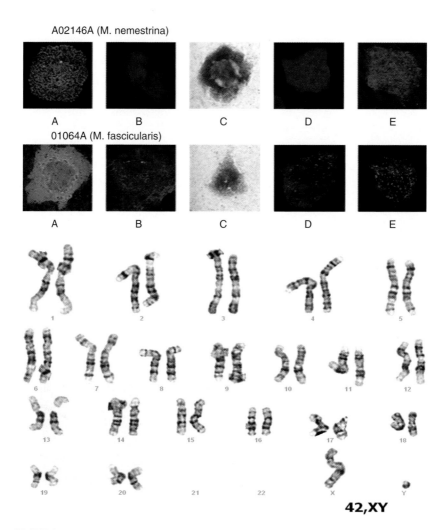

PLATE 8 Expression of pluripotent markers OCT-4 (A), SSEA-4 (B), alkaline phosphatase (AP) (C), TRA-1–81 (D) and TRA-1–60 (E) in *M. nemestrina* animal A02146A and *M. fascicularis* animal 01064A embryonic stem cells lines. Cells were fixed and exposed to primary antibodies directed against the cellular markers of pluripotency and resolved using FITC-conjugated secondary antibodies selective for the primary antibody sequence. Negative controls were exposed to conjugated secondary antibody in the absence of primary antibody (data not shown), positive controls were exposed to nonselective primary antibodies in the presence of FITC-conjugated secondary antibody (data not shown). SSEA-1 was negative for both *M. fascicularis* and *M. nemestrina* embryonic stem cell lines (data not shown). Images were taken at 10× magnification under light and UV microscopy and captured on a digital camera. The karyogram image represents the normal 42,XY karyotype for the 01064A line.

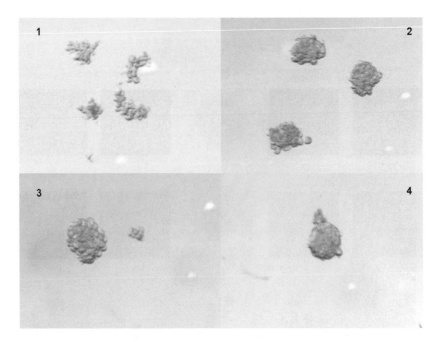

PLATE 9   Embryonic stem cell aggregation with whole embryos to produce chimeric embryos. First embryonic stem cells are labeled with a fluorescent dye that specifically stains mitochondria (1). Compacting morula stage embryos are prepared (2). The embryonic stem cells and embryos are aggregated in the presence of cellular adhesion molecules designed to improve cellular aggregation and prevent cellular apoptosis (3) to produce the chimeric embryo (4).

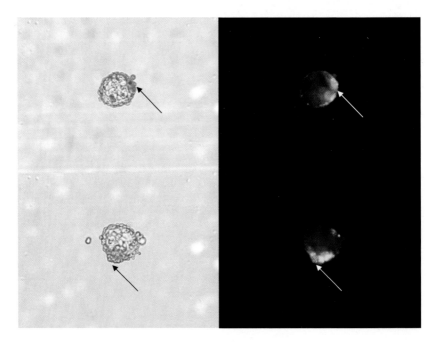

PLATE 10   The ability of labeled embryonic stem cells (orange) to integrate with developing embryos (not labeled) and to allocate in what appears to be the inner cell mass (arrows). Images on the left are light microscope images, images on the right are fluorescent images of the same embryos obtained using filters selective for the mitochondrial dye.

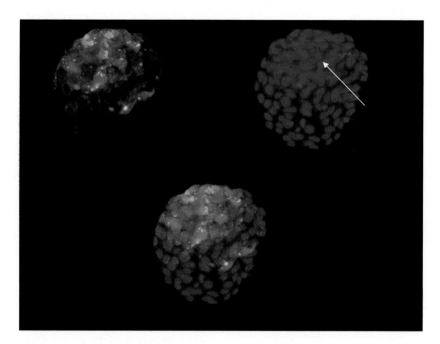

PLATE 11 Confocal microscopy detail of the integration of labeled embryonic stem cells (orange, top left) within the inner cell mass (arrow, top right) of chimeric embryos. The merged image (bottom center) clearly shows the robust overlap of labeled cells within the inner cell mass.

CHAPTER 14

Exposure to Environmental Chemicals and Developmental Risk: Contributions from Studies with Monkeys

Kimberly S. Grant and Deborah C. Rice

INTRODUCTION

For children living in industrialized nations, the world has changed dramatically in the last century. Infant mortality has significantly decreased and the average lifespan of infants born in the United States has increased by two decades since 1900 (Landrigan *et al.*, 2004). The danger that infectious diseases (e.g. smallpox, polio, measles, diphtheria, and cholera) pose to children has been drastically reduced through the development of childhood vaccinations and increased safety of the food and water supply. In certain areas of the world, acquired immune deificiency syndrome (AIDS) and tuberculosis continue to represent a significant risk of infectious disease for children but overall rates of childhood mortality have declined. As the threats of classic pediatric disease have diminished, a subtler threat to children's health has emerged. Over 30 years ago, Haggerty and Rothman (1975) coined the term "new pediatric morbidity" to represent the chronic childhood diseases that pose the greatest risk to children living today. These disorders, which include autism spectrum disorder (ASD), attention deficit hyperactivity disorder (ADHD), learning disabilities, and asthma, have complex etiologies and are frequently associated with injuries to the developing nervous system, impacting school achievement, adaptive behavior, and social competence (Goldman *et al.*, 2004; Pallapies, 2006).

National census data reveal that in the United States, developmental disabilities affect approximately 17% of children aged 18 years old or younger (Bhasin *et al.*, 2006). The most common neurodevelopmental disorders in school-age children

Primate Models of Children's Health and Developmental Disabilities

receiving special education services from public schools are learning disabilities, speech or language impairments, mental retardation and emotional disturbance (U.S. Department of Education, 2005). Whereas the rates of some developmental disabilities are stable or even decreasing, there is accumulating evidence that the prevalence of ASD and ADHD is increasing. In 2007, the Centers for Disease Control and Prevention reported that 1 in every 150 8-year-old children studied had an ASD (Rice, 2007). The reasons behind this increase are not clear, although changes in diagnostic criteria and increasing awareness and recognition of ASD have been very helpful in the identification of these children.

The prevalence of ADHD shows a similar trend. ADHD is the most common neurobehavioral disorder in American schoolchildren. In 2003, approximately 8 in 100 (7.8%) children aged 4–17 years of age were reported to have a history of ADHD diagnosis (MMWR, 2005). This total represents a staggering 4.4 million children and illustrates the widespread nature of this disorder.

DEFINING ENVIRONMENTAL HEALTH RISKS IN CHILDREN

As the rates of certain chronic childhood disabilities increase, there is a growing awareness that exposure to toxic environmental chemicals may be contributing to the increased number of affected children (Goldman *et al.*, 2004). Since World War II, over 70 000 new synthetic chemicals have been developed, and between 2000 and 3000 new chemicals are presented to the Environmental Protection Agency for review each year. Only 7% of these are tested for effects on offspring development (Goldman and Koduru, 2000) (Figure 14.1).

Pregnant women and children are exposed to a vast array of synthetic chemicals in air, water, soil, and food. Effects on exposed children have been documented with a range of environmental pollutants including lead, methylmercury, arsenic, solvents, pesticides, and polychlorinated biphenyls (PCBs) (Grandjean and Landrigan, 2006). The authors posit the existence of a "silent pandemic" associated with early chemical exposure and brain development, emphasizing the vulnerability of the developing nervous system to injury from low-level exposure and the subclinical nature of effects. The level of functional disruption associated with exogenous chemical exposure depends on multiple factors that include timing, route of exposure, and dose (Tilson, 2000). In some cases, prenatal exposure can impair function in the offspring while leaving the mother apparently healthy and without evidence of clinical neurotoxicity.

The study of environmental exposures and child development is now collectively referred to as children's environmental health or environmental pediatrics (Goldman, *et al.*, 2004). Landrigan and colleagues (2002a) estimated the contribution of environmental pollutants to the incidence, prevalence, mortality and costs of four childhood diseases/disabilities: lead poisoning, asthma, childhood cancer, and neurobehavioral disabilities. Using complex statistical modeling techniques,

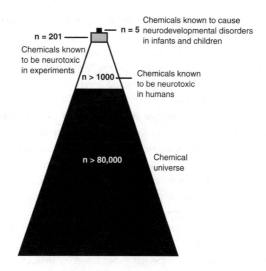

FIGURE 14.1   Only a small number of thousands of known chemicals have been evaluated for effects on the fetus, infant, and child. It is likely that many more will prove to be deleterious to human development. Adapted with permission from P. Grandjean and P. Landrigan (2006), Developmental neurotoxicity of industrial chemicals, *Lancet* **368**, 2167–2178.

the authors conclude that the combined cost of these diseases is US$54.9 billion per year (in 1997 dollars) (2.8% of the total annual cost of illness in the United States), a sum that does not begin to consider the costs of emotional suffering in families with affected children.

The differences between children and adults in response to toxic insult are many and rest in the unique features of development and how children live and play (Faustman *et al.*, 2000).

- **Children often receive higher doses of environmental chemicals** – Based on body weight, children breathe more rapidly and eat and drink more than adults. They also play close to the ground, are often outdoors and engage in frequent hand-to mouth activity (e.g. fingers and toys in the mouth).
- **Breastfeeding may prolong exposure** – Breastfeeding represents an important potential route of early chemical exposure. Breastmilk is an efficient medium for transferring lipid-soluble chemicals from the mother to her infant and contamination of breastmilk is widespread. Residues of PCBs, DDT and metabolites, dioxins, dibenzofurans, polybrominated diphenyl ethers, organochlorine pesticides such as DDT and heavy metals have all been found in breastmilk (Landrigan *et al.*, 2002b).

- **Immaturities of metabolism influence level and duration of exposure** – Infants are not able to eliminate some chemicals from their bodies as efficiently as adults, and thereby may be exposed for longer periods of time (Ginsberg *et al.*, 2004). Impaired ability to metabolize chemicals may also result in higher tissue levels, increasing the likelihood of chemically induced damage.
- **Developing systems are more susceptible to chemically induced injury** – Children may be more susceptible to chemically induced impairment as a result of interference with developmental processes that are ongoing in the developing organism but not in the adult. Development of the central nervous system is characterized by a unique series of stages in which neurons proliferate, migrate to cortical regions, differentiate to mature adult form, form synaptic connections with other neurons, and benefit from support cells and neuronal insulation. Apoptosis, or programmed cell death, is also an important part of normal brain development. These developmental processes may be exquisitely sensitive to disruption (Rice and Barone, 2000).
- **Effects may not be clinically expressed for years and even decades** – There can be long latency periods between exposure and the clinical expression of neurotoxicity (Weiss, 2000). Whereas this principle is commonly recognized in clinical oncology, it is relatively new to neurotoxicology (Reuhl, 1991). Subtle injuries to the central nervous system that alter nervous system development may be expressed much later in the lifespan, perhaps impacting disease onset and behavioral competence during aging. For example, epidemiological and experimental data suggest that methylmercury may accelerate the normal functional declines associated with aging, even though exposure ended years and even decades before (Kinjo *et al.*, 1993; Rice, 1996).

MONKEYS AS MODELS FOR CHILDHOOD CHEMICAL EXPOSURES

Whereas human epidemiology research is important for establishing relationships between chemical exposures and effects in children, comparative work with animals provides a critical link in modeling the developmental consequences of exposure. In humans, it is difficult to make judgments about the relative contribution of any one factor to developmental outcome. Moderating variables such as maternal education, maternal health status, prenatal drug use, socioeconomic status, and levels of environmental enrichment influence the course of childhood development (Sameroff, 1998). Statistical techniques can be applied to human studies to control for the confounding influences of known risk factors but may not control for all relevant variables. Identifying specific causative agents responsible for neurodevelopmental effects is further complicated by the sheer number of exogenous chemicals children are exposed to in daily life (Guillette, 2000). One important advantage of comparative research in the laboratory is the ability to precisely control the exposure history and the rearing environment of the animals, minimizing the impact of many factors that complicate research with human subjects.

Selection of the appropriate animal model for studies of environmental chemicals is generally based on factors such as conditions of exposure (level of contamination, route of exposure, severity of effects), public health significance (extent of exposure in human populations), and economic constraints. Rodents are certainly the animal model of choice for most experiments of this nature but, when special public health considerations exist, various monkey species offer the highest degree of predictability to the human response (Schardein et al., 1985). The brains of monkeys mirror the convoluted morphology of the human brain, in contrast to the lisencephalic (smooth) cortex of rodents. In some cases, the way in which monkeys metabolize xenobiotics is more similar to that in humans than it is in rodents (Tephly, 1991). Vision is the dominant sensory modality for both humans and monkeys and striking similarities exist in key aspects of vision (e.g. De Valois et al., 1974). Monkeys are capable of advanced behaviors that share strong parallels with humans. These parallels include highly developed cognitive skills and binding social relationships. The highly evolved behavioral repertoire of these animals makes them valuable models for research on environmental contaminants and development (Burbacher and Grant, 2000).

The use of the monkey model has provided key insights on the impact that chemical agents can have on the growth and development of species closely related to humans (Hendrickx and Binkerd, 1990; Buse et al., 2003). Most studies of this nature have been conducted with macaque monkeys but baboons, squirrel monkeys, and marmosets have also made valuable contributions (Hamilton and Poswillo, 1972; Hendrickx and Peterson, 1997). This chapter will primarily focus on the relevant literature from *Macaca fascicularis* (cynomolgus, crab-eating or long-tailed macaque) and *Macaca mulatta* (rhesus macaque) monkeys.

Macaque monkeys are Old World primates and share a common evolutionary history with humans, including basic aspects of reproduction and development. Ovarian morphology and physiological control and timing of menses are close to identical in macaques and humans (Hendrickx and Cukierski, 1987). Both have lengthy pregnancies, allowing for protracted CNS development in the fetus, and control the interface between maternal and fetal blood with discoid, hemochorial placentas (King, 1993; Carter, 2007). Similarity in placental architecture is important as it defines transport between the maternal and fetal vascular systems, determining not only the exchange of nutrients and waste but fetal chemical exposure as well. In macaque monkeys and humans, much of the brain growth spurt occurs during fetal development and almost all pregnancies result in a singleton delivery. Monkeys place a great deal of investment in their offspring and spend lengthy periods of time raising their young. In macaques, sexual maturity is not reached until 2–3 years of age. In contrast, rodent dams have short gestations and give birth to litters that typically range in size from 6 to 14 pups. The brain growth spurt occurs principally during postnatal development and pups can reach sexual maturity by five weeks of age.

At birth, monkeys and humans share certain limitations and abilities, particularly during the first months of life. Early parallels in neurobehavioral development have been established for key perceptual-cognitive abilities as well as temperament and spatial vision (Gunderson and Sackett, 1984; Schneider and Suomi, 1992; Kiorpes, 1992; Ha *et al.*, 1997; Heath-Lange *et al.*, 1999). Monkey infants engage in increasingly complex social behaviors and develop strong affiliative bonds with other members of their family/peer groups. Play, exploration, aggression, and withdrawal can be studied in young primates to model social behavior in human infants and children (Worlein and Sackett, 1997). In adolescence, the neuroendocrine pathways that control the onset and timing of puberty are similar between the two species and hallmarks of reproductive maturity include ovulation and menses in females and the adolescent growth spurt in males (Watts and Gavan, 1982; Plant and Barker-Gibb, 2004). These striking interspecies similarities make the macaque monkey an excellent model for studies relevant to human development, offering the opportunity to study biology and behavior in a controlled, laboratory setting (Sackett, 1984). For scientists interested in children's environmental health, the monkey model provides an opportunity to evaluate the long-term consequences of early chemical exposures while minimizing the influence of other environmental risk factors.

Whereas monkeys may provide value to many research applications, the advanced social and cognitive intelligence of these animals mandates that the use of the model be limited and judiciously applied. Strong ethical considerations accompany the use of monkeys in biomedical research. For investigations that require the unique strengths of the monkey model, the financial burden of conducting such research is high and requires specially trained veterinarians and animal caretakers. Federal guidelines require monkeys be housed in facilities that allow for regular exercise and socialization and that all animals be provided an environmental enrichment program (e.g. frozen treats, foraging opportunities, chew toys, and puzzle balls). Given the specialized environments required to successfully breed and care for these animals, research of this type can only be conducted at a limited number of laboratories worldwide. In the United States, there are eight National Primate Research Centers devoted to the study of monkeys in a biomedical research (http://www.ncrr.nih.gov/compmed/cm_nprc.asp). Highly specialized laboratories are also found at the National Center for Toxicology Research, a branch of the Food and Drug Administration that supports many important drug exposure research programs using monkey models (http://www.fda.gov/nctr/index.html).

MEASURING THE EFFECTS OF EXOGENOUS CHEMICAL EXPOSURE

The traditional endpoint in assessing the developmental risks of a chemical or therapeutic agent has been structural malformation in exposed offspring. The prominence of this metric is partially based on the tragic case of human thalidomide poisoning (McBride, 1961). Affected infants, numbering nearly 10 000, showed deformed limbs as well as defects of the eyes, ears and internal organs. Thalidomide-affected infants provided the first clear example of a pharmaceutical product causing severe injury to the developing fetus. In the case of thalidomide teratogenesis, exposed infant monkeys showed limb malformations (phocomelia) characteristic of exposed human infants and displayed similar periods of enhanced vulnerability during organogenesis (Barrow et al., 1969). In an effort to safeguard human pregnancies, monkeys have been used to model the congenital risks associated with prenatal exposure to a number of chemical agents (Schardein et al., 1985). Monkeys have shown sensitivity, in terms of structural malformations, to teratogens such as alcohol (Astley et al., 1999), androgenic hormones (Herman et al., 2000), diethylstilbesterol (Hendrickx et al., 1979; Thompson et al., 1981), anticancer alkylating agents (McClure et al., 1979), methylmercury (Mottet et al., 1985), anticonvulsants (Hendrickx et al., 1988), and vitamin A analogs (Hummler et al., 1990).

As empirical and theoretical models of developmental risk have evolved, so has the conceptualization of what constitutes a chemically induced injury. Contemporary exposure scenarios are typically characterized by chronic, low-dose exposure and the absence of clinical neurotoxicity in both mothers and offspring. Exposure-related effects are likely to originate in the nervous system and be expressed as functional losses in behavior and sensory acuity. In the context of nervous system development, four contaminants have been examined in longitudinal studies with macaque monkeys: lead, methylmercury, polychlorinated biphenyls, and methanol. These studies were designed to investigate the behavioral and sensory consequences of chronic developmental exposure to environmental contaminants at moderate to low doses that, in most cases, mimic relevant exposure scenarios in human populations.

Lead

Lead is probably the most-studied environmental contaminant with respect to the effects of developmental exposure on neuropsychological function in children or animal models. Lead was used in paint in the United States until 1978, and peeling or flaking paint continues to be a major source of lead exposure for children. Lead was added to gasoline in the 1920s, and the body burden of lead in the general population of children (and adults) increased markedly over the next several decades.

Subsequent to lead being removed from gasoline in the 1980s, the body burden of lead in children overall has decreased substantially. Children continue to be at risk from other sources in addition to lead-containing paint in old housing, including ceramics, toys, jewelry, and other imported products containing lead. It has been known since the 1940s that lead poisoning in children may result in permanent behavioral sequelae, including poor school performance, impulsive behavior, and short attention span (Byers and Lord, 1943), observations that were later replicated by other investigators (Thurston, et al., 1955; Jenkins and Mellins 1957; Perlstein and Attala, 1966). Early in the 1970s, deficits in IQ, fine motor performance, and behavioral disorders such as distractibility and constant need for attention were observed in children who had never exhibited overt signs of toxicity (Lin-Fu, 1972; de la Burdé and Choate, 1972). In 1979 Needleman et al. reported decreased IQ and increased incidence of distractibility and inattention in middle-class children with no exposure to lead from paint, alerting the public health community to the possibility of morbidity as a result of environmental exposure to lead.

Developmental lead exposure was associated with decreased IQ in children in numerous studies (Centers for Disease Control and Prevention, 2004) (Table 14.1). Deficits in reading, math, spelling, language, and other academic skills were associated with increased childhood lead exposure (Yule et al., 1981; Fulton et al., 1987; Fergusson et al., 1988a, 1988b, 1988c; Fergusson and Horwood, 1993; Leviton et al., 1993; Canfield et al., 2003a). Effects may be relatively greater at lower blood levels ($1-10\,\mu g/dL$) than at higher levels (Canfield et al., 2003b; Lanphear et al., 2005). The current CDC level of concern is $10\,\mu g/dL$; recently it was suggested that the level should be reduced to $2\,\mu g/dL$ (Gilbert and Weiss, 2006). The experimental literature helped to characterize the behavioral domains affected by lead exposure, including studies in rodents (Rice, 2006).

The bulk of the research on the effects of developmental lead exposure in monkeys was performed at two facilities: the University of Wisconsin with *Macaca mulatta* (rhesus) monkeys, and Health Canada using *Macaca fascicularis* (cynomolgus) monkeys. The Wisconsin studies included either prenatal or postnatal exposure to one year of age, with relatively high blood lead levels during exposure. In some studies at Health Canada, monkeys were exposed over their lifetime beginning at birth. In a study designed to assess possible sensitive periods, monkeys were exposed continuously from birth, during infancy only, or beginning after infancy. This paradigm revealed an early sensitive period for some tasks but not others, suggesting that lead exposure during later childhood could produce deleterious effects. Impairment was observed in the Health Canada studies at blood lead levels as low as $11\,\mu g/dL$ (the lowest exposure group), comparable to the Centers for Disease Control level of concern of $10\,\mu g/dL$. A body burden that did not produce adverse effects was not identified in the monkey studies.

Deficits in acquisition of tasks (learning) have been demonstrated in experimental studies on a variety of tasks (see Table 14.1 for summary of neuropsychological deficits). High doses of lead produced deficits on simple visual discrimination tasks in

TABLE 14.1 Neuropsychological deficits in children and monkeys as a result of developmental lead exposure

Domain	Children		Monkeys	
Deficits on tests of intellectual function, learning	IQ	CDC, 2004	Deficits in acquisition of repeated learning; Learning set	Lilienthal et al., 1986
	Reading, math, spelling, handwriting	Fulton et al., 1987; Yule et al., 1981; Leviton et al., 1993	Concurrent discrimination	Rice, 1992a
	Impaired word recognition	Fergusson and Horwood, 1993	Discrimination reversal, spatial and nonspatial	Rice and Gilbert, 1990a, 1990b; Gilbert and Rice, 1987; Bushnell and Bowman, 1979a, 1979b; Rice and Willes, 1979
	Need for special education, increased grade retention	Bellinger et al., 1984; Lyngbye et al., 1990		
	Deficits in color naming	Canfield et al., 2003a	Concurrent RI-RI	Newland et al., 1994
Increased distractibility, short attention span	Rating scales	Needleman et al., 1979; Yule et al., 1981; Fergusson et al., 1988a, 1988b, 1988c; Thomson et al., 1989; Leviton et al., 1993	Increased attention to irrelevant cues; Nonspatial and spatial discrimination–reversal	Rice, 1985a, 1990; Rice and Gilbert, 1990a, 1987
	Increased reaction time	Needleman et al., 1979; Yule et al., 1981; Hatzakis et al., 1987; Stokes et al., 1998	Hold bar too long, reaction time task	Rice, 1988a
	Decreased number correct, vigilance task	Winneke et al., 1983, 1982, 1989; Winneke and Kraemer, 1984; Hansen et al., 1989; Chiodo et al., 2004; Hatzakis et al., 1987; Walkowiak et al., 1998	Attention to irrelevant positions: nonspatial matching to sample, nonspatial discrimination reversal	Rice, 1984, 1985a, 1990
Perseveration	Wisconsin Card Sort Test	Stiles and Bellinger, 1993; Bellinger et al., 1994; Chiodo et al., 2004	Delayed alternation	Rice and Karpinski, 1998; Rice and Gilbert, 1990b
			Concurrent discrimination	Rice, 1992a
			Nonspatial matching to sample	Rice, 1984

(Continued)

TABLE 14.1   (*Continued*)

Domain	Children		Monkeys	
Inability to inhibit inappropriate responding	DRL increased rate, decreased reinforcement	Stewart et al., 2006	DRL increased rate, decreased reinforcements	Rice, 1992c; Rice and Gilbert, 1985
	Increased errors on vigilance task	Winneke et al., 1989, 1983, 1982; Winneke and Kraemer, 1984; Hatzakis et al., 1987; Hansen et al., 1989	Increased rate, FI	Rice, 1992b, 1988b, 1985b; Rice et al., 1979
			Increased delay responses, delayed alternation	Rice and Gilbert, 1990b
Deficits in changing response strategy	WCST increased errors	Stiles and Bellinger, 1993; Chiodo et al., 2004	Concurrent RI–RI	Newland et al., 1994
	Poorer performance, CANTAB set shift	Canfield et al., 2004	Change in relevant stimulus class, discrimination reversal	Rice, 1985a; Rice and Gilbert, 1990a, 1990b; Gilbert and Rice, 1987
			Delayed alternation, increased perseverative errors	Rice and Gilbert, 1990b; Rice and Karpinski, 1988; Levin and Bowman, 1986
Impairment on tests assessing memory	CANTAB spatial memory	Canfield et al., 2004	Hamilton search task	Levin and Bowman, 1986
	Digit span	Chiodo et al., 2004	Spatial delayed alternation	Levin and Bowman, 1986; Rice and Karpinski, 1988; Rice and Gilbert, 1990b
			Match-to-sample	Rice, 1984
Impaired sensory function	Seashore Rhythm Test	Needleman et al., 1979	Increased auditory thresholds	Rice, 1997
	Word recognition in masking noise or missing frequencies	Dietrich et al., 1992	Auditory electrophysiological studies	Lilienthal et al., 1990; Lilienthal and Winneke, 1996
	Auditory comprehension	Fergusson and Horwood, 1993; Bellinger et al., 1984; Campbell et al., 2000	Ability to discriminate human speech sounds	Molfese et al., 1986
	Visual evoked potentials	Altmann et al., 1998	Visual evoked potentials	Lilienthal et al., 1990, 1988, 1994
			Decreased contrast sensitivity	Bushnell, 1977; Rice, 1998

RI, random interval; DRL, differential reinforcement of low rate; FI, fixed interval; WCST, Wisconsin Card Sort Test.

various species (Carson *et al.*, 1974; Winneke *et al.*, 1977; Zenick *et al.*, 1978). A strategy adopted early in the research on the developmental effects of lead in the monkey was the introduction of two additional requirements to the visual discrimination task: the requirement for reversal performance on an already learned discrimination task and the addition of irrelevant cues. In a discrimination reversal task, the formerly correct stimulus becomes the incorrect one, and vice versa. This task requires extinction of the previously learned response and the learning of a new (opposite) one. The introduction of irrelevant cues assesses reasoning and attentional processes, as well as providing the opportunity to change relevant stimulus dimension, further taxing cognitive abilities. In the nonspatial version of the discrimination reversal task, the relevant stimulus dimension is form or color, for example, rather than the position of stimuli. Nonspatial discrimination reversal was impaired in several cohorts of monkeys exposed to lead postnatally (Bushnell and Bowman, 1979; Rice and Willes, 1979; Rice, 1985; Rice and Gilbert, 1990a). Analysis of the kinds of errors made by treated monkeys in the Health Canada studies revealed that they were attending to irrelevant cues in systematic ways, suggesting that lead-treated monkeys were being distracted by these irrelevant cues to a greater degree than controls. Monkeys exposed only during infancy to moderate lead levels were not impaired on this task, whereas monkeys exposed to the same dose continuously from birth or beginning after infancy were impaired.

Performance on an analogous task was impaired in lead-exposed children. The Cambridge Neuropsychological Testing Automated Battery (CANTAB) was used to assess cognitive function in 5.5-year-old children in relation to average lifetime blood lead concentrations (Canfield *et al.*, 2004). This battery is a computer-based set of cognitive tests, including tests of attention, spatial and nonspatial memory, and executive function. Blood lead concentrations were associated with poorer performance on "intradimensional" and "extradimensional" shift. In this task, the original discrimination required attention to colored (filled) shapes. Following acquisition, a reversal for shape was instituted (intradimensional shift). Irrelevant stimuli (white lines) were then introduced. The stimulus class was then changed from filled shapes to white lines (extradimensional shift). This task is virtually identical to the nonspatial discrimination reversal task with irrelevant cues assessed with monkeys. Similar tasks have not been assessed in rodents, and it is unlikely that rodents could learn these tasks, at least with visual cues.

A spatial version of the discrimination reversal task may assess cognitive processes different from those of the nonspatial version. Spatial discrimination reversal performance was impaired by developmental lead exposure in a number of cohorts (Bushnell and Bowman, 1979; Gilbert and Rice, 1987; Rice, 1990). As in the nonspatial discrimination reversal task, there was evidence that lead-exposed monkeys were attending to the irrelevant stimuli in systematic ways. Unlike the results of the nonspatial version of the task, there was no evidence of a sensitive period for impairment, suggesting that different behavioral mechanisms and brain areas may subserve the two tasks.

Deficits on other cognitive tasks that require the monkey to take advantage of previous experience on cognitive tasks (learning to learn) have also been reported, including learning-set formation (Lilienthal *et al.*, 1986), consecutive form discrimination (Hopper *et al.*, 1986), and concurrent discrimination (Rice, 1992a).

The ability to change response strategy in response to changes in environmental contingencies was assessed in squirrel monkeys exposed in utero using a concurrent random interval/random interval schedule, in which two random interval (RI) schedules operated separately on two levers (Newland *et al.*, 1994). (On an RI schedule, reinforcements are available at unpredictable times, but with some average time such as 15 seconds.) Reinforcement densities were varied across the experiment in such a way that the left or right lever was programed to produce a greater reinforcement density. Under steady state conditions, offspring of mothers with higher blood lead levels were insensitive to the relative "payoff" on the two levers, and exhibited lever bias (responding on a favorite lever irrespective of schedule contingencies). When the relative reinforcement densities on the levers changed, control monkeys gradually switched their responding pattern to the appropriate ratio (e.g. 70% right, 30% left). In contrast, performance of the lead-exposed monkeys changed slowly, not at all, or in the wrong direction. Monkeys whose mothers had lower blood lead concentrations learned to apportion their responses appropriately, but they learned at a slower rate than controls. These results are consistent with results on other tasks, described above, in which lead-treated animals persisted (perseverated) in non-adaptive response patterns, seemingly unresponsive to changing environmental contingencies or the consequences of their own behavior.

Lead also produced impairment on tasks designed to assess memory, but whether the deficits are the result of impairment in memory or deficits in other behavioral domains is unclear (Rice, 2006). In the Hamilton Search Task, which is designed to assess spatial memory, a row of boxes is baited with food and then closed. The monkey lifts the lids to obtain the food. The most efficient performance requires that each box be opened only once, necessitating that the monkey remember which boxes have already been opened. Deficits on this task were observed in monkeys with relatively high blood lead levels (Levin and Bowman, 1986); however, error pattern was not analyzed, so that response strategy could not be determined. Another task designed to assess spatial memory is the delayed spatial alternation task. This task requires alternation of responses between two positions; there are no cues signaling which position is correct on any trial. Delays may be introduced between opportunities to respond to assess spatial memory. Performance on this task was impaired in several cohorts of monkeys (Levin and Bowman, 1986; Rice and Karpinski, 1988; Rice and Gilbert, 1990b). Results from the various studies revealed deficits in acquisition of the task with no delays, poorer performance at shorter compared to longer delays, and/or marked perseveration for position. The types of deficits observed on this task are indicative of associative and other cognitive impairments rather than memory deficits per se.

A delayed matching to sample task was used to assess both spatial and nonspatial memory (Rice, 1984). In the nonspatial version of the task, one of three colors appeared on a sample button on which the monkey responded a specified number of times, which turned off the stimulus and initiated a delay. After a delay period, one of the three colors appeared on each of the three test buttons, and the monkey was required to respond on the button corresponding to the sample color. For the spatial version, one of the three test buttons was lit with the same color; response on that button a specified number of times turned it off and instituted a delay. Following the delay, all three buttons were lit, and the monkey was required to respond on the sample position. Lead-exposed monkeys were not impaired in their ability to learn the matching tasks but were impaired at longer delay values on both the spatial and nonspatial versions of this task. Investigation of the error pattern revealed perseveration for position on the nonspatial version of the task, which may have been responsible for the observed deficit. This was not true for the spatial version of the task, however, suggesting a pure deficit in spatial short-term memory. Rodents have not been assessed on this task, and it is unlikely that they could learn the nonspatial version.

Little attention has been paid to the effects of lead on memory in epidemiological studies. There was little evidence of effect on several tasks, although blood lead levels were marginally associated with poorer performance on the digit span subtest of a version of the Wechsler Intelligence Scale for Children (WISC) (Stiles and Bellinger, 1993; Chiodo et al., 2004). However, performance on digit span reflects attentional and/or higher order sensory processes at least as much as it does memory. Deficits as a function of lead exposure in children were observed on two tests of spatial memory on the CANTAB battery (Canfield et al., 2004). One test was logically equivalent to the Hamilton Search Task, described above, in which impairment was observed in lead-exposed monkeys.

Nonadaptive behavior in children has repeatedly been interpreted as deficits in attention. Increased lead body burden was associated with increased inattentiveness, distractibility, impulsivity, and lack of persistence on teachers' and parents' rating scales (Needleman et al., 1979; Yule et al., 1981; Fergusson et al., 1988a, 1988b, 1988c; Tuthill, 1996; Chiodo et al., 2004). Impairment on the learning and memory studies in monkeys described above may result at least in part from deficits in attentional processes. The increased systematic response to irrelevant cues on discrimination tasks in some studies may reflect attentional deficits. The deficits in ability to change response strategy in response to new schedule contingencies may also be considered to represent an attention deficit. The Wisconsin Card Sort Test (WCST) has been used in lead-exposed children. This is logically equivalent to the discrimination reversal task with irrelevant cues used in monkeys in that it requires the ability to extract general rules and change response strategy. Errors on the WCST are considered to test ability to shift attention. Increased total and/or perseverative errors related to lead body burden were observed in several studies in children (Stiles and Bellinger, 1993; Bellinger et al., 1994; Chiodo et al., 2004).

Longer latencies to respond to presentation of stimuli are also considered indicative of attentional deficits. Increased reaction times were related to lead exposure on a simple reaction time task in children, in which the subject is asked to respond as quickly as possible to a single stimulus (Yule *et al.*, 1981; Needleman, 1987; Hatzakis *et al.*, 1987; Stokes *et al.*, 1998). In contrast, no effect on simple reaction time task was observed in monkeys (Rice, 1988a), although treated monkeys exhibited an increased incidence of holding the bar longer than the maximum 15 seconds allowed. However, the monkeys had a substantial history of performance on a number of behavioral tasks, such that the simple reaction time task may have made minimal demands on attention in such experienced monkeys. Impaired performance on various versions of a vigilance task, in which the subject is required to respond to a target stimulus and refrain from responding to others, were observed in a number of studies in children (Winneke *et al.*, 1982, 1983, 1989; Winneke and Kraemer, 1984; Hatzakis *et al.*, 1987; Hansen *et al.*, 1989; Walkowiak *et al.*, 1998; Chiodo *et al.*, 2004). This task has not been used with monkeys to study the effects of lead.

Simple intermittent schedules of reinforcement may provide information on impulse control, temporal discrimination, and overall activity level. Fixed interval (FI) and differential reinforcement of low rate (DRL) schedules are acquired reasonably rapidly by animals, and performance is similar across species, including humans. Although the FI schedule requires the subject to make only one response at the end of a specified (uncued) interval, FI performance is typically characterized by an initial pause followed by a gradually accelerating rate of response terminating in reinforcement. Moderate doses of lead produced increased response rate on the FI schedule in monkeys (Rice *et al.*, 1979; Rice, 1988b, 1992b, 1992c). There is some evidence that elevated blood lead concentrations in children are associated with an increased incidence of ADHD (Braun *et al.*, 2006). Children with ADHD exhibited increased response rates on the FI, as well as a "bursting" pattern of response produced by a run of closely spaced responses separated by a short pause (Sagvolden *et al.*, 1998). This pattern was also observed in monkeys exposed to lead from birth (Rice *et al.*, 1979). FI performance predicted poorer performance on a test of impulsivity in normal children (Darcheville *et al.*, 1992, 1993): children with high response rates and shorter post-reinforcement pause times chose a smaller immediate reinforcer rather than a larger but delayed reinforcer. This was interpreted as evidence of impulsive behavior in the children with ADHD. In contrast to the FI schedule, the DRL schedule requires a specified time between responses for reinforcement; responding before the specified time resets the contingency. Therefore the DRL schedule punishes failure of response inhibition. Monkeys with moderate blood lead levels exhibited a higher number of nonreinforced responses, a lower number of reinforced responses, and a shorter average time between responses (Rice, 1992b), whereas monkeys with low blood levels learned the task at a slower rate than controls (Rice and Gilbert, 1985). Postnatal blood lead concentrations were associated with failure to inhibit responding on a DRL schedule in 9-year-old children (Stewart *et al.*, 2006). Therefore DRL performance in monkeys predicted the deficit observed on the same schedule in children.

It is clear that lead exposure may result in impairment in visual and auditory function. An inability to perceive or process sensory information would obviously interfere with performance on any particular test. More importantly, however, deficits in higher order sensory processing would make it difficult for the child to learn and respond appropriately to the environment. In fact, it is difficult to define the point at which deficits in sensory processing may be defined as "cognitive" deficits. Monkeys provide a good model for testing effects of toxicant exposure on visual or auditory function. The visual system of macaque monkeys and humans, including spatial and color vision, is virtually identical, whereas rodents have poor spatial vision and almost no color vision. Monkeys can hear about an octave higher than humans; however, auditory thresholds within the range of human detection are the same in Old World monkeys and humans.

Monkeys exposed to lead from birth exhibited impaired detection of pure tones at 13 years of age (Rice, 1997a). A number of electrophysiological studies demonstrated impairment at various parts of the auditory pathway in monkeys and other animals related to lead exposure (Yamamura *et al.*, 1989; Lilienthal *et al.*, 1990, 1988; Otto and Fox, 1993; Lasky *et al.*, 1995; Lilienthal and Winneke, 1996), although electrophysiological changes have not been universally observed (Lasky *et al.*, 2001). Elevated auditory thresholds were observed as a function of increasing blood lead concentrations in children (Schwartz and Otto, 1987; Osman *et al.*, 1999).

Pure-tone thresholds provide only basic, first-level information concerning auditory function. An individual may have normal pure-tone detection and still have difficulty distinguishing speech, for example. Speech is comprised of generally small but rapid changes in frequency and amplitude. A test used clinically to evaluate auditory (language) processing is the determination of the infant's ability to distinguish ba and da, and at a later age bi and di. Monkeys can also discriminate human speech sounds. In a study with rhesus monkeys, there was evidence that developmental lead exposure impaired the ability of young monkeys to discriminate speech sounds (da and pa) based on an electrophysiological procedure (Molfese *et al.*, 1986). Lead-exposed children are impaired on the Seashore Rhythm Test (Needleman *et al.*, 1979; Chiodo *et al.*, 2004), which requires the subject to discriminate whether pairs of tone sequences are the same or different. This is a simplified discrimination compared with analysis of speech sounds. Lead-exposed children also had a decreased ability to identify words when frequencies were filtered out (i.e. when information was missing) (Dietrich *et al.*, 1992). Increased lead body burdens were associated with impaired language processing on difficult but not easy tasks (Campbell *et al.*, 2000), impairment of the development of word recognition (Fergusson and Horwood, 1993), and impaired auditory comprehension (Bellinger *et al.*, 1984). The degree to which the deficits in language development are the result of deficits in higher order auditory processing is unknown.

Lead also produces deficits in visual function. In a study in infant rhesus monkeys with very high lead levels, one infant appeared to develop temporary blindness

(Allen *et al.*, 1974). Rhesus monkeys with high blood lead levels during infancy had impaired scotopic (very low luminance) spatial contrast sensitivity (Bushnell *et al.*, 1977). Both spatial and temporal (motion) contrast sensitivity were examined in cynomolgus monkeys with lifetime exposure to lead (Rice, 1998a). Lead-exposed monkeys exhibited deficits in temporal vision at low and middle frequencies under low luminance conditions, and had decreased dendritic arborization in primary and secondary visual cortex (Reuhl *et al.*, 1989). Lead-induced changes in electrophysiologic responses were observed in rhesus monkeys exposed developmentally to lead, particularly under low-luminance conditions (Lilienthal *et al.*, 1990, 1988, 1994). Altmann *et al.* (1998) reported changes in visual evoked potentials in a cohort of over 3800 4-year-old children, but no differences in visual acuity or spatial contrast sensitivity functions.

Methylmercury

Methylmercury (MeHg) is an environmental pollutant present in many of the world's oceans and waterways. Consumption of predatory fish and marine mammals with high levels of MeHg is the principal means of exposure for both humans and wildlife (National Research Council, 2000). In the last century, episodes of high-dose human exposure occurred in Japan and Iraq (Tokuomi *et al.*, 1961; Bakir *et al.*, 1973). These catastrophic poisonings provided evidence that the fetus is at greatest risk for both functional and structural damage from developmental MeHg exposure. Autopsy data from MeHg-exposed children demonstrated that developmental exposure results in widespread damage to the brain, primarily through hypoplasia and cell loss, and functional effects in highly exposed infants included cerebral palsy-like symptoms, mental retardation, primitive reflexes, dysarthria, and hyperkinesias (Harada, 1978; Kondo, 2000). Significant losses in visual and auditory functioning, including blindness and deafness, have been documented in exposed infants, and sensory disturbances are characteristic of both fetal and adult neurotoxicity (Amin-Zaki *et al.*, 1974, 1981; Harada, 1995). Human epidemiology studies have shown functional losses in the domains of language, attention, memory, visuospatial reasoning, and motor function in infants and children chronically exposed to low levels of this neurotoxicant (Kjellstrom *et al.*, 1986, 1989; Grandjean *et al.*, 1997; Cordier *et al.*, 2002; Debes *et al.*, 2006; Counter *et al.*, 2006). Although the preponderance of data suggest neurocognitive effects are associated with MeHg exposure (National Research Council, 2000), some studies have not found a relationship between developmental exposure and alterations in neurobehavioral outcome (Murata *et al.*, 1999a; Davidson *et al.*, 2006).

The decision to utilize the monkey as a model of developmental MeHg exposure was based on multiple factors such as similarities in brain morphology and toxicokinetics. Certain neuropathological effects of MeHg such as disorganized lamination and ectopic cells have been observed in humans and monkeys but are generally not reported with rodents (Burbacher *et al.*, 1990a). Sensory effects, especially visual, auditory, and somatosensory deficits, are the hallmark of MeHg neurotoxicity in exposed human populations. Sensory processing in macaque monkeys is similar to humans and can be evaluated using procedures that approach human clinical test methods. Important advantages also exist for monkeys in modeling the distribution of MeHg in human tissue (Magos, 1987); current estimates of the blood–brain ratio of mercury in primates (2–5) are much closer to that in humans (6) than in rats (0.06) or mice (1.20) (Rice, 1989, Mottet *et al.*, 1997).

To better understand the relationship between developmental consequences of MeHg exposure, two prospective, longitudinal studies with monkeys were initiated. The Canadian Health Protection Branch Health (Health Canada) in Ottawa initiated the first monkey study of developmental MeHg exposure (Rice, 1989). One cohort of *Macaca fascicularis* monkeys was treated with MeHg for 7 years after birth (50 μg/kg per day) and a second group was exposed in utero to 4–4.5 years after birth with 10, 25, or 50 μg/kg per day. Exposure-related effects were found at all doses used in this study. The second study took place at the University of Washington (UW) to examine the developmental consequences of in utero MeHg exposure in *Macaca fascicularis* monkeys (Burbacher *et al.*, 1984, 1978–88). Adult female monkeys were exposed to 0, 50, 70, or 90 μg/kg per day MeHg prior to and throughout pregnancy and offspring were reared in a specialized primate nursery. Effects on growth and behavior were found at the lowest dose used in this study, 50 μg/kg/day. Results from these studies, as well as other investigations with monkeys, will be explored more fully below.

Methylmercury-related effects on neuropsychological development have been studied from the first days of postnatal life in infant monkeys (see Table 14.2 for summary of neuropsychological deficits). During the neonatal period, animals from the UW cohort were tested on a simian version of the Brazelton Neonatal Behavioral Assessment Scale (Grant *et al.*, 1982). No differences were found between control and MeHg-exposed animals on measures of early reflexes, visual responsivity, and state regulation. This finding differs from a study in two-week-old human infants in which maternal and cord blood mercury concentrations were inversely related to a neurological optimality score (Steuerwald *et al.*, 2000). To evaluate the effects of MeHg on motor function, the development of visually guided reaching was assessed in the UW cohort (Burbacher *et al.*, 1986). Significant delays in the development of reaching behavior were documented in exposed animals. All off-spring were eventually successful in reaching for and retrieving a small attractive toy; it simply took longer for the MeHg-exposed infants to accomplish the task. Delays in the early motor development of the UW monkeys are consistent with recent results from a human study in which higher mercury levels in maternal blood at delivery and infant cord blood were related to lower psychomotor scores on the Bayley Scales of Infant Development at 1 year of age (Jedrychowski *et al.*, 2006).

Early cognitive development was evaluated in the UW monkeys with test measures of object permanence and visual recognition memory. Object permanence is a

TABLE 14.2 Neuropsychological deficits in children and monkeys as a result of developmental methylmercury exposure

Domain	Children		Monkeys	
Clinical signs at high exposures	Cerebral-palsy-like syndrome, mental retardation, primitive reflexes, losses in vision and hearing	Harada, 1978, 1995; Kondo, 2000; Amin-Zaki et al., 1974, 1981	Congenital Minamata disease	Mottet, 1985; Rice, 1989
Deficits on tests of intellectual function and cognition	Decreased IQ	Kjellstrom et al., 1989	Possible disruption of temporal discrimination	Rice, 1992; Gilbert et al., 1996
			Retarded acquisition of response–reinforcer relationship	Newland et al., 1994
	Delayed mental development	Jedrychowski et al., 2005		
	Deficits in visuospatial reasoning	Grandjean et al., 1997, 1999; Cordier et al., 2002		
	Language impairment	Grandjean et al., 1997; Debes et al., 2006		
	Adverse effect on attention (slowed reaction time)	Grandjean et al., 1997; Debes et al., 2006		
Adverse effects on motor development	Delayed psychomotor development	Jedrychowski et al., 2005	Visually guided reaching	Burbacher et al., 1986
	Slowed finger tapping	Grandjean et al., 1997; Dolbec et al., 2000; Debes et al., 2006	Slowed responses on fruit retrieval task, clumsiness	Rice, 1996
	Reduction in fine motor skills and manual dexterity	Lebel et al., 1996, 1998; Grandjean et al., 1999; Dolbec et al., 2000		
	Abnormal reflexes, poor leg coordination	Despres et al., 2005		
	Increased tremor amplitude	Cordier et al., 2002		

Impaired performance on memory tasks	Deficits in visual recognition memory	Oken et al., 2005	Deficits in visual recognition memory	Gunderson et al., 1986, 1988
	Reduced scores on Digit Span (auditory) and California Verbal Learning (auditory)	Grandjean et al., 1997	Deficits in spatial memory	Burbacher et al., 1986
	Deficits in recall	Grandjean et al., 1999		
Impaired sensory function	Impaired spatial vision	Lebel et al., 1996; Lebel et al., 1998	Impaired spatial vision	Rice and Gilbert, 1982, 1990; Burbacher et al., 2005
	Decreased color vision capacity	Lebel et al., 1996	Elevated auditory thresholds	Rice and Gilbert, 1992
	Alterations in visual evoked potentials	Altmann et al., 1998; Saint-Amour et al., 2006; Murata et al., 1999a	Reduced vibration sensitivity	Rice and Gilbert, 1995
	Alterations in auditory evoked potentials	Murata et al., 1999a, 1999b, 2004; Counter et al., 1998; Counter, 2003		

milestone in human cognitive development and based on the infant's knowledge that objects continue to exist when they are removed from sight. Mastery of this concept requires spatial memory as well as competent reasoning about objects. To measure object permanence, subjects were given a series of trials in which they were challenged to look for and retrieve objects (small, brightly colored toys dipped in apple sauce) that were partially or fully hidden from view (Burbacher et al., 1986). MeHg-exposed infants exhibited a significant delay in the attainment of object permanence, showing over a one-month delay in acquisition of this developmental milestone. Visual recognition memory was tested using problems adapted from the original version of the Fagan Test of Infant Intelligence (copyright 1981 by J. F. Fagan III). Using the paired-comparison paradigm, this test makes use of the infant's propensity to explore novel over familiar stimuli and scores are considered a measure of emerging information processing skills (Fagan, 1990). Reduced scores on this test have been linked to high-risk conditions such as prematurity and teratogen exposure in both monkey and human infants and may be related to later intellectual status (e.g. Jacobson et al., 1985; Gunderson et al., 1989; Rose, et al., 2005). MeHg-exposed animals from the UW cohort displayed lower novelty preference scores than controls, suggesting that in utero exposure to MeHg was associated with significant deficits in visual recognition memory (Gunderson et al., 1986, 1988).

This finding has recently been replicated in MeHg-exposed human infants (Oken et al., 2005). Results from a prospective pregnancy and child health study found that while higher maternal fish consumption was associated with better memory scores on a test of visual recognition memory, higher maternal blood mercury levels were related to lower memory scores (reduced novelty preferences). In this case, deficits in visual recognition memory were first identified in MeHg-exposed monkeys and confirmed 20 years later in a human epidemiological study.

Social behavior is an important aspect of development in young monkeys and forms the basis for later reproductive success and placement within the social hierarchy. In the UW cohort, prenatal exposure to MeHg altered the expression of social behavior in infant monkeys such that exposed infants spent more time being passive and nonsocial and less time engaged in play behaviors (Burbacher et al., 1990b). Early differences such as these may translate into enduring social deficits that impair the individual's ability to interact effectively across the lifespan. In humans, the impairment of social competence may have significant effects on academic success, employment, mental health, and life satisfaction. To date, social behavior has not been evaluated in MeHg-exposed children.

Physical growth is frequently interpreted as an overall barometer of health and well-being and is an important marker of developmental neurotoxicity. Although offspring size at birth was not affected in the UW infants (Burbacher et al., 1987–88) and no growth differences were detected during infancy, a significant delay in the male growth spurt was observed in subjects during adolescence (Grant-Webster et al., 1992). Whether this signals a MeHg-related disruption of neuroendocrine development is unknown. Significant alterations in physical growth were noted in highly exposed Japanese children (Harada, 1995) but have not been reported in chronic, low-dose human epidemiology studies.

Monkeys from both longitudinal studies performed competently on tests of learning, demonstrating associative learning skills, cognitive flexibility, and focused attention. Monkeys from the Health Canada studies were evaluated on tests of visual discrimination and discrimination reversals using automated test procedures (see test descriptions in Lead section). No evidence of impaired learning was found on these measures (Rice, 1992d). Exposed animals were able to solve these problems as quickly (in some cases more quickly) than unexposed controls. Similar results were obtained from the UW cohort when, as adults, exposed animals provided evidence of facilitated performance on a test of delayed spatial alternation (see test description in Lead section) (Gilbert *et al.*, 1993). MeHg-exposed monkeys learned the task more quickly than controls and made fewer errors during the initial phase of testing. Findings from the Health Canada and UW monkey studies do not support an association between developmental MeHg exposure and long-term changes in learning abilities.

As noted previously, intermittent schedules of reinforcement have been used in behavioral neurotoxicology studies for over five decades to study cognition in multiple animal species. Evidence from both cohorts of MeHg-exposed monkeys suggests that developmental MeHg exposure may have interfered with temporal discrimination (the ability to judge intervals of time). When Health Canada monkeys were tested on an intermittent schedule of reinforcement, the FI schedule (see test description in Lead section), MeHg-exposed infants received more reinforcements, and had shorter pauses and lower quarter-life values than control monkeys. These results suggest that developmental exposure to MeHg did not result in gross intellectual deficits but may have interfered with temporal discrimination (Rice, 1992d). The UW cohort was tested on a fixed interval/fixed ratio (FI/FR) task to explore differences in pattern and rate of responding in adulthood (Gilbert *et al.*, 1996). Monkeys exposed in utero to MeHg exhibited a sex-specific effect on the FI/FR schedule that could be interpreted as an effect on temporal discrimination. In a study with squirrel monkeys exposed to MeHg during the last half of gestation, adverse changes in learning abilities were documented in exposed offspring (Newland *et al.*, 1994). Using a test in which reinforcement contingencies changed across the test session, monkeys were free to respond to either of two test levers that were programed to deliver reinforcement at different densities (i.e. one lever provided more reinforcement or was "richer" than the other). Unlike controls, exposed monkeys were generally insensitive to differences in reinforcement densities and unable to change their behavior in accordance with shifting environmental contingencies. These studies provide evidence of changes in the learning abilities of exposed animals and suggest that some aspects of basic cognition are not spared by exposure.

Changes in motor function have been documented in infant and adult monkeys after developmental MeHg exposure. Health Canada monkeys displayed slowed responses on a simple fruit retrieval task in adulthood (Rice, 1996). This finding is consistent with the impaired performance of MeHg-exposed children and adults on the finger tapping test, a commonly used metric of motor function in human studies (Grandjean et al., 1997; Dolbec et al., 2000; Debes et al., 2006). Other psychomotor effects such as reduced fine-motor skills, abnormal reflexes, poor leg coordination and increased tremor amplitude have been documented in children living in MeHg-polluted environments (Dolbec et al., 2000; Cordier et al., 2002; Despres et al., 2005). Across species, these studies demonstrate that psychomotor performance may be particularly vulnerable to subclinical MeHg exposure and disorganized or slowed motor responses may represent important functional markers of neurotoxicity.

Strong and compelling evidence of permanent impairments in sensory functioning have been found in both the Health Canada and UW cohorts. Changes in visual function are one of the clinical hallmarks of MeHg neurotoxicity and constriction of visual fields and impaired high-frequency spatial vision have been documented in exposed adults (Mukuno et al., 1981). Results from work with adult macaque monkeys showed constriction of visual fields in MeHg exposed subjects, similar to that observed in humans (Merigan et al., 1983). Decrements in the ability to detect a flickering stimulus were also observed in adult squirrel monkeys where an increase in critical fusion intensity was the earliest sign of MeHg neurotoxicity, occurring months before other symptoms in some animals (Berlin et al., 1975).

Results from monkey studies have provided valuable information on the sensory consequences of developmental MeHg exposure. Impairment in adult spatial vision, as measured by visual contrast sensitivity, has been documented in monkeys after prenatal and/or postnatal exposure to MeHg (Rice and Gilbert, 1982, 1990c; Burbacher et al., 2005). Results from the Health Canada and UW studies provided strong evidence that losses in visual function attributed to developmental MeHg exposure were permanent and did not normalize over time. These results parallel the visual deficits commonly observed in highly exposed humans (Rustam and Hamdi, 1974; Sabeliash and Himli, 1976) and may reflect preferential damage to the parvocellular region of the visual system, known to be responsible for high-frequency spatial vision (Rice, 1996). Interestingly, the ability of developmentally exposed Health Canada monkeys to detect a flickering stimulus over a range of temporal frequencies was superior to that of control animals (Rice and Gilbert, 1990c). The authors posit that this may reflect a remodeling of the visual system wherein the magnocellular system, believed to subserve visual detection of flicker, benefits from MeHg injury to the parvocellular system in the form of expanded function.

Tests of vision, such as contrast sensitivity, are being increasingly used in research to detect the potential health effects of chemical exposure. Studies with infants and young adults have demonstrated an inverse relationship between biomarkers of MeHg exposure and functional (contrast sensitivity) and electrophysiological (visual-evoked potentials) alterations in vision, corroborating the functional losses in spatial vision observed in the Health Canada and UW monkey cohorts (Lebel et al., 1996, 1998; Altmann et al., 1998; Murata et al., 1999b; Saint-Amour et al., 2006).

Further psychophysical testing with the Health Canada monkeys revealed deficits in adult auditory and somatosensory (vibration sensitivity) functioning (Rice and

Gilbert, 1992, 1995). Hearing loss in MeHg-exposed human is a commonly reported symptom in adults and pure-tone thresholds in adult Minamata disease patients revealed impairments in half the ears evaluated (Ino and Mizukoshi, 1977). In utero exposure has been associated with severe hearing impairment, deafness and delayed speech development in humans although methodological detail of test procedures is sparse (Amin-Zaki et al., 1974, 1979). Auditory function was evaluated in the form of pure tone detection in Health Canada monkeys developmentally exposed to MeHg from birth to 7 years of age (Rice and Gilbert, 1992). Results showed that treated monkeys exhibited impaired pure-tone detection thresholds at high frequencies, modeling hearing impairments in humans. Related studies in children have generated evidence that developmental MeHg exposure is associated with abnormal auditory-evoked potentials and in some cases, changes in auditory electrophysiology appear to be permanent (Counter et al., 1998; Murata et al., 1999a, 2004; Counter, 2003). These studies provide evidence of MeHg-related changes in auditory brain processing that is consistent with subtle hearing loss such as that demonstrated in the Health Canada monkeys (Rice and Gilbert, 1992).

Like auditory function, somatosensory functioning (vibration sensitivity) is an important marker of MeHg neurotoxicity and paresthesias are a frequently reported symptom of methylmercury poisoning in adults. Despite this, few objective determinations of somatosensory function have been performed in either MeHg-exposed humans or animals. Following developmental MeHg exposure, somatosensory function was assessed in Health Canada monkeys by measuring sensitivity to vibration applied to the fingertip (Rice and Gilbert, 1995). Evidence showed that exposed animals displayed elevated sensory thresholds (reduced sensitivity) on this test, paralleling clinical finding in highly exposed humans.

Delayed or latent toxicity as a result of developmental MeHg exposure was identified over 25 years ago by Spyker, who observed kyphosis, neuromuscular deficits, and other severe abnormalities in exposed mice as they aged (Spyker et al., 1972). Since that seminal observation in mice, delayed neurotoxicity has also been reported in monkeys, rats, and humans (Rice, 1989, 1996, 1998c; Kinjo et al., 1993; Newland et al., 2004). Data from over 1000 patients with Minamata disease over 40 years old showed that difficulty in performing daily activities increased as a function of age more rapidly than observed in matched controls (Kinjo et al., 1993). Delayed neurotoxicity was observed in Health Canada monkeys treated with MeHg from birth to 7 years of age. When these monkeys reached 13 years of age, individuals began exhibiting clumsiness not previously observed, required more time to retrieve treats than nonexposed controls and displayed abnormalities on a clinical assessment of sense in the hands and feet (Rice, 1996). These results are strongly suggestive of a delayed neurotoxicity that was not clinically apparent until the exposed animals reached middle age. When Health Canada monkeys were evaluated for high-frequency hearing at 19 years of age, a comparison of results with performance at 11 years showed relatively greater deterioration in function in treated animals versus controls (Rice, 1998c). This study provides evidence for the acceleration of impairment of auditory function during aging as a latent consequence of developmental methylmercury exposure.

Polychlorinated biphenyls

Polychlorinated biphenyls (PCBs) are a family of chlorinated hydrocarbons containing 209 different congeners differing in position and degree of chlorine substitution. Their major use was as a dielectric in transformers and capacitors, although they had other industrial uses as well, and they were in widespread use from the 1930s until the 1970s. Although PCBs were banned in the United States in the 1970s and subsequently elsewhere, they are presently a worldwide pollution problem. Residues persist in air, soil, water, and sediment and can be detected in biologic tissue in most residents of industrialized countries. The chemicals are stored in fat, and many congeners are not readily excreted except in breastmilk.

In a tragic epidemic in Japan in 1968, over 1000 people became ill as a result of ingesting rice oil contaminated with PCBs and small amounts of other contaminants. Adults ingesting high levels suffered chloracne, numbness, and weakness of limbs, and decreased peripheral nerve conduction velocities (Kuratsune, 1989). The developing fetus was much more sensitive than the mother; infants born to mothers who consumed the contaminated oil had hyperpigmentation (dark pigmentation of the skin), low birth weight, early eruption of the teeth and swollen gums and eyelids (Kuratsune, 1989). They had decreased reflexes and were dull and apathetic, with IQs of about 70 (Harada, 1976). Children born after a similar incident in Taiwan exhibited delayed developmental milestones (Rogan et al., 1988), cognitive deficits on standard tests of intelligence (IQ) that did not improve over time (Chen et al., 1992; Lai et al., 1994; Guo et al., 1995). Children had overt signs including gum hypertrophy, deformed or pigmented nails, acne, hyperpigmentation, and hair loss (Rogan et al., 1988) as well as poorer health and increased behavior problems (Chen et al., 1994; Yu et al., 1994) and abnormal auditory evoked potentials (Chen and Hsu, 1994). These episodes of human poisoning prompted an exploration of potential developmental neurotoxicity produced by environmental exposure to PCBs.

As is true for lead, the preponderance of research on the effects of developmental PCB exposure in monkeys was performed at the University of Wisconsin and Health Canada. Studies at the University of Wisconsin used two commercial mixtures of PCBs, Aroclor 1248 and Aroclor 1016. (The numbers following the trade name refer to the percentage of chlorine in the mixture, with higher numbers indicating a higher percentage of chlorine.) Rhesus females were exposed to the commercial PCB mixtures in their feed during pregnancy and nursing, and offspring were exposed in utero and through breastmilk until weaning at four months of age.

The study at Health Canada examined the behavioral consequences of low-level PCB exposure during the early postnatal period (Rice, 1999). Cynomolgus infants were separated from their mothers at birth, and dosed from birth to 20 weeks of age with a congener mixture representative of the PCBs found in human breastmilk to assess the potential contribution of nursing to the observed neurotoxic effects in children. Peak blood and fat levels were comparable to those in the general human population (Rice and Hayward, 1997). Monkeys were tested as juveniles (beginning at 3 years of age) on a series of behavioral tasks.

In utero and postnatal exposure to Aroclor 1016 or 1248 produced decreased birth weight of the infants at higher doses, with no difference in head circumference or crown-to-rump length (Allen and Barsotti, 1976; Barsotti and van Miller, 1984) (see Table 14.3 for summary of neuropsychological deficits). Overt signs in the form of hyperpigmentation were present in infants exposed to Aroclor 1248, an effect observed in humans but not produced in rodents. PCB exposure produced hyperactivity during infancy (Bowman et al., 1978, 1981) and hypoactivity at 44 months of age (Bowman and Hieronimus, 1981). In humans, abnormal neurological status and poorer neuropsychological performance during infancy and early childhood were associated with in utero PCB exposure (Jacobson et al., 1984, 1985; Rogan et al., 1986a, 1986b; Gladen and Rogan, 1991; Huisman et al., 1995a, 1995b; Koopman-Esseboom et al., 1996; Stewart et al., 2000). As in monkeys, inconsistent effects on activity were also observed in human studies. The concurrent body burden of the child at 3.5 years was related to more hyperactive and problem behavior on rating scales (Patandin et al., 1999a, 1999c), whereas hypoactivity was predicted by postnatal exposure at 4.0 years in a different study (Jacobson et al., 1990a). In addition, PCB and dioxin levels independently predicted differences in sexually dimorphic play behavior at 7.5 years (Vreugdenhil et al., 2002b).

There is evidence for adverse effects on cognitive function as a result of either prenatal or postnatal exposure to PCBs in monkeys on a number of tasks. In utero exposure to either Aroclor mixture produced deficits in spatial discrimination reversal performance during infancy (Bowman et al., 1978; Schantz et al., 1989, 1991). PCB exposure produced facilitated performance on a shape reversal task following a task in which shape cues were irrelevant (Levin et al., 1988; Schantz et al., 1989, 1991). These findings were interpreted by the authors as a deficit in the treated groups' ability to learn the irrelevance of the shape cue on previous tasks; however, error patterns were not analyzed. In the Health Canada study, the PCB-exposed group was not statistically different from controls on a series of nonspatial (Rice and Hayward, 1997) or spatial (Rice, 1998b) discrimination reversal tasks, although some treated individuals made many more errors than controls over the first several reversals of the experiment. The results from both the Wisconsin and Health Canada studies indicate that PCB-treated monkeys attended to irrelevant cues more than controls, similar to the effects of lead.

Cognitive deficits related to PCB exposure were also observed in children. Deficits in IQ were identified in four longitudinal prospective studies during early childhood (3–4 years of age) (Jacobson et al., 1990b; Patandin et al., 1999b; Walkowiak et al., 2001; Stewart et al., 2003b) but not the fifth (Gladen and Rogan, 1991). Impaired information processing was related to in utero exposure at 4.0 years of age (Jacobson

TABLE 14.3   Neuropsychological deficits in children and monkeys as a result of developmental polychlorinated biphenyl exposure

Domain	Children		Monkeys	
Clinical signs at high exposures	Hyperpigmentation, abnormal dentition	Kuratsune, 1989; Rogan et al., 1988	Hyperpigmentation, abnormal dentition	Barsotti and Miller, 1984
Deficits in tests of intellectual function	Decreased IQ	Harada, 1976; Rogan et al., 1988; Lai et al., 1994; Guo et al., 1995; Chen et al., 1992; Jacobson and Jacobson, 1996; Jacobson et al., 1990b; Stewart et al., 2003b; Patandin et al., 1999c; Walkowiak et al., 2001; Vreugdenhil et al., 2002a	Delayed alternation, retarded acquisition	Schantz et al., 1991; Rice and Hayward, 1997
			Discrimination reversal, increased errors	Rice and Hayward, 1997; Schantz et al., 1989, 1991; Bowman et al., 1978
			FI, retarded acquisition	Rice, 1997b
	Decreased visual processing speed	Jacobson and Jacobson, 1993		
	Reading comprehension	Jacobson and Jacobson, 1996		
	Tower of London	Vreugdenhil et al., 2004		
	Language development	Patandin et al., 1999b; Jacobson and Jacobson, 1996; Jacobson and Jacobson, 2003b		
	Increased reaction time, mental rotation task			
Effects on activity, behavior	Hyperactivity	Patandin et al., 1999c	Hyperactivity	Bowman et al., 1978, 1989
	Hypoactivity	Jacobson et al., 1990a	Hypoactivity	Bowman and Hieronimus, 1981
	Problem behavior	Patandin et al., 1999a		
	Sexually dimorphic play behavior	Vreugdenhil et al., 2002b		
	Decreased complex play	Patandin et al., 1999c		

Impaired performance on memory tasks	Visual recognition	Jacobson et al., 1985; Darville et al., 2000	Delayed alternation (effects not due to impaired memory)	Schantz et al., 1991; Rice and Hayward, 1997
	Verbal memory	Jacobson and Jacobson, 1990b		
	Sternberg memory	Jacobson and Jacobson, 1990b		
	Memory scale, WISC-R	Jacobson and Jacobson, 1996		
Impaired response inhibition, perseveration	DRL, increased rate, decreased reinforcements	Stewart et al., 2006	DRL, increased rate, decreased reinforcements	Rice, 1998b
	Vigilance task, errors of commission	Stewart et al., 2003a, 2005; Patandin et al., 1992c	FI, increased rate	Rice, 1997b
	WCST, perseveration	Jacobson and Jacobson, 2003	Delayed alternation, perseveration	Rice and Hayward, 1997
	Sternberg Memory task, errors of commission	Jacobson and Jacobson, 2003		
Attention, distractibility	Freedom from distractibility, WISC-R	Jacobson and Jacobson, 1996	Attention to irrelevant cues, discrimination reversal	Schantz et al., 1989, 1991; Bowman et al., 1978; Rice and Hayward, 1997
	Digit cancellation	Jacobson and Jacobson, 2003		
	Increased reaction time	Vreugdenhil et al., 2004; Patandin et al., 1999c		

FI, fixed interval; DRL, differential reinforcement of low rate; WCST, Wisconsin Card Sort Test; WISC-R, revised edition of the Wechsler Intelligence Scale for Children.

and Jacobson, 1993). Early effects on IQ attenuated or disappeared at older ages in most (Vreugdenhil *et al.*, 2002a; Winneke *et al.*, 2002; Stewart *et al.*, 2003b) but not all (Jacobson and Jacobson, 2003) studies. Effects on cognition were observed in older children even in the absence of continuing effects on IQ tests. In utero exposure to PCBs was associated with poorer performance on a vigilance task at 4.5 years and again at 8.0 and 9.5 years of age (Stewart *et al.*, 2003a, 2005). Both prenatal and post-natal PCB exposure was associated with poorer performance on one task measuring executive function (Tower of London) but not other cognitive tasks at 9 years of age (Vreugdenhil *et al.*, 2004). Prenatal PCB exposure was associated with poorer reading ability as well as decreased IQ scores at 11 years of age (Jacobson and Jacobson, 1996).

Performance on intermittent schedules has been used to assess learning and response inhibition in the Health Canada monkeys and in children. Early postnatal PCB exposure resulted in an increase in overall response rate in the FI schedule (Rice, 1997b), which may be considered to represent less efficient behavior, since treated monkeys made more responses for the same amount of reinforcement. Treated monkeys also were slower to develop an increase in the initial pause at the beginning of the interval that is characteristic of acquisition of FI performance, sug-gesting a learning deficit. Performance was assessed on a DRL schedule of reinforce-ment (Rice, 1998b) chosen specifically to determine whether PCB-exposed monkeys would inhibit responding when required to do so. The PCB-treated group was markedly impaired on this task, making more nonreinforced responses and fewer reinforced responses than controls, resulting in a higher ratio of nonrein-forced/reinforced responses. This was reflected in a shorter average time between responses (inter-response time or IRT) in the PCB-exposed monkeys. These results clearly demonstrated an inability by the treated monkeys to adapt to the schedule requirement by inhibiting inappropriate (nonreinforced) responding. The robust effects on the DRL schedule in monkeys prompted the investigators one of the lon-gitudinal studies to determine the effects of prenatal PCB exposure in their cohort (Stewart *et al.*, 2006). PCB, lead, and MeHg exposure each independently predicted poorer performance: shorter IRTs and fewer reinforced responses. This effect was independent of the IQ of the child, and in fact there were no differences in IQ related to PCBs at the age of testing. Thus the experimental literature using mon-keys served as a guide to an important finding in an epidemiological study.

Cognitive domains including attention, distractibility, and response inhibition have been assessed on other tasks in some epidemiological studies. Increased reac-tion time and increased errors of commission on a vigilance task were related to the child's body burden (postnatal exposure) at 3.5 years of age (Patandin *et al.*, 1999c), which may represent a cognitive or attentional deficit, as well as failure of response inhibition. Increased reaction time related to prenatal exposure was observed on a simple reaction time task in this cohort at 9 years of age (Vreugdenhil *et al.*, 2004). A parametric analysis of the kinds of errors made on a vigilance task at 8.0 and 9.5 years revealed that impaired response inhibition rather than an attentional deficit was responsible for the observed effects (Stewart *et al.*, 2005). In utero PCB exposure was related to poorer scores on the freedom from distractibility scale on the WISC-R at 11 years (Jacobson and Jacobson, 1996).

The effects of PCB exposure on a task designed to assess memory function were determined in monkeys. As is the case for lead, results suggest deficits in functional domains other than memory. Exposure to Aroclor 1248 produced deficits on a spatial delayed alternation task during adulthood (Schantz et al., 1991); effects were present at all delay values, suggesting an associative rather than a memory deficit. Aroclor 1016 did not produce impairment on this task at the same age (Schantz et al., 1991; Levin et al., 1988). The PCB-treated group in the Health Canada study was clearly impaired on a spatial delayed alternation task, displaying retarded acquisition of the task and an increased number of errors at short delay values (Rice and Hayward, 1997), also suggesting an associative deficit. Treated monkeys engaged in more perseverative responding over the entire experiment, making repeated errors after the first error on a particular trial. Increased perseverative errors were also related to PCB exposure on the WCST in children (Jacobson and Jacobson, 2003).

Memory has been less studied than other cognitive processes in epidemiological studies. Deficits in the memory subscale of the WISC-R were observed in 11-year-old children related to in utero exposure (Jacobson and Jacobson, 1996), as well as deficits in auditory and visual memory at 4 years of age in the same cohort (Jacobson et al., 1990b). Impaired recognition memory during infancy on the Fagan test was observed in two studies (Jacobson et al., 1985; Darvill et al., 2000) but not in a less well-controlled study (Winneke et al., 1998).

Methanol

Methanol is one of the most commonly used chemicals in American industry (National Library of Medicine, Toxicology Information Program) and a recognized neurotoxicant at high levels of exposure. Within the last two decades, the utilization of methanol as an alternative motor fuel has been widely explored. One of the most important characteristics of methanol is that it is a low-emission, high-performance combustible motor fuel. Increased use of methanol as a fuel source could lead to improved air quality by reducing the hydrocarbon emissions responsible for increased atmospheric pollution and, ultimately, global warming (Gold and Moulis, 1988). If methanol-based fuels are adopted as a new energy source, the potential exists for widespread public exposure to vapors, including sensitive subgroups such as pregnant women, infants, and the elderly (Carson et al., 1987).

The hallmark signs of acute methanol toxicity in humans are well documented from cases of poisoning. In brief, the individual typically experiences a short period of intoxication, followed by a period in which no symptoms of intoxication or toxicity are noted. This asymptomatic period is followed by symptoms of poisoning such as headache, nausea, vomiting, loss of equilibrium, severe abdominal pain and difficulty in breathing. These symptoms can be followed by coma and death

(Bennett *et al.*, 1953). Methanol poisoning during human pregnancy has been rarely described. There are four published reports on clinical neurotoxicity in human infants associated with developmental exposure to methanol. In the first case, fetal exposure was associated with maternal solvent abuse (carburetor cleaning fluid) during pregnancy (Bharti, 2003). The infant was born with severe metabolic acidosis, requiring ventilatory support for the first 24 hours of life and abnormalities of muscle tonicity were noted for the first week. Neuroimaging revealed bifrontal cystic leukomalacia with some cortical atrophy. In the second recorded case of gestational methanol exposure, the exposed newborn died due to severe intraventricular bleeding on postnatal day 4 (Belson and Morgan, 2004). A case of postnatal exposure was reported in the literature when a six-week old infant was fed a mixture of formula and windshield cleaner that contained methanol. The infant was hospitalized and appeared to recover without long-term neurological damage (Brent *et al.*, 1991).

Recently, there was a cluster of infant deaths following immunization due to methanol poisoning in Egypt (Darwish *et al.*, 2002). Methanol is an effective anti-inflammatory and anti-pyretic agent and the infant deaths resulted from excessive topical amounts of methanol applied by well-intentioned medical staff.

Methanol is a frank teratogen in rodents and is associated with embryo/fetal death and gross malformations in highly exposed offspring (Rogers *et al.*, 1993; Rogers and Mole, 1997). Given the possible, even pivotal, role that methanol may play in the development of new energy sources, the decision was made to study in utero exposure to inhaled methanol in monkeys. Monkeys show key aspects of human methanol metabolism (Tephly, 1991). Humans and monkeys display similar clinical effects from high-dose methanol exposure due to their limited capability, compared with rodents, to metabolize formate to carbon dioxide (Black *et al.*, 1985). Rodents do not typically display the hallmark signs of methanol toxicity unless they are folate deficient (Makar and Tephly, 1976) whereas monkeys develop metabolic acidosis and visual disturbances that are similar to the clinical profiles of poisoned humans.

Burbacher and colleagues initiated a study to investigate the pharmacokinetics of inhaled methanol in pregnancy in *Macaca fascicularis* monkeys and to evaluate the effects of methanol exposure on female reproduction and offspring development (Burbacher *et al.*, 2004a, 2004b). Adult female *Macaca fascicularis* monkeys were exposed to 0, 200, 600, or 1800 ppm methanol vapor for 2½ hours/day, 7 days/week prior to and during pregnancy. Infants were reared in a specialized nursery and evaluated with a neurobehavioral test battery that included procedures largely adapted from studies with human infants. Methanol exposure was not associated with overt maternal toxicity, reproductive loss, offspring congenital malformations or a reduction in the size of the offspring at birth.

The results of the infancy assessments indicate significant treatment-related effects on visually guided reaching and visual recognition memory, suggesting behavioral deficits in motor and memory development (Burbacher *et al.*, 1999). Prenatal methanol exposure was associated with a delay in early sensorimotor development as measured by the infant's ability to reach for, grasp and retrieve a small object during the first month of life. This motor effect was more prominent in males than females and suggests a sex-specific effect of methanol exposure on the development of visually guided reaching. Methanol intoxication in adult humans is associated with a Parkinsonian-like syndrome that includes rigidity, tremor, and slowness of movement (Ley and Gali, 1983). Visual recognition memory testing revealed that exposed infants generally performed as well as controls on problems using abstract geometric patterns but were unable to solve more difficult test problems using complex social stimuli (monkey faces). Performance on behavioral indices of neonatal reflexes, spatial memory, learning, social behavior, and physical growth was unaffected by exposure. In adulthood, exposed animals showed significant reductions in the amplitude of electroretinograms (ERG) responses under low-light conditions. The ERG results suggest that in utero exposure to methanol is associated with subtle but permanent changes in the electrophysiology of the eye. Disturbances of vision are one of the classic signs of methanol toxicity and permanent blindness and losses in acuity are found in survivors of adult methanol poisoning (Kavet and Nauss, 1990).

Unexpectedly, prenatal methanol exposure was related to a "wasting syndrome" in two of the female offspring in the high dose group after 1 year of age. The syndrome was severe and resulted in the euthanasia of both individuals. Results of assays for simian retroviruses, blood chemistry, CBC, liver, kidney, thyroid, and pancreatic function were unremarkable and veterinarians could not determine the etiology of the condition.

Results from this study demonstrate that exposure to methanol that briefly increases blood methanol levels above background each day is associated with developmental effects in exposed offspring. Although the long-term significance of these effects is unknown, they provide evidence that there are functional consequences of developmental methanol exposure at levels that do not result in the clinical expression of neurotoxicity.

GENERAL CONCLUSIONS

As advances are made in global industrialization, the likelihood of childhood exposures to environment chemicals will increase. Data from the four environmental contaminants reviewed in this chapter demonstrate functional losses in behavior and sensory acuity at levels of exposure that are not associated with overt health effects or clinical neurotoxicity in exposed offspring. In some cases, deficits are permanent and do not appear to normalize over time. These findings underscore the complex and sometimes subtle nature of nervous system injury and provide key insights on the developmental risks associated with environmental chemical exposures.

REFERENCES

Allen, J. R. and Barsotti, D. A. (1976). The effects of transplacental and mammary movement of PCBs on infant Rhesus monkeys. *Toxicology* **6**, 331–340.

Allen, J. R., McWey, P. J., and Suomi, S. J. (1974). Pathobiological and behavioral effects of lead intoxication in the infant Rhesus monkey. *Environ Health Perspect* **7**, 239–246.

Altmann, L., Sveinsson, K., Krämer, U. *et al.* (1998). Visual functions in 6-year-old-children in relation to lead and mercury levels. *Neurotoxicol Teratol* **20**, 9–17.

Amin-Zaki, L., Elhassani, S., Majeed, M. A., Clarkson, T. W., Doherty, R. A., and Greenwood, M. R. (1974). Studies of infants postnatally exposed to methylmercury. *J Pediatr* **85**, 81–84.

Amin-Zaki, L, Majeed, M. A., Elhassani, S. B., Clarkson, T. W., Greenwood, M. R., and Doherty, R. A. (1979). Prenatal methylmercury poisoning. Clinical observations over five years. *Am J Dis Child* **133**, 172–177.

Amin-Zaki, L., Majeed, M. A., Greenwood, M. R., Elhassani, S. B., Clarkson, T. W., and Doherty, R. A. (1981). Methylmercury poisoning in the Iraqi suckling infant: A longitudinal study over five years. *J Appl Toxicol* **1**, 210–214.

Astley, S. J., Magnuson, S. I., Omnell, L. M., and Clarren, S. K. (1999). Fetal alcohol syndrome: changes in craniofacial form with age, cognition, and timing of ethanol exposure in the macaque. *Teratology* **59**, 163–172.

Bakir, F., Damluji, S.F., Amin-Zaki, L. *et al.* (1973). Methylmercury poisoning in Iraq. *Science* **181**, 230–241.

Barrow, M. V., Steffek, A. J., and King, C. T. (1969). Thalidomide syndrome in rhesus monkeys (*Macaca mulatta*). *Folia Primatol (Basel)* **10**, 195–203.

Barsotti, D. A. and van Miller, J. P. (1984). Accumulation of a commercial polychlorinated biphenyl mixture (Aroclor 1016) in adult rhesus monkeys and their nursing infants. *Toxicology* **30**, 31–44.

Belson, M. and Morgan, B. W. (2004). Methanol toxicity in a newborn. *J Toxicol Clin Toxicol* **42**, 673–677.

Bellinger, D., Needleman, H. L., Bromfield, R., and Mintz, M. (1984). A followup study of the academic attainment and classroom behavior of children with elevated dentine lead levels. *Biol Trace Elem Res* **6**, 207–204.

Bellinger, D., Hu, H., Titlebaum, L., and Needleman, H. L. (1994). Attentional correlates of dentin and bone lead levels in adolescents. *Arch Environ Health* **49**, 98–105.

Bennett Jr, I. L., Cary, F. H., Mitchell Jr, G. L., and Cooper, M. N. (1953). Acute methyl alcohol poisoning: a review based on experiences in an outbreak of 323 cases. *Medicine* **32**, 431.

Berlin, M., Grant, C. A. Hellberg, J., Hellstrom, J., and Schultz, A. (1975). Neurotoxicity of methylmercury in squirrel monkeys: cerebral cortical pathology, inference with scotopic vision and changes in operant behavior. *Arch Environ Health* **30**, 340–348.

Bharti, D. (2003). Intrauterine cerebral infarcts and bilateral frontal cortical leukomalacia following chronic maternal inhalation of carburetor cleaning fluid during pregnancy. *J Perinatol* **23**, 693–696.

Bhasin, T. K, Brocksen, S., Avchen, R. N., and Van Naarden Braun, K. (2006). Prevalence of four developmental disabilities among children aged 8 years – Metropolitan Atlanta Developmental Disabilities Surveillance Program, 1996 and 2000. *MMWR Surveill Summ* **55**, 1–9.

Black, K. A., Eells, J. T., Noker, P. E., Hawtrey, C. A., and Tephly, T. R. (1985). Role of hepatic tetrahydrofolate in the species difference in methanol toxicity. *Proc Natl Acad Sci USA* **82**, 3854–3858.

Bowman, R. E. and Hieronimus, M. P. (1981). Hypoactivity in adolescent monkeys perinatally exposed to PCBs and hyperactive as juveniles. *Neurobehav Toxicol Teratol* **3**, 14–18.

Bowman, R. E., Hieronimus, M. P., and Allen, J. R. (1978). Correlation of PCB body burden with behavioral toxicology in monkeys. *Pharmacol Biochem Behav* **9**, 49–56.

Bowman, R. E., Hieronimus, M. P., and Barsotti, D. A. (1981). Locomotor hyperactivity in PCB-exposed rhesus monkeys. *Neurotoxicology* **2**, 251–268.

Braun, J. M., Kahn, R. S., Froelich, T., Auinger, P., and Lanphear, B. P. (2006). Exposures to environmental toxicants and attention deficit hyperactivity disorder in U.S. children. *Environ Health Perspect* **114**, 1904–1909.

Brent, J., Lucas, M., Kulig, K., and Rumack, B. H. (1991) Methanol poisoning in a 6-week-old infant, *J Pediatr* **118**, 644–646.

Burbacher, T. M. and Grant, K. S. (2000). Methods for studying monkeys in neurobehavioral toxicology and teratology. *Neurotoxicol Teratol* **22**, 475–486.

Burbacher, T. M., Monnett, C., Grant, K. S., and Mottet, N. K. (1984). Methylmercury exposure and reproductive dysfunction in the monkey. *Toxicol Appl Pharmacol* **75**, 18–24.

Burbacher, T. M., Grant, K. S., and Mottet, N. K. (1986). Retarded object permanence development in methylmercury exposed *Macaca fascicularis* infants. *Dev Psychol* **22**, 771–776.

Burbacher, T. M, Mohamed, M. K., and Mottett, N. K. (1987–88). Methylmercury effects on reproduction and offspring size at birth. *Reprod Toxicol* **1**, 267–278.

Burbacher, T. M., Rodier, P. M., and Weiss, B. (1990a). Methylmercury developmental neurotoxicity: a comparison of effects in humans and animals. *Neurotoxicol Teratol* **12**, 191–202.

Burbacher, T. M, Sackett, G. P., and Mottet, N. K. (1990b). Methylmercury effects on the social behavior of *Macaca fascicularis* infants. *Neurotoxicol Teratol* **12**, 65–71.

Burbacher, T., Grant, K. S., Shen, D., Damian, D., Ellis, S., and Liberato, N. (1999). Reproductive and offspring developmental effects following maternal inhalation exposure to methanol in nonhuman primates. Part II: Developmental effects in infants exposed prenatally to methanol. *Health Effects Institute Report 89*, 69–117.

Burbacher, T. M., Shen, D. D., Lalovic, B. *et al.* (2004a). Chronic maternal methanol inhalation in monkeys (*Macaca fascicularis*): exposure and toxicokinetics prior to and during pregnancy. *Neurotoxicol Teratol* **26**, 201–221.

Burbacher, T. M., Grant, K. S., Shen, D. D. *et al.* (2004b). Chronic maternal methanol inhalation in monkeys (*Macaca fascicularis*): reproductive performance and birth outcome. *Neurotoxicol Teratol* **26**, 639–650.

Burbacher, T. M., Grant, K. S., Mayfield, D. B., Gilbert, S. G., and Rice, D. C. (2005). Prenatal methylmercury exposure affects spatial vision in adult monkeys. *Toxicol Appl Pharmacol* **208**, 21–28.

Buse, E., Habermann, G., Osterburg, I., Korte, R., and Weinbauer, G. F. (2003) Reproductive/developmental toxicity and immunotoxicity assessment in the monkey model. *Toxicology* **185**, 221–227.

Bushnell, P. J. and Bowman, R. E. (1979). Reversal learning deficits in young monkeys exposed to lead. *Pharmacol Biochem Behav* **10**, 733–742.

Bushnell, P., Bowman, R. H., Allen, J. R., and Marler, R. J. (1977). Scotopic vision deficits in young monkeys exposed to lead. *Science* **196**, 333–335.

Byers, R. K. and Lord, E. E. (1943). Late effects of lead poisoning on mental development. *Am J Dis Child* **66**, 471–494.

Campbell, T. F., Needleman, H. L., Reiss, J. A., and Tobin, M. J. (2000). Bone lead levels and language processing performance. *Dev Neuropsychol* **18**, 171–186.

Canfield, R. L., Kreher, D. A., Cornwell, C., and Henderson, C. R. Jr. (2003a). Low-level lead exposure, executive functioning, and learning in early childhood. *Neuropsychol Dev Cogn C Child Neuropsychol* **9**, 35–53.

Canfield, R. L., Henderson, C. R., Cory-Slechta, D. A., Jusko, T. A., and Lanphear, B. P. (2003b). Intellectual impairment in children with blood concentrations below 10 ug/dL, *N Engl J Med* **348**, 1517–1526.

Canfield, R. L., Gendle, M. H., and Cory-Slechta, D. A. (2004). Impaired neuropsychological functioning in lead-exposed children. *Dev Neuropsychol* **26**, 513–540.

Carson, B. L., McCann, J. L., Ellis, H. V., Ridlen, R. L., Herndon, B. L., and Baker, L. H. (1987). Human health implication of the use of methanol as a gasoline additive, Report to Environmental Health Directorate, Health Protection Branch, Department of National Health and Welfare, Ottawa, Ontario, Canada.

Carson, T. L., Van Gelder, G. A., Karas, G. C., and Buck, W. B. (1974). Slowed learning in lambs prenatally exposed to lead. *Arch Environ Health* **29**, 154–156.

Carter, A. M. (2007). Animal models of human placentation – a review. *Placenta* **28**(suppl A), S41–47.

Centers for Disease Control and Prevention (CDC). (2004). *A Review of Evidence of Health Effects of Blood Lead Levels <10 ug/dl in Children.* Centers for Disease Control and Prevention, National Center for Environmental Health.

Chen, Y. -C. J. and Hsu, C. -C. (1994). Effects of prenatal exposure to PCBs on the neurological function of children: A neuropsychological and neurophysiological study. *Dev Med Child Neurol* **36**, 312–320.

Chen, Y.-C. J., Guo, Y.-L., Hsu, C.-C., and Rogan, W. J. (1992). Cognitive development of yu-cheng ('oil disease') children prenatally exposed to heat-degraded PCBs. *JAMA* **268**, 3213–3218.

Chen, Y.-C., Yu, M.-L., Rogan, W., Gladen, B., and Hsu, C.-C. (1994). A 6-year follow-up of behavior and activity disorders in the Taiwan Yu-cheng children. *Am J Public Health* **84**, 415–421.

Chiodo, L. M., Jacobson, S. W., and Jacobson, J. L. (2004). Neurodevelopmental effects of postnatal lead exposure at very low levels. *Neurotoxicol Teratol* **26**, 359–371.

Cordier, S., Garel, M., Mandereau, L. *et al.* (2002). Neurodevelopmental investigations among methylmercury-exposed children in French Guiana. *Environ Res* **89**, 1–11.

Counter, S. A. (2003).Neurophysiological anomalies in brainstem responses of mercury-exposed children of Andean gold miners. *J Occup Environ Med* **45**, 87–95.

Counter, S. A., Buchanan, L. H., Laurell, G., and Ortega, F. (1998). Blood mercury and auditory neuro-sensory responses in children and adults in the Nambija gold mining area of Ecuador. *Neurotoxicology* **19**, 185–196.

Counter, S. A., Buchanan, L. H., and Ortega, F. (2006). Neurocognitive screening of mercury-exposed children of Andean gold miners. *Int J Occup Environ Health* **12**, 209–214.

Darcheville, J. C., Riviere, V., and Wearden, J. H. (1992). Fixed-interval performance and self-control in children. *J Exp Anal Behav* **57**, 187–199.

Darcheville, J. C., Riviere, V., and Wearden, J. H. (1993). Fixed-interval performance and self-control in infants. *J Exp Anal Behav* **60**, 239–254.

Darvill, T., Lonky, E., Reihman, J., Stewart, P., and Pagano, J. (2000). Prenatal exposure to PCBs and infant performance on the Fagan test of infant intelligence. *Neurotoxicology* **21**, 1029–1038.

Darwish, A., Roth, C. E., Duclos, P. *et al.* (2002) Investigation into a cluster of infant deaths following immunization: evidence for methanol intoxication. *Vaccine* **20**, 29–30.

Davidson, P. W., Myers, G. J., Cox, C. *et al.* (2006). Methylmercury and neurodevelopment: longitudinal analysis of the Seychelles child development cohort. *Neurotoxicol Teratol* **28**, 536–547.

de la Burdé, B. and Choate, M. S. (1972). Early asymptomatic lead exposure and development at school age. *J Pediatr* **87**, 638–642.

De Valois, R. L., Morgan, H., and Snodderly D. M. (1974). Psychophysical studies of monkey vision. 3. Spatial luminance contrast sensitivity tests of macaque and human observers. *Vis Res* **14**, 75–81.

Debes, F., Budtz-Jorgensen, E., Weihe, P., White, R. F., and Grandjean, P. (2006). Impact of prenatal methylmercury exposure on neurobehavioral function at age 14 years. *Neurotoxicol Teratol* **28**, 363–375.

Despres, C., Beuter, A., Richer, F. *et al.* (2005). Neuromotor functions in Inuit preschool children exposed to Pb, PCBs, and Hg. *Neurotoxicol Teratol* **27**, 245–257.

Dietrich, K. N., Succop, P. A., Berger, O. G., and Keith, R. W. (1992). Lead exposure and the central auditory processing abilities and cognitive development of urban children: the Cincinnati lead study cohort at age 5 years. *Neurotoxicol Teratol* **14**, 51–56.

Dolbec, J., Mergler, D., Sousa Passos, C. J., Sousa de Morais, S., and Lebel, J. (2000). Methylmercury exposure affects motor performance of a riverine population of the Tapajos river, Brazilian Amazon. *Int Arch Occup Environ Health* **73**, 195–203.

Fagan, J. F. III (1990). The paired-comparison paradigm and infant intelligence. *Ann N Y Acad Sci* **608**, 337–357.

Faustman, E. M., Silbernagel, S. M., Fenske, R. A., Burbacher, T. M., and Ponce, R. A. (2000). Mechanisms underlying children's susceptibility to environmental toxicants. *Environ Health Perspect* **108**, 13–21.

Fergusson, D. M., Fergusson, J. E., Horwood, L. J., and Kinzett, N. G. (1988a). A longitudinal study of dentine lead levels, intelligence, school performance and behavior. Part I: Dentine lead levels and exposure to environmental risk factors. *J Child Psychol Psychiatr* **29**, 781–792.

Fergusson, D. M., Fergusson, J. E., Horwood, L. J., and Kinzett, N. G. (1988b). A longitudinal study of dentine lead levels, intelligence, school performance and behavior. Part II: Dentine lead and cognitive ability. *J Child Psychol Psychiatr* **29**, 783–809.

Fergusson, D. M., Fergusson, J. E., Horwood, L. J., and Kinzett, N. G. (1988c). A longitudinal study of dentine lead levels, intelligence, school performance and behavior. Part III: Dentine lead levels and attention/activity. *J Child Psychol Psychiatr* **29**, 811–824.

Fergusson, D. M. and Horwood, L. J. (1993). The effects of lead levels on the growth of word recognition in middle childhood. *Int J Epidemiol* **22**, 891–897.

Fulton, M., Raab, G., Thomson, G., Laxen, D., Hunter, R., and Hepburn, W. (1987). Influence of blood lead on the ability and attainment of children in Edinburgh. *Lancet* **8544**, 1221–1226.

Gilbert, S. G. and Rice, D. C. (1987). Low-level lifetime lead exposure produces behavioral toxicity (spatial discrimination reversal) in adult monkeys. *Toxicol Appl Pharmacol* **91**, 484–490.

Gilbert, S. G. and Weiss, B. (2006). A rationale for lowering the blood lead action level from 10 to 2 ug/dL. *Neurotoxicology* **27**, 693–701.

Gilbert, S. G., Burbacher, T. M., and Rice, D. C. (1993). Effects of in utero methylmercury exposure on a spatial delayed alternation task in monkeys. *Toxicol Appl Pharmacol* **123**, 130–136.

Gilbert, S. G., Rice, D. C., and Burbacher, T. M. (1996). Fixed interval/fixed ratio performance in adult monkeys exposed in utero to methylmercury. *Neurotoxicol Teratol* **18**, 539–546.

Ginsberg, G., Hattis, D., and Sonawane, B. (2004). Incorporating pharmacokinetic differences between children and adults in assessing children's risks to environmental toxicants. *Toxicol Appl Pharmacol* **198**, 164–183.

Gladen, B. C. and Rogan, W. J. (1991). Effect of perinatal polychlorinated biphenyls and dichlorodiphenyl dichloroethene on later development. *J Pediatr* **119**, 58–63.

Gold, M. D. and Moulis, C. E. (1988). Effects of emissions standards on methanol vehicle-related ozone, formaldehyde, and methanol exposure. Presentation at 81st annual meeting of the Air Pollution Control Association, Detroit, MI, June 19–24, 1988.

Goldman, L. R. and Koduru, S. (2000). Chemicals in the environment and developmental toxicity to children: a public health and policy perspective. *Environ Health Perspect* **108**, 595–597.

Goldman, L., Falk, H., Landrigan, P. J., Balk, S. J., Reigart, J. R., and Etzel, R. A. (2004). Environmental pediatrics and its impact on government health policy. *Pediatrics* **113**, 1146–1157.

Grandjean, P. and Landrigan, P. J. (2006). Developmental neurotoxicity of industrial chemicals. *Lancet* **368**, 2167–2178.

Grandjean, P., Weihe, P., White, R. F. et al. (1997). Cognitive deficit in 7-year-old children with prenatal exposure to methylmercury. *Neurotoxicol Teratol* **19**, 417–428.

Grant, K., Burbacher, T., Acuna, O., and Mottet, N. K. (1982). Teratogenic effects of low level mercury exposure in the *Cynomolgus* monkey. *Teratology* **24**, 45a.

Grant-Webster, K., Burbacher, T., and Mottet, N. K. (1992). Puberal growth retardation in primates: A latent effect of *in utero* exposure to methylmercury. *The Toxicologist* **12**, 310.

Guillette, E. A. (2000). Examining childhood development in contaminated urban settings. *Environ Health Perspect* **108**(suppl 3), 389–393.

Gunderson, V. M. and Sackett, G. P. (1984). Development of pattern recognition in infant pigtailed macaques (Macaca nemestrina). *Devel Psychol* **20**, 418–426.

Gunderson, V. M., Grant, K. S., Burbacher, T. M., Fagan, J. F. III, and Mottet, N. K. (1986). The effect of low-level prenatal methylmercury exposure on visual recognition memory in infant crab-eating macaques. *Child Dev* **57**, 1076–1083.

Gunderson, V. M., Grant-Webster, K. S., Burbacher, T. M., and Mottet, N. K. (1988). Visual recognition memory deficits in methylmercury-exposed *Macaca fascicularis* infants. *Neurotoxicol Teratol* **10**, 373–379.

Gunderson, V. M., Grant-Webster, K. S., and Sackett, G. P. (1989). Deficits in visual recognition in low birth weight infant pigtailed monkeys (*Macaca nemestrina*). *Child Dev* **60**, 119–127.

Guo, Y. L., Lai, T.-J., Chen, S.-J., and Hsu, C.-C. (1995). Gender-related decrease in Raven=s progressive matrices scores in children prenatally exposed to polychlorinated biphenyls and related contaminants. *Bull Environ Contam Toxicol* **55**, 8–13.

Ha, J. C., Kimpo, C. L., and Sackett, G. P. (1997). Multiple-spell, discrete-time survival analysis of developmental data: object concept in pigtailed macaques. *Dev Psychol* **33**, 1054–1059.

Haggerty, R. and Rothman, J. (1975). *Child Health and the Community*. New York: John Wiley and Sons.

Hamilton, W. J. and Poswillo, D. E. (1972). Limb reduction anomalies induced in the marmoset by thalidomide. *J Anat* **111**, 505–506.

Hansen, O. M., Trillingsgaard, A., Beese, I., Lyngbye, T., and Grandjean, P. (1989). A neuropsychological study of children with elevated dentine lead level: assessment of the effect of lead in different socio-economic groups. *Neurotoxicol Teratol* **11**, 205–214.

Harada, M. (1976). Intrauterine poisoning: clinical and epidemiological studies of the problem. *Bull Inst Constit Med (Kumamoto Univ)* **25**(suppl), 1–60.

Harada, M. (1978). Congenital Minamata disease: intrauterine methylmercury poisoning. *Teratology* **18**, 285–288.

Harada, M. (1995). Minamata disease: methylmercury poisoning in Japan caused by environmental pollution. *Crit Rev Toxicol* **25**, 1–24.

Hatzakis, A., Kokkevi, A., Katsouyanni, K. *et al.* (1987). Psychometric intelligence and attentional performance deficits in lead-exposed children. In: Lindberg, S. E. and Hutchinson, T. C. eds. *Proc. 6th Intl Conf. on Heavy Metals in the Environment*. Edinburgh: CEP Consultants, 204–209.

Heath-Lange, S., Ha, J. C., and Sackett, G. P. (1999). Behavioral measurement of temperament in male nursery-raised infant macaques and baboons. *Am J Primatol* **47**, 43–50.

Hendrickx, A. G. and Binkerd, P. E. (1990). Monkeys and teratological research. *J Med Primatol* **19**, 81–108.

Hendrickx, A. G. and Cukierski, M. A. (1987). Reproductive and developmental toxicology in nonhuman primates. In: Graham, C. R. ed. *Preclinical Safety of Biotechnology Products intended for Human Use*. New York: Alan R. Liss, pp. 73–88.

Hendrickx, A. G. and Peterson, P. E. (1997). Perspectives on the use of the baboon in embryology and teratology research. *Hum Repro Update* **3**, 575–92.

Hendrickx, A. G., Benirschke, K., Thompson, R. S., Ahern, J. K., Lucas, W. E., and Oi, R. H. (1979). The effects of prenatal diethylstilbestrol (DES) exposure on the genitalia of pubertal *Macaca mulatta*. I. Female offspring. *J Reprod Med* **22**, 233–240.

Hendrickx, A. G., Nau, H., Binkerd, P. *et al.* (1988). Valproic acid developmental toxicity and pharmacokinetics in the rhesus monkey: an interspecies comparison. *Teratology* **38**, 329–345.

Herman, R. A., Jones, B., Mann, D. R., and Wallen, K. (2000). Timing of prenatal androgen exposure: anatomical and endocrine effects on juvenile male and female rhesus monkeys. *Horm Behav* **38**, 52–66.

Hopper, D. L., Kernan, W. J., and Lloyd, W. E. (1986). The behavioral effects of prenatal and early postnatal lead exposure in the primate *Macaca fascicularis*. *Toxicol Indust Health* **2**, 1–16.

Huisman, M., Koopman-Esseboom, C., Fidler, V. *et al.* (1995a) Perinatal exposure to polychlorinated biphenyls and dioxins and its effect on neonatal neurological development. *Early Human Dev* **41**, 111–127.

Huisman, M., Koopman-Esseboom, C., Lanting, C. I. *et al.* (1995b). Neurological condition in 18-month-old children perinatally exposed to polychlorinated biphenyls and dioxins. *Early Hum Dev* **43**, 165–176.

Hummler, H., Korte, R., and Hendrickx, A. G. (1990). Induction of malformations in the cynomolgus monkey with 13-cis retinoic acid. *Teratology* **42**, 263–272.

Ino, H. and Mizukoshi, K. (1977). Otorhinolaryngological findings in intoxication by organomercury compounds. In: Tsubaki, T. and Irukayama, K. eds. *Minamata Disease*. Amsterdam: Elsevier, pp. 186–208.

Jacobson, J. L. and Jacobson, S. W. (1993). A 4-year followup study of children born to consumers of Lake Michigan fish. *J Great Lakes Res* **19**, 776–783.

Jacobson, J. L. and Jacobson, S. W. (1996). Intellectual impairment in children exposed to polychlorinated biphenyls in utero. *New Engl J Med* **335**, 783–789.

Jacobson, J. L. and Jacobson, S. W. (2003). Prenatal exposure to polychlorinated biphenyls and attention at school age. *J Pediatr* **143**, 780–788.

Jacobson, J. L., Jacobson, S. W., Fein, G. G., Schwartz, P. M., and Dowler, J. K. (1984). Prenatal exposure to an environmental toxin: a test of the multiple effects model. *Dev Psychol* **20**, 523–532.

Jacobson, S. W., Fein, G. G., Jacobson, J. L., Schwartz, P. M., and Dowler, J. K. (1985). The effect of intrauterine PCB exposure on visual recognition memory. *Child Dev* **56**, 853–860.

Jacobson, J. L., Jacobson, S. W., and Humphrey, H. E. B. (1990a). Effects of exposure to PCBs and related compounds on growth and activity in children. *Neurotoxicol Teratol* **12**, 319–326.

Jacobson, J. L., Jacobson, S. W., and Humphrey, H. E. B. (1990b). Effects of in utero exposure to polychlorinated biphenyls (PCBs) and related contaminants on cognitive functioning in young children. *J Pediatr* **11**, 38–45.

Jedrychowski, W., Jankowski, J., Flak, E. *et al.* (2006). Effects of prenatal exposure to mercury on cognitive and psychomotor function in one-year-old infants: epidemiologic cohort study in Poland. *Ann Epidemiol* **16**, 439–447.

Jenkins, C. D. and Mellins, B. B. (1957). Lead poisoning in children. *AMA Arch Neurol Psychiatr* **77**, 70–78.

Kavet, R. and Nauss, K. M. (1990). The toxicity of inhaled methanol vapors. *Crit Rev Toxicol* **21**, 21–50.

King, B. F. (1993). Development and structure of the placenta and fetal membranes of monkeys. *J Exp Zool* **266**, 528–540.

Kinjo, Y., Higashi, H., Nakano, A., Sakamoto, M., and Sakai R. (1993). Profile of subjective complaints and activities of daily living among current patients with Minamata disease after 3 decades. *Environ Res* **63**, 241–251.

Kiorpes, L. (1992). Development of vernier acuity and grating acuity in normally reared monkeys. *Vis Neurosci* **9**, 243–251.

Kjellstrom, T., Kennedy, P., Wallis, S., and Mantell, C. (1986). Physical and mental development of children with prenatal exposure to mercury from fish. Stage 1: Preliminary tests at age 4. *National Swedish Environmental Protection Board Report 3080*, Solna, Sweden.

Kjellstrom, T., Kennedy, P., Wallis, S., *et al.* (1989). Physical and mental development of children with prenatal exposure to mercury from fish. *National Swedish Environmental Protection Board Report 3642*, Solna, Sweden.

Kondo, K. (2000). Congenital Minamata disease: warnings from Japan's experience. *J Child Neurol* **15**, 458–464.

Koopman-Esseboom, C., Weisglas-Kuperus, N., de Ridder, M. A. J., van der Paauw, C. G., Tuinstra, L. G. M. Th., and Sauer, P. J. J. (1996). Effects of polychlorinated biphenyl/dioxin exposure and feeding type on infants' mental and psychomotor development. *Pediatrics* **97**, 700–706.

Kuratsune, M. (1989). Yusho, with reference to Yu-Cheng. In: Kimbrough, R. D. and Jensen, A.A. eds. *Halogenated Biphenyls, Terphenyls, Naphthalenes, Dibenzodioxins, and Related Products*, 2nd edn. Amsterdam: Elsevier, 381–400.

Lai, T. J., Guo, Y. L., Yu, M. L., Ko, H. C., and Hsu, C. C. (1994). Cognitive development in Yucheng children. *Chemosphere* **29**, 2405–2411.

Landrigan, P. J., Schechter, C. B., Lipton, J. M., Fahs, M. C., and Schwartz, J. (2002a). Environmental pollutants and disease in American children: estimates of morbidity, mortality, and costs for lead poisoning, asthma, cancer, and developmental disabilities. *Environ Health Perspect* **110**, 721–728

Landrigan, P. J., Sonawane, B., Mattison, D., McCally, M., and Garg, A. (2002b). Chemical contaminants in breast milk and their impacts on children's health: an overview. *Environ Health Perspect* **110**, A313–315.

Landrigan, P. J., Kimmel, C. A., Correa, A., and Eskenazi, B. (2004). Children's health and the environment: public health issues and challenges for risk assessment. *Environ Health Perspect* **112**, 257–265.

Lanphear, B. P., Hornung, R., Khoury, J. *et al.* (2005) Low-level environmental lead exposure and children's intellectual function: an international pooled analysis. *Environ Health Perspect* **113**, 894–899.

Lasky, R. E., Maier, M. M., Snodgrass, E. B., Hecox, K. E., and Laughlin, N. K. (1995). The effects of lead on otoacoustic emissions and auditory evoked potentials in monkeys. *Neurotoxicol Teratol* **17**, 633–644.

Lasky, R. E., Luck, M. L., Torre, P. III, and Laughlin, N. (2001). The effects of early lead exposure on auditory function in rhesus monkeys. *Neurotoxicol Tertol* **23**, 639–649.

Lebel, J., Mergler, D., Lucotte, M. *et al.* (1996). Evidence of early nervous system dysfunction in Amazonian populations exposed to low-levels of methylmercury. *Neurotoxicology* **17**, 157–167.

Lebel, J., Mergler, D., Branches, F. *et al.* (1998). Neurotoxic effects of low-level methylmercury contamination in the Amazonian Basin. *Environ Res* **79**, 20–32.

Levin, E. D. and Bowman, R. E. (1986). Long-term lead effects on the Hamilton Search Task and delayed alternation in adult monkeys. *Neurobehav Toxicol Teratol* **8**, 219–224.

Levin, E. D., Schantz, S. L., and Bowman, R. E. (1988). Delayed spatial alternation deficits resulting from perinatal PCB exposure in monkeys. *Arch Toxicol* **62**, 267–273.

Leviton, A., Bellinger, D., Allred, E. N., Rabinowitz, M., Needleman, H., and Schoenbaum, S. (1993). Pre- and postnatal low-level lead exposure and children's dysfunction in school. *Environ Res* **60**, 30–43.

Ley, C. O. and Gali, F. G. (1983). Parkinsonian syndrome after methanol intoxication. *Eur Neurol* **22**, 405–409.

Lilienthal, H. and Winneke, G. (1996). Lead effects on the brain stem auditory evoked potential in monkeys during and after the treatment phase. *Neurotoxicol Teratol* **18**, 17–32.

Lilienthal, H., Winneke, G., Brockhaus, A., and Malik, B. (1986). Pre- and postnatal lead-exposure in monkeys: effects on activity and learning set formation. *Neurobehav Toxicol Teratol* **8**, 265–272.

Lilienthal, H., Lenaerts, C., Winneke, G., and Hennekes, R. (1988). Alteration of the visual evoked potential and the electroretinogram in lead-treated monkeys. *Neurotoxicol Teratol* **10**, 417–422.

Lilienthal, H., Winneke, G., and Ewert, T. (1990). Effects of lead on neurophysiological and performance measures: animal and human data. *Environ Health Perspect* **89**, 21–25.

Lilienthal, H., Kohler, K., Turfeld, M., and Winneke, G. (1994). Persistent increases in scotopic B-wave amplitudes after lead exposure in monkeys. *Exp Eye Res* **59**, 203–209.

Lin-Fu, J. S. (1972). Undue absorption of lead among children – a new look at an old problem. *N Engl J Med* **186**, 702–710.

Magos, L. (1987). The absorption, distribution and excretion of methylmercury. In: Eccles, C. U. and Annau, Z. eds. *The Toxicity of Methylmercury*. Baltimore: Johns Hopkins, pp. 24–44.

Makar, A. B. and Tephly, T. R. (1976). Methanol poisoning in the folate-deficient rat. *Nature* **24**, 715–716.

McBride, W. G. (1961). Thalidomide and congenital abnormalities. *Lancet* **2**, 1358.

McClure, H. M., Wilk, A. L., Horigan, E. A., and Pratt, R. M. (1979). Induction of craniofacial malformations in rhesus monkeys (*Macaca mulatta*) with cyclophosphamide. *Cleft Palate J* **16**, 248–256.

Molfese, D. L., Laughlin, N. K, Morse, P. A., Linnville, S. E., Wetzel, W. F., and Erwin, R. J. (1986). Neuroelectrical correlates of categorical perception for place of articulation in normal and lead-treated rhesus monkeys. *J Clin Exp Neuropsychol* **8**, 680–696.

Mottet, N. K., Shaw, C. M., and Burbacher, T. M. (1985). Health risks from increases in methylmercury exposure. *Environ Health Perspect* **63**, 133–140.

MMWR (Morbidity and Mortality Weekly Report) September (2005). Mental Health in the United States: Prevalence of Diagnosis and Medication Treatment for Attention-Deficit/Hyperactivity Disorder – United States, 2003. **54**, 842–847.

Mottet, N. K., Vahter, M. E., Charleston, J. S., and Friberg, L. T. (1997). Metabolism of methylmercury in the brain and its toxicological significance. *Met Ions Biol Syst* **34**, 371–403.

Merigan, W. H., Maurrisen, J. P., Weiss, B., Eskin, T., and Lapham, L. W. (1983). Neurotoxic actions of methylmercury on the primate visual system. *Neurobehav Toxicol Teratol* **5**, 649–658.

Mukuno, K., Ishikawa, S., and Okamura, R. (1981). Grating test of contrast sensitivity in patients with Minamata disease. *Br J Ophthalmol* **65**, 284–290.

Murata, K., Weihe, P., Renzoni, A., Debes, F. *et al.* (1999a). Delayed evoked potentials in children exposed to methylmercury from seafood. *Neurotoxicol Teratol* **21**, 343–348.

Murata, K., Weihe, P., Araki, S., Budtz-Jorgensen, E., and Grandjean, P. (1999b) Evoked potentials in Faroese children prenatally exposed to methylmercury. *Neurotoxicol Teratol* **21**, 471–472.

Murata, K., Weihe, P., Budtz-Jorgensen, E., Jorgensen, P. J., and Grandjean, P. (2004). Delayed brainstem auditory evoked potential latencies in 14-year-old children exposed to methylmercury. *J Pediatr* **144**, 177–183.

National Research Council (2000). *Toxicological Effects of Methylmercury*. Washington, D.C.: National Academy Press.

Needleman, H. L. (1987). Introduction: Biomarkers in neurodevelopmental toxicology. *Environ Health Perspect* **74**, 149–152.

Needleman, H. L., Gunnoe, C., Leviton, A. *et al.* (1979). Deficits in psychologic and classroom performance of children with elevated dentine lead levels. *N Engl J Med* **300**, 689–695.

Newland, M. C. and Rasmussen, E. B. (2000). Aging unmasks adverse effects of gestational exposure to methylmercury in rats. *Neurotoxicol Teratol* **22**, 819–828.

Newland, M. C., Yezhou, S., Logdberg, B., and Berlin, M. (1994). Prolonged behavioral effects of *in utero* exposure to lead or methyl mercury: reduced sensitivity to changes in reinforcement contingencies during behavioral transitions and in steady state. *Toxicol Appl Pharmacol* **126**, 6–15.

Newland, M. C., Reile, P. A., and Langston, J. L. (2004). Gestational exposure to methylmercury retards choice in transition in aging rats. *Neurotoxicol Teratol* **26**, 179–194.

Oken, E., Wright, R. O., Kleinman, K. P. *et al.* (2005). Maternal fish consumption, hair mercury, and infant cognition in a U.S. Cohort. *Environ Health Perspect* **113**, 1376–1380.

Osman, K., Pawlas, K., Schütz, A., Gazdzik, M., Sokal, J. A., and Vahter, M. (1999). Lead exposure and hearing effects in children in Katowice, Poland. *Environ Res* **80**, 1–8.

Otto, D. A., and Fox, D. A. (1993). Auditory and visual dysfunction following lead exposure. *Neurotoxicology* **14**, 191–207.

Pallapies, D. (2006). Trends in childhood disease. *Mutat Res* **608**, 100–111.

Patandin, S., Koot, H. M., Sauer, P. J. J., and Weisglas-Kuperus, N. (1999a). Problem behavior in Dutch preschool children in relation to background polychlorinated biphenyl and dioxin exposure. In: *Effects of environmental exposure to polychlorinated biphenyls and dioxins on growth and development in young children*. PhD thesis, Erasmus University, Rotterdam, pp. 143–156.

Patandin, S., Lanting, C. I., Mulder, P. G. H., Boersma, E. R., Sauer, P. J. J., and Weisglas-Kuperus, N. (1999b). Effects of environmental exposure to polychlorinated biphenyls and dioxins on cognitive abilities in Dutch children at 42 months of age. *J Pediatr* **134**, 33–41.

Patandin, S., Veenstra, J., Mulder, P. G. H., Sewnaik, A., Sauer, P. J. J., and Weisglas-Kuperus, N. (1999c). Attention and activity in 42-month-old Dutch children with environmental exposure to polychlorinated biphenyls and dioxins. In: *Effects of environmental exposure to polychlorinated biphenyls and dioxins on growth and development in young children*. PhD thesis, Erasmus University, Rotterdam, pp. 123–142.

Perlstein, M. A. and Attala, R. (1966). Neurological sequelae of plumbism in children. *Clin Pediatr* **5**, 282–298.

Plant, T. M. and Barker-Gibb, M. L. (2004). Neurobiological mechanisms of puberty in higher primates. *Hum Reprod Update* **10**, 67–77.

Reuhl, K. R. (1991). Delayed expression of neurotoxicity: the problem of silent damage. *Neurotoxicology* **12**, 341–346.

Reuhl, K. R., Rice, D. C., Gilbert, S. G., and Mallett, J. (1989). Effects of chronic developmental lead exposure on monkey neuroanatomy: visual system. *Toxicol Appl Pharmacol* **99**, 501–509.

Rice, C. (2007). Prevalence of autism spectrum disorders – Autism and Developmental Disabilities Monitoring Network, Six Sites, United States, 2000. *Morbidity and Morality Weekly* **56**, 1–11.

Rice, D. C. (1984). Behavioral deficit (delayed matching to sample) in monkeys exposed from birth to low levels of lead. *Toxicol Appl Pharmacol* **75**, 337–345.

Rice, D. C. (1985). Chronic low-lead exposure from birth produces deficits in discrimination reversal in monkeys. *Toxicol Appl Pharmacol* **77**, 201–210.

Rice, D. C. (1988a). Chronic low-level lead exposure in monkeys does not affect simple reaction time. *Neurotoxicology* **9**, 105–106.

Rice, D. C. (1988b). Schedule-controlled behavior in infant and juvenile monkeys exposed to lead from birth. *Neurotoxicology* **9**, 75–88.

Rice, D. C. (1989). Blood mercury concentrations following methylmercury exposure in adult and infant monkeys. *Environ Res* **49**, 115–126.

Rice, D. C. (1990). Lead-induced behavioral impairment on a spatial discrimination reversal task in monkeys exposed during different periods of development. *Toxicol Appl Pharmacol* **106**, 327–333.

Rice, D. C. (1992a). Effect of lead during different developmental periods in the monkey on concurrent discrimination performance. *Neurotoxicology* **13**, 583–592.

Rice, D. C. (1992b). Behavioral effects of lead in monkeys tested during infancy and adulthood. *Neurotoxicol Teratol* **14**, 235–245.

Rice, D. C. (1992c). Lead exposure during different developmental periods produces different effects in FI performance in monkeys tested as juveniles and adults. *Neurotoxicology* **13**, 757–770.

Rice, D. C. (1992d). Effects of pre- plus postnatal exposure to methylmercury in the monkey on fixed interval and discrimination reversal performance. *Neurotoxicology* **13**, 443–452.

Rice, D. C. (1996). Evidence for delayed neurotoxicity produced by methylmercury. *Neurotoxicology* **17**, 583–596.

Rice, D. C. (1997a). Effects of lifetime lead exposure in monkeys on detection of pure tones. *Fundam Appl Toxicol* **36**, 112–118.

Rice, D. C. (1997b). Effect of postnatal exposure to a PCB mixture in monkeys on multiple fixed interval-fixed ratio performance. *Neurotoxicol Teratol* **19**, 429–434.

Rice, D. C. (1998a). Effects of lifetime lead exposure on spatial and temporal visual function in monkeys. *Neurotoxicology* **19**, 893–902.

Rice, D. C. (1998b). Effects of postnatal exposure of monkeys to a PCB mixture on spatial discrimination reversal and DRL performance. *Neurotoxicol Teratol* **13**, 391–400.

Rice, D. C. (1998c). Age-related increase in auditory impairment in monkeys exposed *in-utero* plus postnatally to methylmercury. *Toxicol Sci* **44**, 191–196.

Rice, D. C. (1999). Behavioral impairment produced by low-level postnatal PCB exposure in monkeys. *Environ Res* **80**, S113–121.

Rice, D. C. (2006). Animal models of cognitive impairment produced by developmental lead exposure. In: Levin, E. D. and Buccafusco, J. J. eds. *Animal Models of Cognitive Impairment*. Boca Raton, FL: CRC Press, pp. 73–100.

Rice, D. and Barone, S. Jr. (2000). Critical periods of vulnerability for the developing nervous system: evidence from humans and animal models. *Environ Health Perspect* **108**, 511–533.

Rice, D. C. and Gilbert, S. G. (1982). Early chronic low-level methylmercury poisoning in monkeys impairs spatial vision. *Science* **216**, 759–761.

Rice, D. C. and Gilbert, S. G. (1985). Low-level lead exposure from birth produces behavioral toxicity (DRL) in monkeys. *Toxicol Appl Pharmacol* **80**, 421–426.

Rice, D. C. and Gilbert, S. G. (1990a). Sensitive periods for lead-induced behavioral impairment (nonspatial discrimination reversal) in monkeys. *Toxicol Appl Pharmacol* **102**, 101–109.

Rice, D. C. and Gilbert, S. G. (1990b). Lack of sensitive period for lead-induced behavioral impairment on a spatial delayed alternation task in monkeys. *Toxicol Appl Pharmacol* **103**, 364–373.

Rice, D. C. and Gilbert, S. G. (1990c). Effects of developmental exposure to methyl mercury on spatial and temporal visual function in monkeys. *Toxicol Appl Pharmacol* **102**, 151–163.

Rice, D. C. and Gilbert, S. G. (1992). Exposure to methyl mercury from birth to adulthood impairs high-frequency hearing in monkeys. *Toxicol Appl Pharmacol* **115**, 6–10.

Rice, D. C. and Gilbert, S. G. (1995). Effects of developmental methylmercury exposure or lifetime lead exposure on vibration sensitivity function in monkeys. *Toxicol Appl Pharmacol* **134**, 161–169.

Rice, D. C. and Hayward, S. (1997). Effects of postnatal exposure to a PCB mixture in monkeys on nonspatial discrimination reversal and delayed alternation performance. *Neurotoxicology* **18**, 479–494.

Rice, D. C. and Karpinski, K. F. (1988). Lifetime low-level lead exposure produces deficits in delayed alternation in adult monkeys. *Neurotoxicol Teratol* **10**, 207–214.

Rice, D. C. and Willes, R. F. (1979). Neonatal low-level lead exposure in monkeys (*Macaca fascicularis*): effect on two-choice nonspatial form discrimination. *J Environ Pathol Toxicol* **2**, 1195–1203.

Rice, D. C., Gilbert, S. G., and Willes, R. F. (1979). Neonatal low-level lead exposure in monkeys (*Macaca fascicularis*): Locomotor activity, schedule-controlled behavior, and the effects of amphetamine. *Toxicol Appl Pharmacol* **51**, 503–513.

Rogan, W. J., Gladen, B. C., McKinney, J. D. *et al.* (1986a). Neonatal effects of transplacental exposure to PCBs and DDE. *J Pediatr* **109**, 335–341.

Rogan, W. J., Gladen, B. C., McKinney, J. D. *et al.* (1986b). Polychlorinated biphenyls (PCBs) and dichlorodiphenyl dichloroethene (DDE) in human milk: effects of maternal factors and previous lactation. *Am J Public Health* **76**, 172–177.

Rogan, W. J., Gladen, B. C., Hung, K. L. *et al.* (1988). Congenital poisoning by polychlorinated biphenyls and their contaminants in Taiwan. *Science* **241**, 334–336.

Rogers, J. M. and Mole, M. L. (1997). Critical periods of sensitivity to the developmental toxicity of inhaled methanol in the CD-1 mouse. *Teratology* **55**, 364–372.

Rogers, J. M., Mole, M. L., Chernoff, N. *et al.* (1993). The developmental toxicity of inhaled methanol in the CD-1 mouse, with quantitative dose-response modeling for estimation of benchmark doses, *Teratology* **47**, 175–188.

Rose, S. A., Feldman, J. F., Jankowski, J. J., and Van Rossem, R. (2005). Pathways from prematurity and infant abilities to later cognition. *Child Dev* **76**, 1172–1184.

Rustam, H. and Hamdi, T. (1974). Methyl mercury poisoning in Iraq. A neurological study. *Brain* **97**, 500–510.

Sackett, G. P. (1984). A monkey model of risk for deviant development. *Am J Ment Defic* **88**, 469–476.

Sabeliash, S. and Himli, G. (1976). Ocular manifestations of mercury poisoning. *Bull WHO Suppl* **53**, 83–86.

Sagvolden, T., Aase, H., Zeiner, P., and Berger, D. (1998). Altered reinforcement mechanisms in attention-deficit/hyperactivity disorder. *Behav Brain Res* **94**, 61–71.

Saint-Amour, D., Roy, M. S., Bastien, C. *et al.* (2006). Alterations of visual evoked potentials in preschool Inuit children exposed to methylmercury and polychlorinated biphenyls from a marine diet. *Neurotoxicology* **27**, 567–578.

Sameroff, A. J. (1998). Environmental risk factors in infancy. *Pediatrics* **102**, 1287–1292.

Schantz, S. L., Levin, E. D., Bowman, R. E., Hieronimus, M., and Laughlin, N. K. (1989). Effects of perinatal PCB exposure on discrimination-reversal learning in monkeys. *Neurotoxicol Teratol* **11**, 243–250.

Schantz, S. L., Levin, E. D., and Bowman, R. E. (1991). Long-term neurobehavioral effects of perinatal polychlorinated biphenyl (PCB) exposure in monkeys. *Environ Toxicol Chem* **10**, 747–756.

Schardein, J. L., Schwetz, B. A., and Kenel, M. F. (1985). Species sensitivities and prediction of teratogenic potential. *Environ Health Perspect* **61**, 55–67.

Schneider, M. L. and Suomi, S. J. (1992). Neurobehavioral assessment in rhesus monkey neonates (Macaca mulatta): Developmental changes, behavioral stability, and early experience. *Infant Behav Dev* **15**, 155–177.

Schwartz, J. and Otto, D. (1987). Blood lead, hearing thresholds, and neurobehavioral development in children and youth. *Arch Environ Health* **42**, 153–160.

Spyker, J. M., Sparber, S. B., and Goldberg, A. M. (1972). Subtle consequences of methylmercury exposure: behavioral deviations in offspring of treated mothers. *Science* **177**, 621–623.

Steuerwald, U., Weihe, P., Jorgensen, P. J. *et al.* (2000). Maternal seafood diet, methylmercury exposure, and neonatal neurologic function. *J Pediatr* **136**, 599–605.

Stewart, P., Reihman, J., Lonky, E., Darvill, T., and Pagano, J. (2000). Prenatal PCB exposure and neonatal behavioral assessment scale (NBAS) performance. *Neurotoxicol Teratol* **22**, 21–29.

Stewart, P., Fitzgerald, S., Reihman, J. *et al.* (2003a). Prenatal PCB exposure, the corpus callosum, and response inhibition. *Environ Health Perspect* **111**, 1670–1677.

Stewart, P. W., Reihman, J., Lonky, E. I., Darvill, T. J., and Pagano, J. (2003b). Cognitive development in preschool children prenatally exposed to PCBs and MeHg. *Neurotoxicol Teratol* **25**, 11–22.

Stewart, P., Reihman, J., Gump, B., Lonky, E., Darvill, T., and Pagano, J. (2005). Response inhibition at 8 and 9½ years of age in children prenatally exposed to PCBs. *Neurotoxicol Teratol* **27**, 771–780.

Stewart, P. W., Sargent, D. M., Reihman, J. *et al.* (2006). Response inhibition during differential reinforcement of low rates (DRL) schedules may be sensitive to low-level polychlorinated biphenyl, methylmercury, and lead exposure in children. *Environ Health Perspect* **114**, 1923–1929.

Stiles, K. M. and Bellinger, D. C. (1993). Neuropsychological correlates of low-level lead exposure in school-age children: a prospective study. *Neurotoxicol Teratol* **15**, 27–35.

Stokes, L., Letz, R., Gerr, F. *et al.* (1998). Neurotoxicity in young adults 20 years after childhood exposure to lead: the Bunker Hill experience. *Occup Environ Med* **55**, 507–516.

Tephly, T. R. (1991). The toxicity of methanol. *Life Sci* **48**, 1031–1041.

Tilson, H. A. (2000). Neurotoxicology risk assessment guidelines: developmental neurotoxicology. *Neurotoxicology* **21**, 189–194.

Thompson, R. S., Hess, D. L., Binkerd, P. E., and Hendrickx, A. G. (1981). The effects of prenatal diethylstilbestrol exposure on the genitalia of pubertal Macaca mulatta. II. Male offspring. *J Reprod Med* **26**, 309–316.

Thurston, D. L., Middelkamp, J. N., and Mason, E. (1955). The late effects of lead poisoning. *J Pediatr* **47**, 413–423.

Tokuomi, H., Okajima, T., Kanai, J. *et al.* (1961). Minamata disease. *World Neurol* **2**, 536–545.

Tuthill, R. W. (1996). Hair lead levels related to children's classroom attention-deficit behavior. *Arch Environ Health* **51**, 214–220.

U.S. Department of Education (2005). Office of Special Education & Rehabilitative Services, Office of Special Education, 26th Annual (2004) Report to Congress on the Implementation of the Individuals with Disabilities Education Act, Vol 1, Washington, D.C.

Vreugdenhil, H. J. I., Lanting, C. I., Mulder, P. G. H., Boersma, R., and Weisglas-Kuperus, N. (2002a). Effects of prenatal PCB and dioxin background exposure on cognitive and motor abilities in Dutch children at school age. *J Pediatr* **140**, 48–56.

Vreugdenhil, H. J. I., Slijper, F. M. E., Mulder, P. G. H., and Weisglas-Kuperus, N. (2002b). Effects of perinatal exposure to PCBs and dioxins on play behavior in Dutch children at school age. *Environ Health Perspect* **110**, A593–A598.

Vreugdenhil, H. J., Mulder, P. G., Emmen, H. H., and Weisglas-Kuperus, N. (2004). Effects of perinatal exposure to PCBs on neuropsychological functions in the Rotterdam cohort at 9 years of age. *Neuropsychology* **18**, 185–193.

Walkowiak, J., Altmann, L., Krämer, U. *et al.* (1998). Cognitive and sensorimotor functions in 6-year-old children in relation to lead and mercury levels: adjustment for intelligence and contrast sensitivity in computerized testing. *Neurotoxicol Teratol* **20**, 511–521.

Walkowiak, J., Wiener, J.-A., Fastabend, A. *et al.* (2001). Environmental exposure to polychlorinated biphenyls and quality of the home environment: effects on psychodevelopment in early childhood. *Lancet* **358**, 1602–1607.

Watts, E. S. and Gavan, J. A. (1982). Postnatal growth of monkeys: the problem of the adolescent spurt. *Hum Biol* **54**, 53–70.

Weiss, B. (2000). Vulnerability of children and the developing brain to neurotoxic hazards. *Environ Health Perspect* **108**, 375–381.

Winneke, G. and Kraemer, V. (1984). Neuropsychological effects of lead in children: interaction with social background variables. *Neuropsychobiology* **11**, 195–202.

Winneke, G., Brockhaus, A., and Baltissen, R. (1977). Neurobehavioral and systemic effects of long-term blood lead elevation in rats. I: Discrimination learning and open-field behavior. *Arch Toxicol* **37**, 247–263.

Winneke, G., Hrdina, K., and Brockhaus, A. (1982). Neuropsychological studies in children with elevated tooth-lead concentration. *Int Arch Occup Environ Health* **51**, 169–183.

Winneke, G., Kraemer, V., Brockhaus, A. *et al.* (1983). Neuropsychologic studies in children with elevated tooth-lead concentrations. II: Extended study. *Int Arch Occup Environ Health* **51**, 231–252.

Winneke, G., Brockhaus, A., Collet, W., and Kraemer, V. (1989). Modulation of lead-induced performance deficit in children by varying signal rate in a serial choice reaction task. *Neurotoxicol Teratol* **11**, 587–592.

Winneke, G., Bucholski, A., Heinzow, B. *et al.* (1998). Developmental neurotoxicity of polychlorinated biphenyls (PCBs): Cognitive and psychomotor functions in 7-month old children. *Toxicol Lett* **102/103**, 423–428.

Winneke, G., Kraemer, U., Walkowiak, J. *et al.* (2002). Delay of neurobehavioral development following pre- and postnatal PCB exposure: Persistent or reversible? The Second PCB Workshop – Recent advances in the environmental toxicology and health effects of PCBs. Brno, Czech Republic, May 2002. Abstract published in *Naunyn-Schmiedeberg's Arch Pharmacol* **365** (suppl), Heidelberg: Springer-Verlag.

Worlein, J. M. and Sackett, G. P. (1997). Social development in nursery-reared pigtailed macaques (*Macaca nemestrina*). *Am J Primatol* **41**, 23–35.

Yamamura, K., Terayama, K., Yamamoto, N., Kohyama, A., and Kishi, R. (1989). Effects of acute lead acetate exposure on adult guinea pigs: electrophysiological study of the inner ear. *Fundam Appl Toxicol* **13**, 509–515.

Yu, M. L., Hsu, C. C., Guo, Y. L., Lai, T. J., Chen, S. J., and Luo, J. M. (1994). Disordered behavior in the early-born Taiwan Yucheng children. *Chemosphere* **29**, 2413–2422.

Yule, W., Lansdown, R., Millar, I., and Urbanowicz, M. (1981). The relationship between blood lead concentration, intelligence, and attainment in a school population: a pilot study. *Dev Med Child Neurol* **23**, 567–576.

Zenick, H., Rodriquez, W., Ward, J., and Elkington, B. (1978). Influence of prenatal and postnatal lead exposure on discrimination learning in rats. *Pharmacol Biochem Behav* **8**, 347–350.

CHAPTER 15

Future Directions: Assisted Reproductive Technologies as Tools for Creating Nonhuman Primate Models of Developmental Disability

Eric S. Hayes, Eliza C. Curnow, and Jennifer C. Potter

INTRODUCTION

Biological model systems that support descriptive pathology based on gene–environment interactions and span the spectrum from pathogenesis to clinical phenotype are required for basic scientific and clinically meaningful study of developmental disabilities. Developmental disabilities are often complex pathologies that exhibit significant genetic, epigenetic and environmental variation. Because no one model system can adequately address all input and output variables, a wide variety of model systems are used to dissect out specific mechanisms relevant to a given affliction.

Simple organisms such as *Saccharomyces cerevisiae, Caenorhabditis elegans* and *Drosophila melanogaster* are very useful for understanding molecular and biochemical features of developmental disabilities that exhibit genetic abnormalities in one or a limited number of highly conserved genes (Balakumaran *et al.*, 2000; Menzel *et al.*, 2004; Zarnescu *et al.*, 2005). Rodent models amenable to gene knockin, knockout, and knockdown on a variety of homogeneous genetic backgrounds have proven extremely useful in generating phenotypic and modifier gene data for a variety of developmental disorders (Bakker and Oostra, 2003; Errijgers and Kooy, 2004). Nonhuman primates represent exceptional clinically relevant model systems with which to study complex behavioral consequences of developmental disabilities and potential therapies. Primate models are also useful for studying susceptibility to epigenetic and environmental influences on disability.

Primate Models of Children's Health and Developmental Disabilities
Copyright © 2008 by Elsevier Inc. All rights of reproduction in any form reserved.

Despite their unique status as models of human developmental disabilities, non-human primates exist largely as outbred populations and are currently not amenable to genetic modifications using techniques widely available in rodents and other mammalian species. Experimental procedures that can (a) reduce or elimi-nate background genetic variation between individual nonhuman primates and (b) support selected genetic modifications of the nonhuman primate genome that are transmissible through the germline will help expand the scope and relevance of nonhuman primate model systems used to study the pathogenesis, management and treatment of human developmental disabilities.

Assisted reproductive technologies (ARTs) encompass an enormous array of skills from both basic sciences and clinical medicine, span the spectrum of most species used for scientific experimentation and cover molecular to integrated sys-tems approaches to reproductive biology. Advances in embryology and stem cell-based ARTs are directly responsible for the generation of genetically modified and genetically identical mammals (Meissner and Jaenisch, 2006) and have had a large impact on progress in rodent models of developmental disability (Bakker and Oostra, 2003). Thus development and application of ARTs in nonhuman primates represents a promising avenue for expanded use of nonhuman primate models of developmental disabilities. Herein we describe the current state of the nonhuman primate embryology and embryonic stem cell-based ARTs, our own work with embryo twinning and embryonic stem cells and the potential impact of these non-human primate ARTs on the field of developmental disability research.

BRIEF HISTORY AND STATUS OF NONHUMAN PRIMATE ARTS

Embryology and stem cell-based ARTs in nonprimate mammalian species long predated (Meissner and Jaenisch, 2006) the birth of Louise Brown in 1978 (Steptoe and Edwards, 1978), the first human baby produced by *in vitro* fertilization (IVF) (Figure 15.1). In 1984, 6 years after Louise Brown, the first nonhuman primate derived from IVF-produced embryos was born (Bavister *et al.*, 1984). Since 1984 the progress of nonhuman primate ARTs has followed progress of human ARTs related to embryo production, *in vitro* culture, and cryopreservation. Live-born nonhuman primates were produced from frozen–thawed embryos and the use of intracytoplasmic sperm injection (ICSI), a technique whereby sperm are injected directly into mature oocytes using a fine glass pipette, in 1988 and 1998, respec-tively 4 and 6 years after successful conduct of the same procedures in humans (Figure 15.1).

There are, however, two notable exceptions. First, in 1995–1996 embryonic stem cells were derived from blastocyst stage embryos of two species of nonhuman primate (Thomson *et al.*, 1995, 1996), one of which is an Old World species of monkey sharing greater than 95% genetic identity with humans. Human embryonic

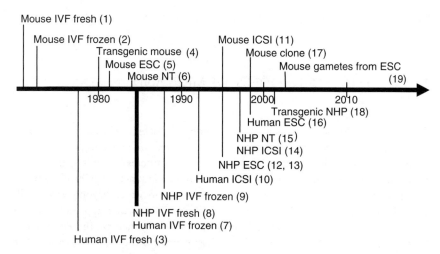

FIGURE 15.1   A brief history of nonhuman primate (NHP) assisted reproductive technologies (ARTs) including *in vitro* fertilization (IVF), intracytoplasmic sperm injection (ICSI), embryonic stem cell (ESC) development, nuclear transfer (NT), and transgenesis. "Fresh" indicates the use of fresh embryos. "Frozen" indicates the use of frozen/thawed embryos. Selected mouse and human ARTs are included for comparative purposes. Numbers in parentheses indicate the relative order of ART occurrence over time.

stem cells were derived by the same group using similar techniques, but not until 1998 (Thomson *et al.*, 1998). Second, in 1997, live born nonhuman primate offspring were produced using nuclear transfer (NT), a technique that involves injection of a diploid cell into an oocyte that has had the genetic material removed (Meng *et al.*, 1997). The oocyte is believed to reprogram the nucleus of the injected cell back to its embryonic state. Where successful reprogramming has occurred, the donated cell then acts as a full diploid content of DNA, replacing DNA that would normally be provided by sperm and oocyte. This technique serves as the basis of animal cloning (Wilmut *et al.*, 1997). This technique can also be used to produce transgenic animals in situations where a genetic modification can be made to the donor cell and maintained throughout subsequent development following nuclear transfer (Landry *et al.*, 2005).

Ethical and legal considerations dictate that NT procedures will not be applied to humans in the near future, if at all. Therefore, although advances in human ARTs continue to serve as the model for basic gamete biology and embryology that support nonhuman primate ARTs (e.g. ovarian stimulation, embryo culture and embryo cryopreservation) application of advanced ARTs in nonhuman primates is now poised to parallel advances in other domestic species and rodents. To this end a transgenic nonhuman primate was produced in 2001 using virus-mediated gene transfer (Chan *et al.*, 2001) and several groups are now actively involved in developing methods that aim to support nonhuman primate cloning and transgenesis using NT (Mitalipov *et al.*, 2002a, 2002b; Ng *et al.*, 2004; Simerly *et al.*, 2004; Zhou *et al.*, 2006).

ARTS AND DISEASE MODELS: OF MICE AND MONKEYS

The utility of rodents as models of developmental disabilities is largely driven by two key factors: (a) reduced genetic variation in inbred rodent strains and (b) introduction of gene modifications that are expressed in gametes (germline) and can be passed onto the next generation using normal breeding practices. Germline transgenesis is conducted using pronuclear microinjection or embryonic stem cell-derived chimeras (Sigmund, 1993; Stewart, 1993). The former approach involves injection of modified DNA directly into the zygote formed by the coupling of sperm and oocyte DNA before cellular division within the embryo begins. The latter approach involves aggregation of embryonic stem cells that have been genetically modified with embryos that have been rendered to contain twice the normal DNA content (tetraploid) to produce a chimeric embryo. Under these conditions the embryonic stem cells generate all of the cells that will contribute to the fetus whereas the tetraploid cells will only contribute to extra-embryonic anatomical structures that support embryo implantation (e.g. placenta).

Although both wild-type and transgenic cloned mice have been produced using NT techniques (Meissner and Jaenisch, 2006), when compared with pronuclear microinjection and embryonic stem cell chimeras this approach is considered relatively inefficient for routine production of models of genetic disease (Wakayama, 2007; Melo *et al.*, 2007).

Inbreeding can and does occur in both wild and captive nonhuman primate populations (Williams–Blangero *et al.*, 2002; Bolter and Zihlman, 2003). Inbreeding is used infrequently on a very small scale in captive situations to generate animals with known genotypes (Rogers and Hixson, 1997). However, this practice is not routinely employed on a larger scale given the deleterious effect of inbreeding depression on reproductive fitness (Williams–Blangero *et al.*, 2002). Although pronuclear microinjection is theoretically possible in nonhuman primates, to date this has not been attempted. It is not considered practical given the low efficiency of germline transmission of functional genes using this approach in large mono-ovulatory species (Melo *et al.*, 2007) and the relatively long delay to sexual maturity in nonhuman primates (~4 years) compared with rodents (~28 days) (Karsch *et al.*, 1973). In rodent species such as mice uniparental inheritance of the centrosomes that control proper allocation of DNA to sister cells during cell division (Schatten *et al.*, 1985) allows for production of true tetraploid embryos and ensures that selectivity of embryonic stem cell contribution to the fetus can be achieved by production of embryonic stem cell-tetraploid chimeras (Stewart, 1993). Higher mammalian species including nonhuman primates exhibit biparental inheritance of centrosomes (Sathananthan *et al.*, 1997; Sathananthan, 1997) and are thus less likely to form true tetraploids (Curnow *et al.*, 2000) and subsequent chimeric embryos that are capable of full-term development. Although NT has been attempted with limited success in nonhuman primates, functional transgenic and cloned nonhuman primates have not yet been produced (Wolf *et al.*, 1999; Chan *et al.*, 2001).

Despite the seemingly insurmountable obstacles that limit experimental reduction in background genetic variation and introduction of defined genetic modifications in nonhuman primates, recent advances in nonhuman primate ARTs hold promise for production of identical animals and effective gene targeting. The latter will be required for improving the quality of nonhuman primate models of developmental disability. Advances in embryo and embryonic stem cell production and manipulation are at the heart of nonhuman primate ARTs and further progress in both these areas will be required for large-scale production of identical and genetically modified nonhuman primates.

IDENTICAL ANIMALS: WHY CLONE, WHEN YOU CAN TWIN?

Since the birth of Dolly in 1997 (Wilmut *et al.*, 1997) more than 11 mammalian species have been cloned using NT techniques (Fulka and Fulka, 2007). The promise of cloning for large-scale production of genetically identical animals has not been realized and today cloning efficiencies in mice remain below 5% (Wakayama, 2007). Nonhuman primates are no exception and appear to be less well suited to cloning than other mammalian species (Simerly *et al.*, 2003; Chen *et al.*, 2006). There are only a handful of groups world-wide that have the skill and resources required to routinely perform NT and cloning experiments in nonhuman primates (Mitalipov *et al.*, 2002a, 2002b; Simerly *et al.*, 2003; Ng *et al.*, 2004; Zhou *et al.*, 2006). A review of NT and cloning efficiencies by these groups over the past decade indicates approximately 50% cloned embryo production per oocyte, less than 10% pregnancy rate for surrogate embryo recipients, less than 1% live born per embryo transferred and no live-born clones produced to date.

Technical difficulties and efficiency rates are only two of the limitations to widespread use of cloning. In species where true cloned animals can be produced, the cloned offspring normally exhibit heteroplasmy for mitochondrial DNA content (donor cell and recipient cytoplast), a situation that may produce abnormalities in cellular energetics and metabolism (St John *et al.*, 2004). Furthermore, individual donor cells used for NT may not be "reprogrammed" to the same extent and differences in methylation status or "imprinting" of genes in batches of clones has been observed (Mann *et al.*, 2003). Cloned embryos exhibit very low implantation rates as a result of problems with placentation and are often born with gross physical abnormalities (Constant *et al.*, 2006). Very recent studies have shown that the very subtle genetic and epigenetic changes in otherwise healthy cloned offspring may have a large impact on phenotypic variation (Landry *et al.*, 2005; Tamashiro *et al.*, 2007). Taken together, the limitations of cloning at its current level suggest that this will not be a viable approach for production of identical nonhuman primates in the foreseeable future.

Our philosophy has been that monozygotic twin nonhuman primates represent an ideal model system for the study of human disease. Monozygotic twinning occurs naturally in primate species including humans. Live-born twin offspring have been produced from mouse, goat, pig, sheep, and cow embryos produced and manipulated in an *in vitro* setting (Tsunoda and McLaren, 1983; Willadsen and Godke, 1984; Nagashima *et al.*, 1989; Nowshari and Holtz, 1993). It can be argued that monozygotic twins exhibit phenotypic variance (Singh *et al.*, 2002) and often complete discordance with respect to heritable diseases (Weksberg *et al.*, 2002; Bestor, 2003). However, the vast majority of literature relating to monozygotic twins indicate high levels of genetic similarity, high levels of concordance for genetic traits and low levels of discordance (Gringras and Chen, 2001). In many cases discordance is attributable to epigenetic or environmental factors as opposed to genetic factors (Kato *et al.*, 2005) and/or the developmental stage at which twinning takes place (Singh *et al.*, 2002). Some ARTs employ gametes from known genetic stocks for the *in vitro* production of monozygotic twin embryos at defined developmental stages and defined embryo culture and transfer regimens. These represent a novel approach for development of nonhuman primate model systems for the study of experimental manipulations related to developmental disability.

MONOZYGOTIC TWIN NONHUMAN PRIMATES

The techniques employed to produce twin monkeys are usually one of two varieties: (a) disaggregation of cleavage stage embryos followed by re-aggregation of individual blastomeres into twin sets and (b) splitting of blastocyst stage embryos to produce twin pairs (Figure 15.2). The former approach offers the benefits of twin embryo production at a defined developmental stage with known equivalence of cell content in twin pairs. The drawbacks to this approach include *in vitro* culture and transfer of zona pellucida-free embryos. The latter approach benefits from robust culture of zona-intact embryos and the known developmental competence of the embryo producing the twin pairs. However, the latter approach suffers a significant drawback in terms of unknown equivalence in cellular content in twin pairs as well as the same limitations in zona-free embryo transfer observed for the former approach.

To date there are only three published reports of monozygotic twinning efforts in nonhuman primates (Chan *et al.*, 2000; Mitalipov *et al.*, 2002a; Schramm and Paprocki, 2004). All of those efforts were conducted in a single species of Old World monkey, *Macaca mulatta*, with transfer of twin embryos occurring in only two of the three studies. The studies by Chan *et al.* (2000) and Mitalipov *et al.* (2002a)

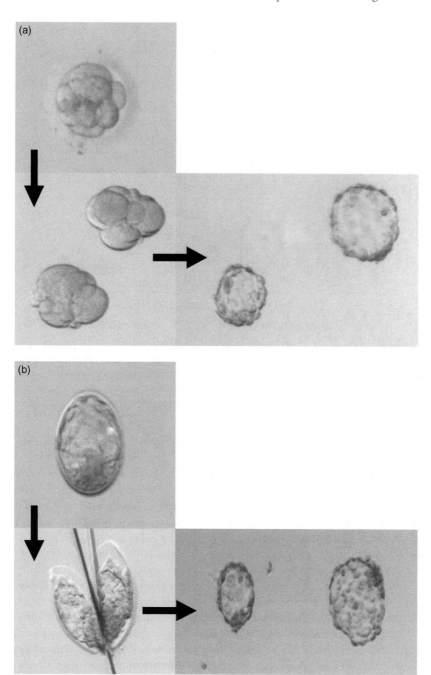

FIGURE 15.2   Two common methods for producing identical twin nonhuman primate embryos. (a) Embryo disaggregation and re-aggregation involves the separation of a single embryo into individual blastomeres, re-aggregation of individual blastomeres into twin pairs and culture to the blastocyst stage prior to transfer. (b) Embryo splitting involves bisection of a single blastocyst stage embryo through the middle of the inner cell mass to produce twin pairs that are allowed to re-expand in culture prior to transfer. (See Plate 5 for the color version of this figure.)

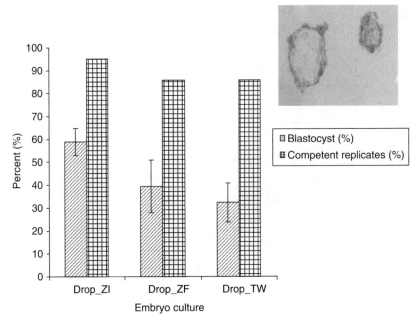

FIGURE 15.3 The effects of micro-drop culture (drop) of twin embryos on blastocyst development rates (% of cleaved embryos; diagonal stripe) of zona-intact (ZI), zona-free (ZF), and twin (TW) embryos produced by *in vitro* fertilization. Data are expressed as mean ± SEM for 57–399 embryos from 7–21 replicates. The proportion of blastocyst competent replicates is expressed as a percentage (cross-hatch). Inset shows the discordant development of identical twin embryo pairs using these techniques. (See Plate 6 for the color version of this figure.)

employed embryo transfer with twin embryos derived from early cleavage stage embryos that were cultured in homologous or heterologous zona to facilitate embryo transfer to the oviducts while avoiding the potential for ectopic pregnancy. Mitalipov *et al.* (2002b) also employed blastocyst splitting and transfer to the uterus. This method was associated with higher pregnancy and live-born rates than the studies with early cleavage embryos and oviductal transfer. The study by Schramm and Paprocki (2004) utilized early embryo disaggregation and re-aggregation but did not involve transfer of twin embryos to recipients. Twin embryos were cultured as aggregates with presumed tetraploid or asynchronous embryos in an attempt to drive cell allocation and increase cell numbers in resulting twin embryos. However, given that mammals with biparental inheritance of centrosomes do not form true tetraploids (see above) the rationale for that approach is not obvious.

Our own work involves the use of *Macaca fascicularis* monkeys and early cleavage embryo disaggregation and re-aggregation techniques to produce twin embryo pairs. Much of our work has been focused on the development of *in vitro* embryo culture techniques that support robust development of zona-intact whole embryos (ZI), zona-free whole embryos (ZF), and zona-free twin embryo pairs (TW) to the blastocyst stage and techniques for transfer of blastocyst stage twin embryos to the uterus of surrogate recipient females. As a summary of our experience, we found that our best protocol for embryo production using IVF and our best culture system-drop culture in sequential culture medium worked very well for normal zona-intact whole embryos. This produced a 55% blastocyst rate with 90% blastocyst competent replicates. The same culture techniques were less useful for zona-free control whole embryos and twin embryos produced by blastomere disaggregation and re-aggregation (Figure 15.3). Under these conditions we often observed very discordant size development of twin embryo pairs, with high levels of blastomere fragmentation and apoptosis (Figure 15.3, inset).

Therefore, we set out to develop a novel embryo production and culture system that would improve twin embryo derivation rates and morphological quality to rival control zona-intact embryos. The approach addressed four key issues. First, to improve the numbers of early cleavage embryos available for twinning, we employed ICSI in preference to IVF to avoid potential male factor effects causing fertilization failure. Second, we added a novel combination of cell surface adhesion molecules to the isolated blastomeres to improve re-aggregation and prevent blastomere fragmentation and apoptosis. Third, we examined the utility of exogenous cellular mitogens to stimulate cell growth in the twin embryo pairs. Finally, we developed and employed a novel synthetic micro-well culture system to provide a "pseudo zona-like" environment for each embryo during subsequent culture. The results of those efforts are summarized in Figure 15.4. The key outcome of those studies was that we were able to (a) generate blastocyst development rates that were equivalent to or greater than zona-intact and zona-free whole embryo control blastocyst rates and (b) improve the percentage of blastocyst competent replicate experiments in which pairs of viable twin embryos were obtained. Furthermore, twin embryo morphology was improved to resemble control embryos (Figure 15.5a–c). Dual staining of control and twin embryos to facilitate cell counts (Figure 15.5d) indicated that twin embryos showed good inner cell mass development and, on average, had more than half the expected number of the cells found in control zona intact whole embryos (Table 15.1).

The only reliable test of twin embryo viability and quality is production of live-born offspring. In developing intrauterine blastocyst embryo transfer techniques for *Macaca fascicularis* we found that target serum hormone profiles, estradiol below 100 pg/mL and progesterone at or above 3.0 ng/mL, at the time of embryo transfer provide the best indication of ovulatory and pregnancy competent cycles in recipient females. We also found that in the absence of daily serum hormone profiles, the surrogate measure of ovulation using the day of ovulation/cycle length ratio (Dukelow et al., 1979) did not accurately predict ovulatory cycles (59%). Thus, target serum hormone profiles and pregnancies with twin embryo transfers were difficult to achieve using this approach (Table 15.2). To circumvent this problem we developed a modified approach to urinary estrone–glucuronide measurements using a human urinary dipstick test kit.

Application of these methods resulted in very accurate detection of ovulatory cycles with the desired serum hormone profiles and an accompanying increase in

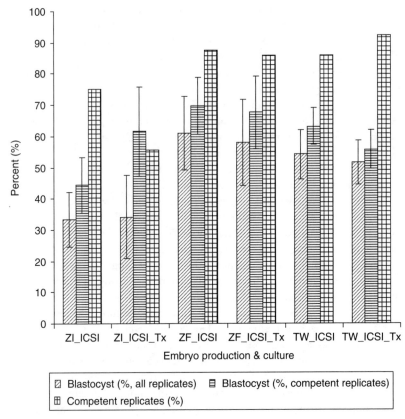

FIGURE 15.4   The effects of embryo culture media supplemented with pharmacological agents designed to increase cell numbers (Tx) on blastocyst development rates (% of cleaved embryos) of zona-intact (ZI), zona-free (ZF), and twin (TW) embryos produced by intracytoplasmic sperm injection (ICSI). All embryos were cultured in a novel synthetic micro-well device, in culture medium supplemented with a novel combination of cellular adhesion molecules designed to improve blastomere re-aggregation and prevent blastomere apoptosis. Data are expressed as mean ± SEM for 27–70 embryos from 7–14 replicates. Blastocyst development rates are expressed for all replicates (diagonal stripe) and for blastocyst competent replicates only (horizontal stripe). The proportion of blastocyst competent replicates is expressed as a percentage (cross-hatch).

pregnancy rates for twin embryos (Table 15.2). We are currently awaiting the birth of two animals that may be the first live-born identical twin primates produced using these techniques. Although live-born identical twins are not yet on the ground, pregnancy and live birth rates for demi-embryos are 6-fold and 20-fold higher, respectively, compared with the same measures obtained for NT-derived nonhuman primate embryos (Wolf *et al.*, 2004). Thus, improvements to nonhuman primate embryology-based ARTs will ensure that larger scale production of live-born identical twins is achieved in the foreseeable future.

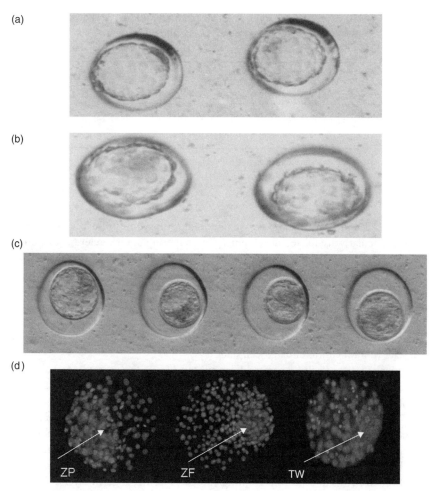

FIGURE 15.5   Size and morphology of twin blastocyst embryos cultured using a novel synthetic micro-well device in the absence (a) or presence (b) of mitogen, and (c) zona-intact control embryos cultured in the absence of mitogen. Although the image sizes are different the micro-well dimensions are the same in each image (200 μm). Cellular development of zona-intact (ZP), zona-free (ZF), and twin (TW) embryos produced using the novel embryo production platform is indicated in (d). Arrows indicate inner cell mass cells as determined by differential staining with Hoescht and propidium iodide. (See Plate 7 for the color version of this figure.)

NONHUMAN PRIMATE EMBRYONIC STEM CELLS

Many of the common mechanisms for production of transgenic rodents are not applicable to nonhuman primates and somatic cell NT has many limitations and potential confounders. Thus, other methods of producing gene modifications related to developmental disabilities are required for nonhuman primate species.

TABLE 15.1   Total (inner cell mass and trophectoderm) cell
counts for zona-intact and twin embryos cultured in a novel
synthetic micro-well system

Embryo	Control		Treated	
	N	Total cells	N	Total cells
Zona–intact	10	148 ± 13	7	148 ± 9
Twin	11	88 ± 12	8	80 ± 7

Data are expressed as mean ± SEM for a given number of embryos (N).

Self-renewal and pluripotency are attributes of embryonic stem cells that make
them particularly useful for developing gene targeting studies relevant to human
disease (Friel *et al.*, 2006). Self-renewal of embryonic stem cells ensures that experimentally induced gene modifications can be actively selected for and monitored
for proper expression/function in the absence of genetic changes related to cellular
differentiation and/or senescence. The pluripotent nature of embryonic stem cells
allows for detailed study and manipulation of gene function and susceptibility to
epigenetic and environmental control during directed differentiation from the stem
cell state to a fully differentiated cell state.

Embryonic stem cells generated from whole *Macaca mulatta* and *Macaca fascicularis* embryos have played a critical role in developing nonhuman primate stem cell
sciences (Umeda *et al.*, 2006; Fujimoto *et al.*, 2006; Byrne *et al.,* 2006; Rajesh *et al.*,
2007). We have generated embryonic stem cell lines from whole embryos of *Macaca
fascicularis,* and for the very first time *Macaca nemestrina*, using standard techniques
for embryonic stem cell derivation. The cell lines express the standard battery of
cellular markers associated with cellular pluripotency (Figure 15.6), and on differentiation from tissue types representing the three primary germ layers (data not
shown). We were pleasantly surprised by the ability of inner cell masses isolated
from zona-free and twin *Macaca fascicularis* embryos cultured in our novel micro-
well format to develop into embryonic stem cell lines at very high rates compared
with pronase-treated whole embryos (Figure 15.7). Embryonic stem cell lines generated from twin embryos also exhibited the cellular markers characteristic of cellular pluripotency (data not shown).

One of our goals was to use nonhuman primate embryonic stem cells to generate transgenic animals without using NT. We initially conducted proof of principle
experiments to determine the ability of embryonic stem cells to contribute to the
inner cell mass of chimeric embryos produced by aggregation. First we labeled the
embryonic stem cells with a mitochondrial specific marker dye (panel 1, Figure
15.8) and aggregated the marked cells with normally developing zona-free
embryos (panel 2, Figure 15.8) using the same techniques for cell aggregation and

TABLE 15.2   Improvements in twin embryo transfer outcomes for whole and twin embryos in *Macaca fascicularis* when recipient females are screened based on urinary estrone-conjugate measurements as opposed to use of surrogate measures of ovulation and receptivity

	Embryos transferred	Transfer (day of cycle)	Estradiol (pg/mL)	Progesterone (ng/mL)	Ovulatory cycles (%)	Pregnant cycles (%)	Live born
Whole embryo[a] (n = 22)	2.1 ± 0.1	17 ± 0.3	118 ± 17	2.5 ± 0.4	13/22 (59)	4/13 (31)	4
Twin embryo[a] (n = 5)	2.2 ± 0.2	17 ± 0.2	150 ± 20	1.5 ± 2	3/5 (60)	0/3 (0)	0
Twin embryo[b] (n = 11)	2.5 ± 0.1	17 ± 0.4	44 ± 7	4.1 ± 0.6	11/11 (100)	4/6 (75)*	NA

Data are expressed as mean ± SEM or proportion (percentage).

Based on indirect measures of ovulation and receptivity (a) and for twin embryo transfers based on quantitative screening methods (b). The asterisk (*) indicates that four of six recipients exhibited implantation bleeding (15–21 days). Two recipients may carry identical twins and one recipient may have a fetus with an MHC-compatible embryonic stem cell line, with term delivery still pending.

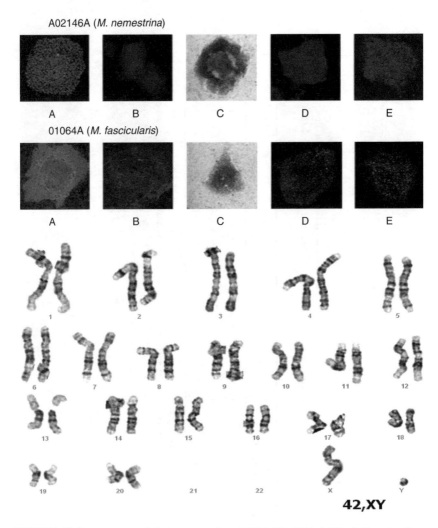

FIGURE 15.6   Expression of pluripotent markers OCT-4 (A), SSEA-4 (B), alkaline phosphatase (AP) (C), TRA-1–81 (D) and TRA-1–60 (E) in *M. nemestrina* animal A02146A and *M. fascicularis* animal 01064A embryonic stem cells lines. Cells were fixed and exposed to primary antibodies directed against the cellular markers of pluripotency and resolved using FITC-conjugated secondary antibodies selective for the primary antibody sequence. Negative controls were exposed to conjugated secondary antibody in the absence of primary antibody (data not shown), positive controls were exposed to nonselective primary antibodies in the presence of FITC-conjugated secondary antibody (data not shown). SSEA-1 was negative for both *M. fascicularis* and *M. nemestrina* embryonic stem cell lines (data not shown). Images were taken at 10× magnification under light and UV microscopy and captured on a digital camera. The karyogram image represents the normal 42,XY karyotype for the 01064A line. (See Plate 8 for the color version of this figure.)

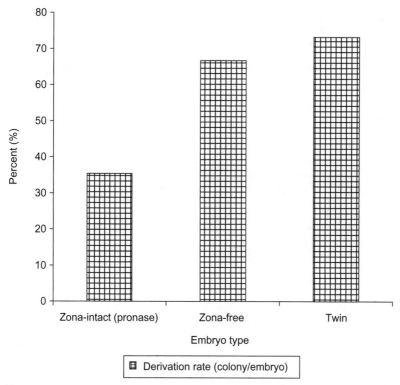

FIGURE 15.7 Efficiency of embryonic stem cell line derivation using whole zona-intact embryos subjected to pronase treatment or zona-free and twin embryos grown in the absence of zonae and spared treatment with pronase prior to inner cell mass isolation. Data are expressed as the proportion (3–34 embryos) of embryonic stem cell lines forming per embryo subjected to inner cell mass isolation.

embryo culture developed for the production of twin embryos (panels 3–4, Figure 15.8). Fluorescent microscopic images of aggregated embryos that developed to the blastocyst stage indicated that the marked embryonic stem cells were integrating with the developing embryo (Figure 15.9). Subsequent analysis using confocal microscopy indicated that the embryonic stem cells had integrated to the desired location within the inner cell mass of the chimeric embryo (Figure 15.10). These experiments demonstrated high blastocyst development rates (53%) and a high proportion of blastocyst competent replicates (100%). This indicates that this approach has good potential for use in nonhuman primate gene manipulation experiments. Thus, the ability to generate twin embryos and embryonic stem cell lines from one half of a twin embryo pair opens a wide range of possibilities for modeling developmental disorders in nonhuman primates.

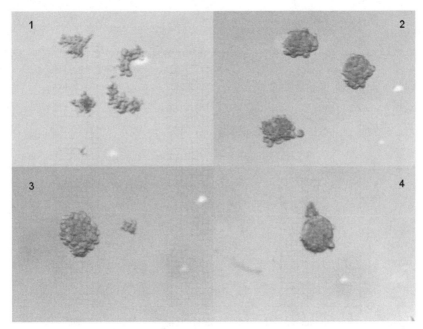

FIGURE 15.8 Embryonic stem cell aggregation with whole embryos to produce chimeric embryos. First embryonic stem cells are labeled with a fluorescent dye that specifically stains mitochondria (1). Compacting morula stage embryos are prepared (2). The embryonic stem cells and embryos are aggregated in the presence of cellular adhesion molecules designed to improve cellular aggregation and prevent cellular apoptosis (3) to produce the chimeric embryo (4). (See Plate 9 for the color version of this figure.)

TWIN AND EMBRYONIC STEM CELL-BASED MODELS OF DEVELOPMENTAL DISORDERS

There are at least four model scenarios where twin and embryonic stem cell-based ARTs may be useful for modeling developmental disorders in nonhuman primates. The first scenario involves the use of identical twin animals. Exposure of dams carrying twin embryos to various teratogens would be a very useful model to study environmental and epigenetic mechanisms responsible for alteration in fetal gene expression and the developmental consequences of those exposures. Similar experiments conducted in post-natal twin pairs could be useful for defining specific developmental periods where sensitivity to a particular teratogen is altered and to study therapeutic approaches to environmental and epigenetic causes of developmental disorders (see Chapters 4, 6, and 8).

The second scenario involves the use of embryonic stem cells to study gene expression on cellular phenotypes in undifferentiated and differentiated states. By producing embryonic stem cell lines from each half of a twin embryo pair one gains

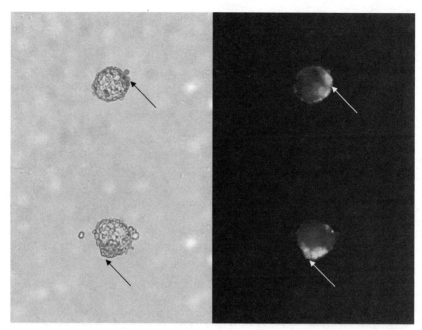

FIGURE 15.9   The ability of labeled embryonic stem cells (orange) to integrate with developing embryos (not labeled) and to allocate in what appears to be the inner cell mass (arrows). Images on the left are light microscope images, images on the right are fluorescent images of the same embryos obtained using filters selective for the mitochondrial dye. (See Plate 10 for the color version of this figure.)

the opportunity to make genetic modifications to one line while maintaining the other line in its wild-type state. The gene modification can then be compared to wild-type during extended undifferentiated culture or examined in detail follow-ing directed differentiation into generalized (e.g. embryoid body) or specific cell types (e.g. neurons). This type of model system will be particularly useful to study the molecular biology of trinucleotide repeat disorders such as spinocerebellar ataxia, fragile-X, and Huntington's disease (Lorincz *et al.*, 2004). Using this system, modifier genes and epigenetic controls that regulate trinucleotide repeat stability and expansion can be examined, as well as potential therapeutic strategies aimed at controlling repeat expansion and methylation status.

A third modeling scenario involves the use of twin embryo pairs to produce major histocompatibility complex (MHC)-compatible live-born offspring and embryonic stem cells. This type of model system would be particularly useful to study cell-based gene therapies for developmental disorders such as Cockayne and fragile-X syndromes where loss of protein expression/function is associated with the clinical phenotype (Hoogeveen *et al.*, 2002; Newman *et al.*, 2006). In this sce-nario the desired abnormality could be induced in the live-born offspring using gene/protein silencing technologies (e.g. small interfering RNA). The abnormality

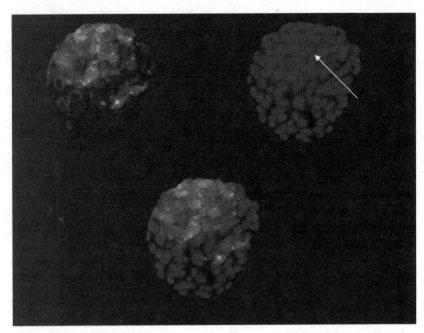

FIGURE 15.10 Confocal microscopy detail of the integration of labeled embryonic stem cells (orange, top left) within the inner cell mass (arrow, top right) of chimeric embryos. The merged image (bottom center) clearly shows the robust overlap of labeled cells within the inner cell mass. (See Plate 11 for the color version of this figure.)

could then be rescued by transfer of undifferentiated embryonic stem cells or differentiated cell types derived from embryonic stem cells that produce and express the protein of interest. This type of model system would also be useful for tolerability, long-term safety, and efficacy testing of artificial chromosome-mediated gene delivery and organ-selective gene targeting through the use of tissue-specific promoters and enhancers (Pimenta and Levitt, 2005).

A fourth experimental scenario would use genetically modified embryonic stem cells to introduce germline-stable genetic modifications related to a given developmental disorder. In this example a live-born animal would be produced with one-half of a twin embryo pair, while the other half would be used to create genetically modified embryonic stem cells (knockin, knockout, knockdown). Those stem cells would then be aggregated with a developing embryo (see above) to produce a chimeric embryo harboring the affected gene. Ideally both control and genetically modified infants would be generated from embryonic stem cells aggregated with embryos produced by the same mother–father pairs to minimize potential procedural confounders and ensure homogeneity of genetic background. As an example, this system would be well suited for genomic, proteomic, morphological, and developmental comparisons of MHC-compatible wild-type animals with animals harboring selected loss-of-function genetic modifications such as fragile-X. The additional benefit of this approach is that when germline-stable genetic modifications are obtained, the changes could be maintained through normal breeding practices.

LIMITATIONS AND SUPPORT FOR THE ASSISTED REPRODUCTIVE TECHNOLOGIES

Advances in nonhuman primate ARTs can enhance the utility of nonhuman primates as one of the best preclinical models of developmental disabilities. However, there are limitations to the use of embryology and embryonic stem cell-based ARTs for the routine production of nonhuman primate models of developmental disorders. Application of advances in related ARTs and other fields of basic research and clinical medicine will be required to fulfill the potential of current ART practices.

One of the most obvious limitations to current practices is the low numbers of live-born offspring produced per embryo transfer despite very reasonable rates of embryo production. Better embryo transfer and surrogate recipient screening and management procedures will be required to increase production of live-born animals. Pharmacological manipulation of the recipient endometrium to ensure high rates of term delivery of multiple gestations is an avenue that we are pursuing to address this problem (Hayes *et al.*, 2004). In situations where small numbers of recipient animals are available for embryo transfer, development of twin embryo cryopreservation protocols will be required to ensure that all available transfer cycles are accompanied by viable twin embryo pairs at the appropriate time.

Many developmental disorders exhibit a sex bias (Bartley, 2006). Therefore, development of nonhuman primate model systems for these disorders should be accompanied by the ability to predetermine the sex of embryos produced for embryology and embryonic stem cell-based ARTs. Sex sorting of sperm is the most efficient way to achieve this goal. Sperm sex sorting has been successfully applied to domestic animal breeding programs (de Graaf *et al.*, 2007) and has been investigated for application to nonhuman primate captive breeding and conservation programs (O'Brien *et al.*, 2005a, 2005b). Successful development of these techniques, in combination with the application of ICSI to ensure selected sperm delivery to the oocyte, will have a great impact on our ability to produce gender specific models of developmental disorders. Long-term cryobanking of male genetic resources will also be required to ensure that transport-ready sources of sperm from normal animals and animals with naturally occurring genetic abnormalities (Garcia Arocena *et al.*, 2003) are available for ART applications at primate facilities throughout the world (VandeVoort, 2004).

Embryonic stem cells are the key to successful germline-stable gene targeting in nonhuman primates. Therefore, advances in gene targeting strategies that have been developed in other model systems and that address the issues of (a) positional effect, (b) gene silencing, (c) gene copy number, and (d) host–vector interactions will be crucial to advancing ART-derived nonhuman primate models of human developmental disabilities. Other related technologies such as small interfering RNA (Aigner, 2006) and inducible gene knockin and knockout may also prove useful for gene regulation in embryonic stem cells and for temporal and reversible gene regulation to facilitate the study of gene function during specific developmental periods (Pimenta and Levitt, 2005). Comparisons of embryonic stem cell aggregation chimeras and embryonic stem cell-based NT should be conducted and refined to determine an optimal system for stable germline transgenesis that can be managed with normal breeding practices.

SUMMARY

Developmental disorders encompass a broad range of genetic abnormalities that are subject to epigenetic and environmental modification. Simple nonmammalian organism and rodent model systems have proven extremely useful for the study of gene function related to developmental disability. However, for some developmental disorders, nonprimate orthologs of the affected human gene(s) may not exist. Furthermore, sensory modalities and functionally integrated physiological systems (e.g. immune system) that respond to and are affected by epigenetic and environmental influences are known to be quite different in primate than in nonprimate species. Given these differences, nonprimate models of developmental disabilities may exhibit vastly different phenotypes compared with the human condition.

Nonhuman primates share a high degree of genetic similarity to humans and are exceptional models for human physiology and disease. Unlike many nonprimate species, nonhuman primates also serve as outstanding models for complex behavioral analysis. Despite these attributes, copulation breeding of nonhuman primates, unlike inbred nonprimate species, does not allow for rigorous control of background genetic variation. Furthermore, selective modifications to the primate genome that allows for unambiguous study of developmental disabilities are not easily conducted in nonhuman primate species. ARTs represent novel tools that can be used to overcome these hurdles.

Twinning can be used to limit background genetic variation between control and experimental subjects. Although ART-derived live-born identical twins have not yet been produced, more than 20 live-born nonhuman primate offspring have been produced from half-embryos. Improvements in ART-based twin embryo production and recipient receptivity to twin embryo implantation will be required to ensure routine production of large numbers of viable identical twin animals. Nuclear transfer represents a promising approach for larger scale production of identical animals but currently suffers from a lack of efficiency and will require further development. Embryonic stem cells have been produced from three species of Old World nonhuman primates. Such cells represent the key to successful targeted gene modifications related to developmental disabilities. Advances in gene targeting for nonhuman primate embryonic stem cells, coupled with advances in embryology-based ART methods that support efficient introduction of selected gene modifications to the germline of nonhuman primate offspring, will provide novel clinically relevant tools for the study of developmental disabilities.

REFERENCES

Aigner, A. (2006). Delivery systems for the direct application of siRNAs to induce RNA interference (RNAi) in vivo. *J Biomed Biotechnol* **2006**, 71659.

Bakker, C. E. and Oostra, B. A. (2003). Understanding fragile X syndrome: insights from animal models. *Cytogenet Genome Res* **100**, 111–123.

Balakumaran, B. S., Freudenreich, C. H., and Zakian, V. A. (2000). CGG/CCG repeats exhibit orientation-dependent instability and orientation-independent fragility in *Saccharomyces cerevisiae*. *Hum Mol Genet* **9**, 93–100.

Bartley, J. J. (2006). An update on autism: science, gender, and the law. *Gend Med* **3**, 73–78.

Bavister, B. D., Boatman, D. E., Collins, K., Dierschke, D. J., and Eisele, S. G. (1984). Birth of rhesus monkey infant after in vitro fertilization and nonsurgical embryo transfer. *Proc Natl Acad Sci USA* **81**, 2218–2222.

Bestor, T. H. (2003). Imprinting errors and developmental asymmetry. *Philos Trans R Soc Lond B Biol Sci* **358**, 1411–1415.

Bolter, D. R. and Zihlman, A. L. (2003). Morphometric analysis of growth and development in wild-collected vervet monkeys (*Cercopithecus aethiops*) with implications for growth patterns across Old World monkeys, apes, and humans. *J Zool (Lond)* **260**, 99–110.

Byrne, J. A., Mitalipov, S. M., Clepper, L., and Wolf, D. P. (2006). Transcriptional profiling of rhesus monkey embryonic stem cells. *Biol Reprod* **75**, 908–915.

Chan, A. W., Dominko, T., Luetjens, C. M. *et al.* (2000). Clonal propagation of primate offspring by embryo splitting. *Science* **287**, 317–319.

Chan, A. W., Chong, K. Y., Martinovich, C., Simerly, C., and Schatten, G. (2001). Transgenic monkeys produced by retroviral gene transfer into mature oocytes. *Science* **291**, 309–312.

Chen, N., Liow, S. L., Yip, W. Y., Tan, L. G., Tong, G. Q., and Ng, S. C. (2006). Early development of reconstructed embryos after somatic cell nuclear transfer in a non-human primate. *Theriogenology* **66**, 1300–1306.

Constant, F., Guillomot, M., Heyman, Y. *et al.* (2006). Large offspring or large placenta syndrome? Morphometric analysis of late gestation bovine placentomes from somatic nuclear transfer pregnancies complicated by hydrallantois. *Biol Reprod* **75**, 122–130.

Curnow, E. C., Gunn, I. M., and Trounson, A. O. (2000). Electrofusion of two-cell bovine embryos for the production of tetraploid blastocysts in vitro. *Mol Reprod Dev* **56**, 372–377.

de Graaf, S. P., Evans, G., Maxwell, W. M., Cran, D. G., and O'Brien, J. K. (2007). Birth of offspring of pre-determined sex after artificial insemination of frozen-thawed, sex-sorted and re-frozen-thawed ram spermatoza. *Theriogenology* **67**, 391–398.

Dukelow, W. R., Grauwiler, J., and Bruggemann, S. (1979). Characteristics of the menstrual cycle in nonhuman primates. I. Similarities and dissimilarities between *Macaca fascicularis* and *Macaca arctoides*. *J Med Primatol* **8**, 39–47.

Errijgers, V. and Kooy, R. F. (2004). Genetic modifiers in mice: the example of the fragile X mouse model. *Cytogenet Genome Res* **105**, 448–454.

Friel, R., Fisher, D., and Hook, L. (2006). Embryonic stem cell technology: applications and uses in functional genomic studies. *Stem Cell Rev* **2**, 31–35.

Fujimoto, A., Mitalipov, S. M., Kuo, H. C., and Wolf, D. P. (2006). Aberrant genomic imprinting in rhesus monkey embryonic stem cells. *Stem Cells* **24**, 595–603.

Fulka, J. Jr and Fulka, H. (2007). Somatic cell nuclear transfer (SCNT) in mammals: the cytoplast and its reprogramming activities. *Adv Exp Med Biol* **591**, 93–102.

Garcia Arocena, D., Breece, K. E., and Hagerman, P. J. (2003). Distribution of CGG repeat sizes within the fragile X mental retardation 1 (FMR1) homologue in a non-human primate population. *Hum Genet* **113**, 371–376.

Gringras, P. and Chen, W. (2001). Mechanisms for differences in monozygous twins. *Early Hum Dev* **64**, 105–117.

Hayes, E. S., Curnow, E. C., Trounson, A. O., Danielson, L. A., and Unemori, E. N. (2004). Implantation and pregnancy following in vitro fertilization and the effect of recombinant human relaxin administration in *Macaca fascicularis*. *Biol Reprod* **71**, 1591–1597.

Hoogeveen, A. T., Willemsen, R. and Oostra, B. A. (2002). Fragile X syndrome, the fragile X related proteins, and animal models. *Microsc Res Tech* **57**, 148–155.

Karsch, F. J., Dierschke, D. J., and Knobil, E. (1973). Sexual differentiation of pituitary function: apparent difference bewteen primates and rodents. *Science* **179**, 484–486.

Kato, T., Iwamoto, K., Kakiuchi, C., Kuratomi, G., and Okazaki, Y. (2005). Genetic or epigenetic difference causing discordance between monozygotic twins as a clue to molecular basis of mental disorders. *Mol Psychiatry* **10**, 622–630.

Landry, A. M., Landry, D. J., Gentry, L. R. *et al.* (2005). Endocrine profiles and growth patterns of cloned goats. *Cloning Stem Cells* **7**, 214–225.

Lorincz, M. T., Detloff, P. J., Albin, R. L., and O'Shea, K. S. (2004). Embryonic stem cells expressing expanded CAG repeats undergo aberrant neuronal differentiation and have persistent Oct-4 and REST/NRSF expression. *Mol Cell Neurosci* **26**, 135–143.

Mann, M. R., Chung, Y. G., Nolen, L. D., Verona, R. I., Latham, K. E., and Bartolomei, M. S. (2003). Disruption of imprinted gene methylation and expression in cloned preimplantation stage mouse embryos. *Biol Reprod* **69**, 902–914.

Meissner, A. and Jaenisch, R. (2006). Mammalian nuclear transfer. *Dev Dyn* **235**, 2460–2469.

Melo, E. O., Canavessi, A. M., Franco, M. M., and Rumpf, R. (2007). Animal transgenesis: state of the art and applications. *J Appl Genet* **48**, 47–61.

Meng, L., Ely, J. J., Stouffer, R. L., and Wolf, D. P. (1997). Rhesus monkeys produced by nuclear transfer. *Biol Reprod* **57**, 454–459.

Menzel, O., Vellai, T., Takacs-Vellai, K. *et al.* (2004). The *Caenorhabditis elegans* ortholog of C21orf80, a potential new protein O-fucosyltransferase, is required for normal development. *Genomics* **84**, 320–330.

Mitalipov, S. M., Yeoman, R. R., Kuo, H. C., and Wolf, D. P. (2002a). Monozygotic twinning in rhesus monkeys by manipulation of in vitro-derived embryos. *Biol Reprod* **66**, 1449–1455.

Mitalipov, S. M., Yeoman, R. R., Nusser, K. D., and Wolf, D. P. (2002b). Rhesus monkey embryos produced by nuclear transfer from embryonic blastomeres or somatic cells. *Biol Reprod* **66**, 1367–1373.

Nagashima, H., Kato, Y., and Ogawa, S. (1989). Microsurgical bisection of porcine morulae and blastocysts to produce monozygotic twin pregnancy. *Gamete Res* **23**, 1–9.

Newman, J. C., Bailey, A. D., and Weiner, A. M. (2006). Cockayne syndrome group B protein (CSB) plays a general role in chromatin maintenance and remodeling. *Proc Natl Acad Sci USA* **103**, 9613–9618.

Ng, S. C., Chen, N., Yip, W. Y. *et al.* (2004). The first cell cycle after transfer of somatic cell nuclei in a non-human primate. *Development* **131**, 2475–2484.

Nowshari, M. A. and Holtz, W. (1993). Transfer of split goat embryos without zonae pellucidae either fresh or after freezing. *J Anim Sci* **71**, 3403–3408.

O'Brien, J. K., Stojanov, T., Crichton, E. G. *et al.* (2005a). Flow cytometric sorting of fresh and frozen-thawed spermatozoa in the western lowland gorilla (*Gorilla gorilla gorilla*). *Am J Primatol* **66**, 297–315.

O'Brien, J. K., Stojanov, T., Heffernan, S. J. *et al.* (2005b). Flow cytometric sorting of non-human primate sperm nuclei. *Theriogenology* **63**, 246–259.

Pimenta, A. F. and Levitt, P. (2005). Applications of gene targeting technology to mental retardation and developmental disability research. *Ment Retard Dev Disabil Res Rev* **11**, 295–302.

Rajesh, D., Chinnasamy, N., Mitalipov, S. M. *et al.* (2007). Differential requirements for hematopoietic commitment between human and rhesus embryonic stem cells. *Stem Cells* **25**, 490–499.

Rogers, J. and Hixson, J. E. (1997). Baboons as an animal model for genetic studies of common human disease. *Am J Hum Genet* **61**, 489–493.

Sathananthan, A. H. (1997). Mitosis in the human embryo: the vital role of the sperm centrosome (centriole). *Histol Histopathol* **12**, 827–856.

Sathananthan, A. H., Tatham, B., Dharmawardena, V., Grills, B., Lewis, I., and Trounson, A. (1997). Inheritance of sperm centrioles and centrosomes in bovine embryos. *Arch Androl* **38**, 37–48.

Schatten, G., Simerly, C., and Schatten, H. (1985). Microtubule configurations during fertilization, mitosis, and early development in the mouse and the requirement for egg microtubule-mediated motility during mammalian fertilization. *Proc Natl Acad Sci USA* **82**, 4152–4156.

Schramm, R. D. and Paprocki, A. M. (2004). In vitro development and cell allocation following aggregation of split embryos with tetraploid or developmentally asynchronous blastomeres in rhesus monkeys. *Cloning Stem Cells* **6**, 302–314.

Sigmund, C. D. (1993). Major approaches for generating and analyzing transgenic mice. An overview. *Hypertension* **22**, 599–607.

Simerly, C., Dominko, T., Navara, C. *et al.* (2003). Molecular correlates of primate nuclear transfer failures. *Science* **300**, 297.

Simerly, C., Navara, C., Hyun, S. H. *et al.* (2004). Embryogenesis and blastocyst development after somatic cell nuclear transfer in nonhuman primates: overcoming defects caused by meiotic spindle extraction. *Dev Biol* **276**, 237–252.

Singh, S. M., Murphy, B., and O'Reilly, R. (2002). Epigenetic contributors to the discordance of monozygotic twins. *Clin Genet* **62**, 97–103.

St John, J. C. and Schatten, G. (2004). Paternal mitochondrial DNA transmission during nonhuman primate nuclear transfer. *Genetics* **167**, 897–905.

Steptoe, P. C. and Edwards, R. G. (1978). Birth after the reimplantation of a human embryo. *Lancet* **2**, 366.

Stewart, C. L. (1993). Production of chimeras between embryonic stem cells and embryos. *Methods Enzymol* **225**, 823–855.

Tamashiro, K. L., Sakai, R. R., Yamazaki, Y., Wakayama, T., and Yanagimachi, R. (2007). Developmental, behavioral, and physiological phenotype of cloned mice. *Adv Exp Med Biol* **591**, 72–83.

Thomson, J. A., Kalishman, J., Golos, T. G. *et al.* (1995). Isolation of a primate embryonic stem cell line. *Proc Natl Acad Sci USA* **92**, 7844–7888.

Thomson, J. A., Kalishman, J., Golos, T. G., Durning, M., Harris, C. P., and Hearn, J. P. (1996). Pluripotent cell lines derived from common marmoset (*Callithrix jacchus*) blastocysts. *Biol Reprod* **55**, 254–259.

Thomson, J. A., Itskovitz-Eldor, J., Shapiro, S. S. *et al.* (1998). Embryonic stem cell lines derived from human blastocysts. *Science* **282**, 1145–1147.

Tsunoda, Y. and McLaren, A. (1983). Effect of various procedures on the viability of mouse embryos containing half the normal number of blastomeres. *J Reprod Fertil* **69**, 315–322.

Umeda, K., Heike, T., Yoshimoto, M. *et al.* (2006). Identification and characterization of hemoangiogenic progenitors during cynomolgus monkey embryonic stem cell differentiation. *Stem Cells* **24**, 1348–1358.

VandeVoort, C. A. (2004). High quality sperm for nonhuman primate ART: production and assessment. *Reprod Biol Endocrinol* **16**, 2–33.

Wakayama, T. (2007). Production of cloned mice and ES cells from adult somatic cells by nuclear transfer: how to improve cloning efficiency? *J Reprod Dev* **53**, 13–26.

Weksberg, R., Shuman, C., Caluseriu, O. *et al.* (2002). Discordant KCNQ1OT1 imprinting in sets of monozygotic twins discordant for Beckwith-Wiedemann syndrome. *Hum Mol Genet* **11**, 1317–1325.

Willadsen, S. M. and Godke, R. A. (1984). A simple procedure for the production of identical sheep twins. *Vet Rec* **14**, 240–243.

Williams-Blangero, S., VandeBerg, J. L., and Dyke, B. (2002). Genetic management of nonhuman primates. *J Med Primatol* **31**, 1–7.

Wilmut, I., Schnieke, A. E., McWhir, J., Kind, A. J., and Campbell, K. H. (1997). Viable offspring derived from fetal and adult mammalian cells. *Nature* **385**, 810–813.

Wolf, D. P., Meng, L., Ouhibi, N., and Zelinski-Wooten, M. (1999). Nuclear transfer in the rhesus monkey: practical and basic implications. *Biol Reprod* **60**, 199–204.

Wolf, D. P., Thormahlen, S., Ramsey, C., Yeoman, R. R., Fanton, J., and Mitalipov, S. (2004). Use of assisted reproductive technologies in the propagation of rhesus macaque offspring. *Biol Reprod* **71**, 486–493.

Zarnescu, D. C., Shan, G., Warren, S. T., and Jin, P. (2005). Come FLY with us: toward understanding fragile X syndrome. *Genes Brain Behav* **4**, 385–392.

Zhou, Q., Yang, S. H., Ding, C. H. *et al.* (2006). A comparative approach to somatic cell nuclear transfer in the rhesus monkey. *Hum Reprod* **21**, 2564–2571.

Index